D1597575

CARDIAC REPOLARIZATION

CONTEMPORARY CARDIOLOGY

CHRISTOPHER P. CANNON, MD
SERIES EDITOR

CARDIAC REPOLARIZATION
BRIDGING BASIC AND CLINICAL SCIENCE

Edited by

IHOR GUSSAK, MD, PhD

eResearch Technology Inc., Bridgewater, NJ

CHARLES ANTZELEVITCH, PhD

Masonic Medical Research Laboratory, Utica, NY

Co-Edited by

STEPHEN C. HAMMILL, MD

Mayo Clinic, Rochester, MN

WIN-KUANG SHEN, MD

Mayo Clinic, Rochester, MN

PREBEN BJERREGAARD, MD, DMSc

St. Louis University Health Sciences Center, St. Louis, MO

Foreword by

DOUGLAS P. ZIPES, MD

Indiana University School of Medicine, Indianapolis, IN

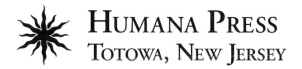

HUMANA PRESS
TOTOWA, NEW JERSEY

© 2003 Humana Press Inc.
999 Riverview Drive, Suite 208
Totowa, New Jersey 07512

www.humanapr.com

For additional copies, pricing for bulk purchases, and/or information about other Humana titles, contact Humana at the above address or at any of the following numbers: Tel.: 973-256-1699; Fax: 973-256-8341, E-mail: humana@humanapr.com; or visit our website.

The content and opinions expressed in this book are the sole work of the authors and editors, who have warranted due diligence in the creation and issuance of their work. The publisher, editors, and authors are not responsible for errors or omissions or for any consequences arising from the information or opinions presented in this book and make no warranty, express or implied, with respect to its contents.

Due diligence has been taken by the publishers, editors, and authors of this book to assure the accuracy of the information published and to describe generally accepted practices. The contributors herein have carefully checked to ensure that the drug selections and dosages set forth in this text are accurate and in accord with the standards accepted at the time of publication. Notwithstanding, as new research, changes in government regulations, and knowledge from clinical experience relating to drug therapy and drug reactions constantly occurs, the reader is advised to check the product information provided by the manufacturer of each drug for any change in dosages or for additional warnings and contraindications. This is of utmost importance when the recommended drug herein is a new or infrequently used drug. It is the responsibility of the treating physician to determine dosages and treatment strategies for individual patients. Further it is the responsibility of the health care provider to ascertain the Food and Drug Administration status of each drug or device used in their clinical practice. The publisher, editors, and authors are not responsible for errors or omissions or for any consequences from the application of the information presented in this book and make no warranty, express or implied, with respect to the contents in this publication.

Production Editor: Mark J. Breaugh.

Cover design by Patricia F. Cleary.

This publication is printed on acid-free paper. ∞
ANSI Z39.48-1984 (American National Standards Institute) Permanence of Paper for Printed Library Materials.

Printed in the United States of America. 10 9 8 7 6 5 4 3 2 1

Library of Congress Cataloging-in-Publication Data

Dedication

FOREWORD

I once wrote, paraphrasing Churchill's description of Stalin, that "The AV node is an enigma in an island of whimsy surrounded by a sea of uncertainty." I could easily substitute the T wave for the AV node in that statement. Despite intense study for 100 years, unanswered questions about the T wave abound. Some of these important questions are relatively pedestrian and include how to accurately measure the QT interval when the end of the T wave is blurred or merged with the U wave, or the T wave contour is distorted; how to correct for rate changes (Bazett's formula is most commonly used despite its under correction at slow rates and over correction at fast rates and the fact that Bazett applied it only in normal, relatively young, drug-free individuals); the relation of the T wave to the U wave, what causes the U wave, and what the importance of the QU interval is; the meaning of T wave lability (for the clinician: just what does "nonspecific T wave change" really mean?); the mechanism of broad negative T waves in non-Q-wave myocardial infarction and CNS injury; how to measure T wave dispersion accurately and what does it mean; the impact of autonomic and hormonal alterations; and the true upper limit of normal for the QT and QTc intervals for men and women.

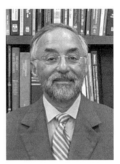

Douglas P. Zipes, MD
*Indiana University
School of Medicine,
Indianapolis, IN*

Then, probing deeper, what is the relationship of the long QT syndrome (LQTS) to the sudden infant death syndrome; do all patients who develop drug-induced LQTS start with a congenital abnormality; do early after-depolarizations precipitate or maintain *torsades de pointes*; can *torsades de pointes* occur in the atria; and do patients who prolong ventricular repolarization after cardiac remodeling from heart failure or ventricular hypertrophy really die from *torsades de pointes*?

And then, at a basic level, how relevant are data from models such as the left ventricular wedge, isolated myocytes and membrane patches, and computer simulations? What is the role of M cells in repolarization, the U wave, and *torsades de pointes*? How do the intracellular Ca^{2+}/calmodulin-dependent processes regulate the development of *torsades de pointes*?

While it seems we have more questions than answers—and indeed the questions I have asked are only a partial list—*Cardiac Repolarization: Bridging Basic and Clinical Science* attempts to answer some of those questions. From basic electrophysiology, pharmacology, and molecular biology to clinical physiology and pathophysiology and a consideration of specific electrocardiographic phenomena and syndromes, world-class experts give their views on these and related topics.

The study of cardiac repolarization is an area of intense interest, but an evolving field. As new knowledge accumulates, our concepts are certain to change, but that is the challenge and fun of what we do. Hopefully, in several years, we will be reading a much updated second edition.

Douglas P. Zipes, MD
Indiana, IN

PREFACE

There are a number of excellent books on molecular biology, single-channel electrophysiology, animal experimentation, and clinical electrophysiology. However, the past decade has seen an explosion of knowledge and radical changes in our understanding of ventricular repolarization as an integral part of the cardiac electrophysiologic matrix; a topic which, until now, has not been covered in depth. *Cardiac Repolarization: Bridging Basic and Clinical Science* presents comprehensively the latest developments in the field of cardiac electrophysiology with a focus on the clinical and experimental aspects of ventricular repolarization, newly discovered clinical repolarization syndromes, electrocardiographic phenomena, and their correlation with the most recent advances in basic science.

Repolarization has distinct adaptive mechanisms that are responsible for maintenance of electrophysiological equilibrium and electrical stability of the heart under normal and pathophysiological conditions. Both congenital and acquired abnormalities of ventricular repolarization have recently received significant recognition because these are major contributors of life-threatening cardiac arrhythmias and are an important target for anti-arrhythmic drugs and interventions. We have aimed to provide unique prospective views on ventricular repolarization by emphasizing the clinical and basic aspects of physiology and pathophysiology in conjunction with new clinical findings and research discoveries. The authors have provided a thought-provoking and enlightening review of the latest research and clinical accomplishments in their areas of expertise. Each chapter is outlined with objectives, key points, current perspectives, and recommendations for future investigations. Each chapter includes established and evidence-based knowledge, the authors' personal opinions, areas of controversy, and future trends. We aimed to provide a contemporary and succinct distillation of the current status of cardiac repolarization. Although some of the areas are highly subspecialized, this book has been designed for a broad audience ranging from medical and graduate students to clinicians and scientists.

Cardiac Repolarization: Bridging Basic and Clinical Science is organized so as to make the large volume of rapidly evolving information understandable and easy to assimilate, with each section focusing on a theme of cardiac repolarization. The spectrum of ventricular repolarization, historical milestones of electrical signal recording, and their relevance to clinical arrhythmias and sudden cardiac death syndromes are presented as an introduction. Part II focuses on the theme of basic mechanisms underlying ventricular repolarization. In addition to an overview of electrophysiology, pharmacology, and molecular biology underlying ventricular repolarization, basic mechanisms have been integrated with specific disease conditions, including heart failure, ischemia, long QT syndrome, and Brugada syndrome. The theme of Part III includes clinical physiology and pathophysiology of ventricular repolarization; state-of-the-art information on human cardiac repolarization with an emphasis on clinical application; challenges and clinical relevance of the dynamic interactions of neurohumeral and pharmacological factors; and a peek into the future of antiarrhythmic drug development based on molecular and electrophysiological properties. Part IV of the book provides a comprehensive review of the clinical presentation and management of specific cardiac repolarization conditions, including early repolarization and short QT interval, Brugada syndrome, long QT syndrome, and sudden infant death syndrome.

The editors of *Cardiac Repolarization: Bridging Basic and Clinical Science* wish to recognize the significant contribution made by all of the authors. The book is the result of a collaboration that has brought together the skills and perspectives of researchers, scientists, and clinicians. We also wish to thank all of our mentors, without whom the work presented in the book would not have been realized. Finally, we are grateful to our colleagues, trainees, and students for stimulating interactions that have served as the basis for many innovative ideas and investigations.

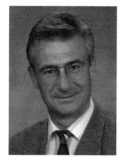

Ihor Gussak, MD, PhD

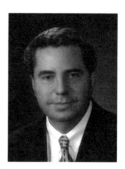

Charles Antzelevitch, PhD

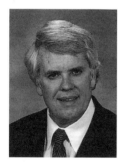

Stephen C. Hammill, MD

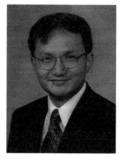

Win-Kuang Shen, MD

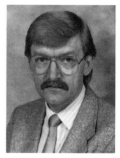

Preben Bjerregaard,
MD, DMSc

CONTENTS

CONTRIBUTORS

MICHAEL J. ACKERMAN, MD, PhD • *Assistant Professor of Medicine, Pediatrics, and Molecular Pharmacology; Director, Long QT Syndrome Clinic and Sudden Death Genomics Laboratory, Mayo Clinic, Rochester, MN, USA*

CHARLES ANTZELEVITCH, PhD, FACC, FAHA • *Professor of Pharmacology, Upstate Medical University, Syracuse, NY; Executive Director and Director of Research, Gordon K. Moe Scholar, Experimental Cardiology Program Director, Masonic Medical Research Laboratory, Utica, NY, USA*

ANTONIS A. ARMOUNDAS, PhD • *Postdoctoral Fellow, Institute of Molecular Cardiobiology, Division of Molecular Cardiology, Department of Medicine, Johns Hopkins University, Baltimore, MD, USA*

MORTON F. ARNSDORF, MD, MACC • *Professor of Medicine (Cardiology), Section of Cardiology, Department of Medicine, The Pritzker School of Medicine, The University of Chicago, Chicago, IL, USA*

CONNIE R. BEZZINA, PhD • *Post-Doctorate Fellow, Experimental and Molecular Cardiology Group, Laboratory of Experimental Cardiology, Academic Medical Center, University of Amsterdam, The Netherlands*

PREBEN BJERREGAARD, MD, DMSc, FACC • *Professor of Medicine, Director, Electrophysiology and Pacemaker Service, St. Louis University Hospital, St. Louis, MO, USA*

JOSEP BRUGADA, MD, PhD • *Associate Professor of Medicine, Director of the Arrhythmia Section, Cardiovascular Institute, Hospital Clínic of the University of Barcelona, and Vice President-Elect of the Spanish Society of Cardiology, Barcelona, Spain*

PEDRO BRUGADA, MD, PhD, FESC, FAHA • *Professor of Cardiology, Cardiovascular Center Aalst, Co-Founder and CEO of the Cardiovascular Research and Teaching Institute Aalst and of the Ramon Brugada Senior Foundation, Aalst, Belgium*

RAMON BRUGADA, MD • *Director, Molecular Genetics Program, Masonic Medical Research Laboratory, Utica, NY, USA*

ALEXANDER BURASHNIKOV, PhD • *Research Scientist, Department of Experimental Cardiology, Masonic Medical Research Laboratory, Utica, NY, USA*

PHILIPPE COUMEL, MD, FESC • *Professor of Cardiology, Department of Cardiology, Lariboisiére University Hospital, Paris, France*

JOSE M. DI DIEGO, MD • *Research Scientist, Department of Experimental Cardiology, Masonic Medical Research Laboratory, Utica, NY, USA*

ROBERT DUMAINE, PhD • *Research Scientist, Department of Experimental Cardiology, Masonic Medical Research Laboratory, Utica, NY, USA*

JEFFREY FISH, DVM • *Research Scientist, Department of Experimental Cardiology, Masonic Medical Research Laboratory, Utica, NY, USA*

DANIEL GOODMAN, MD • *Director of Medical Affairs, Covance Central Diagnostics, Reno, NV, USA*

IHOR GUSSAK, MD, PhD, FACC • *Clinical Associate Professor of Medicine,UMDNJ-Robert Wood Johnson Medical School, New Brunswick, NJ; Vice President of Global Medical Affairs, eResearchTechnology, Inc.; Associate Editor, Journal of Electrocardiology, Bridgewater, NJ, USA*

STEPHEN C. HAMMILL, MD • *Professor of Medicine, Director, Heart Rhythm Services; Division of Cardiovascular Diseases, Department of Internal Medicine, Mayo Clinic, Rochester, MN, USA*

ARSHAD JAHANGIR, MD, FACC • *Senior Associate Consultant, Division of Cardiovascular Diseases, Department of Internal Medicine, Mayo Clinic, Rochester, MN, USA*

MICHIEL J. JANSE, MD, PhD • *Professor Emeritus of Experimental Cardiology, University of Amsterdam; Editor-in-Chief, Cardiovascular Research, Academic Medical Center, Amsterdam, The Netherlands*

ROBERT S. KASS, PhD • *David Hosack Professor of Pharmacology, Chairman, Center for Neurobiology & Behavior, Columbia University College of Physicians and Surgeons, New York, NY, USA*

ANANT KHOSITSETH, MD • *Fellow, Department of Pediatric Cardiology, Mayo Clinic, Rochester, MN, USA*

ANDRÉ G. KLÉBER, MD • *Professor of Physiology, Department of Physiology, Faculty of Medicine, University of Bern, Bern, Switzerland*

THORSTEN LEWALTER, MD • *Associate Professor of Medicine, Department of Medicine-Cardiology, University of Bonn, Bonn, Germany*

BERNDT LÜDERITZ, MD, FESC, FACC, FAHA • *Professor of Medicine, Head of Department of Medicine-Cardiology, University of Bonn, Bonn, Germany*

PIERRE MAISON-BLANCHE, MD • *Professor of Cardiology, Department of Cardiology, Lariboisiére University Hospital, Paris, France*

ARTHUR J. MOSS, MD, FACC • *Professor of Medicine (Cardiology), Director of Heart Research Follow-up Program, University of Rochester Medical Center, Rochester, NY, USA*

KOONLAWEE NADEMANEE, MD • *Professor of Medicine, Director of Electrophysiology, University of Southern California, Los Angeles, CA, USA*

CARLO NAPOLITANO, MD, PhD • *Senior Scientist, Department of Molecular Cardiology, Fondazione Salvatore Maugeri, Pavia, Italy*

JAN NĚMEC, MD • *Cardiologist, 2nd Dept. Internal Medicine, 1st Faculty of Medicine, Charles University, Prague, Czech Republic*

JEANNE M. NERBONNE, PhD • *Alumni Endowed Professor, Department of Molecular Biology and Pharmacology, Washington University School of Medicine, St. Louis, MO, USA*

VLADISLAV V. NESTERENKO, PhD • *Research Scientist, Department of Experimental Cardiology, Masonic Medical Research Laboratory, Utica, NY, USA*

GUILLERMO PEREZ, PhD • *Research Scientist, Department of Experimental Cardiology, Masonic Medical Research Laboratory, Utica, NY, USA*

SILVIA G. PRIORI, MD, PhD, FESC • *Associate Professor of Cardiology, Director of Molecular Cardiology, University of Pavia, Fondazione Salvatore Maugeri, Pavia, Italy*

ETIENNE PRUVOT, MD • *Visiting Scientist, Heart & Vascular Research Center, Case Western Reserve University, Cleveland, OH, USA*

DAVID S. ROSENBAUM, MD, FACC • *Associate Professor of Medicine, Biomedical Engineering, Physiology, and Biophysics; Director, Heart & Vascular Research Center, Case Western Reserve University, Cleveland, OH, USA*

PHILIP T. SAGER, MD, FACC, FAHA • *Clinical Professor of Medicine, UMDNJ-New Jersey Medical School, Newark, NJ; Director, Cardiac Research, Schering-Plough Research Institute, Kenilworth, NJ, USA*

PETER J. SCHWARTZ, MD, FACC, FESC, FAHA • *Professor and Chairman, Department of Cardiology, University of Pavia and Policlinico S. Matteo, IRCCS, Pavia, Italy*

FABIANA SCORNIK, PhD • *Research Scientist, Department of Experimental Cardiology, Masonic Medical Research Laboratory, Utica, NY, USA*

WIN-KUANG SHEN, MD, FACC, FAHA • *Professor of Medicine, Mayo Medical School, Consultant, Division of Cardiovascular Diseases, Mayo Clinic, Rochester, MN, USA*

ANDRE TERZIC, MD, PhD • *Professor of Medicine and Pharmacology, and Vice-Chair Cardiovascular Research, Department of Internal Medicine and Department of Molecular Pharmacology and Experimental Therapeutics, Mayo Clinic, Rochester, MN, USA*

GORDON F. TOMASELLI, MD • *Director, Molecular Cardiology, Professor of Medicine, Cellular and Molecular Medicine, Institute of Molecular Cardiobiology, Johns Hopkins University, Baltimore, MD, USA*

JEFFREY TOWBIN, MD, PhD • *Professor of Pediatric Cardiology, Departments of Pediatrics (Cardiology), Cardiovascular Sciences, and Molecular and Human Genetics Texas Children's Hospital, Baylor College of Medicine, Houston, TX, USA*

HEIN J. WELLENS, MD • *Professor Emeritus of Cardiology, The Interuniversity Cardiology Institute of the Netherlands, Utrecht, The Netherlands*

ARTHUR A. M. WILDE, MD, PhD, FESC, FAHA • *Professor of Cardiology, Experimental and Molecular Cardiology Group, Laboratory of Experimental Cardiology, Academic Medical Center, University of Amsterdam, The Netherlands*

WOJCIECH ZAREBA, MD, PhD, FACC • *Associate Professor of Medicine (Cardiology), Associate Director of Heart Research Follow-up Program, Director of Clinical Research, Cardiology Unit, University of Rochester Medical Center, Rochester, NY, USA*

DOUGLAS P. ZIPES, MD • *Director, Krannert Institute of Cardiology, Distinguished Professor of Medicine, Pharmacology, and Toxicology, Indiana University School of Medicine, Indianapolis, IN, USA*

ANDREW C. ZYGMUNT, PhD • *Research Scientist, Department of Experimental Cardiology, Masonic Medical Research Laboratory, Utica, NY, USA*

PART I

INTRODUCTION

1

Ventricular Repolarization and the Identification of the Sudden Death Candidate

Hype or Hope?

Hein J. Wellens, MD *and Douglas P. Zipes,* MD

In 1940 Wiggers described disparity in repolarization times across the ventricles as a marker of susceptibility for ventricular arrhythmias *(1)*. This observation was followed by many attempts to quantify those differences and to determine their prognostic significance. Several techniques were used to measure duration and disparity of repolarization such as body surface mapping *(2,3)*, endocardial monophasic action potential recordings *(4)*, and epicardial *(5–7)* recordings. This was followed by endeavors to obtain that information from the 12–lead electrocardiogram by measuring the QT interval. This brought the suggestion and hope that measuring the QT interval in different ECG leads looking for QT dispersion could be of help to identify cardiac patients at increased risk of dying suddenly *(8–14)*. However, the idea could not be confirmed in prospective studies by Zabel et al. *(15)* in patients after a myocardial infarction and by Brendorp et al. *(16)* in patients with heart failure.

What are the possible causes for the discrepancy between the initial and subsequent studies? The ST segment and the T wave on the surface ECG represent an integrated signal from multiple repolarization wave fronts *(4,17)*. Ventricular repolarization is a complex series of events occurring in a nonlinear and inhomogeneous fashion. Therefore, as pointed out by Surawicz *(18)*, of the different components of the 12-lead electrocardiogram, the ST segment and the T wave have the greatest potential for misinterpretation.

Willems et al. *(19)* showed that measurements of the QT interval using surface ECG leads were frought with a large intra- and interobserver variability even when supported by computer algorithms; the problem being the identification of the end of the T wave *(20,21)*.

Secondly, the QT interval does not represent ventricular repolarization only but is a reflection of the entire ventricular depolarization and repolarization process. Especially

From: *Contemporary Cardiology: Cardiac Repolarization: Bridging Basic and Clinical Science*
Edited by: I. Gussak et al. © Humana Press Inc., Totowa, NJ

the precordial leads present the local de- and repolarization process. Duration of repolarization may truly differ between precordial leads but may also seem to differ because of isoelectric portions of the QRS complex, falsely suggesting QT disparity between the precordial leads.

Thirdly, prolongation of the QT interval does not necessarily mean increased disparity in ventricular repolarization and increased risk for an arrhythmic death. The prime example is amiodarone which uniformly prolongs repolarization resulting in QT prolongation but with anti-arrhythmic and not pro-arrhythmic consequences *(9)*. In the congenital and acquired long QT it was shown that the prolonged QT interval was accompanied by arrhythmias based upon early after depolarizations *(10)*. However as recently shown by Van Opstal et al. *(22)* amiodarone induced QT prolongation is not accompanied by the emergence of early after depolarizations.

Differences in QT interval may have an arrhythmogenic meaning favoring re-entry, but only when these differences are present in ventricular areas located close to each other. When areas with repolarization disparity are far apart they may not predispose to ventricular arrhythmias. The widely spaced bipolar extremity leads give global information about de- and repolarization of the ventricles whereas the unipolar leads reflect more local events occurring under the electrode. But unfortunately even the 6 precordial leads of the 12-lead ECG give limited information of adjacent heterogeneity in repolarization duration because those 6 leads reflect only small and relatively widely spaced precordial areas.

This may be the reason why in the presence of global repolarization disparity in the ventricular muscle wall, as in the long QT syndrome *(10,23)* the 12-lead ECG can correctly pick up the patients at risk for dying suddenly. However, in local disparity, such as after a myocardial infarction, this may only be possible when many closely spaced precordial leads as in precordial mapping reveal QT disparity of the underlying cardiac area. Finally, the scalar ECG provides no information specifically about transmural heterogeneity, shown by Antzelevitch and his group to be an important predictor in animal studies *(23)*. All these considerations should be taken into account when using QT interval differences as a marker for increased risk of dying suddenly.

The differences in outcome of these studies on QT dispersion as a surface ECG marker of vulnerability to ventricular arrhythmias and cardiovascular mortality, which took place during the past two decades, prompted a search for other methods to document repolarization abnormalities and their prognostic significance. Several of these methods are discussed in the different chapters of this book. They include: QT dynamicity; T wave alternans, both during rate increase or following premature beats; temporal complexity of repolarization; 12–lead T wave morphology; T wave loop morphology; T wave projection; and Total Cosine between R and T (TCRT) which uses the concept of the ventricular gradient.

Many of these approaches are now being prospectively evaluated in patients with cardiac disease such as after a myocardial infarction or with congestive heart failure. Time will tell what their value is in the recognition of the patient at high risk of a life threatening ventricular arrhythmia. It is likely that the absence of an abnormality in one of these tests will have a high negative predictive accuracy.

The key question however will be how high is the positive predictive accuracy of the test. Will it be better than a left ventricular ejection fraction, heart rate variability or baroreflex sensitivity?

What will be the best combination of tests? At this point in time only 10% of people dying suddenly out of hospital can be recognized as being at high risk for such an event *(24)*. There can be no discussion that abnormalities in ventricular repolarization increase the risk of dying suddenly. Let us hope that easily obtainable, reproducible markers of ventricular repolarization will be developed with sufficiently high positive predictive accuracy to better identify the high risk candidate to be able to start preventive measures on time.

REFERENCES

1. Wiggers CJ. The mechanism and nature of ventricular fibrillation. Am Heart J 1940;20:399–412.
2. Mirvis DM. Spatial variation of QT intervals in normal persons and patients with acute myocardial infarction. Am Coll Cardiol 1985;5:625–631.
3. De Ambroggi L, Bertoni T, Locati E, Stramba-Badiale M, Schwartz PJ. Mapping of body surface potentials in patients with the idiopathic long QT syndrome. Circulation 1986;74:1334–1345.
4. Franz MR, Bragheer K, Rafflenbeul W, Haverich A, Lichtlen PR. Monophasis action potential mapping human subjects with normal electrocardiograms: direct evidence for the genisis of the T wave. Circulation 1987;75:379–386.
5. Cowan JC, Hilton CJ, Griffiths CJ, et al. Sequence of epicardial repolarization and configuration of the T wave. Brit Heart J 1988;60:424–433.
6. Misier AR, Opthof T, van Hemel NM, et al. Dispersion of refractoriness in noninfarcted myocardium of patients with ventricular tachycardia or ventricular fibrillation after myocardial infarction. Circulation 1995;91:2566–2572.
7. Zabel M, Portnoy S, Franz MR. Electrocardiographic indexes of dispersion of ventricular repolarization: an isolated heart validation study. J Amer Coll Cardiol 1995;25:746–752.
8. Day CP, McComb JM, Campbell RW. QT dispersion: an indication of arrhythmia risk in patients with long QT intervals. Brit Heart J 1990;63:342–344.
9. Hii JT, Wyse DG, Gillis AM, Duff HJ, Solylo MA, Mitchell LB. Precordial QT interval dispersion as a marker of torsade de pointes. Disparate effects of class la antiarrhythmic drugs and amiodarone. Circulation 1992;86:1376–1382.
10. Priori SG, Napolitano C, Diehl L, Schwartz PJ. Dispersion of the QT interval. A marker of therapeutic efficacy in the idiopathic long QT syndrome. Circulation 1994;89:1681–1689.
11. Barr CS, Naas A, Freeman M, Lang CC, Struthers AD. QT dispersion and sudden unexpected death in chronic heart failure. Lancet 1994;343:327–329.
12. Zareba W, Moss AJ, Le Cessie S. Dispersion of ventricular repolarization and arrhythmic cardiac death in coronary artery disease. Am J Cardiol 1994;74:550–553.
13. de Bruyne MC, Hoes AW, Kors JA, Hofman A, van Bemmel JH, Grobbe DE. QTc dispersion predicts cardiac mortality in the elderly: the Rotterdam study. Circulation 1998;97:467–472.
14. Okin PM, Devereux RB, Howard BV, Fabsitz RR, Lee ET, Welty TK. Assessment of QT dispersion for prediction of all-cause and cardiovascular mortality in American Indians: the Strong Heart Study. Circulation 2000;101:61–66.
15. Zabel M, Klingenheben T, Frantz MR, Hohnloser SH. Assessment of QT dispersion for prediction of mortality of arrhythmic events after myocardial infarction: results of a prospective, long-term follow-up study. Circulation 1998;97:2543–2550.
16. Brendorp B, Elming H, Jung L, et al. QT dispersion has no prognostic information for patients with advanced congestive heart failure and reduced left ventricular systolic function. Circulation 2001;103:831–835.
17. Merri M, Benhorn J, Alberti M, et al. Electrocardiographic quantitation of ventricular repolarization. Circulation 1989;80:1301–1308.
18. Surawicz, B. Electrophysiologic basis of ECG and cardiac arrhythmias. Williams & Wilkins, Malvern, 1995. p. 192.
19. Willems JL, Abreu-Lima C, Arnaud P, et al. The diagnostic performance of computer programs for the interpretations of electrocardiograms. N Engl J Med 1991;325:1767–1773.
20. Malik M, Batchvarov VN. Measurement, interpretation and clinical potential of QT dispersion. Am J Cardiol 2000;36:1749–1766.

21. Xue Q, Reddy S. Computerized QT analysis algorithms. J. Electrocardiol 1997;30(Suppl):181–186.
22. Van Opstal JM, Schoenmakers M, Verduyn SC, et al. Chronic amiodarone evokes no torsade de pointes arrhythmias despite QT lengthening in an animal model of acquired long-QT syndrome. Circulation 2001;104:2722–2730.
23. Antzelevitch C, Sicouri S, Litovsky SH, et al. Heterogeneity within the ventricular wall: Electrophysiology and pharmacology of epicardial, endocardial, and M cells. Circ Res 1991;69:1427–1449.
24. Zipes DP, Wellens HJJ. Sudden cardiac death. Circulation 1998;98:2334–2351.

2

Historical Milestones of Electrical Signal Recording and Analysis

Thorsten Lewalter, MD
and Berndt Lüderitz, MD

CONTENTS

HISTORY OF THE HUMAN ELECTROCARDIOGRAM AND VENTRICULAR REPOLARIZATION

The Human Electrocardiogram

Aside from the discovery of the cardiac conduction system (Table 1) and advancements in the electrotherapy of cardiac arrhythmias (Table 2), the development of electrocardiography was the key issue for a more detailed understanding of arrhythmogenesis as a cause and correlate of cardiac disorders (Table 3). After the first documentation of a cardiac action potential by *Rudolph von Koelliker* and *Heinrich Müller* in 1856, two decades later *Augustus Desiré Waller* (Fig. 1) recorded the first human electrocardiogram. After qualifying as a medical doctor Waller joined the department of physiology at the University of London where he studied in *John Burdon Sanderson's* laboratories the electrical activity of the excised mammalian heart. In 1884 he was appointed lecturer in physiology at St. Mary's Hospital London where he used a capillary electrometer, an instrument invented 15 yr earlier by the French scientist *Gabriel Lippmann*, to record cardiac potentials in animals (Fig. 2). In 1887, he was able to obtain the first human electrocardiogram from the body surface and published his findings in the *Journal of Physiology*: "A demonstration on man of electromotive changes accompanying the hearts beat *(45)*." Waller also proved that the electrical phenomenon preceded the muscle contraction, thus excluding the possibility that the recorded activity was only an artifact. Furthermore, he recognized that it was not essential for the recording that the electrodes

From: *Contemporary Cardiology: Cardiac Repolarization: Bridging Basic and Clinical Science*
Edited by: I. Gussak et al. © Humana Press Inc., Totowa, NJ

Table 1
Discovery of the Sinus Node and the Cardiac Conduction System

1845	Purkinje fibers	J.E. Purkinje (1)
1865/1893	Bundle of Kent	G. Paladino and A.F.S. Kent (2)
1893	Bundle of His	W. His, Jr. (3)
1906	AV node	L. Aschoff and S. Tawara (4)
1906/1907	Wenckebach bundle	K.F. Wenckebach (5)
1907	Sinus node	A.B. Keith and M.W. Flack (6)
1916	Bachmann bundle	J.G. Bachmann (7)
1932	Mahaim fibers	I. Mahaim (8)
1961	Bundle of James	T.N. James (9)

Table 2
Historical Perspectives on Electrotherapy of Cardiac Arrhythmias

1580	Mercuriale, G. (1530–1606): Ubi pulsus sit rarus semper expectanda est syncope (10)
1717	Gerbezius, M. (1658–1718): Constitutio Anni 1717 a.A.D. Marco Gerbezio Labaco 10. Decem. descripta. Miscellanea Emphemerides Academiae Naturae (11)
1761	Morgagni, G.B. (1682–1771): De sedibus et causis morborum per anatomen indagatis (12)
1791	Galvani L., (1737–1798): De viribus electricitatis in motu musculari commentarius (13)
1800	Bichat, M.F.X. (1771–1802): Recherches physiologiques sur la vie et la mort (14) (Physiologic study on life and death)
1804	Aldini G. (1762–1834): Essai theorique et experimental sur le galvanisme, avec une serie d'experiences faites en presence des commissaires de l'institut national de France, et en divers amphitheatres de Londres (15) (Theoretical and experimental essay on galvanism with a series of experiments conducted in the presence of representatives of the National Institute of France at various amphitheatres in London)
1827/1846	Adams R. (1791–1875); Stokes, W. (1804–1878): Cases of diseases of the heart accompanied with pathological observations; Observations of some cases of permanently slow pulse (16,17)
1872	Duchenne de Bologne, G.B.A. (1806–1875): De l'ectrisation localisée et de son application à la pathologie et à la thérapeutique par courants induits et par courants galvaniques interrompus et continues (18) (On localized electrical stimulation and its pathological and therapeutic application by induced and galvanized current, both interrupted and continuous)
1882	von Ziemssen, H. (1829–1902): Studien über die Bewegungsvorgänge am menschlichen Herzen sowie über die mechanische und elektrische Erregbarkeit des Herzens und des Nervus phrenicus, angestellt an dem freiliegenden Herzen der Catharina Serafin (19) (Studies on the motions of the human heart as well as the mechanical and electrical excitability of the heart and phrenic nerve, observed in the case of the exposed heart of Catharina Serafin)
1890	Huchard, H.: La maladie de Adams-Stokes (Adams-Stokes Syndrome)
1932	Hyman, A.S.: Resuscitation of the stopped heart by intracardial therapy. II. Experimental use of an artificial pacemaker (20)
1952	Zoll, P.M.: Resuscitation of heart in ventricular standstill by external electrical stimulation (21) (Continued)

Table 2 (*Continued*)
Historical Perspectives on Electrotherapy of Cardiac Arrhythmias

1958	Elmquist, R., Senning A.: An implantable pacemaker for the heart *(22)*
1958	Furman S., Robinson G.: The use of an intracardiac pacemaker in the correction of total heart block *(23)*
1961	Bouvrain, Y., Zacouto, F.: L'entrainment électrosystolique du coeur *(24)* (Electrical capture of the heart)
1962	Lown, B. et al.: New method for terminating cardiac arrhythmias *(25)*
1969	Berkovits, B.V. et al.: Bifocal demand pacing *(26)*
1972	Wellens, H.J.J. et al.: Electrical stimulation of the heart in patients with ventricular tachycardia *(27)*
1975	Zipes, D.P. et al.: Termination of ventricular fibrillation in dogs by depolarizing a critical amount of myocardium *(28)*
1978	Josephson, M.E. et al.: Recurrent sustained ventricular tachycardia *(29)*
1980	Mirowski, M. et al.: Termination of malignant ventricular arrhythmias with an implanted automatic defibrillator in human beings *(30)*
1982	Gallagher, J.J. et al.: Catheter technique for closed-chest ablation of the atrio-ventricular conduction system: A therapeutic alternative for the treatment of refractory supraventricular tachycardia *(31)*
1982	Scheinman, M.M. et al.: Transvenous catheter technique for induction of damage to the atrioventricular conduction system *(32)*
1982	Lüderitz, B. et al.: Therapeutic pacing in tachyarrhythmias by implanted pacemakers *(33)*
1985	Manz, M. et al.: Antitachycardia pacemaker (Tachylog) and automatic implantable defibrillator (AID): Combined use in ventricular tachyarrhythmias *(34)*
1987	Borggrefe, M. et al.: High frequency alternating current ablation of an accessory pathway in humans *(35)*
1988	Saksena, S., Parsonnet, V.: Implantation of a cardioverter-defibrillator without thoracotomy using a triple electrode system *(36)*
1991	Jackman, W.M. et al.: Catheter ablation of accessory atrioventricular pathways (Wolff-Parkinson-White syndrome) by radiofrequency current *(37)*
1991	Kuck, K.H. et al.: Radiofrequency current catheter ablation of accessory pathways *(38)*
1994	Daubert, C. et al.: Permanent atrial resynchronisation by syncronous bi-atrial pacing in the preventive treatment of atrial flutter associated with high degree interatrial block *(39)*
1994	Cazeau, S. et al.: Four chamber pacing in dilated cardiomyopathy *(40)*
1995	Camm, A.J. et al.: Implantable atrial defibrillator *(41)*
1997	Jung, W. et al.: First worldwide implantation of an arrhythmia management system *(42)*
1998	Haissaguerre, M. et al.: Spontaneous initiation of atrial fibrillation by ectopic beats originating in the pulmonary veins *(43)*
1999	Josephson, M. et al: Hybrid pharmacologic and ablative therapy: a novel and effective approach for the management of atrial fibrillation *(44)*

are applied to the subject's chest, he wrote: "if the two hands or one hand and one foot be plunged into two dishes of salt solution connected with the two sides of the electrometer, the column of though less than when the electrodes are strapped to the chest." Waller demonstrated his recording technique at the First International Congress of Physiologists in Basel, Switzerland 1889 where young researchers like *William Bayliss, Edward Star-*

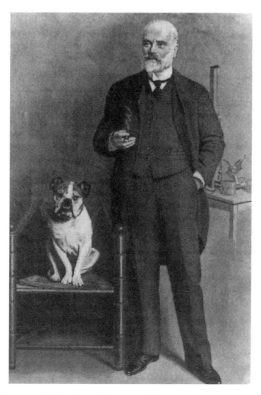

Fig. 1. Augustus Desiré Waller (1856–1922) with his laboratory dog named Jimmie. Augustus Desiré Waller was born in Paris as the son of the celebrated British physiologist Augustus Volney Waller, discoverer of the Wallerian degeneration of nerves. After qualifying in medicine at Aberdeen, Scotland and post-graduate studies under Carl Ludwig in Leipzig and John Burdon Sanderson in London he became lecturer in physiology at St. Mary's Hospital in London in 1884. He was Fellow and Croonian lecturer of the Royal Society of London and Laureat of the Institute of France and awarded the Montyon Medal of the French Academy of Science. A.D. Waller is buried in Finchley cemetery, London.

Table 3
Chronology of Electrocardiography

1887	First human ECG	A.D. Waller (45)
1902	Surface lead ECG	W. Einthoven (46)
1906	Esophageal ECG	M. Cremer (47)
1933	Unipolar chest wall leads	F.N. Wilson (48)
1936	Vector electrocardiography	F. Schellong (49)
1938	Small triangle F" (RA, LA, RL)	W. Nehb (50)
1942	Unipolar amplified extremity leads	E. Goldberger (51)
1956	Corrected orthogonal lead systems	E. Frank (52)
1960	Intracardial leads	G. Giraud and P. Puech (53)
1969	His bundle ECG	B.J. Scherlag (54)

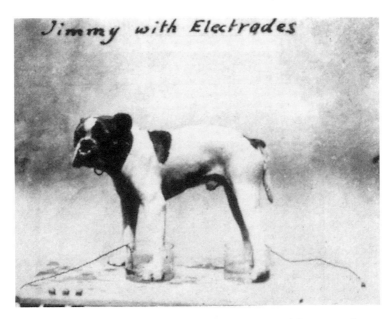

Fig. 2. Dog "Jimmie" on the Waller table. Waller's experiments and demonstrations were in part done with his pet bulldog "Jimmie" who was trained to stand quietly with two legs in pots of normal saline.

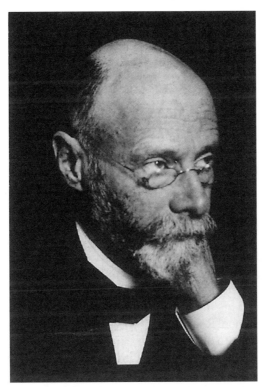

Fig. 3. Willem Einthoven (1860–1927) was born on May 21, 1860, the son of a military doctor in Semarang on the island of Java. After the death of his father, the family returned to the Netherlands in 1870, where Einthoven finished school and started medical school at the University of Utrecht in 1879. There he earned his doctorate in 1885. The same year he became a professor of physiology and histology at the University of Leiden. Einthoven held that position until his death on September 28, 1927.

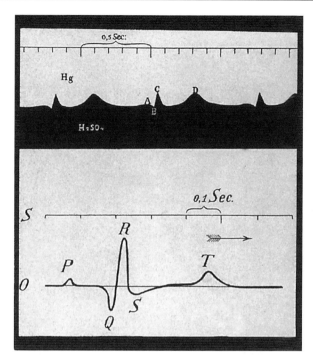

Fig. 4. Einthoven's first ECG tracings. Recording of an ECG with A, B, C and D wave using a capillary electrometer (upper registration). The lower ECG registration is Einthoven's first published electrocardiographic tracing using a string galvanometer and a different nomenclature with P, Q, R, S, and T wave.

ling, and *Willem Einthoven* were in the audience. *Willem Einthoven* (Fig. 3), a Dutch physiologist was stimulated by the presentation of Waller to further investigate cardiac electrical activity. Owing to the poor frequency response of the Lippmann capillary electrometer, Einthoven tried to refine this method for the application in cardiac electrophysiology. Using complex mathematical and physical maneuvers he succeeded in recording higher frequency curves and described the results in his first paper on the subject in 1895 *(55)*. Initially Einthoven identified four distinct waves on the electrocardiogram (Fig. 4, A–D). However, he finally turned to another technical approach and modified the string galvanometer, an apparatus recently and independently invented by the French physicist *Arsène D'Arsonval* and the engineer *Clement Ader (56)*. Einthoven's string galvanometer and his first recording were described in 1902 in a "Festschrift" for the Dutch physician Samuel Rosenstein (Fig. 4) *(57)*. In the following years he published several papers coming from his early experiences in recordings from 6 persons to a first structured overview about normal and abnormal electrocardiograms in patients from the University Hospital Leiden including atrial fibrillation, ventricular premature contractions, ventricular bigemini, and atrial flutter *(58–60)*.

Even though Einthoven's 600-pound apparatus was large and cumbersome, clinical researchers like *Thomas Lewis* quickly started to use it for the study and characterization of disorders in cardiac impulse formation and conduction including measurements of the myocardial depolarization and repolarization (Fig. 5). Parameters like PQ-, QRS- or QT-interval were investigated and in part identified as rate dependent *(61)*. *Bernhard*

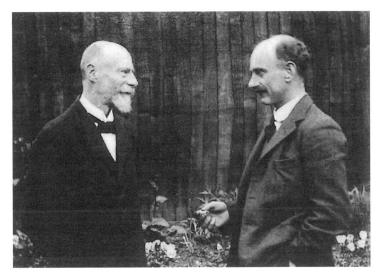

Fig. 5. Willem Einthoven and Sir Thomas Lewis in 1921.

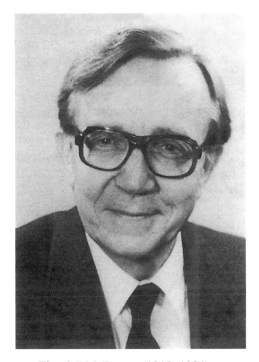

Fig. 6. Dirk Durrer (1918–1984).

Lüderitz for example analyzed in 1938 the QRS duration in relationship to the actual heart rate in 500 electrocardiograms in control subjects *(62)*.

A more detailed approach to arrhythmias became available with the introduction of invasive electrophysiologic procedures which base as a heart catheter technique on the historical maneuver performed by *Werner Forssmann (63)*. Following this pioneer, *Scherlag* described the first intracardiac catheter recordings of the His-bundle in 1969 *(64)*,

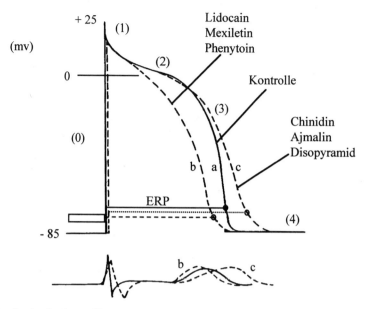

Fig. 7. Antiarrhythmic drug effects on the ventricular action potential. Effects of various antiarrhythmic drugs on the ventricular action potential. The unbroken line (a) represents the control state. The circles indicate the level of repolarization at which the fiber becomes reexcitable (ERP = effective refractory period). Action potential duration and the QT-interval are prolonged in b under the effect of Quinidine or Procainamide and shortened when exposed to Lidocain (c) *(73–75)*.

whereas *Dirk Durrer* and *Henrick JJ Wellens* were the first who executed programmed stimulation in men (Fig. 6) *(65,66)*. The programmed stimulation technique has in first-line been used to induce ventricular tachycardia and to elucidate the mechanisms of tachycardias in the Wolff-Parkinson-White-Syndrome *(67)*. Electrophysiologic testing was then more and more used to guide pharmacological therapy and to delineate the electrophysiologic effects of drugs on the normal and diseased myocardium *(68)*. The registration of the action potential in the experimental laboratory and in the intact human heart via catheter technique did substantially change our mechanisms in cellular de- and repolarization *(69–71)*, antiarrhythmic drug effects (Fig. 7) *(72–75)*, and arrhythmogenesis *(76,77)*.

History of Repolarization

In the late 18th century the Italian scientist *Felice Fontana* described a phenomenon later called the refractory period while he was investigating irregular impulses of the heart *(78)*. Subsequently, *Moritz Schiff*, a German physiologist (Fig. 8), reported in 1850 that a strong electrical stimulus that has been delivered during the late refractory period of cardiac muscle could induce a contraction. Confirmation of these findings was achieved by *Hugo Kronecker* and the French physiologist *Etienne Jules Marey*, who performed a first documentation of phenomenons like premature ventricular beats using a polygraph recording of the radial and apical impulse simultaneously *(79)*. Schiff's, Kroneckers's, and Marey's experiments have been completed by the work of *Anton Carlson*, an American physiologist, who established the still accepted concept of absolute and relative

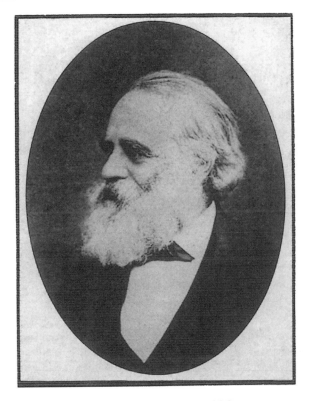

Fig. 8. Moritz Schiff (1823–1896).

refractory periods in cardiac tissue *(80)*. In 1920 *Bazett* described the relationship between rate and the duration of the QT-interval in 39 normal subjects *(81)*. He summarized, that the QT interval varies with the square root of the cycle length:

$$QT\ (s) = k(_{constant}) \times \sqrt{R\text{-}R}\ (s)$$

The constant k has been fixed to 0.37 in men and 0.4 in women by *Bazett*. Later on *Shipley* and coworkers changed these values to 0.397 and 0.415 respectively after investigating 200 normal subjects *(82)*. Today, the Bazett calculation is generally used as QT_c = $QT\sqrt{R\text{-}R}$. Thus the QT_c-interval is corrected or normalized to the QT interval at a heart rate of 60 beats/min. Several attempts have been made since to modify or substitute the Bazett calculation to gain a still better expression of the cardiac physiology. *Fridericia* for example proposed a cube root formula in 1920 after analyzing 50 normal subjects where $QT = k(_{constant}) \times \sqrt[3]{R\text{-}R}$ *(82)*. However, comparing the cube root formula to the normal range of the QT interval, this calculation gives too short intervals at low rates and too long intervals at high rates. Subsequently, *Ashman* proposed a logarithmic formula in 1942 with $QT = k_1 \times \log\ (10 \times [R\text{-}R + k_2])$ with the disadvantage of this type of calculation again exhibiting too low intervals at low heart rates *(83)*. A straight-line formula has also been discussed by various investigators *(84–88)*, however the Bazett calculation is still the most widely accepted. It has also been Ashman who investigated the relationship of heart rate and the refractory period; he described first that aberration can be induced by prolongation of the preceding cycle, an observation which is commonly referred to as the Ashman phenomenon *(89)*.

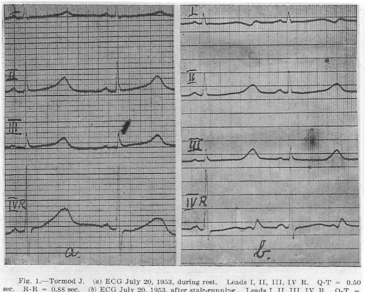

Fig. 1.—Tormod J.   (a) ECG July 20, 1953, during rest.   Leads I, II, III, IV R.   Q-T = 0.50
sec.   R-R = 0.88 sec.   (b) ECG July 20, 1953, after stair-running.   Leads I, II, III, IV R.   Q-T =
0.60 sec.   R-R = 0.86 sec.

Fig. 9. Jervell and Lange-Nielsen syndrome. A combination of deaf-mutism and a peculiar heart disease has been observed in 4 children in a family of 6. The parents were not related, and were, as the other 2 children, who otherwise seemed quite healthy and had normal hearing. The deaf-mute children, who otherwise seemed quite healthy, suffered from fainting attacks "occurring from the age to 3 to years. By clinical and roentgen examination, which was performed in 3 of the children, no signs of heart disease could be discovered. The electrocardiograms, however, revealed a pronounced prolongation of the QT interval in all cases. Three of the deaf-mute children died suddenly at the ages of 4, 5, and 9 years respectively."

Reproduced from Jervell A, Lange-Nielsen F: Congenital deaf mutism, functional heart disease with prolongation of the QT interval, and sudden death. Am Heart J 1957;54:59–68 with permission.

Lepeschkin and *Surawicz* described in 1952 QT interval differences among the 12 leads of the surface ECG as a possible expression of spatial inhomogeneity of ventricular repolarization *(90)*. However, it lasted until the mid-80s until systematic investigations of the spatial inhomogeneity of repolarization were performed: *Mirvis* and colleagues studied the difference between the longest and shortest QT interval using body surface mapping in normals and patients after myocardial infarction *(91)*. The term "QT dispersion" as an expression of regional differences in myocardial repolarization has been established in clinical cardiology by *Ronald WF Campbell* and coworkers *(92)*. Even if in our days the relevance of the QT dispersion for clinical decision making is very limited owing to methodological problems and contradicting study results, it served as an important step for a better understanding of the spatial aspects of repolarization.

HISTORY OF THE "LONG QT SYNDROME" AND "TORSADES DE POINTES" TACHYCARDIA

The *long QT syndrome* is characterized by QT interval prolongation and syncope or sudden cardiac death owing to ventricular tachyarrhythmias. The congenital form can either be familial or idiopathic *(93,94)*. The familial type consists of two subgroups:

**La tachycardie ventriculaire
à deux foyers opposés variables**

Par F. DESSERTENNE (*)

L'étude que nous avons faite d'un certain nombre de tracés de fibrillation ventriculaire recueillis dans le service de réanimation de l'hôpital
Lariboisière comportait une description et une hypothèse.
Pour le cardiologue habitué à reconnaître des ventriculogrammes
et à ne rencontrer que des variations brusques de l'amplitude du tracé,
lors de l'extra-systole par exemple, la description mettait l'accent sur la
succession ininterrompue d'oscillations irrégulières présentant dans
l'ensemble des variations progressives d'amplitude autour d'une ligne
de référence, en fuseaux.
L'hypothèse était qu'un tel aspect évoque un phénomène de batte-
ment produit par les combinaisons de l'activité électrique de plusieurs
centres, tantôt en phase et tantôt en opposition de phase.
Or, il s'en faut que toutes les variations progressives d'amplitude
d'un tracé relèvent de la fibrillation des ventricules.
Nous en avons rencontré au cours des accidents syncopaux du
bloc complet du faisceau de His, dont l'aspect en torsades de pointes
paraît relever d'une tachycardie ventriculaire à deux foyers opposés
variables.
C'est une observation clinique récente qui nous a mis sur cette voie.

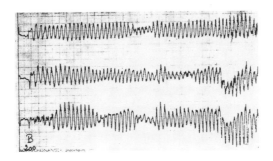

Fig. 10. Torsades de pointes tachycardia. Dessertenne first described this form of polymorphic tachycardia in 1966 when he observed this rhythm disorder in an 80-year old female patient with complete AV block *(46)*.

1. The Jervell and Lange-Nielsen which is associated with deafness.
2. The Romano-Ward syndrome with normal hearing. Two classical descriptions of these functional, hereditary syncopal cardiac disorders exist *(95–98)*.

Jervell and Lange-Nielsen Syndrome. In 1957 *Anton Jervell* and *Fred Lange-Nielsen* described a case of syncopal arrhythmia and QT prolongation combined with a profound congenital deafness in a Norwegian family with six children *(95)*. Four of the children were deaf-mutes, suffered from syncopal episodes with loss of consciousness and demonstrated a clear QT interval prolongation on their surface electrocardiograms (Fig. 9). Three of the four children with the disease died suddenly. Interestingly the parents of those children were healthy as an indicator for the recessive genetics in the Jervell and Lange-Nielsen syndrome.

Romano-Ward Syndrome. Cesarino Romano was born in Voghera, Italy in 1924. After his study of medicine at the University of Pavia, he worked in pediatrics at the University of Genoa. In 1961 he became a professor for pediatrics and later he served as the director of the First Pediatric Department and the Scientific Institute of the Pediatric Clinics at the University of Genoa. Among numerous publications dealing with hereditary hypothyroidism, cystic fibrosis, and cardiac disorders, he described in 1963 an inherited functional syncopal heart disorder with prolonged QT interval in a 3-mo-old female patient

("Aritmie cardiache rare dell'eta'pediatrica") *(96)*. Two brothers of his patient had exhibited the same symptoms and died suddenly at a young age. Independently of Romano, *Owen Conor Ward*, professor for clinical pediatrics at the University of Dublin, published one year later a work in Ireland entitled "*A New Familial Cardiac Syndrome in Children*." He also described syncopal attacks and a prolonged QT interval in both a young female patient and her brother *(97)*. Ward was born in Monaghan, Ireland on August 27, 1923. After completing St. Macarten's College in Monaghan, Ward studied medicine at the University College of Dublin where he passed his examinations in 1947. After his internship in various Irish hospitals, Ward specialized in pediatric medicine in 1949 and earned his doctorate in 1951 with a thesis on hypoglycemia in neonates. After that, Ward worked for a few years in a Dublin pediatric clinic. In 1972, he was made a professor of clinical pediatrics at the University of Dublin, where he has served as first professor for pediatrics since 1983.

The typical arrhythmia of patients with congenital or acquired long QT syndrome is the *torsades de pointes tachycardia*. This specific form of a dangerous polymorphic ventricular tachyarrhythmia is characterized by a repetitive change of the main QRS vector during tachycardia in the presence of a prolonged repolarization. *Dessertenne* first described the torsades de pointes morphology in an 80-yr-old female patient with intermittent AV block (Fig. 10) *(99)*. The cause of her recurring syncopal episodes was the torsades de pointes tachycardia rather than the bradycardia, as it has primarily been suspected. Dessertenne himself suggested in his description that two competing foci were responsible for the typical torsades de pointes morphology. This hypothesis has been tested in experimental animal studies, one using a porcine Langendorff heart technique by *Christoph Naumann d'Alnoncourt* and *Berndt Lüderitz* and in a canine heart *in situ* experiment from *Gust H Bardy* and *Raymond E Idecker (100,101)*. In both studies pacing from the left and right ventricular site at a similar but periodically changing rate resulted in an electrocardiogram with torsades de pointes configuration.

REFERENCES

1. Purkinje JE. Mikroskopisch-neurologische Beobachtungen. Arch Anat Physiol Wiss Med II/III:281–295.
2. Paladino G. Contribuzione all'Anatomia, Istologia e Fisilogia del Cuore. Napoli: Movim Med Chir, 1876.
3. His W Jr. Die Tätigkeit des embryonalen Herzens und deren Bedeutung für die Lehre von der Herzbewegung beim Erwachsenen. Arb Med Klin 1893;14–49.
4. Aschoff L, Tawara S. Die heutige Lehre von den pathologisch-anatomischen Grundlagen der Herzschwäche. Kritische Bemerkungen auf Grund eigener Untersuchungen. Jena, Fischer, 1906.
5. Wenckebach KF. Beiträge zur Kenntnis der menschlichen Herztätigkeit. Arch Anat Physiol 1906; 297–354.
6. Keith A, Flack M. The form and nature of the muscular connections between the primary divisions of the vertebrate heart. J Anat Physiol 1907;41:172–189.
7. Bachmann G. The inter-auricular time interval. Am J Physiol 1916;41:309–320.
8. Mahaim I. Kent fibers and the AV paraspecific conduction through the upper connections of the bundle of His-Tawara. Am Heart J 1947;33:651–653.
9. James TN. Morphology of the human atrioventricular node with remarks pertinent to its electrophysiology. Am Heart J 1961;62:756–771.
10. Hirsch A, ed. Biographisches Lexikon der hervorragenden Ärzte aller Zeiten und Völker. 3.Aufl. Bd. IV. München, Urban & Schwarzenberg, 1929.
11. Volavsek B, ed. Marko Gerbec. Marcus Gerbezius 1658–1718. Syndroma Gerbezius-Morgagni-Adams-Stokes. Ljubljana, 1977.

12. Cammilli L, Feruglio GA. Breve cronistoria della cardiostimolazione elettrica date, uomini e fatti da ricordare. Publicazione Distribuita in Occcasione des Secondo Simposio Europeo di Cardiostimolazione. Firenze, 3–6 Maggio, 1981.
13. Galvani L. De viribus electricitatis in motu musculari commentarius. Bologna Inst Sci, 1791.
14. Bichat MFX. Recherches physiologiques sur la vie et la mort. Paris, Fournier, 1804.
15. Aldini G. Essai theorique et experimental sur le galvanisme, avec une serie d'experiences faites en presence des commissaires de l'institut national de France, et en divers amphitheatres de Londres. Paris, Fournier, 1804.
16. Adams R. Cases of diseases of the heart accompanied with pathological observations. Dublin Hosp Rep 1827;4:353–453.
17. Stokes W. Observations of some cases of permanently slow pulse. Dublin Q J Med Sci 1846;2:73–85.
18. Duchenne de Bologne GBA. De l'ectrisation localisée et de son application à la pathologie et à la thérapeutique par courants induits et par courants galvaniques interrompus et continues. Paris, Bailliére, 1872.
19. von Ziemssen H. Studien über die Bewegungsvorgänge am menschlichen Herzen sowie über die mechanische und elektrische Erregbarkeit des Herzens und des Nervus phrenicus, angestellt an dem freiliegenden Herzen der Catharina Serafin. Arch Klin Med 1882;30:270–303.
20. Hyman AS. Resuscitation of the stopped heart by intracardial therapy. II. Experimental use of an artificial pacemaker. Arch Intern Med 1932;50:283–305.
21. Zoll PM. Resuscitation of heart in ventricular standstill by external electrical stimulation. N Engl J Med 1952;247:768–771.
22. Elmquist R, Senning A. An implantable pacemaker for the heart. In: Smyth CN, ed. Medical Electronics. Proceedings of the Second International Conference on Medical Electronics, Paris 1959. London, Iliffe & Sons, 1960.
23. Furman S, Robinson G. The use of an intracardiac pacemaker in the correction of total heart block. Surg Forum 1958;9:245–248.
24. Bouvrain Y, Zacouto F. L'entrainment électrosystolique du coeur. Presse Med 1961;69:525–528.
25. Lown B, Amarasingham R, Neumann J. New method for terminating cardiac arrhythmias. Use of synchronized capacitor discharge. JAMA 1962;182:548–555.
26. Berkovits BV, Castellanos A Jr, Lemberg L. Bifocal demand pacing. Circulation 1969;40(Suppl):III44.
27. Wellens HJJ. Electrical stimulation of the heart in the study and treatment of tachycardias. Leiden, Kroese, 1971.
28. Zipes DP, Fischer J, King RM, et al. Termination of ventricular fibrillation in dogs by depolarizing a critical amount of myocardium. Am J Cardiol 1975;36:37–44.
29. Josephson ME, Horowitz LN, Farshidi A, et al. Recurrent sustained ventricular tachycardia. Circulation 1978;57:431–440.
30. Mirowski M, Reid PR, Mower MM, et al. Termination of malignant ventricular arrhythmias with an implanted automatic defibrillator in human beings. New Engl J Med 1980;303:322–324.
31. Gallagher JJ, Svenson RH, Kasell JH, et al. Catheter technique for closed-chest ablation of the atrioventricular conduction system: A therapeutic alternative for the treatment of refractory supraventricular tachycardia. N Engl J Med 1982;306:194–200.
32. Scheinmann MM, Morady F, Hess DS, et al. Transvenous catheter technique for induction of damage to the atrioventricular junction in man. Am J Cardiol 1982;49:1013.
33. Lüderitz B, Naumann d'Alnoncourt C, Steinbeck G, et al. Therapeutic pacing in tachyarrhythmias by implanted pacemakers. PACE 1982;5:366–371.
34. Manz M, Gerckens U, Lüderitz B. Antitachycardia pacemaker (Tachylog) and automatic implantable defibrillator (AID): Combined use in ventricular tachyarrhythmias. Circulation 1985;72(Suppl):III383.
35. Borggrefe M, Budde T, Podczek A, et al. High frequency alternating current ablation of an accessory pathway in humans. J Am Coll Cardiol 1987;10:576–582.
36. Saksena S, Parsonnet V. Implantation of a cardioverter-defibrillator without thoracotomy using a triple electrode system. JAMA 1988;259:69–72.
37. Jackman WM, Wang X, Friday KJ, et al. Catheter ablation of accessory atrioventricular pathways (Wolff-Parkinson-White syndrome) by radiofrequency current. N Engl J Med 1991;324:1605–1611.
38. Kuck KH, Schlüter M, Geiger M, et al. Radiofrequency current catheter ablation of accessory pathways. Lancet 1991;337:1557–1561.
39. Daubert C, Gras D, Berder V, et al. Permanent atrial resynchronisation by syncronous bi-atrial pacing in the preventive treatment of atrial flutter associated with high degree interatrial block. Arch Mal Coeur Vaiss 1994;11:1535–1546

40. Cazeau S, Ritter P, Bakdach S, et al. Four chamber pacing in dilated cardiomyopathy. PACE 1994;17:1974–1979.

41. Lau CP, Tse HF, Lee K, et al. Initial clinical experience of a human implantable atrial defibrillator. PACE 1996;19:625.

42. Jung W, Lüderitz B. First worldwide implantation of an arrhythmia management system for ventricular and supraventricular tachyarrhythmias. Lancet 1997;349:853–854.

43. Haissaguerre M, Jais P, Shah DC, et al. Spontaneous initiation of atrial fibrillation by ectopic beats originating in the pulmonary veins. N Engl J Med 1998;339:659–666.

44. Huang DT, Monahan KM, Zimetbaum P, et al. Hybrid pharmacologic and ablative therapy: a novel and effective approach for the management of atrial fibrillation. J Cardiovasc Electrophysiol 1999;9:462–469.

45. Waller AG. A demonstration on man of electromotive changes accompanying the heart's beat. J Physiol 1887;8:229–234.

46. Einthoven W. Ein neues Galvanometer. Ann Phys 1903;12:1059–1071.

47. Cremer M. Über die direkte Ableitung der Aktionsströme des menschlichen Herzens vom Oesophagus und über das Elektrokardiogramm des Fötus. Münch Med Wschr 1906;53:811–813.

48. Wilson FN, Johnston FD, MacLeod AG, Barker PS. Electrocardiograms that represent the potential variations of a single electrode. Am Heart J. 1933;9:447–458.

49. Schellong F, Heller S, Schwingel E. Das Vektorkardiogramm, eine Untersuchungsmethode des Herzens. I. Mitteilung Z Kreislaufforsch 1937;29:497.

50. Nehb W. Zur Standardisierung der Brustwandableitungen des Elektrokardiogramms. Klin Wochenschr 1938;17:1807.

51. Goldberger E. A simple indifferent, electrocardiographic electrode of zero potential and a technique of obtaining augmented unipolar, extremity leads. Am Heart J 1942;23:483–492.

52. Frank E. An accurate, clinically practical system for spatial vectorcardiography. Circulation 1956;13:737–749.

53. Giraud G, Puech P, Latour H, Hertault J. Variations de potentiel liées à l'activité du systéme de conduction auricula-ventriculaire chez l'homme. Arch Mal Coeur 1960;53:757–776.

54. Scherlag BJ, Lau SH, Helfant RH, Berkowitz WD, Stein E, Damato AN. Catheter technique for recording His bundle activity in man. Circulation 1969;39:13–18.

55. Einthoven W. Über die Form des menschlichen Elektrocardiogramms. Arch f d Ges Physiol 1895;60:101–123.

56. Ader C. Sur un nouvel appareil enregistreur pour cables sous-marins. Compt Rend Acad Sci 1897;124:1440–1442.

57. Einthoven W. Galvanometrische registratie van het menschelijk electrocardiogram. In: Herinnerings-bundel Professor S.S. Rosenstein. Leiden: Eduard Ijdo.1902:101–107

58. Einthoven W. Die galvanometrische Registrierung des menschlichen Elektrokardiogramms, zugleich eine Beurteilung der Anwendung des Kapillar-Elektrometers in der Physiologie. Pflügers Arch 1903;99:472–480.

59. Einthoven W. The string galvanometer and the human electrocardiogram. Proc Kon Akademie voor Wetenschappen 1903;6:107–115.

60. Einhoven W. Le télécardiogramme. Arch Int de Physiol 1906;4:132–164.

61. Pardée HEB. Clinical aspects of the electrocardiogram. New York, London, Paul B Hoeber Inc, 1942, pp 32–76.

62. Lüderitz B. Über die Beziehung zwischen der Breite von QRS und der Form des ST-Stückes im menschlichen EKG. Arch f Kreislaufforsch 1939;5:223–238.

63. Forssmann W. Die Sondierung des rechten Herzens. Klin Wochenschr 1929;8:2085–2087.

64. Scherlag BJ, Lau SH, Helfant RH, et al. Catheter technique for recording His bundle activity in man. Circulation 1969;39:13–18.

65. Durrer D, Ross JP. Epicardial excitation of the ventricles in a patient with Wolff-Parkinson-White-Syndrome. Circulation 1967;35:15–21.

66. Wellens HJJ, Schuilenburg RM, Durrer D. Electrical stimulation of the heart in patients with ventricular tachycardia. Circulation 1972;46:216–226.

67. Gallagher JJ, Pritchett ELC, Sealy WC, et al. The preexcitation syndromes. Prog Cardiovasc Dis 1978;20:285–327.

68. Horowitz LN, Josephson ME, Farshidi Λ, et al. Recurrent sustained ventricular tachycardia: role of the electrophysiologic study in selection of antiarrhythmic regimens. Circulation 1978;58:986–997.

69. Burdon-Sanderson J, Page FJM. On the time-relations of the excitatory process in the ventricle of the heart of the frog. J Physiol 1882;2:385–412.
70. Schütz E. Einphasische Aktionsströme vom in situ durchbluteten Säugetierherzen. Z Biol 1932;92: 441–425.
71. Franz MR. Monophasic action potentials. Armonk, NY, Futura Publishing Co, 2000, pp 149–363.
72. Vaughan Williams EM. Classification of antiarrhythmic drugs. In: Sandoe E, Flensted-Jensen E, Olesen KH, eds. Cardiac Arrhythmias. Astra Södertälje, 1970, pp 449–469.
73. Gettes LS. The electrophysiologic effects of antiarrhythmic drugs. Am J Cardiol 1971;28:526–535.
74. Davis LD, Temte JV. Electrophysiological actions of lidocaine on canine ventricular muscle and Purkinje fibers. Circ Res 1969;24:639–655.
75. Bigger JT, Mandel WJ. Effect of lidocaine on the electrophysiological properties of ventricular muscle and Purkinje fibers. J Clin Invest 1970;49:63–77.
76. Task Force of the Working Group on Arrhythmias of the European Society of Cardiology. The Sicilian Gambit. Circulation 1991;84:1831–1851.
77. Lüderitz B. Herzrhythmusstörungen. 5. Aufl., Berlin Heidelberg New York, Springer-Verlag, 1998.
78. Hoff HE. The history of the refractory period: a neglected contribution of Felice Fontana. Yale J Biol Med 1942;14:635–672.
79. Marey EJ. Des excitations electriques due coeur. Physiologie Experimentale. Travaux du Labaratorie de M Marey. Paris, G. Masson, 1876;2:63–86.
80. Shapiro E. The electrocardiogram and the arrhythmias: historical insights. In: Mandel WJ, ed. Cardiac Arrhythmias: Their Mechanism, Diagnosis and Management. Philadelphia, J. B. Lippincott, 1980, pp 1–11.
81. Bazett HC. An analysis of the time-relations of electrocardiograms. Heart 1920;7:353–386.
82. Shipley RA, Hallaran WR. The four-lead electrocardiogram in two hundred normal men and women. Am Heart J 1936;11:325–329.
83. Fridericia LS. Die Systolendauer im Elektrokardiogramm bei normalen Menschen und bei Herzkranken. Acta Med Scand 1920;53:469–486.
84. Ashman R. The normal duration of the QT interval. Am Heart J 1942;23:522–533.
85. Adams W. The normal duration of the electrocardiographic ventricular complex. J Clin Invest 1936;15:335–342.
86. Ljung O. A simple formula for clinical interpretation of the QT interval. Acta Med Scand 1949;134: 79–86.
87. Schlamowitz I. An analysis of the time relationship within the cardiac cycle in electrocardiograms of normal men. Am Heart J 1946;31:329–342.
88. Simonson E, Cady LD, Woodbury M. The normal QT interval. Am Heart J 1962:63:747–753.
89. Gouaux JL, Ashman R. Auricular fibrillation with aberration simulating ventricular paroxysmal tachycardia. Am Heart J 1947;34:366.
90. Lepeschkin E, Surawicz B. The measurement of the QT interval of the electrocardiogram. Circulation 1952;6:378–388.
91. Mirvis DM. Spatial variation of QT intervals in normal persons and patients with acute myocardial infarction. J Am Coll Cardiol 1985;5:625–631.
92. Day CP, McComb JM, Campbell RWF. QT-dispersion: an indication of arrhythmia risk in patients with long QT intervals. Br Heart J 1990;63:342–344.
93. Jackman WM, Friday KJ, Anderson JL, et al. The long QT syndromes: a critical review, new clinical observations and a unifying hypothesis. Prog Cardiovasc Dis 1988;31:118–172.
94. Roden DM, Spooner PN. Inherited long QT syndrome: a paradigm for understanding arrhythmogenesis. J Cardiovasc Electrophysiol 1999;10:1664–1683.
95. Jervell A, Lange-Nielsen F. Congenital deaf mutism, functional heart disease with prolongation of the QT interval, and sudden death. Am Heart J 1957;54:59–68.
96. Romano C, Gemme G, Pongiglione R. Aritmie cardiache rare dell'eta' pediatrica. Clin Pediatr 1963;45:656–683.
97. Ward OC. A new familial cardiac syndrome in children. J Irish Med Assoc 1964;54:103–107.
98. Lüderitz B. History of the Disorders of Cardiac Rhythm. Armonk, NY, Futura, 1998.
99. Dessertenne F. La Tachycardie ventriculaire a deux foyers opposes variables. Arch Mal Couer 1966;59:263–272.
100. Naumann d'Alnoncourt C, Zierhut W, Lüderitz B. "Torsade de pointes" tachycardia: reentry or focal activity? Br Heart J 1982;48:213–216.
101. Bardy GH, Ungerleider RM, Smith WM, et al. A mechanism of torsades de pointes in a canine model. Circulation 1983;67:52–59.

PART II

BASIC ELECTROPHYSIOLOGY, PHARMACOLOGY, AND MOLECULAR BIOLOGY OF VENTRICULAR REPOLARIZATION

Edited by Charles Antzelevitch

3

Physiology and Molecular Biology of Ion Channels Contributing to Ventricular Repolarization

Jeanne M. Nerbonne, PhD, and Robert S. Kass, PhD

CONTENTS

INTRODUCTION

Ventricular action potential waveforms reflect the coordinated activity of multiple ion channels that open, close, and inactivate on different time scales (Fig. 1). The rapid upstroke of the action potential (phase 0) is caused by a large inward current through voltage-gated Na^+ channels, and is followed by a transient repolarization (phase 1), reflecting Na^+ channel inactivation and the activation of voltage-gated outward K^+ currents (Fig. 1). This transient repolarization or "notch" influences the height and duration of the plateau phase (phase 2) of the action potential, which depends on the delicate balance of inward (Ca^{2+} and Na^+) currents and outward (K^+) currents. Although Ca^{2+} influx through high threshold, L-type voltage-gated Ca^{2+} channels is the main contributor of inward current during the plateau phase, this current declines during phase 2 as the (L-type Ca^{2+}) channels undergo Ca^{2+} and voltage-dependent inactivation. The driving

From: *Contemporary Cardiology: Cardiac Repolarization: Bridging Basic and Clinical Science*
Edited by: I. Gussak et al. © Humana Press Inc., Totowa, NJ

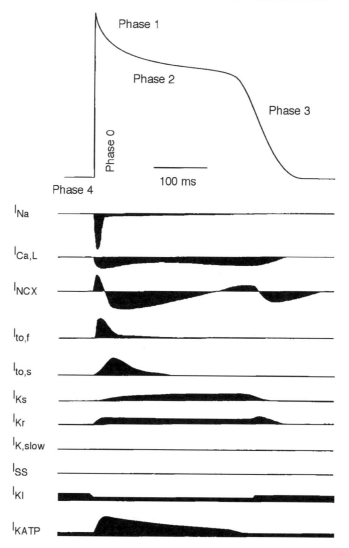

Fig. 1. Schematic of the action potential and underlying ionic currents in adult human ventricular myocytes. The contributions of some K^+ currents, such as $I_{K,slow}$ and I_{ss}, which are expressed in other species, have not been defined in human ventricular cells.

force for K^+ efflux through the voltage-gated (and other) K^+ channels, however, is high during the plateau and, as the Ca^{2+} channels inactivate, the outward K^+ currents predominate resulting in a second, rapid phase (phase 3) of repolarization back to the resting potential (Fig. 1). The height and the duration of the action potential plateau, as well as the time- and voltage-dependent properties of the underlying voltage-gated Na^+, Ca^{2+}, and K^+ currents, therefore, also influence action potential durations. As a result, modifications in the properties or the densities of any of these channels could have dramatic effects on ventricular action potential waveforms, refractory periods, and cardiac rhythms.

Electrophysiological studies have detailed the properties of the major voltage-gated inward Na^+ and Ca^{2+} and outward K^+ currents (Table 1) that determine the heights and

Table 1
Ionic Currents Contributing to Ventricular Action Potential Repolarization

Current	Activation	Inactivation	Recovery	Blocker*	Species
I_{Na}	fast	fast	fast	TTX	cat, dog, ferret, human, mouse, rat
$I_{Ca(L)}$	fast	Ca^{2+}-dep	fast	DHP Cd^{2+}	cat, dog, ferret, human, mouse, rat
$I_{to,f}$	fast	fast	fast	mM 4-AP Flecainide HaTX HpTX	cat, dog, ferret, human, mouse, rat
$I_{to,s}$	fast	slow	slow	mM 4-AP	ferret, human, mouse, rat, rabbit
I_{Kr}	moderate	fast	slow	E-4031 Dofetilide Lanthanum	cat, dog, guinea pig, human, mouse rabbit, rat
I_{Ks}	very slow	no	—	NE-10064 NE-10133	dog, guinea pig, human, rabbit rabbit
I_{Kp}	fast	no	—	Ba^{2+}	guinea pig
I_K	slow	slow	slow	mM TEA	rat
$I_{K,slow1}$	fast	slow	slow	mM 4-AP	mouse
$I_{K,slow2}$	fast	very slow	slow	mM TEA	mouse
I_{ss}	slow	no	—	mM TEA	dog, human, mouse, rat
I_{Kl}	—	—	—	Ba^{2+}	cat, dog, ferret, human, mouse, rabbit, rat
$I_{K(ATP)}$	—	—	—	SUR	cat, dog, ferret, human, mouse, rabbit, rat

*TTX = tetrodotoxin; DHP = dihydropyridine; 4-AP = 4-aminopyridine; HATX = hanatoxin; HpTX = heteropodatoxin; α-DTX = α-dendrotoxin; SUR = sulfonylurea; TEA = tetraethylammonium;

the durations of ventricular action potentials. In contrast to the Na^+ and Ca^{2+} currents, there are multiple types of K^+ currents in ventricular myocytes, and, of the various K^+ currents, the voltage-gated K^+ currents are the most numerous and diverse. At least two types of transient outward currents, $I_{to,f}$ and $I_{to,s}$, and several components of delayed rectification, including I_{Kr} ($I_{K(rapid)}$) and I_{Ks} ($I_{K(slow)}$), for example, have been distinguished in ventricular myocytes in a variety of different species (Table 1). In addition, there are marked regional differences in the expression patterns of these (voltage-gated) K^+ currents, and these differences contribute to the observed variability in ventricular action potential waveforms (1–4). Importantly, however, the time- and voltage-dependent properties of the various repolarizing currents in myocytes isolated from different species and/or from different regions of the ventricles in the same species are similar, suggesting that the molecular correlates of the underlying channels are also the same (5). A rather large number of pore forming (α) and accessory (β, δ, and γ) subunits encoding Na^+, Ca^{2+}, and K^+ channels have been identified in mammalian ventricles, and considerable progress has been made in defining the relationships between these subunits and functional ventricular Na^+, Ca^{2+}, and K^+ channels. Importantly, these studies have revealed that distinct molecular entities underlie the various ion channels contributing to ventricular action potential repolarization.

The densities and the properties of voltage-gated Na^+, Ca^{2+}, and K^+ currents change during normal ventricular development, reshaping ventricular action potential waveforms (6) and modifying the sensitivity to antiarrhythmics. In addition, alterations in the densities and properties of voltage-gated Na^+, Ca^{2+}, and K^+ currents occur in a number of myocardial disease states (7–16), changes that can lead to the generation of life threatening ventricular arrhythmias. As a result, there is considerable interest in defining the molecular mechanisms controlling the regulation, modulation, and functional expression of the channels underlying action potential repolarization in the ventricles.

INWARD NA⁺ AND CA²⁺ CURRENTS IN MAMMALIAN VENTRICLES

Voltage-Gated Ventricular Na⁺ Currents

Voltage-gated Na^+ channels open rapidly on membrane depolarization and underlie the rapid rising phases of the action potentials in mammalian ventricular myocytes (Fig. 1). The threshold for activation of these channels is quite negative (≈ -55 mV) and activation is steeply voltage-dependent. The inward movement of Na^+ through open voltage-gated Na^+ channels underlies impulse conduction in ventricular muscle, as well as in the specialized conducting network of Purkinje fibers in the ventricle (17). Voltage-gated Na^+ channels also inactivate rapidly and, during the plateau phase of the ventricular action potential, most of the Na^+ channels are in an inactivated and nonconducting state (17). There is, however, a finite probability of channel reopening at voltages corresponding to the action potential plateau (Fig. 1) and present estimates are that approx 99% of the channels are inactivated and 1% of the channels are open during the plateau phase (18–20). Although the magnitude of the Na^+ current is small during the plateau phase (particularly when compared with phase 0) of the action potential (Fig. 1), this inward current contributes to maintaining the depolarized state and, therefore, also plays a role in repolarization of the ventricular action potential.

The probability of Na^+ channel reopening at depolarized voltages (i.e., during phase 2) is determined by the overlap of the curves describing the voltage-dependences of channel activation (a measure of the probability of the channel transitioning from a closed, but available, to an open state) and steady-state inactivation (a measure of the availability of channels in the closed state). This overlap has been termed the "window" current because it is conducted over a "window" of voltages where the two curves overlap (21). At the molecular level, the fact that some channels can reopen over this voltage range implies that there is a finite probability that inactivation is reversible even at depolarized voltages. Although the Na^+ channel "window" current has been recognized as an important determinant of action potential duration in the heart for many years (21,22), recent studies focused on exploring the mechanisms underlying inherited cardiac arrhythmias have shown that voltage-gated Na^+ channels play an important role in ventricular action potential repolarization. In addition, there are regional differences in the expression of the persistent component of the voltage-gated Na^+ current in the ventricles (23). Together with the marked differences in voltage-gated outward K^+ current densities and properties, differences in Na^+ current densities may contribute to observed regional heterogeneities in ventricular action potential amplitudes and durations *(4)*.

Voltage-Gated Ventricular Ca^{2+} Currents

A number of different subtypes of voltage-gated calcium (Ca^{2+}) currents/channels have been distinguished in neurons and in muscle cells based on differences in time- and voltage-dependent properties and pharmacological profiles, and two (somewhat similar) classification schemes have evolved to describe the voltage-gated Ca^{2+} currents/channels in a variety of different cell types, including mammalian ventricular myocytes. In the first system, voltage-gated Ca^{2+} channels are referred to as low-voltage-activated (LVA) and high-voltage-activated (HVA) Ca^{2+} channels based primarily on differences in the (voltage) threshold of channel activation. Similar to voltage-gated Na^+ channels, for example, the LVA Ca^{2+} activate at relatively hyperpolarized membrane potentials, i.e., ≈-50 mV. In addition, LVA Ca^{2+} channels activate and inactivate rapidly. HVA Ca^{2+} channels, in contrast, open on depolarization to membrane potentials more positive than -20 mV, and inactivate over a time course of several hundred milliseconds to seconds. Only HVA Ca^{2+} currents are evident in mammalian ventricular myocytes (Fig. 1).

There is considerable variability in the detailed kinetic and pharmacological properties of the HVA Ca^{2+} channels expressed in different cell types, and it is now clear that HVA Ca^{2+} are considerably more heterogeneous than LVA Ca^{2+} channels. In the alternate Ca^{2+} channel nomenclature the various HVA channels are referred to by a single letter designation, i.e., L, N, P, Q, or R. In this scheme, LVA channels are referred to as T (transient) type Ca^{2+} channels. Although all HVA Ca^{2+} channels exhibit relatively large single channel conductances (13 to 25 pS) and have similar permeation properties, the electrophysiological and pharmacological properties of L- (long lasting), N- (Neither L- nor T-), P- (Purkinje), Q- and R- (Remaining) type channels are distinct.

In mammalian ventricular myocytes, the HVA current is through L-type voltage-gated Ca^{2+} channels, and the densities of the L-type Ca^{2+} channel currents do not vary appreciably in different species and/or in myocytes isolated from different region of the ventricles of the same species. These channels require strong depolarization for activation, generate relative long lasting calcium currents, $I_{Ca(L)}$, when Ba^{2+} is the charge carrier and are selectively blocked by dihydropyridine Ca^{2+} channel antagonists, such as nifedipine and nitrendipine (Table 1). The opening of L-type voltage-gated Ca^{2+} channels in response to membrane depolarization in ventricular myocytes is delayed relative to the voltage-gated Na^+ channels (Fig. 1). As a result, the L-type Ca^{2+} channels contribute little to the rapid rising phase (phase 0) of ventricular action potentials (Fig. 1). Ca^{2+} influx through the L-type Ca^{2+} channels triggers Ca^{2+} release from intracellular Ca^{2+} stores and contributes importantly, therefore, to excitation-contraction coupling. In addition, the inward Ca^{2+} current through these channels counters outward K^+ efflux and contributes importantly, therefore, to the prominent plateau phase of the action potential in ventricular myocytes (Fig. 1). Nevertheless, at positive potentials, L-type Ca^{2+} channels do inactivate and the inactivation of these channels is voltage- and Ca^{2+}-dependent. Under normal physiological conditions with Ca^{2+} as the charge carrier, inactivation of ventricular L-type voltage-gated Ca^{2+} currents is rapid owing to Ca^2-dependent channel inactivation. In addition to contributing to the termination of the action potential plateau and action potential repolarization, the spontaneous closing (inactivation) of ventricular $I_{Ca(L)}$ channels functions as a negative feedback system that is critical in governing intracellular Ca^{2+} concentration.

DIVERSITY OF VOLTAGE-GATED, OUTWARD K⁺ CURRENTS IN MAMMALIAN VENTRICLES

Voltage-gated K^+ channel currents influence the amplitudes and durations of ventricular action potentials and, in most cells, two broad classes of voltage-gated K^+ currents have been distinguished: transient outward K^+ currents, I_{to}; and delayed, outwardly rectifying K^+ currents, I_K (Table 1).

The transient currents (I_{to}) activate and inactivate rapidly and underlie the early phase (phase 1) of repolarization, whereas the delayed rectifiers (I_K) determine the latter phase (phase 3) of action potential repolarization in the ventricular myocardium (Fig. 1). These are broad classifications, however, and there are actually multiple types of I_{to} and of I_K (Table 1) expressed in ventricular cells. In addition, there are species and regional differences in the densities, as well as the detailed biophysical properties, of these currents, and these are evident in the waveforms of ventricular action potentials recorded in different cell types/species *(1–4)*.

Transient Outward K^+ Current Channels, I_{to}

Although two transient outward current components, referred to as I_{to1} and I_{to2}, were originally distinguished in cardiac Purkinje fibers and assumed to reflect distinct K^+ conductance pathways *(24–26)* the Ca^{2+}-dependent I_{to2} appears to be a Cl^- (not a K^+) current *(24–27)*. The Ca^{++}-independent, 4-aminopyridine (4-AP)-sensitive I_{to1} in cardiac Purkinje fibers, in contrast, is K^+-selective *(25,26)*. Numerous studies have described the properties of Ca^{++}-independent, 4-AP-sensitive transient outward K^+ currents in ventricular cells (Table 1), although the currents have been variably referred to as I_{to}, I_{to1}, or I_t *(5,30,31)*. Electrophysiological and pharmacological studies, however, have now clearly demonstrated that there are two distinct transient outward K^+ currents, $I_{to,fast}$ ($I_{to,f}$) and $I_{to,slow}$ ($I_{Ito,s}$), in ventricular cells and that these currents are differentially distributed *(2,3,32–35)*.

The rapidly activating and inactivating transient outward K^+ currents that are also characterized by rapid recovery from steady-state inactivation are referred to as $I_{to,fast}$ ($I_{to,f}$) and the rapidly activating and inactivating transient outward K^+ currents that recover slowly from inactivation are referred to as $I_{to,slow}$ ($I_{Ito,s}$) (Table 1) following the nomenclature suggested by Xu and colleagues *(33)*. Although prominent in ventricular myocytes from most species including cat *(36)*, dog *(37,38)*, ferret *(30)*, human *(39–41)*, mouse *(33,42–44)*, and rat *(39,45)* (Table 1), $I_{to,f}$ is recorded in guinea pig ventricular myocytes only when extracellular Ca^{2+} is removed *(46)*. The time- and voltage-dependent properties of ventricular $I_{to,f}$ in different species (Table 1) are similar in that activation, inactivation, and recovery from steady-state inactivation are all rapid *(30,33,37–41,45,47)*. In addition, $I_{to,f}$ is readily distinguished from other voltage-gated outward K^+ currents including $I_{to,s}$ using the spider K^+ channel toxins *Heteropoda* toxin-2 or -3 *(32–34,48)*. The fact that the properties of ventricular $I_{to,f}$ in different species are similar (Table 1) led to the hypothesis that the molecular correlates of functional ventricular $I_{to,f}$ channels in different species are the same *(5)*, and considerable experimental evidence in support of this hypothesis has now been provided. Indeed, all available evidence suggests that members of the Kv4 subfamily of α subunits encode functional ventricular $I_{to,f}$ channels *(2,3)*. Nevertheless, there are differences in the biophysical properties of ventricular $I_{to,f}$ channels, suggesting that there are subtle, albeit important, differences in the molecular correlates of these channels in different species.

The transient outward K^+ currents in rabbit ventricular myocytes (originally referred to as I_t) inactivate slowly and recover from steady-state inactivation very slowly, with complete recovery requiring seconds *(49–51)*. The properties of rabbit ventricular I_t are similar to the slow transient K^+ current, referred to as $I_{to,slow}$ or $I_{to,s}$, that was distinguished (from $I_{to,f}$) in mouse ventricular myocytes by the slow rates of inactivation and recovery from inactivation *(33)*. In adult mouse ventricle, $I_{to,f}$ and $I_{to,s}$ are differentially distributed *(33–35)*. In all cells isolated from the wall of the right (RV) and left (LV) ventricles, for example, $I_{to,f}$ is expressed and $I_{to,s}$ is undetectable *(33–35)*. There are, however, differences in $I_{to,f}$ densities in RV and LV cells *(33–35)*. In the ventricular septum, the currents are more heterogeneous: $\approx 80\%$ of the cells express $I_{to,f}$ and $I_{to,s}$ and the remaining ($\approx 20\%$) express $I_{to,s}$ alone. In addition, when present, $I_{to,f}$ density is significantly ($p < .001$) lower in septum, than in RV or LV, cells *(33,34)*.

The rates of inactivation and recovery from inactivation of the transient outward K^+ currents are significantly slower in ferret LV endocardial than epicardial cells *(32)*. Interestingly, the time- and voltage-dependent properties and the pharmacological sensitivities of the transient outward K^+ current in these cells are similar to mouse ventricular $I_{to,s}$ and $I_{to,f}$, respectively. The properties of I_{to} (I_t) in rabbit ventricular myocytes, in contrast, appear to be analogous to mouse ventricular $I_{to,s}$ (Table 1).

Delayed Rectifier K^+ Currents/Channels, I_K

Delayed rectifier K^+ currents, I_K, have been characterized extensively in myocytes isolated from canine *(38,47,52,53)*, feline *(54,55)*, guinea pig *(56–62)*, human *(63,64)*, mouse *(33,34,44,65,66)*, rabbit *(67,68)*, and rat *(45,69,70)* hearts and, in most cells, multiple components of I_K (Table 1) are co-expressed. In guinea pig ventricular myocytes, for example, two prominent components of I_K, I_{Kr} ($I_{K,rapid}$) and I_{Ks} ($I_{K,slow}$), were distinguished based on differences in time- and voltage-dependent properties *(59)*. I_{Kr} activates rapidly, inactivates very rapidly, displays marked inward rectification and is selectively blocked by several class III anti-arrhythmics, including dofetilide, E-4031 and sotalol *(59)*. No inward rectification is evident for I_{Ks} and this current is blocked by class III compounds, including NE-10064 and NE-10133, which do not affect I_{Kr} *(71)*. In human *(63,64,72,73)*, canine *(47,52)*, and rabbit *(68,74)* ventricular cells, both I_{Kr} and I_{Ks} are expressed and are prominent repolarizing currents. In feline *(54)* and rat *(70)* ventricular myocytes, however, only I_{Kr} is detected. I_{Kr} and I_{Ks} are also readily distinguished at the microscopic level *(56,57,67,68)*, and molecular genetic studies suggest that the molecular correlates of these channels are distinct *(2,3)*.

In rodent ventricles, there are additional components of I_K with properties different from I_{Ks} and I_{Kr} (Table 1). In rat ventricular myocytes, for example, there are novel delayed rectifier K^+ currents, referred to as I_K and I_{ss} (Table 1) *(45,75)*. In mouse ventricular myocytes, two voltage-gated K^+ currents, $I_{K,slow}$ and I_{ss}, have also been identified *(33,44,65,66,76)*. $I_{K,slow}$ is rapidly activating and slowly inactivating K^+ current with kinetic and pharmacological properties distinct from $I_{to,f}$ and $I_{to,s}$ (and I_{ss}); in addition, $I_{K,slow}$ is blocked effectively and selectively by μM concentrations of 4-AP *(65,66,76)* which do not affect $I_{to,f}$ or $I_{to,s}$ in the same cells *(33,44)*. The current, I_{ss}, remaining at the end of long (up to 10 s) depolarizing voltage steps, in contrast, is slowly activating and 4-AP insensitive *(33,44)*. In contrast to the differential distribution of $I_{to,f}$ and $I_{to,s}$, however, $I_{K,slow}$ and I_{ss} appear to be expressed in all mouse ventricular myocytes *(33,34,44)*.

Developmental Changes in Voltage-Gated K^+ Channel Expression

During postnatal development, ventricular action potentials shorten, phase 1 repolarization (Fig. 1) becomes more pronounced, and functional $I_{to,f}$ density is increased (75,77–86). In neonatal canine ventricular myocytes, for example, the "notch" and the rapid (phase 1) repolarization that are typical in adult cells are not clearly evident (78). Action potentials in neonatal cells are insensitive to 4-AP, and voltage-clamp recordings reveal that $I_{to,f}$ is undetectable (78). In cells from two-mo-old animals, $I_{to,f}$ is present and phase 1 repolarization is clearly evident (78).

The density of $I_{to,f}$ density is also low in neonatal mouse (79,85) and rat (75,77,80,82–84,86) ventricular myocytes and increases several (5–6) fold during early postnatal development. In rat, the properties of the currents in 1–2 day ventricular myocytes (86) are also distinct from those of $I_{to,f}$ in postnatal day 5 to adult cells (75) in that inactivation and recovery from inactivation are slower in postnatal day 1–2 cells. Indeed, the properties of the transient outward currents in postnatal day 1–2 rat ventricular cells (86) more closely resemble $I_{to,s}$ than $I_{to,f}$. Neither $I_{to,s}$ nor $I_{to,f}$, however, is detectable in embryonic ventricular myocytes (87).

In rabbit ventricular myocytes, transient outward K^+ current density increases and the kinetic properties of the currents also change during postnatal development (81). In contrast to rat, however, the rate of recovery of the currents (mean recovery time ≈ 100 ms) is ten times faster in neonatal than in adult (mean recovery time ≈ 1300 ms) cells (81). The slow recovery of the transient outward currents underlies the marked broadening of action potentials at high stimulation frequencies in adult (but not in neonatal) rabbit ventricular myocytes (81,88). In rabbit ventricular cells, therefore, it appears that the change in the transient outward K^+ currents is opposite to that seen in other species, i.e., $I_{to,f}$ is expressed in the neonate, whereas $I_{to,s}$ is prominent in the adult.

The expression patterns of delayed rectifier K^+ currents also change during postnatal development. Both I_{Kr} and I_{Ks}, for example, are readily detected in fetal/neonatal mouse ventricular myocytes (79,89,90), whereas these currents are difficult to detect in adult cells (33,34,44). Although I_{Kr} appears to be the predominant repolarizing K^+ current in fetal mouse ventricular cells, I_{Kr} density decreases with age (33,34,89,90). The density of I_{Ks} increases during late embryonic development (89), and subsequently decreases during postnatal development (79,85,89). Because I_{Kr} and I_{Ks} are prominent repolarizing K^+ currents in adult cardiac cells in several species, changes in the expression and/or the properties of these conductance pathways must be distinct from those observed in the mouse heart. In contrast to the marked changes in $I_{to,f}$, the density of I_K does not change significantly in rat ventricular cells after postnatal day 5 (75,84).

Regional Differences in K^+ Current Expression

There are marked differences in $I_{to,f}$ densities in different regions of the ventricles in canine (37,91), cat (55), ferret (32), human (40; but, see also 41), mouse (33,34) and rat (92). In canine left ventricle, for example, $I_{to,f}$ density is 5–6-fold higher in epicardial and midmyocardial, than in endocardial cells (91). $I_{to,s}$ density is also variable in mouse and ferret left ventricles (32–34), being detected only in (ferret) endocardial (32) and (mouse) septum (33,34) ventricular cells.

The densities of ventricular I_{Ks} and I_{Kr} are also variable. In dog, for example, I_{Ks} density is higher in epicardial and endocardial cells than in M cells (52). There are also regional differences I_{Kr} and I_{Ks} expression in guinea pig LV (93,94). In cells isolated from the LV free wall, for example, the density of I_{Kr} is higher in subepicardial, than in midmyocardial or subendocardial, myocytes (94). At the base of the LV, in contrast, I_{Kr} and I_{Ks} densities are significantly lower in endocardial than in midmyocardial or epicardial cells. These differences in voltage-gated K^+ current densities contribute to the variations in action potential waveforms recorded in different regions (right vs left; apex vs base) and layers (epicardial, midmyocardial, and endocardial) of the ventricles (1,2,4,30,37,52,93,94).

OTHER IONIC CURRENTS CONTRIBUTING TO REPOLARIZATION IN MAMMALIAN VENTRICLES

In addition to the voltage-gated K^+ channels, there are other K^+ channels that play a role in action potential repolarization in mammalian ventricles. These are the inwardly rectifying K^+ channels which are readily distinguished biophysically from the voltage-gated, outwardly rectifying K^+ channels because these channels carry inward K^+ current better than outward K^+ current. This biophysical property of these channels, however, is of no functional importance because the membrane potential of cardiac myocytes never reaches values more negative than the reversal potential for K^+ (around –90 mV). It is the outward K^+ currents through these channels that are important physiologically, and these currents also play a role in action potential repolarization. Two types of inwardly rectifying K^+ channel currents have been described in the mammalian ventricular myocytes: the cardiac inward rectifier current, I_{K1}, and the ATP-dependent K^+ current, I_{KATP}. Although the densities of these currents vary in different regions (atria, ventricles, and conducting tissue) of the heart, in the ventricles, these currents appear to be uniformly expressed.

In mammalian ventricular myocytes, I_{K1} plays a role in establishing the resting membrane potential, the plateau potential and contributes to phase 3 repolarization (Fig. 1). The strong inward rectification evident in these channels is attributed to block by intracellular Mg^{2+} (95) and by polyamines (96–98). The fact that the conductance of these channels is high at negative membrane potentials underlies the contribution of I_{K1} to ventricular resting membrane potentials (98). The voltage dependent properties of I_{K1} channels, however, are such that the conductance is very low at potentials positive to approx –40 mV (98). Nevertheless, because the driving force on K^+ is markedly increased at depolarized potentials, these channels do contribute outward K^+ current during the plateau phase of the action potential in ventricular cells, as well as during phase 3 repolarization (Fig. 1).

The weakly inwardly rectifying ATP-dependent K^+ channels, first identified in cardiac muscle, are inhibited by increased intracellular ATP and activated by nucleotide diphosphates (99). These channels are thought, therefore, to provide a link between cellular metabolism and membrane potential. In ventricular myocytes, activation of I_{KATP} channels has been suggested to play a role in the shortening of action potential durations and the loss of K^+ that occurs in various myocardial disease states, including ischemia and hypoxia, which are associated with altered metabolism or metabolic stress (100). The opening of I_{KATP} channels has also been suggested to contribute to the cardioprotection resulting from ischemic preconditioning (101,102). Unlike the voltage-gated K^+ channels expressed in the ventricular myocardium, I_{KATP} channels appear to be distributed uniformly through the right and left ventricles and through the thickness of the ventricular wall. The I_{KATP} channels, however, are expressed at much higher density than other sarcolemmal K^+ channels *(102)*. Although these channels are inhibited under normal physiological conditions, the high density suggests that action potentials will be shortened markedly when only a small number of I_{KATP} channels is activated *(103)*.

MOLECULAR CORRELATES OF VOLTAGE-GATED NA⁺ AND CA²⁺ CURRENTS IN MAMMALIAN VENTRICLE

Voltage-Gated Na⁺ Channel (Na_v) Pore-Forming α Subunits

Voltage-gated Na^+ (Na_v) channel pore-forming (α) subunits (Fig. 2A) belong to the "S4" superfamily of genes encoding voltage-gated ion channels. Although a number of Na_v α subunits (Fig. 2A) have been identified to date (Table 2), only one of these, Na_v1.5 (SCN5A) appears to be expressed in mammalian ventricular myocardium (Table 2). Each Na_v α subunit, which forms the ion-conducting pore and contains channel gating components, consists of four homologous domains (I to IV) (Fig. 2). Each domain contains six α-helical transmembrane repeats (S1–S6), for which mutagenesis studies have revealed key functional roles. The cytoplasmic linker between domains III and IV, for example, is an integral component underlying voltage-dependent inactivation *(104)*, and a critical isoleucine, phenylalanine, and methionine (IFM) motif within this linker *(105– 107)*, has been identified as the inactivation gate *(108–110)*. Na^+ channel inactivation is due to rapid block of the inner mouth of the channel pore by the cytoplasmic linker between domains III and IV that occurs within milliseconds of membrane depolarization *(111)*. NMR analysis of this linker (gate) in solution has revealed a rigid helical structure that is positioned such that it can block the pore, providing a structural interpretation of the functional studies *(112)*.

During the plateau phase of the ventricular action potential, more than 99% of the voltage-gated Na^+ channels are in an inactivated, nonconducting state in which the inactivation gate occludes the inner mouth of the conducting pore through specific interactions with sites on the S6 segment of domain IV *(113)* or the S4–S5 loop of domain IV *(114)*. Inherited mutations (i.e., ΔKPQ) in the linker between domains III and IV in SCN5A disrupt inactivation and cause one form of Long QT syndrome, LQT3 *(115)*. The mutation-induced enhancement of sustained Na^+ current activity measured during prolonged depolarization is caused by altering modes of channel gating. In a gating mode in which sustained current is enhanced, single channel recordings revealed that channels do not enter an absorbing inactivated state but instead reopen. Enhanced sustained current caused by bursting is sufficient to prolong cellular action potentials in theoretical models *(116)* and in genetically-modified mice *(117)*. Subsequent analysis of additional SNC5A mutations, linked both to LQT-3 and another inherited arrhythmia, the Brugada Syndrome, however, has revealed that this is not the only mechanism by which altered Na^+ channel function can prolong the cardiac action potential.

Several studies have revealed a critical role for the carboxy (C)-terminal tail of the Na_v channel α subunit in the control of channel inactivation *(118–122)*. Point mutations in the C-terminus, for example, can shift the voltage-dependence of inactivation, promote sustained Na^+ channel activity, change the kinetics of both the onset of and recovery from inactivation, and alter drug-channel interactions *(123–127)*. In an investigation into the secondary structure of the Na^+ channel C-terminus and the roles of possible tail structures

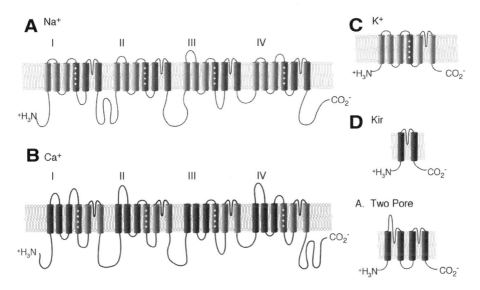

Fig. 2. Pore-forming (α) subunits of cardiac ion channels. Comparisons of primary sequences and the membrane topologies of the α subunits encoding voltage-gated Na^+ (Na_v) (**A**), voltage-gated Ca^{2+} (Ca_v) (**B**), voltage-gated (Kv) K^+ (**C**) and inwardly rectifying (Kir) K^+ channels (**D**) are illustrated. A schematic of a four transmembrane, two-pore domain K^+ channel α subunit is also presented.

in the control of inactivation, single channel data revealed that the C-terminus has pronounced effects on repetitive channel openings that occur in bursts during prolonged depolarization *(128)*. Homology modeling of the C-terminus, assuming similarity to the N-terminal domain of calmodulin, predicted that the C-terminus would adopt a predominantly α-helical structure, a prediction verified by circular dichroism (CD) of a purified C-terminus fusion protein. Only the proximal region of the C-terminus, which contains all of the helical structure, markedly modulates channel inactivation, but not activation. The distal C-terminal tail, which is largely unstructured, does not affect channel gating, but affects the density of functional Na^+ channels in the surface membrane. Taken together, these experiments suggest that interactions occur between the structured region of the C-terminus and other components of the channel protein and that these interactions function to stabilize the channel in a pore-blocked inactivated state during membrane depolarization.

The structural data also provide a framework to interpret the mechanistic basis of a large number of mutations linked either to LQT-3 or Brugada Syndrome that occur within the structured and charged proximal region of the C-terminus of the channel *(129–132)*. All inherited mutations linked to LQT-3, for example, alter Na^+ channel activity in a manner that prolongs the QT interval of the electrocardiogram (EKG) in mutation carriers, but at least three different mutations, discovered by linkage to LQT-3, have now been reported that do not result in increased sustained inward Na^+ current. The first mutation, D1790G, was discovered in a large Israeli family *(133)*. Initial expression studies revealed that this mutation changed the voltage-dependence and kinetics of inactivation of mutant channels but did not promote sustained current *(134)*, a finding questioned by subsequent investigations *(135)*. Computer based simulations suggest that this

Table 2
Diversity of Voltage-Gated Na$^+$ and Ca^{2+} α Subunits

Subfamily	Protein	Gene	Location Human	Mouse	Cardiac	Current
Na$^+$						
Na$_V$1	Na$_V$1.1	SCN1A	2q24	2		
	Na$_V$1.2	SCN2A	2q23	2		
	Na$_V$1.3	SCN3A	2q24	2		
	Na$_V$1.4	SCN4A	17q21	11		
	Na$_V$1.5	SCN5A	3p21	9		I$_{Na}$
	Na$_V$1.6	SCN8A	2q13	12		
	Na$_V$1.7	SCN9A	2q24	2		
	Na$_V$1.8	SCN10A	3p22	9		
	Na$_V$1.9	SCN11A	3p21	9		
Na$_X$	Na$_V$2.1	SCN7A	2q21-23	2		
Ca^{2+}						
Ca$_V$1	Ca$_V$1.1 ($\alpha_1$1.1) (α_{1S})	CACNA1S	1q31-32	1		
	Ca$_V$1.2 ($\alpha_1$1.2) (α_{1C})	CACNA1C	12p13.3			I$_{Ca(L)}$
	Ca$_V$1.3 ($\alpha_1$1.3) (α_{1D})	CACNA1D	3p14.3	3		
	Ca$_V$1.4 ($\alpha_1$1.4) (α_{1F})	CACNA1F	Xp11.23	X		
Ca$_V$2	Ca$_V$2.1 ($\alpha_1$2.1) (α_{1A})	CACNA1A	19p13	19		
	Ca$_V$2.2 ($\alpha_1$2.2) (α_{1B})	CACNA1B	9q34			
	Ca$_V$2.3 ($\alpha_1$2.3) (α_{1E})	CACNA1E	1q25-31	1		I$_{Ca(R)}$
Ca$_V$3	Ca$_V$3.1 ($\alpha_1$3.1) (α_{1G})	CACNA1G	17q21	17		
	Ca$_V$3.2 ($\alpha_1$3.2) (α_{1H})	CACNA1H	16p13.3	16		
	Ca$_V$3.3 ($\alpha_1$3.3) (α_{1I})	CACNA1I	22q13	22		

☐ Denotes ventricular expression

Table 3
Diversity of Na^+ and Ca^{2+} Channel Accessory Subunits

Subfamily	Protein	Gene	Location Human	Mouse	Cardiac Current
Na^+					
β	β_1	SCN1B		7	
	$\boxed{\beta_2}$	SCN2B	11q24		
	$\boxed{\beta_3}$	SCN3B		9	
Ca^{2+}					
β	β_1	CACNB1		17	
	$\boxed{\beta_2}$	CACNB2		10	$I_{Ca(L)}$
	β_3	CACNB3		12	
	β_4	CACNB4	2q23	3	
$\alpha_2\delta$	$\boxed{\alpha_2\delta\text{-}1}$	CACNA2D1	7q11.2	7	$I_{Ca(L)}$
	$\boxed{\alpha_2\delta\text{-}2}$	CACNA2D2	3p14	3	?
	$\alpha_2\delta\text{-}3$	CACNA2D3	3p13		
γ	γ_1	CACNG1			
	γ_2	CACNG2	22q13	22	
	γ_3	CACNG3		16	
	γ_4	CACNG4			
	γ_5	CACNG5			
	γ_6	CACNG6	19q13.4	19	
	γ_7	CACNG7	19q13.4	19	

$\boxed{}$ Denotes ventricular expression

mutation may prolong action potential duration through an indirect effect on the control of cytoplasmic calcium concentrations *(136),* a result that awaits testing in animal models.

Another LQT-3 mutation has also been reported that does not appear to result in enhanced sustained current *(137).* In this case, the mutation (E1295K) alters both activation and inactivation gating by causing small but significant shifts in the voltage-dependence of gating. As a result, although there is no enhanced sustained Na^+ current, the voltage-dependence of the "window" current is changed. The peak of the "window" current is shifted in the positive direction such that the background currents against which it is expressed are different than in the case of wild type channels *(137)*. As a result, window current of the same amplitude will have a greater effect on net membrane currents and, because the currents flowing during the plateau phase are so small, the net result will be increased inward current and action potential prolongation *(103,138,139)*. More recently, a similar mechanism has been proposed to explain the cellular consequences of another Na^+ channel mutation linked to sudden infant death syndrome *(140)*.

Voltage-Gated Na⁺ Channel (Na) Accessory β Subunits

Functional voltage-gated Na^+ channels appear to be multi-subunit complexes consisting of a central pore-forming α subunit (Fig. 2A) and one to two auxiliary β subunits *(141)*. There are at least three different β subunit genes, SCN1b *(142,143)*, SCN2b *(144,145)*, and SCN3b *(146)* (Table 3). In the heart, the functional role of these subunits remains controversial. Most studies have focused on the role of SCN1b, which has relatively minor effects on channel gating in heart compared with its effects on gating in skeletal muscle *(147)*. Nevertheless, it has been shown that co-expression of SCN1b affects inactivation kinetics and current densities *(134,148)*. Although relatively few functional effects have been reported for SCN2b *(149)*, it has been reported that this subunit plays a role in controlling the Ca^{2+} permeability of voltage-gated Na^+ channels *(150)*. Recently, SCN3b has been reported to also be expressed in the heart with predominant expression in the Purkinje fibers and ventricles, but little expression in the atria *(148)*. In addition, like SCN1b, co-expression of SCN3b increases current density, and may affect inactivation gating *(148)*.

Voltage-Gated Ca²⁺ Channel (Ca_v) Pore-Forming α-Subunits

Voltage-gated Ca^{2+} (Ca_v) channel pore-forming (α) subunits (Fig. 2B) belong to the "S4" superfamily of voltage-gated ion channel genes that also includes voltage-gated Na^+ (Fig. 2A) and K^+ (Fig. 2C–E) channel α subunits. Structurally, functional voltage-gated Ca^{2+} (Ca_v) channels consist of a $Ca_v\alpha_1$ subunit, with a predicted mass of 212~273 kDa, and auxiliary, Ca_v β and Ca_v $\alpha_2\delta$, subunits (Fig. 3). In most voltage-gated Ca^{2+} channels, the α_1 subunit determines the properties of the resulting channels. The transmembrane topology of $Ca_v\alpha_1$ subunits is similar to the $Na_v\alpha_1$ subunits in that $Ca_v\alpha_1$ subunits comprise four homologous domains (domain I–IV), each of which is composed of six putative transmembrane segments (S1–S6), one of which is the "S4" voltage sensing domain, and a region between S5 and S6 that contributes to the Ca^{2+} selective pore (Fig. 2B). Also similar to voltage-gate $Na_v\alpha_1$ subunits (Fig. 2A), the N- and C-termini of $Ca_v\alpha_1$ subunits are intracellular (Fig. 2B). Activation of voltage-gated Ca^{2+} channels by membrane depolarization is attributed to the movement of the positively charged "S4" segment in each of the four domains.

To date, four distinct subfamilies of Ca_v channel pore-forming α_1 subunits, Ca_v1, Ca_v2, Ca_v3 and Ca_v4 *(151)*, have been identified and in each case there are many subfamily members (Table 2). The various Ca_v α subunits are differentially expressed, and heterologous expression studies have revealed that these genes encode voltage-gated Ca^{2+} channels with distinct time- and voltage-dependent properties and pharmacological sensitivities. Functional expression of any one of the four members of the Ca_v1 subfamily, $Ca_v1.1$, $Ca_v1.2$, $Ca_v1.3$ or $Ca_v1.4$ (Table 2), for example, reveals L-type Ca^{2+} channel currents, which are long lasting when Ba^{2+} is the charge carrier. These channels activate

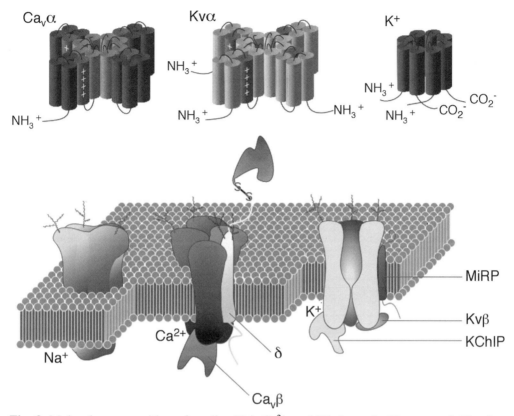

Fig. 3. Molecular composition of cardiac Na^+, Ca^{2+}, and K^+ channels. Upper panel: The four domains of the Ca_v (or Na_v) α subunit form monomeric Ca^{2+} (or Na^+) channels, whereas four Kv or Kir α subunits combine to form tetrameric K^+ channels. Lower panel: Schematic illustrating functional cardiac Na^+, Ca^{2+}, and K^+ channels, composed of the pore-forming α subunits and a variety of accessory subunits.

at relative high voltages ($\geq$–20 mV) and are selectively blocked by dihydropyridine (DHP) Ca^{2+} channel antagonists.

One member of this subfamily, $Ca_v1.2$, which encodes the widely expressed voltage-gated Ca^{2+} channel α subunit, α_{1C} ($\alpha_1 1.2$), is composed of 44 invariant and six alternative exons *(152)*, and three different isoforms of the α_{1C} protein, $\alpha_1 1.2a$, $\alpha_1 1.2b$, and $\alpha_1 1.2c$ *(153,154)*, have been identified. Although nearly identical (> 95%) in amino acid sequences, these isoforms are differentially expressed, and the cardiac specific isoform is $\alpha_1 1.2a$ *(153)*. This subunit encodes the voltage-gated L-type Ca^{2+} channel currents that are prominent in adult mammalian ventricular myocytes.

Ca_v Channel Accessory Subunits

There are at least two distinct types of accessory subunits of voltage-gated Ca^{2+} (Ca_v) channels, $Ca_v\beta$ and $Ca_v\alpha_2\delta$ subunits (Table 3). The β subunits are cytosolic proteins that are believed to form part of each functional voltage-gated L-type Ca^{2+} channel protein complex (Fig. 3). Four different $Ca_v\beta$ subunit genes, $Ca_v\beta_1$ *(155,156)*, $Ca_v\beta_2$ *(157,158)*, $Ca_v\beta_3$ *(157–159)*, and $Ca_v\beta_4$ *(159,160)* have been identified to date (Table 3). There are three variable regions flanking two highly conserved domains in each of the $Ca_v\beta$ subunits.

Table 4
Voltage-Gated K⁺ α Subunits

Voltage-Gated K^+ α Subunits

Family	Subfamily	Protein	Gene	Human	Mouse	Cardiac Current
				Location		
Family	*Subfamily*	*Protein*	*Gene*	*Human*	*Mouse*	*Cardiac Current*
Kv						
	Kv1					
		Kv1.1	KCNA1	12p13	6	
		Kv1.2	KCNA2	1p11	3	$I_{K,slow\,(rat)}$ ($I_{K,DTX}$)
		Kv1.3	KCNA3	1p21	3	
		Kv1.4	KCNA4	11p14	2	$I_{to,s}$
		Kv1.5	KCNA5	12p13	6	I_{Kur} (human/rat) $I_{K,slow}$ (mouse)
		Kv1.6	KCNA6	12p13	6	
		Kv1.7	KCNA7	19q13	7	
		Kv1.10	KCNA10	1p11		
	Kv2					
		Kv2.1	KCNB1	20q13.1	2	$I_{K,slow}$ (mouse)
		Kv2.2	KCNB2	8q13		??
	Kv3					
		Kv3.1	KCNC1	11p15	7	I_{Kur} (canine)
		Kv3.2	KCNC2			
		Kv3.3	KCNC3	19q13.4	7	
		Kv3.4	KCNC4	1p11		
	Kv4					
		Kv4.1	KCND1	Xp11.2	X	??
		Kv4.2	KCND2	7q32	6	$I_{to,f}$
		Kv4.3	KCND3	1p11	3	$I_{to,f}$
	Kv5					
		Kv5.1	KCNF1	2p25		??
	Kv6					
		Kv6.1	KCNG1	20q13.1		
		Kv6.2	KCNG2	18q23		
	Kv8					
		Kv8.1	KCN?			
	Kv9					
		Kv9.1	KCNS1	20q12	2	
		Kv9.2	KCNS2			
		Kv9.3	KCNS3	2p25		
EAG						
	eag					
		eag	KCNH1	1q32	1	
		erg1	KCNH2	7q36	5	I_{Kr}
		erg2	KCNH3		15	
		erg3	KCNH4	17q21		
		elk				
	KvLQT					
		KvLQT1	KCNQ1	11p15		I_{Ks}
		KCNQ2	KCNQ2	20p11.1	2	
		KCNQ3	KCNQ3	8q24.3		
		KCNQ4	KCNQ4	1p34.3		

☐ Denotes ventricular expression.

The variable regions are the carboxyl terminus, the amino terminus and small (~ 100 amino acids) region in the center of the linear protein sequence between the two conserved domains. The conserved domains of the $Ca_V\beta$ subunits mediate interactions with the pore-forming $Ca_V\alpha_1$ subunits, and the variable domains influence the functional effects of $Ca_V\beta$ subunit co-expression on the properties of the resulting Ca^{2+} channels (161).

In heterologous expression systems, all four $Ca_V\beta$ subunits associate with $Ca_V\alpha_1$ subunits (Fig. 3) and modify the time- and voltage-dependent properties, as well as the magnitude, of the expressed currents. It has been suggested that co-expression of $Ca_V\beta$ subunits with $Ca_V\alpha_1$ subunits increases the number of functional cell surface membrane channels, resulting in increases in Ca^{2+} current amplitudes and densities (162–165). Alternatively, the association of $Ca_V\beta$ subunits and the resulting increases in current amplitudes/densities could reflect increased expression of the $Ca_V\alpha_1$ subunit, an increase the channel open probability (163) and/or the stabilization of channel complex in the cell membrane (163,166–168). In addition to increasing current amplitudes, co-expression of $Ca_V\beta$ subunits modifies the kinetics and the voltage-dependences of current activation and inactivation (169–172).

Detailed analysis of different $Ca_V\alpha_1$ subunits has revealed that a highly conserved sequence motif, called the alpha subunit interaction domain (or AID), mediates the interaction(s) with $Ca_V\beta$ subunits (161). The AID sequence, QqxExxLxGYxxWIxxxE is located 24 amino acids from the S6 transmembrane region of domain I (Fig. 2B) of the $Ca_V\alpha_1$ subunit (154,173–175). Regions outside of AID, including low affinity binding sites in the C-termini of the $Ca_V\alpha_1$ subunits, have also been suggested to participate in the $Ca_V\beta$ - $Ca_V\alpha_1$ subunit-subunit interactions (176–178). Nevertheless, it appears that these C-terminal regions in $Ca_V\alpha_1$ also interact specifically with the second (internal) highly conserved domain of the $Ca_V\beta$ subunits to induce the observed modulatory effects (179,180).

In addition to $Ca_V\beta$ subunits, a disulfide-linked, transmembrane accessory subunit, referred to as $Ca_V\alpha_2\delta$, is also found in the complex of functional Ca^{2+} channels (Fig. 3). The first $Ca_V\alpha_2\delta$ subunit was cloned from skeletal muscle (181), and, to date, five different isoforms of $Ca_V\alpha_2\delta$-1 have been identified (Table 3). In addition, two homologous $Ca_V\alpha_2\delta$ genes, $Ca_V\alpha_2\delta$-2 and $Ca_V\alpha_2\delta$-3, have been identified in brain (182). Sequence comparison revealed ≈ 55% amino acid identity between $Ca_V\alpha_2\delta$-1 and $Ca_V\alpha_2\delta$-2 and ≈ 30% identity between $Ca_V\alpha_2\delta$-1 and $Ca_V\alpha_2\delta$-3 (182). The $Ca_V\alpha_2\delta$ $\alpha_2\delta$ subunits are heavily glycosylated proteins that are cleaved posttranslationally to yield disulfide-linked α_2 and δ proteins (Fig. 3). The $Ca_V\alpha_2$ domain is located extracellularly, whereas the $Ca_V\delta$ domain has a large hyrophobic region, which inserts into the membrane and serves as an anchor to secure the $Ca_V\alpha_2\delta$ complex (183–185).

In contrast to the accessory $Ca_V\beta$ subunits, the functional roles of $Ca_V\alpha_2\delta$ are somewhat variable and depend, at least in part, on the identities of the co-expressed $Ca_V\alpha_1$ and $Ca_V\beta$ subunits and the expression environment. In general, co-expression of $Ca_V\alpha_2\delta$-1 shifts the voltage-dependence of channel activation, accelerates the rates of current activation and inactivation, and increases current amplitudes, compared with the currents produced on expression of $Ca_V\alpha_1$ and $Ca_V\beta$ subunits alone (182,183,185–188). The increase in current density reflects improved targeting of $Ca_V\alpha_1$ subunits to the membrane (189). This effect is attributed to α_2, whereas the changes in channel kinetics reflect the expression of the δ protein (189).

MOLECULAR BASIS OF VOLTAGE-GATED K⁺ CURRENT DIVERSITY IN MAMMALIAN VENTRICLE

Voltage-Gated K^+ (Kv) Channel Pore-Forming α Subunits

Voltage-gated K^+ channel (Kv) pore-forming (α) subunits are six transmembrane spanning domain proteins (Fig. 2C) with a region between the fifth and sixth transmembrane domains that contributes to the K^+-selective pore *(2)*. The positively charged fourth transmembrane domain in the Kv α subunits (Fig. 2C) is homologous to the corresponding region in voltage-gated Na^+ (Fig. 2A) and Ca^{++} (Fig. 2B) channel α subunits, placing them in the "S4" superfamily of voltage-gated channels *(190)*. In contrast to voltage-gated Na^+ and Ca^{2+} channels, however, functional voltage-gated K^+ channels comprise four α subunits (Fig. 3). In addition, in contrast to Na^+ and Ca^{2+} α subunits (Table 2), but similar to the diversity of functional voltage-gated K^+ channels (Table 1), there are multiple Kv α subunits (Table 4). Several homologous Kv α subunit subfamilies, Kv1.x, Kv2.x, Kv3.x, Kv4.x, for example, have been identified and many of these are expressed in mammalian ventricles (Table 4). In addition to the multiplicity of Kv α subunits (Table 4), further functional K^+ channel diversity can arise through alternative splicing of transcripts, as well as through the formation of heteromultimeric channels *(191)* between two or more Kv α subunit proteins in the same Kv subfamily *(2)*.

In contrast to the Kv1.x – Kv4.x α subunit subfamilies, heterologous expression of Kv5.x – Kv9.x (Table 4) α subunits alone does not reveal functional voltage-gated K^+ channels *(192–195)*. Interestingly, however, coinjection of any of these (Kv5.1, Kv6.1, Kv8.1, or Kv9.1) subunits with Shab (Kv2.x) subfamily members attenuates the amplitudes of the Shab- (Kv2.x-) induced currents *(195)*. These observations have been interpreted as suggesting that the Kv5.x – Kv9.x subunits are regulatory Kv α subunits of the Kv2.x subfamily *(194)*, although the roles of these "silent" subunits in the generation of functional voltage-gated K^+ channels in cardiac cells remain to be determined.

Another subfamily of voltage-gated K^+ channel α subunit genes was revealed with the cloning of the Drosophila ether-a-go-go (eag) locus *(196)*. Homology screening led to the identification of human eag, as well as the human eag-related gene, referred to as HERG *(197)*, which was subsequently identified as the locus of mutations leading to one form of familial long QT-syndrome, LQT2 *(198)*. Expression of HERG (human ERG1) in Xenopus oocytes reveals inwardly rectifying voltage-gated, K^+-selective currents *(199,200)* with properties similar to cardiac I_{Kr} (Table 4). Related ERG genes, ERG2 and ERG3, have also been identified (Table 4), although these appear to be nervous system-specific and are not expressed in the mammalian heart *(201)*. Alternatively processed forms of ERG1, however, have been cloned from mouse and human heart cDNA libraries and postulated to contribute to cardiac I_{Kr} *(202–204)*.

Another subfamily of voltage-gated K^+ channel α subunits was revealed with the cloning of KvLQT1 *(205)*, the loci of mutations in another inherited form of long-QT syndrome (LQT1) (Table 4). Although expression of KvLQT1 (KCNQ1) alone reveals rapidly activating and noninactivating K^+ currents, co-expression with minK (I_{sK}) produces slowly activating K^+ currents that resemble the slow component of cardiac delayed rectification, I_{Ks} *(206,207)*. Additional KCNQ subfamily members, KCNQ2 and KCNQ3, although not expressed in heart, have been identified *(208–210)*. Interestingly, however, KCNQ2 and KCNQ3 have been identified as loci of mutations leading to benign familial neonatal convulsions *(208,210)*. Heterologous expression of KCNQ2 or KCNQ3 pro-

Table 5
Auxiliary K$^+$ Channel Subunits

| Family | Subunit | Gene | Chromosome | | Cardiac Current |
			Human	Mouse	
Kvβ					
	Kvβ1	KCNAB1	3q25	3	??
	Kvβ2	KCNAB2		4	??
	Kvβ3	KCNAB3	17p13	11	
	Kvβ4				
KCNE					
	Mink	KCNE1	21q22	16	I_{Ks}
	MiRP1	KCNE2	21q22		I_{Kr}??, $I_{to,f}$??
	MiRP2	KCNE3	11q13		
	MiRP3	KCNE4			
KChAP					
	KChAP				Ito,f??, IK??
KChIP					
	KChIP1	KCNIP1	5q35		
	KChIP2	KCNIP2	10q25		$I_{to,f}$
	KChIP3	KCNIP3			
	KChIP4				
NCS					
	NCS-1	FREQ	9q34		$I_{to,f}$
SUR					
	SUR1	ABCC8	11p15		??
	SUR2	ABCC9	12p11.1	6	$I_{K(ATP)}$

☐ Expressed in ventricle.

duces slowly activating, noninactivating K$^+$-selective currents that deactivate very slowly on membrane repolarization *(210,211)*. The unique kinetic and pharmacological properties of the expressed currents suggest that functional neuronal M channels reflect the heteromeric assembly KCNQ2 and KCNQ3 *(211)*.

Voltage-Gated K$^+$ (Kv) Channel Accessory Subunits

A number of voltage-gated K$^+$ (Kv) channel accessory subunits have now been identified (Table 5). The first of these, minK (or I_{sK}), encodes a small (130 amino acids) protein with a single membrane spanning domain *(212–214)*. As expected for an accessory Kv channel subunit, minK does not produce functional voltage-gated K$^+$ channels when expressed alone in heterologous systems *(207)*. Rather, I_{sK} appears to co-assemble with KvLQT1 to form functional I_{Ks} channels *(206,207)*. Additional minK homologues, MiRP1 (KCNE2), MiRP2 (KCNE3), and MiRP3 (KCNE4) have also been identified (Table 5), and it has been suggested that MiRP1 functions as an accessory subunit of

ERG1 in the generation of (cardiac) I_{Kr} *(215,216)*. Although it is unclear whether minK, MiRP1 or other KCNE subfamily members *(215)* contribute to the formation of voltage-gated K$^+$ channels in addition to I_{Ks} and I_{Kr} in the myocardium, it has been reported that that MiRP2 assembles with Kv3.4 in mammalian skeletal muscle *(217)* and with Kv4.x α subunits in heterologous expression systems *(218)*. These observations suggest the interesting possibility that members of the KCNE subfamily of accessory subunits can assemble with multiple Kv α subunits and contribute to the formation of multiple types of voltage-gated myocardial K$^+$ channels. Direct experimental support for this hypothesis, however, has not been provided to date, and the roles of the KCNE family of accessory subunits in the generation of functional ventricular K$^+$ channels need to be defined.

Another type of Kv accessory subunit was revealed with the identification of low molecular weight ($\approx$ 45 kD) cytosolic β subunits in brain *(219,220)*. Four homologous Kv β subunits, Kv β1, Kv β2, Kv β3, and Kv β4 (Table 5), as well as alternatively spliced transcripts, have been identified *(221–226)*, and both Kv β1 and Kv β2 are expressed in heart *(226)*. The Kvβ subunits interact with the intracellular domains of the Kv α subunits of the Kv1 subfamily in assembled voltage-gated K$^+$ channels, and heterologous expression studies suggest that Kvβ subunit co-expression affects the functional properties and the cell surface expression of Kv α subunit-encoded K$^+$ currents *(221–225,227–229)*. Because Kv α and β subunits co-assemble in the endoplasmic reticulum *(230)*, the increase in functional channel expression suggests that the Kv β subunits affect channel assembly, processing or stability or, function as chaperon proteins.

Heterologous co-expression studies suggest that the effects of the Kv β subunits are subfamily specific, i.e., Kv β1, Kv β2, and Kv β3 interact only with the Kv 1 subfamily of α subunits *(231,232)*, whereas Kv β4 is specific for the Kv2 subfamily *(233)*. Nevertheless, it is not known which Kv α subunit(s) the Kv β1 and Kv β2 subunits associate with in the myocardium, and the roles of these (Kvβ) subunits in the generation of functional cardiac K$^+$ channels remain to be determined.

Using a yeast two-hybrid screen, Wible and colleagues (1998) identified a novel voltage-gated K$^+$ channel regulatory protein, KChAP (K$^+$ channel accessory protein) (Table 5) *(234)*. Sequence analysis of KChAP revealed a 574 amino acid protein with no transmembrane domains and no homology to Kv α or Kvβ subunits *(234)*. Co-expression of KChAP with Kv2.1 (or Kv2.2) in Xenopus oocytes, however, markedly increases functional Kv2.x-induced current densities without measurably affecting the time- and/or the voltage-dependent properties of the currents *(234)* suggesting that KChAP functions as a chaperon protein. Yeast two-hybrid assays also revealed that KChAP interacts with the N-termini of Kv1.x α subunits and with the C-termini of Kv β1.x subunits *(234)*.

Using the intracellular N-terminus (amino acids 1 – 180) of Kv4.2 as the "bait" in a yeast two-hybrid screen, An and colleagues (2000) identified three novel Kv Channel Interacting Proteins, KChIP1, KChIP2, and KChIP3 (Table 5) *(235)*. Of these, only KChIP2 appears to be in heart *(235,236)*, although there are several splice variants of KChIP2 expressed *(236–238)*. Sequence analysis revealed that the KChIPs belong to the recoverin family of neuronal Ca^{2+}-sensing (NCS) proteins, particularly in the "core" regions, which contain multiple EF-hand domains *(239)*. Unlike other NCS-1 proteins, however, KChIP2 and KChIP3 lack N-terminal myristoylation sites, and the N-termini of the KChIP proteins are unique *(235)*. Interestingly, KChIP3 is identical to the NCS protein calsenilin, a Ca^{2+}-binding protein that interacts with the presenilin proteins and regulates proteolytic processing *(240)*. In addition, the nucleotide sequence of KChIP3 is 99% identical to the Ca^{2+}-regulated transcriptional repressor, DREAM *(241)*. The expression of several genes has been shown to be regulated by downstream regulatory elements (DRE) and, importantly, the DREAM protein binds to DRE elements in the absence of Ca^{2+} and dissociates when Ca^{2+} is elevated *(241)*. Thus, DREAM is thought to act as an activity-dependent regulator of gene expression *(241)*. It should be noted, however, that DREAM is predicted to have an alternative start codon resulting in a twenty amino acid N-terminal extension not present in KChIP3 *(235,241)*. Nevertheless, these findings suggest the interesting possibility that the KChIP proteins may be expressed in different cellular compartments and may subserve multiple cellular functions.

When expressed in CHO cells with Kv4.2, the KChIPs increase the functional cell surface expression of Kv4.2 encoded K^+ currents, slow current inactivation, speed recovery from inactivation and shift the voltage-dependence of activation *(235)*. Similar effects are observed when Kv4.2 or Kv4.3 is expressed with the KChIPs in Xenopus oocytes *(235)* or HEK-293 cells *(242,243)*. In contrast, KChIP expression does not affect the properties or the densities of Kv1.4- or Kv2.1-encoded K^+ currents, suggesting that the modulatory effects of the KChIP proteins are specific for α subunits of the Kv4 subfamily *(235)*. In addition, although the binding of the KChIP proteins to Kv4 α subunits is not Ca^{2+}-dependent, mutations in EF hand domains 2, 3, and 4 eliminate the modulatory effects of KChIP1 on Kv4.2-induced K^+ currents in CHO cells *(235)*. It has recently been shown that KChIP2 co-immunoprecipitates with Kv4.2 and Kv4.3 α subunits from adult mouse ventricles, consistent with a role for this subunit in the generation of Kv4-encoded mouse ventricular $I_{to,f}$ channels *(242)*. Interestingly, a gradient in KChIP2 message expression is observed through the thickness of the ventricular wall in canine and human heart, suggesting that KChIP2 underlies the observed differences in $I_{to,f}$ densities in the epicardium and endocardium in human and canine ventricles *(236)*. In rat and mouse, however, there is no gradient in KChIP2 expression *(236,242)*, and it appears that differences in Kv4.2 underlie the regional variations in $I_{to,f}$ densities in rodents *(242,244)*.

Relation between Kv Subunits and Ventricular Transient Outward K^+ Channels

Considerable experimental evidence has accumulated documenting a role for Kv α subunits of the Kv4 subfamily in the generation of ventricular $I_{to,f}$ channels. In rat ventricular myocytes exposed to antisense oligodeoxynucleotides (AsODNs) targeted against Kv4.2 or Kv4.3, for example, $I_{to,f}$ density is reduced by ~ 50% *(245)*. Similar results have recently been obtained in studies on mouse ventricular $I_{to,f}$ *(242)*. Reductions in rat ventricular $I_{to,f}$ density are also seen in cells exposed to adenoviral constructs encoding a truncated Kv4.2 subunit (Kv4.2ST) that functions as a dominant negative *(246)*. In ventricular myocytes isolated from transgenic mice expressing a dominant negative pore mutant of Kv4.2 (Kv4.2W362F) in the myocardium, $I_{to,f}$ is eliminated *(247)*. Taken together, these results demonstrate that members of the Kv4 subfamily underlie $I_{to,f}$ in mouse and rat ventricles. In addition, biochemical and electrophysiological studies suggest that Kv4.2 and Kv4.3 are associated in adult mouse ventricles and that functional mouse ventricular $I_{to,f}$ are heteromeric *(242)*. Given the similarities in the properties of $I_{to,f}$ (Table 1), it seems reasonable to suggest that Kv 4 α subunits also underlie $I_{to,f}$ in other species. In dog and human, however, the candidate subunit is Kv4.3 because Kv4.2 appears not to be expressed *(248)*. Two splice variants of Kv4.3 have been identified in human *(249)* and rat *(250,251)* heart. Although the longer version of Kv4.3, which contains a 19 amino acid insert in the carboxy tail, is the more abundant message *(249–251)*, the expression levels of the two Kv4.3 proteins, as well as the roles of these subunits in the generation of functional cardiac $I_{to,f}$ channels have been determined.

The kinetic and pharmacological properties of the slow transient outward K^+ currents, $I_{to,s}$, in ventricular myocytes are distinct from $I_{to,f}$ (Table 1), suggesting that the molecular correlates of ventricular $I_{to,s}$ and $I_{to,f}$ channels. Direct experimental support for this hypothesis has now been provided in studies completed on ventricular myocytes isolated from (C57BL6) mice with a targeted deletion in the Kv1.4 gene, Kv1.4$^{-/-}$ animals *(252)*. The waveforms of the outward K^+ currents in cells isolated from the RV or from the LV apex of Kv1.4$^{-/-}$ animals are indistinguishable from those recorded in wild-type (right ventricle and left ventricular apex) cells which lack $I_{to,s}$ *(34)*. In cells isolated from the septum of Kv1.4$^{-/-}$ animals, $I_{to,s}$ is undetectable, demonstrating that Kv1.4 underlies $I_{to,s}$ *(34)*.

Interestingly, $I_{to,s}$ (and Kv1.4 protein) is upregulated in left ventricular apex and in right ventricular cells in the Kv4.2W362F-expressing transgenics *(35)*, suggesting that electrical remodeling occurs when $I_{to,f}$ is eliminated. When the dominant negative Kv4.2W362F transgene is expressed in the Kv1.4$^{-/-}$ null background, both $I_{to,f}$ and $I_{to,s}$ are eliminated, although no further electrical remodeling is evident *(35)*. Indeed, electro-physiological recordings from Kv4.2W362F-expressing Kv1.4$^{-/-}$ cells revealed that the waveforms of the outward K^+ currents in all right and left ventricular cells are indistinguishable *(35)*. Given the similarities in the time- and voltage-dependent properties of the slow transient outward K^+ currents in other species *(32,51)*, it seems reasonable to suggest that Kv1.4 also encodes $I_{to,s}$ in ferret rabbit and human left ventricular myocytes. Direct experimental support for this hypothesis, however, has not been provided to date.

Relation between Kv Subunits and Ventricular Delayed Rectifier K^+ Channels

Human ERG1 was identified as the locus of one form of long QT-syndrome, LQT2 *(198)*, and heterologous expression of ERG1 in Xenopus oocytes reveals voltage-gated, inwardly rectifying K^+-selective channels that are similar to cardiac I_{Kr} *(199,200)*. Although these observations suggest that ERG1 encodes functional cardiac I_{Kr} channels *(199)*, AsODNS targeted against minK attenuate I_{Kr} in AT-1 (an atrial tumor line) cells *(253)* and heterologously expressed ERG1 and I_{sK} co-immunoprecipitate *(254)*. Although these observations might be interpreted as suggesting that I_{Kr} channels are multimeric, comprising the protein products of KCNH2 and KCNE1 *(253,254)*, to date, it has not been shown directly that ERG1 and minK are associated in mammalian cardiac cells.

Alternatively processed forms of HERG1 and MERG1 with unique N- and C-termini have also been identified in mouse and human heart *(202–204)*, and suggested to be important in the generation of functional I_{Kr} channels *(202,203)*. Western blot analysis of ERG1 protein expression in the myocardium, however, revealed that only the full-length ERG1 proteins are detected in rat, mouse, and human ventricles, suggesting that alternatively spliced (ERG1) variants do not play a role in the generation of functional I_{Kr} channels *(70)*.

Although heterologous expression of KCNQ1, the locus of mutations leading to LQT1 *(205)*, reveals rapidly activating, noninactivating voltage-gated K^+ currents, co-expression with minK produces slowly activating K^+ currents similar to I_{Ks} *(206,207)*. These observations, together with biochemical data demonstrating that heterologously expressed KvLQT1 and minK associate *(206)*, have been interpreted as suggesting that minK coassembles with KvLQT1 form functional cardiac I_{Ks} channels *(206,207)*. In addition, the finding that mutations in the transmembrane domain of minK alter the properties of the resulting I_{Ks} channels suggests that the transmembrane segment of I_{sK} contributes to the I_{Ks} channel pore *(255–258)*. Nevertheless, direct biochemical evidence for co-assembly of KvLQT1 and minK in mammalian ventricles has yet to be provided, and the stoichiometry of functional I_{Ks} channels has not been determined. In addition, the functional role of N-terminal splice variants of KvLQT1, which exert a dominant negative effect when co-expressed with full-length KvLQT1 *(259)*, in the generation of I_{Ks} channels in vivo remains to be determined.

Alternative experimental strategies, primarily in mice, have been exploited in studies focused on defining the molecular correlates of several of the other delayed rectifier K^+ currents in mammalian ventricles (Table 1). A role for Kv1 α subunits in the generation of mouse ventricular $I_{K,slow}$, for example, was revealed with the demonstration that $I_{K,slow}$ is selectively attenuated in ventricular myocytes isolated from transgenic mice expressing a truncated Kv1.1 α subunit, *Kv1.1N206Tag*, that functions as a dominant negative *(76)*. It was subsequently shown, however, that $I_{K,slow}$ is also reduced in ventricular myocytes expressing a dominant negative mutant of Kv 2.1, Kv2.1N216 *(260)*. Further analyses revealed that there are actually two distinct components of wild-type mouse ventricular $I_{K,slow}$: one that is sensitive to μM concentrations of 4-aminopyridine and encoded by Kv1 α subunits; and, another that is sensitive to TEA and encoded by Kv2 α subunits *(260)*. Subsequent studies revealed that the μM 4-aminopyridine-sensitive component of $I_{K,slow}$ is eliminated in ventricular myocytes isolated from mice in which Kv1.5 has been deleted suggest that Kv1.5 encodes the μM 4-AP-sensitive component of mouse ventricular $I_{K,slow}$ *(261)*. In addition, however, these findings, together with the previous results obtained on cells isolated from Kv1.4$^{-/-}$ animals, in which $I_{to,s}$ is eliminated *(34)*, suggesting that, in contrast to the Kv 4 α subunits *(242)*, the Kv 1 α subunits, Kv1.4 and Kv1.5 do not associate in adult mouse ventricles *in situ*. Rather, functional Kv1 α subunit-encoded K^+ channels in mouse ventricular myocytes are homomeric, composed of Kv1.4 α subunits ($I_{to,s}$) or Kv1.5 α subunits (the μM 4-AP-sensitive component of $I_{K,slow}$).

MOLECULAR CORRELATES
OF OTHER VENTRICULAR K⁺ CURRENTS

Subunits Encoding Inwardly Rectifying Ventricular K⁺ Channels

In cardiac and other cells, the inwardly rectifying K^+ channels are encoded by a large and diverse subfamily of inward rectifier K^+ (Kir) channel pore-forming α subunit genes (Table 6), each of which encodes a protein with two transmembrane domains (Fig. 2D). The Kir subunits assemble as tetramers to form K^+ selective pores (Fig. 3). Based on the properties of the currents produced in heterologous expression systems, Kir2 α subunits have been suggested to encode the strong inwardly rectifying cardiac I_{K1} channels *(262)* and, several members of the Kir 2 subfamily (Table 6) are expressed in the myocardium *(263)*. Direct insights into the role(s) of Kir 2 α subunits in the generation of ventricular I_{K1} channels was provided in studies completed on myocytes isolated from mice with a targeted deletion of the coding region of Kir2.1 (Kir2.1$^{-/-}$) or Kir 2.2 (Kir2.2$^{-/-}$) *(264,265)*.

Table 6
Inward Rectifier and Two-Pore K⁺ Channel α Subunits

Family	Subfamily	Protein	Gene	Human	Mouse	Cardiac Current
				Location		
Kir						
	Kir1					
		Kir1.1	*KCNJ1*	11q25		??
	Kir2					
		Kir2.1	*KCNJ2*	17q23	11	I_{K1}
		Kir2.2	*KCNJ12*	17p11.2	11	I_{K1}
		Kir2.3	*KCNJ4*	22U		??
		Kir2.4	*KCNJ14*	19q13.4		??
	Kir3					
		Kir3.1	*KCNJ3*		2	I_{KACh}
		Kir3.2	*KCNJ6*	21q22		
			KCNJ7		16	
		Kir3.3	*KCNJ9*	1q21	1	
		Kir3.4	*KCNJ5*	11q25	9	I_{KACh}
	Kir4					
		Kir4.1	*KCNJ10*	1q21	1	
		Kir4.2	*KCNJ15*	21q22	16	
	Kir5					
		Kir5.1	*KCNJ16*	17q25		
	Kir6					
		Kir6.1	*KCNJ8*	12p11.1	6	
		Kir6.2	*KCNJ11*	11p15		I_{KATP}
Two-Pore						
	TWIK					
		TWIK-1	*KCNK1*	1q42	8	??
		TWIK-2	*KCNK6*	19q11	7	??
		TWIK-3	*KCNK7*			
		TWIK-4	*KCNK8*	11q12	19	
	TREK					
		TREK-1	*KCNK2*		1	??
		TREK-2	*KCNK10*	14q32		
	TASK					
		TASK-1	*KCNK3*	2p24		I_{Kp} ??
		TASK-2	*KCNK5*	6p21.1	14	
		TASK-3	*KCNK9*	8q24.3		
		TASK-4	*KCNK14*			
		TASK-5	*KCNK15*	20q12		
	TRAAK					
		TRAAK-1	*KCNK4*	11q12	19	
	THIK					
		THIK-1	*KCNK13*	14q32		
		THIK-2	*KCNK12*	2p21		??
	TALK					
		TALK-1	*KCNK16*	6p21		
		TALK-2	*KCNK17*	6p21		??

☐ Expressed in ventricle.

The Kir2.1$^{-/-}$ mice have cleft palate and die shortly after birth, thereby precluding electrophysiological studies on adult animals *(264)*. Nevertheless, voltage-clamp recordings from isolated newborn Kir2.1$^{-/-}$ ventricular myocytes revealed that I_{K1} is absent *(265)*. Interestingly, a small, slowly activating inward rectifier current, distinct from I_{K1}, is evident in Kir2.1$^{-/-}$ myocytes *(265)*. The phenotypic consequences of deletion of Kir 2.2 are less dramatic and voltage-clamp recordings from adult Kir2.2$^{-/-}$ ventricular myocytes reveal a quantitative reduction in IK1 *(265)*. Taken together, these results suggest that both Kir2.1 and Kir2.2 contribute to (mouse) ventricular I_{K1} channels. The observation that Kir2.2 does not generate I_{K1} channels in the absence of Kir2.1, however, further suggests that functional cardiac I_{K1} channels are heteromeric.

In the heart, I_{KATP} channels are involved in myocardial ischemia and preconditioning *(101,102)*. In heterologous systems, I_{KATP} channels can be reconstituted by co-expression of Kir6.x subunits with ATP-binding cassette proteins that encode sulfonylurea receptors, SURx *(266)*. Although pharmacological and (mRNA) expression data suggest that cardiac sarcolemmal I_{KATP} channels are likely encoded by Kir6.2 and SUR2A, Kir6.1 is also expressed in heart *(267)* and antisense oligodeoxynucleotides against SUR1 reduce ventricular I_{KATP} channel densities *(268)*. Nevertheless, the essential role of the Kir6.2 subunit in the generation of cardiac I_{KATP} channels was documented with the demon-stration that I_{KATP} channel activity is absent in ventricular myocytes isolated from Kir6.2$^{-/-}$ animals *(269,270)*. The role of SUR2 in the generation of cardiac I_{KATP} channels is suggested by the finding that I_{KATP} channel density is reduced in myocytes from SUR2$^{-/-}$ animals *(271)*, whereas there are no cardiac effects of deleting SUR1 *(272)*. Interestingly, the properties of the residual I_{KATP} channels in SUR2$^{-/-}$ myocytes are similar to those seen on co-expression of Kir6.2 and SUR1 *(271)*, suggesting that SUR1 may also coassemble with Kir 6.2.

As might be expected, action potentials in Kir6.2$^{-/-}$ ventricular myocytes are indistinguishable from those seen in wild-type cells *(270)*. Importantly, however, the action potential shortening observed in wild-type cells during ischemia or metabolic blockade is abolished in the Kir6.2$^{-/-}$ cells *(270)*, consistent with the hypothesis that cardiac I_{KATP} channels play an important physiological role under pathophysiological conditions, particularly those involving metabolic stress *(101,102)*. It is also interesting to note, however, that action potential durations are largely unaffected in transgenic animals expressing mutant I_{KATP} channels with markedly (40-fold) reduced ATP sensitivity *(273)*. This observation suggests that there likely are additional inhibitory mechanisms that regulate cardiac I_{KATP} channel activity in vivo *(273)*.

Two Pore Domain K$^+$ Channels

In addition to the many voltage-gated K$^+$ (Table 4) and the inwardly rectifying K$^+$ (Table 6) channel α subunits, a novel type of K$^+$ α subunit with four transmembrane spanning regions and two pore domains (Fig. 2E) was identified with the cloning of TWIK-1 *(274)*. Both pore-domains contribute to the formation of the K$^+$ selective pore and functional TWIK channels assemble as dimers, rather than tetramers as is the case for other K$^+$ channels *(275)*. Subsequent to the identification of TWIK-1, a rather large number of four transmembrane and two pore domain K$^+$ channel α subunit genes have been identified and a number of these have been shown to be expressed in the myocardium (Table 6). Heterologous expression studies reveal that the members of various two pore domain subunit subfamilies give rise to currents that display distinct current-voltage-relations and differential sensitivities to a variety of modulators, including pH and fatty acids *(275)*.

The facts that there are so many of these subunits, that many of them appear to be ubiquitously expressed and that the properties of the channels encoded by these subunits are regulated by relevant physiological stimuli suggest that the two-pore domain K$^+$ channels likely subserve a variety of important physiological functions. To date, however, the physiological roles of these subunits/channels in the myocardium, as well as in other cell types, remain to be determined. Both TREK-1 and TASK-1, however, are expressed in the heart and heterologous expression of either of these subunits gives rise to instantaneous, noninactivating K$^+$ currents that display little or no voltage-dependence *(275)*. These properties have led to suggestions that these subunits contribute to "background" or "leak" currents *(276)*. To date, however, there has been no direct experimental evidence to support this hypothesis. Nevertheless, it is interesting to note that the properties of the currents produced on expression of TREK-1 or TASK-1 are similar to those of the current referred to as I$_{Kp}$ identified in guinea pig ventricular myocytes *(277,278)*.

SUMMARY AND CONCLUSIONS

Electrophysiological studies have clearly identified multiple types of voltage-gated inward and outward currents that contribute to action potential repolarization in mammalian ventricular myocardium (Table 1). Interestingly, the outward currents are more numerous and more diverse than the inward currents, and mammalian ventricular myocytes express a repertoire of voltage-gated and inwardly rectifying K$^+$ channels (Table 1) that all contribute importantly to shaping the waveforms of action potentials, as well as influencing automaticity and refractoriness. Nevertheless, the voltage-gated inward Ca^{2+} channel currents and the Na$^+$ channel "window" current *(21,22,279)* also contribute to ventricular repolarization. The pivotal role played by the Na$^+$ channel "window" current has been elegantly demonstrated in studies characterizing mutations in SCN5A that underlie Long QT-3. These studies have revealed novel mechanisms whereby altered Na$^+$ channel function impacts ventricular action potential durations. Computer-based simulations of cellular electrical activity have also been helpful in linking altered Na$^+$ (and other) channel functioning to possible/likely effects on action potential waveforms *(117,138,139,280)*. The results of these studies demonstrate that subtle changes in Na$^+$ channel gating can have profound effects on repolarization because the plateau phase of the action potential is maintained by the balance of very small currents, a lesson learned more than 50 yr ago from the elegant experiments of Silvio Weidmann *(281)*. The insights gleaned from the analysis of inherited Na$^+$ (and other) channel mutations also underscores the importance of the interplay of all of the ionic currents contributing to repolarization in determining ventricular action potential waveforms.

Molecular cloning studies have revealed an unexpected diversity of voltage-gated ion channel pore-forming α subunits (Tables 2, 4, and 6) and accessory subunits (Tables 3 and 5) that contribute to the formation of the various inward and outward current channels (Table 1) identified electrophysiologically. Similar to the electrophysiological diversity of ventricular K$^+$ channels (Table 1), the molecular analyses has revealed that multiple voltage-gated (Kv) (Table 4) and inwardly rectifying (Kir) (Table 6) K$^+$ channel pore-forming α subunits, as well as the accessory subunits of these channels (Table 5), are expressed in the myocardium, and a variety of in vitro and in vivo experimental approaches have been exploited to probe the relationship(s) between these subunits and functional ventricular K^+ channels. Important insights into these relationships have been provided through molecular genetics and the application of techniques that allow functional channel expression to be manipulated in vitro and in vivo, and the results of these efforts have led to the identification of the pore-forming α subunits contributing to the formation of most of the K^+ channels expressed in mammalian ventricular myocytes (Tables 4–6).

In contrast to the progress made in defining the Kv and the Kir α subunits encoding the functional voltage-gated and inwardly rectifying K^+ currents expressed in mammalian ventricular myocytes, there is presently very little is known about the functional roles of the two-pore domain K^+ channel α subunits (Table 6). In addition, the roles of the various accessory subunits (Table 5) in the generation of functional cardiac K^+ channels remain to be clarified.

It seems reasonable to suggest that defining the molecular correlates/compositions of the channels underlying ventricular action potential repolarization will facilitate future efforts focused on delineating the molecular mechanisms controlling the properties and the functional expression of these channels. Numerous studies have documented changes in functional ion channel expression during normal ventricular development, as well as in damaged or diseased ventricular myocardium. Importantly, it has also been shown that electrical remodeling occurs in the ventricles in response to changes in cardiac electrical activity or cardiac output, and most of the effects observed can be attributed to changes in the expression and/or the properties of the channels underlying ventricular repolarization. Although there are numerous possible (transcriptional, translational, and posttranslational) mechanisms that could be involved in regulating the expression and the properties of the inward and outward current channels underlying repolarization, little is presently known about the underlying molecular mechanisms that are important in mediating the changes in channel expression evident during normal development, as well as in conjunction with myocardial damage, disease and/or electrical remodeling. Clearly, a major focus of future research will be on exploring these mechanisms in detail.

REFERENCES

1. Antzelevitch C, Dumaine R. Electrical heterogeneity in the heart: physiological, pharmacological and clinical implications. In: Solaro RJ, ed. Handbook of Physiology. Vol. 1. New York: Oxford, 2002: 654–692.
2. Nerbonne JM. Molecular basis of functional voltage-gated K^+ channel diversity in the mammalian myocardium. J Physiol 2000;525 Pt 2:285–298.
3. Nerbonne JM. Molecular analysis of voltage-gated K^+ channel diversity and functioning in the mammalian heart. In: Solaro RJ, ed. Handbook of Physiology. Vol. 1. New York: Oxford, 2002:568–594.
4. Nerbonne JM, Guo W. Heterogeneous expression of voltage-gated potassium channels in the heart: Roles in normal excitation and arrhythmias. J Cardiovasc Electrophysiol 2002;13:406–409.
5. Barry DM, Nerbonne JM. Myocardial potassium channels: electrophysiological and molecular diversity. Annu Rev Physiol 1996;58:363–394.
6. Wetzel GT, Klitzner TS. Developmental cardiac electrophysiology recent advances in cellular physiology. Cardiovasc Res 1996;31 Spec No:E52–E60.
7. Benitah JP, Gomez AM, Bailly P, et al. Heterogeneity of the early outward current in ventricular cells isolated from normal and hypertrophied rat hearts. J Physiol 1993;469:111–138.
8. Beuckelmann DJ, Nabauer M, Erdmann E. Alterations of K^+ currents in isolated human ventricular myocytes from patients with terminal heart failure. Circ Res 1993;73:379–385.
9. Nabauer M, Beuckelmann DJ, Erdmann E. Characteristics of transient outward current in human ventricular myocytes from patients with terminal heart failure. Circ Res 1993;73:386–394.

10. Boyden PA, Jeck CD. Ion channel function in disease. Cardiovasc Res 1995;29:312–318.
11. Kaab S, Nuss HB, Chiamvimonvat N, et al. Ionic mechanism of action potential prolongation in ventricular myocytes from dogs with pacing-induced heart failure. Circ Res 1996;78:262–273.
12. Potreau D, Gomez JP, Fares N. Depressed transient outward current in single hypertrophied cardiomyocytes isolated from the right ventricle of ferret heart. Cardiovasc Res 1995;30:440–448.
13. Bailly P, Benitah JP, Mouchoniere M, Vassort G, Lorente P. Regional alteration of the transient outward current in human left ventricular septum during compensated hypertrophy. Circulation 1997;96:1266–1274.
14. Freeman LC, Pacioretty LM, Moise NS, Kass RS, Gilmour RF, Jr. Decreased density of I_{to} in left ventricular myocytes from German shepherd dogs with inherited arrhythmias. J Cardiovasc Electrophysiol 1997;8:872–883.
15. Gomez AM, Benitah JP, Henzel D, Vinet A, Lorente P, Delgado C. Modulation of electrical heterogeneity by compensated hypertrophy in rat left ventricle. Am J Physiol 1997;272:H1078–H1086.
16. Nabauer M, Kaab S. Potassium channel down-regulation in heart failure. Cardiovasc Res 1998;37: 324–334.
17. Catterall WA. From ionic currents to molecular mechanisms: the structure and function of voltage-gated sodium channels. Neuron 2000;26:13–25.
18. Bennett P B. Long QT syndrome: biophysical and pharmacologic mechanisms in LQT3. J Cardiovasc Electrophysiol 2000;11:819–822.
19. Rivolta I, Clancy CE, Tateyama M, Liu H, Priori SG, Kass RS. A novel SCN5A mutation associated with long QT-3; altered inactivation kinetics and channel dysfunction. Physiol Genomics 2002;10: 191–197.
20. Wang DW, Yazawa K, George A LJ, Bennett PB. Characterization of human cardiac Na^+ channel mutations in the congenital long QT syndrome. PNAS, USA 1996;93:13200–13205.
21. Attwell D, Cohen I, Eisner D, Ohba M, Ojeda C. The steady state TTX-sensitive ("window") sodium current in cardiac Purkinje fibres. Pflugers Arch 1979;379:137–142.
22. Salata JJ, Wasserstrom JA. Effects of quinidine on action potentials and ionic currents in isolated canine ventricular myocytes. Circ Res 1988;62:324–337.
23. Sakmann BF, Spindler AJ, Bryant SM, Linz KW, Noble D. Distribution of a persistent sodium current across the ventricular wall in guinea pigs. Circ Res 2000;87:910–914.
24. Kenyon JL, Gibbons WR. Influence of chloride, potassium, and tetraethylammonium on the early outward current of sheep cardiac Purkinje fibers. J Gen Physiol 1979;73:117–138.
25. Kenyon JL, Gibbons WR. 4-Aminopyridine and the early outward current of sheep cardiac Purkinje fibers. J Gen Physiol 1979;73:139–157.
26. Coraboeuf E, Carmeliet E. Existence of two transient outward currents in sheep cardiac Purkinje fibers. Pflugers Arch 1982;392:352–359.
27. Zygmunt AC, Gibbons WR. Calcium-activated chloride current in rabbit ventricular myocytes. Circ Res 1991;68:424–437.
28. Zygmunt AC, Gibbons WR. Properties of the calcium-activated chloride current in heart. J Gen Physiol 1992;99:391–414.
29. Zygmunt AC. Intracellular calcium activates a chloride current in canine ventricular myocytes. Am J Physiol 1994;267:H1984–H1995.
30. Campbell DL, Rasmusson RL, Qu Y, Strauss HC. The calcium-independent transient outward potassium current in isolated ferret right ventricular myocytes. I. Basic characterization and kinetic analysis. J Gen Physiol 1993;101:571–601.
31. Nerbonne JM. Regulation of voltage-gated K^+ channel expression in the developing mammalian myocardium. J Neurobiol 1998;37:37–59.
32. Brahmajothi MV, Campbell DL, Rasmusson RL, et al. Distinct transient outward potassium current (Ito) phenotypes and distribution of fast-inactivating potassium channel alpha subunits in ferret left ventricular myocytes. J Gen Physiol 1999;113:581–600.
33. Xu H, Guo W, Nerbonne JM. Four kinetically distinct depolarization-activated K^+ currents in adult mouse ventricular myocytes. J Gen Physiol 1999;113:661–678.
34. Guo W, Xu H, London B, Nerbonne JM. Molecular basis of transient outward K^+ current diversity in mouse ventricular myocytes. J Physiol 1999;521 Pt 3:587–599.
35. Guo W, Li H, London B, Nerbonne JM. Functional consequences of elimination of $I_{(to,f)}$ and $I_{(to,s)}$: early afterdepolarizations, atrioventricular block, and ventricular arrhythmias in mice lacking Kv1.4 and expressing a dominant-negative Kv4 alpha subunit. Circ Res 2000;87:73–79.

36. Furukawa T, Myerburg RJ, Furukawa N, Bassett AL, Kimura S. Differences in transient outward currents of feline endocardial and epicardial myocytes. Circ Res 1990;67:1287–1291.

37. Litovsky SH, Antzelevitch C. Transient outward current prominent in canine ventricular epicardium but not endocardium. Circ Res 1988;62:116–126.

38. Tseng GN, Hoffman BF. Two components of transient outward current in canine ventricular myocytes. Circ Res 1989;64:633–647.

39. Wettwer E, Amos G, Gath J, Zerkowski HR, Reidemeister JC, Ravens U. Transient outward current in human and rat ventricular myocytes. Cardiovasc Res 1993;27:1662–1669.

40. Wettwer E, Amos GJ, Posival H, Ravens U. Transient outward current in human ventricular myocytes of subepicardial and subendocardial origin. Circ Res 1994;75:473–482.

41. Konarzewska H, Peeters GA, Sanguinetti MC. Repolarizing K+ currents in nonfailing human hearts. Similarities between right septal subendocardial and left subepicardial ventricular myocytes. Circulation 1995;92:1179–1187.

42. Benndorf K, Markwardt F, Nilius B. Two types of transient outward currents in cardiac ventricular cells of mice. Pflugers Arch 1987;409:641–643.

43. Benndorf K, Nilius B. Properties of an early outward current in single cells of the mouse ventricle. Gen Physiol Biophys 1988;7:449–466.

44. Xu H, Barry DM, Li H, Brunet S, Guo W, Nerbonne JM. Attenuation of the slow component of delayed rectification, action potential prolongation, and triggered activity in mice expressing a dominant-negative Kv2 alpha subunit. Circ Res 1999;85:623–633.

45. Apkon M, Nerbonne JM. Characterization of two distinct depolarization-activated K+ currents in isolated adult rat ventricular myocytes. J Gen Physiol 1991;97:973–1011.

46. Inoue M, Imanaga I. Masking of A-type K+ channel in guinea pig cardiac cells by extracellular Ca2+. Am J Physiol 1993;264:C1434–C1438.

47. Yue L, Feng J, Li GR, Nattel S. Transient outward and delayed rectifier currents in canine atrium: properties and role of isolation methods. Am J Physiol 1996;270:H2157–H2168.

48. Sanguinetti MC, Johnson JH, Hammerland LG, et al. Heteropodatoxins: peptides isolated from spider venom that block Kv4.2 potassium channels. Mol Pharmacol 1997;51:491–498.

49. Giles WR, Imaizumi Y. Comparison of potassium currents in rabbit atrial and ventricular cells. J Physiol 1988;405:123–145.

50. Fedida D, Giles WR. Regional variations in action potentials and transient outward current in myocytes isolated from rabbit left ventricle. J Physiol 1991;442:191–209.

51. Wang Z, Feng J, Shi H, Pond A, Nerbonne JM, Nattel S. Potential molecular basis of different physiological properties of the transient outward K+ current in rabbit and human atrial myocytes. Circ Res 1999;84:551–561.

52. Liu DW, Antzelevitch C. Characteristics of the delayed rectifier current (I$_{Kr}$ and I$_{Ks}$) in canine ventricular epicardial, midmyocardial, and endocardial myocytes. A weaker I$_{Ks}$ contributes to the longer action potential of the M cell. Circ Res 1995;76:351–365.

53. Yue L, Feng J, Li GR, Nattel S. Characterization of an ultrarapid delayed rectifier potassium channel involved in canine atrial repolarization. J Physiol 1996;496 (Pt 3):647–662.

54. Follmer CH, Colatsky TJ. Block of delayed rectifier potassium current, IK, by flecainide and E-4031 in cat ventricular myocytes. Circulation 1990;82:289–293.

55. Furukawa T, Kimura S, Furukawa N, Bassett AL, Myerburg RJ. Potassium rectifier currents differ in myocytes of endocardial and epicardial origin. Circ Res 1992;70:91–103.

56. Hume JR, Uehara A. Ionic basis of the different action potential configurations of single guinea-pig atrial and ventricular myocytes. J Physiol 1985;368:525–544.

57. Balser JR, Bennett PB, Roden DM. Time-dependent outward current in guinea pig ventricular myocytes. Gating kinetics of the delayed rectifier. J Gen Physiol 1990;96:835–863.

58. Horie M, Hayashi S, Kawai C. Two types of delayed rectifying K+ channels in atrial cells of guinea pig heart. Jpn J Physiol 1990;40:479–490.

59. Sanguinetti MC, Jurkiewicz NK. Delayed rectifier outward K+ current is composed of two currents in guinea pig atrial cells. Am J Physiol 1991;260:H393–H399.

60. Walsh KB, Arena JP, Kwok WM, Freeman L, Kass RS. Delayed-rectifier potassium channel activity in isolated membrane patches of guinea pig ventricular myocytes. Am J Physiol 1991;260:H1390–H1393.

61. Anumonwo JM, Freeman LC, Kwok WM, Kass RS. Delayed rectification in single cells isolated from guinea pig sinoatrial node. Am J Physiol 1992;262:H921–H925.

62. Freeman LC, Kass RS. Delayed rectifier potassium channels in ventricle and sinoatrial node of the guinea pig: molecular and regulatory properties. Cardiovasc Drugs Ther 1993;7 Suppl 3:627–635.
63. Wang Z, Fermini B, Nattel S. Rapid and slow components of delayed rectifier current in human atrial myocytes. Cardiovasc Res 1994;28:1540–1546.
64. Li GR, Feng J, Yue L, Carrier M, Nattel S. Evidence for two components of delayed rectifier K+ current in human ventricular myocytes. Circ Res 1996;78:689–696.
65. Fiset C, Clark RB, Larsen TS, Giles WR. A rapidly activating sustained K+ current modulates repolarization and excitation-contraction coupling in adult mouse ventricle. J Physiol 1997;504 (Pt 3):557–563.
66. Zhou J, Jeron A, London B, Han X, Koren G. Characterization of a slowly inactivating outward current in adult mouse ventricular myocytes. Circ Res 1998;83:806–814.
67. Shibasaki T. Conductance and kinetics of delayed rectifier potassium channels in nodal cells of the rabbit heart. J Physiol 1987;387:227–250.
68. Veldkamp MW, van Ginneken AC, Bouman LN. Single delayed rectifier channels in the membrane of rabbit ventricular myocytes. Circ Res 1993;72:865–878.
69. Boyle WA, Nerbonne JM. Two functionally distinct 4-aminopyridine-sensitive outward K+ currents in rat atrial myocytes. J Gen Physiol 1992;100:1041–1067.
70. Pond AL, Scheve BK, Benedict AT, et al. Expression of distinct ERG proteins in rat, mouse, and human heart. Relation to functional $I_{(Kr)}$ channels. J Biol Chem 2000;275:5997–6006.
71. Busch AE, Malloy K, Groh WJ, Varnum MD, Adelman JP, Maylie J. The novel class III antiarrhythmics NE-10064 and NE-10133 inhibit IsK channels expressed in Xenopus oocytes and I_{Ks} in guinea pig cardiac myocytes. Biochem Biophys Res Commun 1994;202:265–270.
72. Wang Z, Fermini B, Nattel S. Sustained depolarization-induced outward current in human atrial myocytes. Evidence for a novel delayed rectifier K+ current similar to Kv1.5 cloned channel currents. Circ Res 1993;73:1061–1076.
73. Wang Z, Fermini B, Nattel S. Delayed rectifier outward current and repolarization in human atrial myocytes. Circ Res 1993;73:276–285.
74. Salata JJ, Jurkiewicz NK, Jow B, et al. I_K of rabbit ventricle is composed of two currents: evidence for IKs. Am J Physiol 1996;271:H2477–H2489.
75. Xu H, Dixon JE, Barry DM, et al. Developmental analysis reveals mismatches in the expression of K+ channel alpha subunits and voltage-gated K+ channel currents in rat ventricular myocytes. J Gen Physiol 1996;108:405–419.
76. London B, Jeron A, Zhou J, et al. Long QT and ventricular arrhythmias in transgenic mice expressing the N terminus and first transmembrane segment of a voltage-gated potassium channel. Proc Natl Acad Sci USA 1998;95:2926–2931.
77. Kilborn MJ, Fedida D. A study of the developmental changes in outward currents of rat ventricular myocytes. J Physiol 1990;430:37–60.
78. Jeck CD, Boyden PA. Age-related appearance of outward currents may contribute to developmental differences in ventricular repolarization. Circ Res 1992;71:1390–1403.
79. Nuss HB, Marban E. Electrophysiological properties of neonatal mouse cardiac myocytes in primary culture. J Physiol 1994;479 (Pt 2):265–279.
80. Wahler GM, Dollinger SJ, Smith JM, Flemal KL. Time course of postnatal changes in rat heart action potential and in transient outward current is different. Am J Physiol 1994;267:H1157–H1166.
81. Sanchez-Chapula J, Elizalde A, Navarro-Polanco R, Barajas H. Differences in outward currents between neonatal and adult rabbit ventricular cells. Am J Physiol 1994;266:H1184–H1194.
82. Guo W, Kamiya K, Toyama J. Modulated expression of transient outward current in cultured neonatal rat ventricular myocytes: comparison with development in situ. Cardiovasc Res 1996;32:524–533.
83. Guo W, Kamiya K, Toyama J. Roles of the voltage-gated K+ channel subunits, Kv 1.5 and Kv 1.4, in the developmental changes of K+ currents in cultured neonatal rat ventricular cells. Pflügers Arch 1997;434:206–208.
84. Shimoni Y, Fiset C, Clark RB, Dixon JE, McKinnon D, Giles WR. Thyroid hormone regulates postnatal expression of transient K+ channel isoforms in rat ventricle. J Physiol 1997;500 (Pt 1):65–73.
85. Wang L, Duff HJ. Developmental changes in transient outward current in mouse ventricle. Circ Res 1997;81:120–127.
86. Wickenden AD, Kaprielian R, Parker TG, Jones OT, Backx PH. Effects of development and thyroid hormone on K+ currents and K+ channel gene expression in rat ventricle. J Physiol 1997;504 (Pt 2):271–286.

87. Petersen KR, Nerbonne JM. Expression environment determines K$^+$ current properties: Kv1 and Kv4 alpha-subunit-induced K$^+$ currents in mammalian cell lines and cardiac myocytes. Pflugers Arch 1999;437:381–392.

88. Fermini B, Wang Z, Duan D, Nattel S. Differences in rate dependence of transient outward current in rabbit and human atrium. Am J Physiol 1992;263:H1747–H1754.

89. Davies MP, An RH, Doevendans P, Kubalak S, Chien KR, Kass RS. Develomental changes in ionic channel activity in the embryonic murine heart. Circ Res 1996;78:15–25.

90. Wang L, Feng Z, Kondo C, Sheldon RS, Duff HJ. Developmental changes in the delayed rectifier K$^+$ channels in mouse heart. Circ Res 1996;79:79–85.

91. Liu DW, Gintant GA, Antzelevitch C. Ionic basis for electrophysiological distinctions among epicardial, midmyocardial, and endocardial myocytes from the free wall of the canine left ventricle. Circ Res 1993;72:671–687.

92. Clark RB, Bouchard RA, Salinas-Stefanon E, Sanchez-Chapula J, Giles WR. Heterogeneity of action potential waveforms and potassium currents in rat ventricle. Cardiovasc Res 1993;27:1795–1799.

93. Bryant SM, Wan X, Shipsey SJ, Hart G. Regional differences in the delayed rectifier current (I_{Kr} and I_{Ks}) contribute to the differences in action potential duration in basal left ventricular myocytes in guinea-pig. Cardiovasc Res 1998;40:322–331.

94. Main MC, Bryant SM, Hart G. Regional differences in action potential characteristics and membrane currents of guinea-pig left ventricular myocytes. Exp Physiol 1998;83:747–761.

95. Vandenberg CA. Inward rectification of a potassium channel in cardiac ventricular cells depends on internal magnesium ions. Proc Natl Acad Sci USA 1987;84:2560–2564.

96. Ficker E, Taglialatela M, Wible BA, Henley CM, Brown AM. Spermine and spermidine as gating molecules for inward rectifier K$^+$ channels. Science 1994;266:1068–1072.

97. Lopatin AN, Makhina EN, Nichols CG. Potassium channel block by cytoplasmic polyamines as the mechanism of intrinsic rectification. Nature 1994;372:366–369.

98. Nichols CG, Lopatin AN. Inward rectifier potassium channels. Annu Rev Physiol 1997;59:171–191.

99. Noma A. ATP-regulated K$^+$ channels in cardiac muscle. Nature 1983;305:147–148.

100. Findlay I. The ATP sensitive potassium channel of cardiac muscle and action potential shortening during metabolic stress. Cardiovasc Res 1994;28:760–761.

101. Downey JM. Ischemic preconditioning: Nature's own cardio-protective intervention. Trends Cardiovasc Med 1992;2:170–176.

102. Grover GJ, Garlid KD. ATP-Sensitive potassium channels: a review of their cardioprotective pharmacology. J Mol Cell Cardiol 2000;32:677–695.

103. Shaw RM, Rudy Y. Ionic mechanisms of propagation in cardiac tissue. Roles of the sodium and L-type calcium currents during reduced excitability and decreased gap junction coupling. Circ Res 1997;81:727–741.

104. Patton DE, West JW, Catterall WA, Goldin AL. Amino acid residues required for fast Na+ -channel inactivation: charge neutralizations and deletions in the III–IV linker. PNAS, USA 1992;89:10905–10909.

105. Catterall WA. Molecular mechanisms of inactivation and modulation of sodium channels. Renal Physiol Biochem 1994;17:121–125.

106. Catterall WA. From ionic currents to molecular mechanisms: the structure and function of voltage-gated sodium channels. Neuron 2000;26:13–25.

107. Fozzard HA, Hanck DA. Structure and function of voltage-dependent sodium channels: comparison of brain II and cardiac isoforms. Physiol Rev 1996;76:887–926.

108. Vassilev PM, Scheuer T, Catterall WA. Identification of an intracellular peptide segment involved in sodium channel inactivation. Science 1988;241:1658–1661.

109. Vassilev P, Scheuer T, Catterall WA. Inhibition of inactivation of single sodium channels by a site-directed antibody. Proc Natl Acad Sci USA 1989;86:8147–8151.

110. West JW, Patton DE, Scheuer T, Wang Y, Goldin AL, Catterall WA. A cluster of hydrophobic amino acid residues required for fast Na($^+$)-channel inactivation. Proc Natl Acad Sci USA 1992;89:10910–10914.

111. Stuhmer W, Conti F, Suzuki H, et al. Structural parts involved in activation and inactivation of the sodium channel. Nature 1989;339:597–603.

112. Rohl CA, Boeckman FA, Baker C, Scheuer T, Catterall WA, Klevit RE. Solution structure of the sodium channel inactivation gate. Biochemistry 1999;38:855–861.

113. McPhee JC, Ragsdale DS, Scheuer T, Catterall WA. A critical role for transmembrane segment IVS6 of the sodium channel alpha subunit in fast inactivation. Journal of Biological Chemistry 1995;270:12025–12034.

114. McPhee JC, Ragsdale DS, Scheuer T, Catterall WA. A critical role for the S4–S5 intracellular loop in domain IV of the sodium channel alpha-subunit in fast inactivation. Journal of Biological Chemistry 1998;273:1121–1129.

115. Bennet PB, Yazawa K, Makita N, George AL. Molecular mechanism for an inherited cardiac arrhythmia. Nature 1995;376:683–685.

116. Clancy CE, Rudy Y. Linking a genetic defect to its cellular phenotype in a cardiac arrhythmia. Nature 1999;400:566–569.

117. Nuyens D, Stengl M, Dugarmaa S, et al. Abrupt rate accelerations or premature beats cause life-threatening arrhythmias in mice with long-QT3 syndrome. Nat Med 2001;7:1021–1027.

118. Balser JR. Inherited sodium channelopathies: models for acquired arrhythmias? Am J Physiol 2002;282:H1175–1180.

119. Bennet PB. Long QT syndrome: biophysical and pharmacologic mechanisms in LQT3. J Cardiovasc Electrophysiol 2000;11:819–822.

120. Keating MT, Sanguinetti MC. Molecular and cellular mechanisms of cardiac arrhythmias. 2001;104:569–580.

121. Kambouris NG, Nuss HB, Johns DC, Marban E, Tomaselli G, Balser JR. A revised view of cardiac sodium channel "blockade" in the long-QT syndrome. J Clin Invest 2000;105:1133–1140.

122. Viswanathan PC, Bezzina CR, George AL, Jr, Roden DM, Wilde AA, Balser JR. Gating-dependent mechanisms for flecainide action in SCN5A-linked arrhythmia syndromes. Circulation 2001; 104:1200–1205.

123. Abriel H, Wehrens XH, Benhorin J, Kerem B, Kass RS. Molecular pharmacology of the sodium channel mutation D1790G linked to the long-QT syndrome. Circulation 2000;102:921–925.

124. Benhorin J, Taub R, Goldmit M, Kerem B, Kass RS, Windman I, Medina A. Effects of flecainide in patients with new SCN5A mutation: mutation-specific therapy for long-QT syndrome? Circulation 2000;101:1698–1706.

125. Liu H, Tateyama M, Clancy CE, Abriel H, Kass RS. Channel openings are necessary but not sufficient for use-dependent block of cardiac Na$^+$ channels by flecainide: Evidence from the analysis of disease-linked mutations. J Gen Physiol 2002;120:39–51.

126. Keating MT, Atkinson D, Dunn C, Timothy K, Vincent GM, Leppert M. Evidence of genetic heterogeneity in the long QT syndrome. Science 1993;260:1960–1961.

127. Moss AJ, Robinson JL. The long-QT syndrome: genetic considerations. Trends Cardiovasc Med 1993;2:81–83.

128. Cormier JW, Rivolta I, Tateyama M, Yang AS, Kass RS. Secondary structure of the human cardiac Na+ channel C terminus. Evidence for a role of helical structures in modulation of channel inactivation. J Biol Chem 2002;277:9233–9241.

129. Bezzina C, Veldkamp MW, van Den Berg MP, et al. A single Na($^+$) channel mutation causing both long-QT and Brugada syndromes. Circ Res 1999;85:1206–1213.

130. Wei J, Wang DW, Alings M, et al. Congenital long-QT syndrome caused by a novel mutation in a conserved acidic domain of the cardiac Na$^+$ channel. Circulation 1999;99:3165–3171.

131. Veldkamp MW, Viswanathan PC, Bezzina C, Baartscheer A, Wilde AA, Balser JR. Two distinct congenital arrhythmias evoked by a multidysfunctional Na$^+$ channel. Circ Res 2000;86:E91–E97.

132. Rivolta I, Abriel H, Tateyama M, et al. Inherited Brugada and long QT-3 syndrome mutations of a single residue of the cardiac sodium channel confer distinct channel and clinical phenotypes. J Biol Chem 2001;276:30623–30630.

133. Benhorin J, Goldmit M, MacCluer JW, et al. Identification of a new SCN5A mutation, D1840G, associated with the long QT syndrome. Mutations in brief no. 153. Online. Hum Mutat 1998;12:72.

134. An RH, Wang XL, Kerem B, et al. Novel LQT-3 mutation affects Na$^+$ channel activity through interactions between alpha- and beta1-subunits. Circ Res 1998;83:141–146.

135. Baroudi G, Chahine M. Biophysical phenotypes of SCN5A mutations causing long QT and Brugada syndromes. FEBS Lett 2000;487:224–228.

136. Wehrens XH, Abriel H, Cabo C, Benhorin J, Kass RS. Arrhythmogenic mechanism of an LQT-3 mutation of the human heart Na$^+$ channel alpha-subunit: A computational analysis. Circulation 2000;102:584–590.

137. Abriel H, Cabo C, Wehrens XH, et al. Novel arrhythmogenic mechanism revealed by a long-QT syndrome mutation in the cardiac Na$^+$ channel. Circ Res 2001;88:740–745.

138. Luo CH, Rudy Y. A dynamic model of the cardiac ventricular action potential. I. Simulations of ionic currents and concentration changes. Circ Res 1994;74:1071–1096.

139. Luo CH, Rudy Y. A dynamic model of the cardiac ventricular action potential. II. After depolarizations, triggered activity, and potentiation. Circ Res 1994;74:1097–1113.
140. Wedekind H, Smits JP, Schulze-Bahr E, et al. De novo mutation in the SCN5A gene associated with early onset of sudden infant death. Circulation 2001;104:1158–1164.
141. Isom LL, De Jongh KS, Catterall WA. Auxiliary subunits of voltage-gated ion channels. Neuron 1994;12:1183–1194.
142. Isom LL, De Jongh KS, Patton DE, et al. Primary structure and functional expression of the beta 1 subunit of the rat brain sodium channel. Science 1992;256:839–842.
143. Makita N, Sloan-Brown K, Weghuis DO, Ropers HH, George AL, Jr. Genomic organization and chromosomal assignment of the human voltage-gated Na$^+$ channel beta 1 subunit gene (SCN1B). Genomics 1994;23:628–634.
144. Isom LL, Ragsdale DS, De Jongh KS, et al. Structure and function of the beta 2 subunit of brain sodium channels, a transmembrane glycoprotein with a CAM motif. Cell 1995;83:433–442.
145. Jones JM, Meisler MH, Isom LL. Scn2b, a voltage-gated sodium channel beta2 gene on mouse chromosome 9. Genomics 1996;34:258–259.
146. Morgan K, Stevens EB, Shah B, et al. beta 3: an additional auxiliary subunit of the voltage-sensitive sodium channel that modulates channel gating with distinct kinetics. Proc Natl Acad Sci USA 2000;97:2308–2313.
147. Makita N, Bennett PB, George AL, Jr. Molecular determinants of beta 1 subunit-induced gating modulation in voltage-dependent Na$^+$ channels. J Neurosci 1996;16:7117–7127.
148. Fahmi AI, Patel M, Stevens EB, et al. The sodium channel beta-subunit SCN3b modulates the kinetics of SCN5a and is expressed heterogeneously in sheep heart. J Physiol 2001;537:693–700.
149. Dhar Malhotra J, Chen C, Rivolta I, et al. Characterization of sodium channel alpha- and beta-subunits in rat and mouse cardiac myocytes. Circulation 2001;103:1303–1310.
150. Santana LF, Gomez AM, Lederer WJ. Ca^{2+} flux through promiscuous cardiac Na$^+$ channels: slip-mode conductance. Science 1998;279:1027–1033.
151. Ertel EA, Campbell KP, Harpold MM, et al. Nomenclature of voltage-gated calcium channels. Neuron 2000;25:533–535.
152. Soldatov NM. Genomic structure of human L-type Ca^{2+} channel. Genomics 1994;22:77–87.
153. Mikami A, Imoto K, Tanabe T, et al. Primary structure and functional expression of the cardiac dihydropyridine-sensitive calcium channel. Nature 1989;340:230–233.
154. Biel M, Ruth P, Bosse E, et al. Primary structure and functional expression of a high voltage activated calcium channel from rabbit lung. FEBS Lett 1990;269:409–412.
155. Ruth P, Rohrkasten A, Biel M, et al. Primary structure of the beta subunit of the DHP-sensitive calcium channel from skeletal muscle. Science 1989;245:1115–1118.
156. Pragnell M, Sakamoto J, Jay SD, Campbell KP. Cloning and tissue-specific expression of the brain calcium channel beta-subunit. FEBS Lett 1991;291:253–258.
157. Perez-Reyes E, Castellano A, Kim HS, et al. Cloning and expression of a cardiac/brain beta subunit of the L-type calcium channel. J Biol Chem 1992;267:1792–1797.
158. Hullin R, Singer-Lahat D, Freichel M, et al. Calcium channel beta subunit heterogeneity: functional expression of cloned cDNA from heart, aorta and brain. Embo J 1992;11:885–890.
159. Castellano A, Wei X, Birnbaumer L, Perez-Reyes E. Cloning and expression of a neuronal calcium channel beta subunit. J Biol Chem 1993;268:12359–12366.
160. Vance CL, Begg CM, Lee WL, Haase H, Copeland TD, McEnery MW. Differential expression and association of calcium channel alpha1B and beta subunits during rat brain ontogeny. J Biol Chem 1998;273:14495–14502.
161. Pragnell M, De Waard M, Mori Y, Tanabe T, Snutch TP, Campbell KP. Calcium channel beta-subunit binds to a conserved motif in the I-II cytoplasmic linker of the alpha 1-subunit. Nature 1994;368:67–70.
162. Gregg RG, Messing A, Strube C, et al. Absence of the beta subunit (cchb1) of the skeletal muscle dihydropyridine receptor alters expression of the alpha 1 subunit and eliminates excitation-contraction coupling. Proc Natl Acad Sci USA 1996;93:13961–13966.
163. Yamaguchi H, Hara M, Strobeck M, Fukasawa K, Schwartz A, Varadi G. Multiple modulation pathways of calcium channel activity by a beta subunit. Direct evidence of beta subunit participation in membrane trafficking of the alpha1C subunit. J Biol Chem 1998;273:19348–19356.
164. Beurg M, Sukhareva M, Strube C, Powers PA, Gregg RG, Coronado R. Recovery of Ca^{2+} current, charge movements, and Ca^{2+} transients in myotubes deficient in dihydropyridine receptor beta 1 subunit transfected with beta 1 cDNA. Biophys J 1997;73:807–818.

165. Wei SK, Colecraft HM, DeMaria CD, et al. Ca^{2+} channel modulation by recombinant auxiliary beta subunits expressed in young adult heart cells. Circ Res 2000;86:175–184.

166. Chien AJ, Zhao X, Shirokov RE, et al. Roles of a membrane-localized beta subunit in the formation and targeting of functional L-type Ca^{2+} channels. J Biol Chem 1995;270:30036–30044.

167. Chien AJ, Gao T, Perez-Reyes E, Hosey MM. Membrane targeting of L-type calcium channels. Role of palmitoylation in the subcellular localization of the beta2a subunit. J Biol Chem 1998;273:23590–23597.

168. Brice NL, Berrow NS, Campbell V, et al. Importance of the different beta subunits in the membrane expression of the alpha1A and alpha2 calcium channel subunits: studies using a depolarization-sensitive alpha1A antibody. Eur J Neurosci 1997;9:749–759.

169. Lacerda AE, Kim HS, Ruth P, et al. Normalization of current kinetics by interaction between the alpha 1 and beta subunits of the skeletal muscle dihydropyridine-sensitive Ca^{2+} channel. Nature 1991;352:527–530.

170. Varadi G, Lory P, Schultz D, Varadi M, Schwartz A. Acceleration of activation and inactivation by the beta subunit of the skeletal muscle calcium channel. Nature 1991;352:159–162.

171. Bourinet E, Charnet P, Tomlinson WJ, Stea A, Snutch TP, Nargeot J. Voltage-dependent facilitation of a neuronal alpha 1C L-type calcium channel. Embo J 1994;13:5032–5039.

172. Jones LP, Wei SK, Yue DT. Mechanism of auxiliary subunit modulation of neuronal alpha1E calcium channels. J Gen Physiol 1998;112:125–143.

173. De Waard M, Witcher DR, Pragnell M, Liu H, Campbell KP. Properties of the alpha 1–beta anchoring site in voltage-dependent Ca^{2+} channels. J Biol Chem 1995;270:12056–12064.

174. Hohaus A, Poteser M, Romanin C, et al. Modulation of the smooth-muscle L-type Ca^{2+} channel alpha1 subunit (alpha1C-b) by the beta2a subunit: a peptide which inhibits binding of beta to the I-II linker of alpha1 induces functional uncoupling. Biochem J 2000;348 Pt 3:657–665.

175. Bichet D, Lecomte C, Sabatier JM, Felix R, De Waard M. Reversibility of the Ca^{2+} channel alpha(1)-beta subunit interaction. Biochem Biophys Res Commun 2000;277:729–735.

176. Qin N, Platano D, Olcese R, Stefani E, Birnbaumer L. Direct interaction of gbetagamma with a C-terminal gbetagamma-binding domain of the Ca^{2+} channel alpha1 subunit is responsible for channel inhibition by G protein-coupled receptors. Proc Natl Acad Sci USA 1997;94:8866–8871.

177. Tareilus E, Roux M, Qin N, et al. A Xenopus oocyte beta subunit: evidence for a role in the assembly/expression of voltage-gated calcium channels that is separate from its role as a regulatory subunit. Proc Natl Acad Sci USA 1997;94:1703–1708.

178. Walker D, Bichet D, Campbell KP, De Waard M. A beta 4 isoform-specific interaction site in the carboxyl-terminal region of the voltage-dependent Ca^{2+} channel alpha 1A subunit. J Biol Chem 1998;273:2361–2367.

179. De Waard M, Pragnell M, Campbell KP. Ca^{2+} channel regulation by a conserved beta subunit domain. Neuron 1994;13:495–503.

180. Gao T, Chien AJ, Hosey MM. Complexes of the alpha1C and beta subunits generate the necessary signal for membrane targeting of class C L-type calcium channels. J Biol Chem 1999;274:2137–2144.

181. Ellis SB, Williams ME, Ways NR, et al. Sequence and expression of mRNAs encoding the alpha 1 and alpha 2 subunits of a DHP-sensitive calcium channel. Science 1988;241:1661–1664.

182. Klugbauer N, Marais E, Lacinova L, Hofmann F. A T-type calcium channel from mouse brain. Pflugers Arch 1999;437:710–715.

183. Gurnett CA, De Waard M, Campbell KP. Dual function of the voltage-dependent Ca^{2+} channel alpha 2 delta subunit in current stimulation and subunit interaction. Neuron 1996;16:431–440.

184. Gurnett CA, Felix R, Campbell KP. Extracellular interaction of the voltage-dependent Ca^{2+} channel alpha2delta and alpha1 subunits. J Biol Chem 1997;272:18508–18512.

185. Wiser O, Trus M, Tobi D, Halevi S, Giladi E, Atlas D. The alpha 2/delta subunit of voltage sensitive Ca^{2+} channels is a single transmembrane extracellular protein which is involved in regulated secretion. FEBS Lett 1996;379:15–20.

186. Singer D, Biel M, Lotan I, Flockerzi V, Hofmann F, Dascal N. The roles of the subunits in the function of the calcium channel. Science 1991;253:1553–1557.

187. Bangalore R, Mehrke G, Gingrich K, Hofmann F, Kass RS. Influence of L-type Ca channel alpha 2/delta-subunit on ionic and gating current in transiently transfected HEK 293 cells. Am J Physiol 1996;270:H1521–H1528.

188. Felix R, Gurnett CA, De Waard M, Campbell KP. Dissection of functional domains of the voltage-dependent Ca^{2+} channel alpha2delta subunit. J Neurosci 1997;17:6884–6891.

189. Shistik E, Ivanina T, Puri T, Hosey M, Dascal N. Ca^{2+} current enhancement by alpha 2/delta and beta subunits in Xenopus oocytes: contribution of changes in channel gating and alpha 1 protein level. J Physiol 1995;489 (Pt 1):55–62.

190. Pongs O. Molecular biology of voltage-dependent potassium channels. Physiol Rev 1992;72:S69–S88.

191. Covarrubias M, Wei AA, Salkoff L. Shaker, Shal, Shab, and Shaw express independent K$^+$ current systems. Neuron 1991;7:763–773.

192. Drewe JA, Verma S, Frech G, Joho RH. Distinct spatial and temporal expression patterns of K+ channel mRNAs from different subfamilies. J Neurosci 1992;12:538–548.

193. Hugnot JP, Salinas M, Lesage F, et al. Kv8.1, a new neuronal potassium channel subunit with specific inhibitory properties towards Shab and Shaw channels. Embo J 1996;15:3322–3331.

194. Castellano A, Chiara MD, Mellstrom B, et al. Identification and functional characterization of a K$^+$ channel alpha-subunit with regulatory properties specific to brain. J Neurosci 1997;17:4652–4661.

195. Salinas M, Duprat F, Heurteaux C, Hugnot JP, Lazdunski M. New modulatory alpha subunits for mammalian Shab K$^+$ channels. J Biol Chem 1997;272:24371–24379.

196. Warmke J, Drysdale R, Ganetzky B. A distinct potassium channel polypeptide encoded by the Drosophila eag locus. Science 1991;252:1560–1562.

197. Warmke JW, Ganetzky B. A family of potassium channel genes related to eag in Drosophila and mammals. Proc Natl Acad Sci USA 1994;91:3438–3442.

198. Curran ME, Splawski I, Timothy KW, Vincent GM, Green ED, Keating MT. A molecular basis for cardiac arrhythmia: HERG mutations cause long QT syndrome. Cell 1995;80:795–803.

199. Sanguinetti MC, Jiang C, Curran ME, Keating MT. A mechanistic link between an inherited and an acquired cardiac arrhythmia: HERG encodes the I$_{Kr}$ potassium channel. Cell 1995;81:299–307.

200. Trudeau MC, Warmke JW, Ganetzky B, Robertson GA. HERG, a human inward rectifier in the voltage-gated potassium channel family. Science 1995;269:92–95.

201. Shi W, Wymore RS, Wang HS, et al. Identification of two nervous system-specific members of the erg potassium channel gene family. J Neurosci 1997;17:9423–9432.

202. Lees-Miller JP, Kondo C, Wang L, Duff HJ. Electrophysiological characterization of an alternatively processed ERG K$^+$ channel in mouse and human hearts. Circ Res 1997;81:719–726.

203. London B, Trudeau MC, Newton KP, et al. Two isoforms of the mouse ether-a-go-go-related gene coassemble to form channels with properties similar to the rapidly activating component of the cardiac delayed rectifier K$^+$ current. Circ Res 1997;81:870–878.

204. Kupershmidt S, Snyders DJ, Raes A, Roden DM. A K$^+$ channel splice variant common in human heart lacks a C-terminal domain required for expression of rapidly activating delayed rectifier current. J Biol Chem 1998;273:27231–27235.

205. Wang Q, Curran ME, Splawski I, et al. Positional cloning of a novel potassium channel gene: KVLQT1 mutations cause cardiac arrhythmias. Nat Genet 1996;12:17–23.

206. Barhanin J, Lesage F, Guillemare E, Fink M, Lazdunski M, Romey G. K(V)LQT1 and lsK (minK) proteins associate to form the I$_{(Ks)}$ cardiac potassium current. Nature 1996;384:78–80.

207. Sanguinetti MC, Curran ME, Zou A, et al. Coassembly of KvLQT1 and minK (IsK) proteins to form cardiac I$_{(Ks)}$ potassium channel. Nature 1996;384:80–83.

208. Biervert C, Schroeder BC, Kubisch C, et al. A potassium channel mutation in neonatal human epilepsy. Science 1998;279:403–406.

209. Wang Z, Yue L, White M, Pelletier G, Nattel S. Differential distribution of inward rectifier potassium channel transcripts in human atrium versus ventricle. Circulation 1998;98:2422–2428.

210. Schroeder BC, Kubisch C, Stein V, Jentsch TJ. Moderate loss of function of cyclic-AMP-modulated KCNQ2/KCNQ3 K$^+$ channels causes epilepsy. Nature 1998;396:687–690.

211. Wang HS, Pan Z, Shi W, et al. KCNQ2 and KCNQ3 potassium channel subunits: molecular correlates of the M-channel. Science 1998;282:1890–1893.

212. Murai T, Kakizuka A, Takumi T, Ohkubo H, Nakanishi S. Molecular cloning and sequence analysis of human genomic DNA encoding a novel membrane protein which exhibits a slowly activating potassium channel activity. Biochem Biophys Res Commun 1989;161:176–181.

213. Folander K, Smith JS, Antanavage J, Bennett C, Stein RB, Swanson R. Cloning and expression of the delayed-rectifier IsK channel from neonatal rat heart and diethylstilbestrol-primed rat uterus. Proc Natl Acad Sci USA 1990;87:2975–2979.

214. Lesage F, Attali B, Lazdunski M, Barhanin J. IsK, a slowly activating voltage-sensitive K$^+$ channel. Characterization of multiple cDNAs and gene organization in the mouse. FEBS Lett 1992;301:168–172.

215. Abbott GW, Goldstein SA. A superfamily of small potassium channel subunits: form and function of the MinK-related peptides (MiRPs). Q Rev Biophys 1998;31:357–398.

216. Abbott GW, Sesti F, Splawski I, et al. MiRP1 forms I_{Kr} potassium channels with HERG and is associated with cardiac arrhythmia. Cell 1999;97:175–187.

217. Abbott GW, Butler MH, Bendahhou S, Dalakas MC, Ptacek LJ, Goldstein SA. MiRP2 forms potassium channels in skeletal muscle with Kv3.4 and is associated with periodic paralysis. Cell 2001;104:217–231.

218. Zhang M, Jiang M, Tseng GN. minK-related peptide 1 associates with Kv4.2 and modulates its gating function: potential role as beta subunit of cardiac transient outward channel? Circ Res 2001;88:1012–1019.

219. Muniz ZM, Parcej DN, Dolly JO. Characterization of monoclonal antibodies against voltage-dependent K^+ channels raised using alpha-dendrotoxin acceptors purified from bovine brain. Biochemistry 1992;31:12297–12303.

220. Rettig J, Heinemann SH, Wunder F, et al. Inactivation properties of voltage-gated K^+ channels altered by presence of beta-subunit. Nature 1994;369:289–294.

221. Castellino RC, Morales MJ, Strauss HC, Rasmusson RL. Time- and voltage-dependent modulation of a Kv1.4 channel by a beta-subunit (Kv beta 3) cloned from ferret ventricle. Am J Physiol 1995;269:H385–H391.

222. England SK, Uebele VN, Kodali J, Bennett PB, Tamkun MM. A novel K^+ channel beta-subunit (hKv beta 1.3) is produced via alternative mRNA splicing. J Biol Chem 1995;270:28531–28534.

223. England SK, Uebele VN, Shear H, Kodali J, Bennett PB, Tamkun MM. Characterization of a voltage-gated K^+ channel beta subunit expressed in human heart. Proc Natl Acad Sci USA 1995;92:6309–6313.

224. Majumder K, De Biasi M, Wang Z, Wible BA. Molecular cloning and functional expression of a novel potassium channel beta-subunit from human atrium. FEBS Lett 1995;361:13–16.

225. Morales MJ, Castellino RC, Crews AL, Rasmusson RL, Strauss HC. A novel beta subunit increases rate of inactivation of specific voltage-gated potassium channel alpha subunits. J Biol Chem 1995;270:6272–6277.

226. Deal KK, England SK, Tamkun MM. Molecular physiology of cardiac potassium channels. Physiol Rev 1996;76:49–67.

227. Shi G, Nakahira K, Hammond S, Rhodes KJ, Schechter LE, Trimmer JS. Beta subunits promote K^+ channel surface expression through effects early in biosynthesis. Neuron 1996;16:843–852.

228. Accili EA, Kiehn J, Wible BA, Brown AM. Interactions among inactivating and noninactivating Kvbeta subunits, and Kvalpha1.2, produce potassium currents with intermediate inactivation. J Biol Chem 1997;272:28232–28236.

229. Accili EA, Kiehn J, Yang Q, Wang Z, Brown AM, Wible BA. Separable Kvbeta subunit domains alter expression and gating of potassium channels. J Biol Chem 1997;272:25824–25831.

230. Nagaya N, Papazian DM. Potassium channel alpha and beta subunits assemble in the endoplasmic reticulum. J Biol Chem 1997;272:3022–3027.

231. Nakahira K, Shi G, Rhodes KJ, Trimmer JS. Selective interaction of voltage-gated K^+ channel beta-subunits with alpha-subunits. J Biol Chem 1996;271:7084–7089.

232. Sewing S, Roeper J, Pongs O. Kv beta 1 subunit binding specific for shaker-related potassium channel alpha subunits. Neuron 1996;16:455–463.

233. Fink M, Duprat F, Lesage F, et al. A new K^+ channel beta subunit to specifically enhance Kv2.2 (CDRK) expression. J Biol Chem 1996;271:26341–26348.

234. Wible BA, Yang Q, Kuryshev YA, Accili EA, Brown AM. Cloning and expression of a novel K+ channel regulatory protein, KChAP. J Biol Chem 1998;273:11745–11751.

235. An WF, Bowlby MR, Betty M, et al. Modulation of A-type potassium channels by a family of calcium sensors. Nature 2000;403:553–556.

236. Rosati B, Pan Z, Lypen S, et al. Regulation of KChIP2 potassium channel beta subunit gene expression underlies the gradient of transient outward current in canine and human ventricle. J Physiol 2001;533:119–125.

237. Bahring R, Dannenberg J, Peters HC, Leicher T, Pongs O, Isbrandt D. Conserved Kv4 N-terminal domain critical for effects of Kv channel-interacting protein 2.2 on channel expression and gating. J Biol Chem 2001;276:23888–23894.

238. Decher N, Uyguner O, Scherer CR, et al. hKChIP2 is a functional modifier of hKv4.3 potassium channels: cloning and expression of a short hKChIP2 splice variant. Cardiovasc Res 2001;52:255–264.

239. Burgoyne RD, Weiss JL. The neuronal calcium sensor family of Ca^{2+}-binding proteins. Biochem J 2001;353:1–12.
240. Buxbaum JD, Choi EK, Luo Y, et al. Calsenilin: a calcium-binding protein that interacts with the presenilins and regulates the levels of a presenilin fragment. Nat Med 1998;4:1177–1181.
241. Carrion AM, Link WA, Ledo F, Mellstrom B, Naranjo JR. DREAM is a Ca^{2+}-regulated transcriptional repressor. Nature 1999;398:80–84.
242. Guo W, Li H, Aimond F, et al. Role of heteromultimers in the generation of myocardial transient outward K^+ currents. Circ Res 2002;90:586–593.
243. Guo W, Malin SA, Johns DC, Jeromin A, Nerbonne JM. Modulation of Kv4–encoded K^+ currents in the mammalian myocardium by neuronal calcium sensor-1. J Biol Chem 2002;277:26436–26444.
244. Dixon JE, McKinnon D. Quantitative analysis of potassium channel mRNA expression in atrial and ventricular muscle of rats. Circ Res 1994;75:252–260.
245. Fiset C, Clark RB, Shimoni Y, Giles WR. Shal-type channels contribute to the Ca^{2+}-independent transient outward K+ current in rat ventricle. J Physiol 1997;500 (Pt 1):51–64.
246. Johns DC, Nuss HB, Marban E. Suppression of neuronal and cardiac transient outward currents by viral gene transfer of dominant-negative Kv4.2 constructs. J Biol Chem 1997;272:31598–31603.
247. Barry DM, Xu H, Schuessler RB, Nerbonne JM. Functional knockout of the transient outward current, long-QT syndrome, and cardiac remodeling in mice expressing a dominant-negative Kv4 alpha subunit. Circ Res 1998;83:560–567.
248. Dixon JE, Shi W, Wang HS, et al. Role of the Kv4.3 K^+ channel in ventricular muscle. A molecular correlate for the transient outward current. Circ Res 1996;79:659–668.
249. Kong W, Po S, Yamagishi T, Ashen MD, Stetten G, Tomaselli GF. Isolation and characterization of the human gene encoding Ito: further diversity by alternative mRNA splicing. Am J Physiol 1998;275:H1963–H1970.
250. Takimoto K, Li D, Hershman KM, Li P, Jackson EK, Levitan ES. Decreased expression of Kv4.2 and novel Kv4.3 K^+ channel subunit mRNAs in ventricles of renovascular hypertensive rats. Circ Res 1997;81:533–539.
251. Ohya S, Tanaka M, Oku T, et al. Molecular cloning and tissue distribution of an alternatively spliced variant of an A-type K^+ channel alpha-subunit, Kv4.3 in the rat. FEBS Lett 1997;420:47–53.
252. London B, Wang DW, Hill JA, Bennett PB. The transient outward current in mice lacking the potassium channel gene Kv1.4. J Physiol 1998;509 (Pt 1):171–182.
253. Yang T, Kupershmidt S, Roden DM. Anti-minK antisense decreases the amplitude of the rapidly activating cardiac delayed rectifier K^+ current. Circ Res 1995;77:1246–1253.
254. McDonald TV, Yu Z, Ming Z, et al. A minK-HERG complex regulates the cardiac potassium current I(Kr). Nature 1997;388:289–292.
255. Goldstein SA, Miller C. Site-specific mutations in a minimal voltage-dependent K^+ channel alter ion selectivity and open-channel block. Neuron 1991;7:403–408.
256. Takumi T, Ohkubo H, Nakanishi S. Cloning of a membrane protein that induces a slow voltage-gated potassium current. Science 1988;242:1042–1045.
257. Wang KW, Tai KK, Goldstein SA. MinK residues line a potassium channel pore. Neuron 1996;16:571–577.
258. Tai KK, Goldstein SA. The conduction pore of a cardiac potassium channel. Nature 1998;391:605–608.
259. Jiang M, Tseng-Crank J, Tseng GN. Suppression of slow delayed rectifier current by a truncated isoform of KvLQT1 cloned from normal human heart. J Biol Chem 1997;272:24109–24112.
260. Xu H, Li H, Nerbonne JM. Elimination of the transient outward current and action potential prolongation in mouse atrial myocytes expressing a dominant negative Kv4 alpha subunit. J Physiol 1999; 519:11–21.
261. London B, Guo W, Pan X, et al. Targeted replacement of KV1.5 in the mouse leads to loss of the 4-aminopyridine-sensitive component of $I_{(K,slow)}$ and resistance to drug-induced QT prolongation. Circ Res 2001;88:940–946.
262. Takahashi N, Morishige K, Jahangir A, et al. Molecular cloning and functional expression of cDNA encoding a second class of inward rectifier potassium channels in the mouse brain. J Biol Chem 1994;269:23274–23289.
263. Liu GX, Derst C, Schlichthorl G, et al. Comparison of cloned Kir2 channels with native inward rectifier K^+ channels from guinea-pig cardiomyocytes. J Physiol 2001;532:115–126.
264. Zaritsky JJ, Eckman DM, Wellman GC, Nelson MT, Schwarz TL. Targeted disruption of Kir2.1 and Kir2.2 genes reveals the essential role of the inwardly rectifying K^+ current in K^+-mediated vasodilation. Circ Res 2000;87:160–166.

265. Zaritsky JJ, Redell JB, Tempel BL, Schwarz TL. The consequences of disrupting cardiac inwardly rectifying K⁺ current (I_{K1}) as revealed by the targeted deletion of the murine Kir2.1 and Kir2.2 genes. J Physiol 2001;533:697–710.

266. Babenko AP, Aguilar-Bryan L, Bryan J. A view of sur/KIR6.X, KATP channels. Annu Rev Physiol 1998;60:667–687.

267. Pountney DJ, Sun ZQ, Porter LM, et al. Is the molecular composition of K(ATP) channels more complex than originally thought? J Mol Cell Cardiol 2001;33:1541–1546.

268. Yokoshiki H, Sunagawa M, Seki T, Sperelakis N. Antisense oligodeoxynucleotides of sulfonylurea receptors inhibit ATP-sensitive K⁺ channels in cultured neonatal rat ventricular cells. Pflugers Arch 1999;437:400–408.

269. Li RA, Leppo M, Miki T, Seino S, Marban E. Molecular basis of electrocardiographic ST-segment elevation. Circ Res 2000;87:837–839.

270. Suzuki M, Li RA, Miki T, et al. Functional roles of cardiac and vascular ATP-sensitive potassium channels clarified by Kir6.2-knockout mice. Circ Res 2001;88:570–577.

271. Pu J, Wada T, Valdivia C, Chutkow WA, Burant CF, Makielski JC. Evidence of KATP channels in native cardiac cells without SUR. Biophys J 2001;80:625–626.

272. Seghers V, Nakazaki M, DeMayo F, Aguilar-Bryan L, Bryan J. Sur1 knockout mice. A model for K(ATP) channel-independent regulation of insulin secretion. J Biol Chem 2000;275:9270–9277.

273. Koster JC, Knopp A, Flagg TP, et al. Tolerance for ATP-insensitive K(ATP) channels in transgenic mice. Circ Res 2001;89:1022–1029.

274. Lesage F, Guillemare E, Fink M, et al. TWIK-1, a ubiquitous human weakly inward rectifying K⁺ channel with a novel structure. Embo J 1996;15:1004–1011.

275. Lesage F, Lazdunski M. Potassium channels with two P domains. In: Jan LY, ed. Current Topics in Membranes. Vol. 46. San Diego: Academic Press, 1999:199–222.

276. Goldstein SA, Bockenhauer D, O'Kelly I, Zilberberg N. Potassium leak channels and the KCNK family of two-P-domain subunits. Nat Rev Neurosci 2001;2:175–184.

277. Yue DT, Marban E. A novel cardiac potassium channel that is active and conductive at depolarized potentials. Pflugers Arch 1988;413:127–133.

278. Backx PH, Marban E. Background potassium current active during the plateau of the action potential in guinea pig ventricular myocytes. Circ Res 1993;72:890–900.

279. Wasserstrom JA, Salata JJ. Basis for tetrodotoxin and lidocaine effects on action potentials in dog ventricular myocytes. Am J Physiol 1988;254:H1157–H1166.

280. Clancy CE, Rudy Y. Na⁺ channel mutation that causes both Brugada and long-QT syndrome phenotypes: a simulation study of mechanism. Circulation 2002;105:1208–1213.

281. Weidmann S. Effect of current flow on the membrane potential of cardiac muscle. J Physiol 1951;115:227–236.

4

Electrophysiology and Pharmacology of Ventricular Repolarization

Charles Antzelevitch, PhD,
Andrew C. Zygmunt, PhD,
and Robert Dumaine, PhD

CONTENTS

INTRODUCTION

Repolarization of the ventricular action potential is responsible for the inscription of the T wave and definition of the QT interval in the electrocardiogram (ECG). Repolarization forces play a determining role in the normal function of the myocardium and when defective are often responsible for the development of life-threatening arrhythmias. Thus, our understanding of the electrocardiographic representation of the electrical activity of the heart and appreciation of the mechanisms of arrhythmogenesis requires a fundamental knowledge of the mechanisms of repolarization and the degree to which they differ among the various cell types present within the ventricle of the heart.

The diversity of repolarization characteristics among the myocardial cells that comprise the ventricles of the heart has been highlighted in recent years (reviews *1–8*). Prominent among the heterogeneities uncovered are electrical and pharmacologic distinctions between endocardium and epicardium of the canine, feline, rabbit, rat, and human heart *(9–18)*, as well as differences in the electrophysiologic characteristics and pharmacologic responsiveness of M cells located in the deep structures of the canine,

From: *Contemporary Cardiology: Cardiac Repolarization: Bridging Basic and Clinical Science*
Edited by: I. Gussak et al. © Humana Press Inc., Totowa, NJ

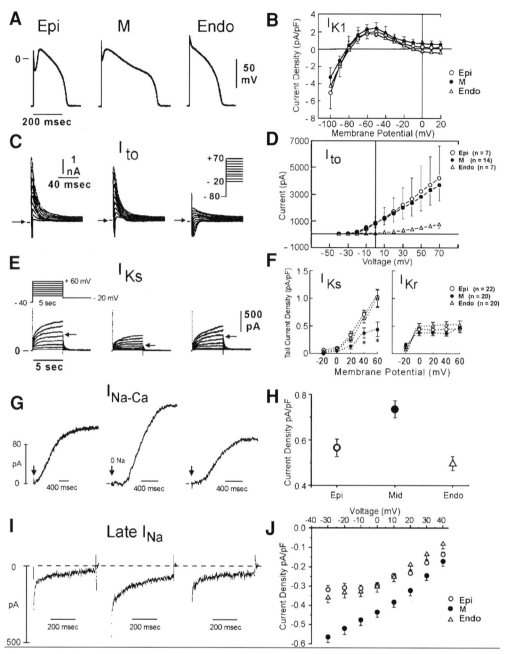

Fig. 1. (A) Action potentials recorded from myocytes isolated from the epicardial (Epi), endocardial (Endo) and M regions of the canine LV. **(B)** I-V relations for I_{K1} in Epi, Endo and M region myocytes. Values are mean ± S.D. **(C)** Transient outward current (I_{to}) recorded from the three cell types (current traces recorded during depolarizing steps from a holding potential of –80 mV to test potentials ranging between –20 and +70 mV). **(D)** The average peak current-voltage relationship for I_{to} for each of the three cell types. Values are mean ± S.D. **(E)** Voltage-dependent activation of the slowly activating component of the delayed rectifier K^+ current (I_{Ks}) (currents were elicited by the voltage pulse protocol shown in the inset; Na^+-, K^+- and Ca^{2+}- free solution). **(F)** Voltage dependence of I_{Ks} (current remaining after exposure to E-4031) and I_{Kr} (E-4031-sensitive current). Values are mean ± S.E. * $p<0.05$ compared with Epi or Endo. From references *(15,24,47)* with permission. **(G)** Reverse-mode sodium-calcium exchange currents recorded in potassium- and chloride-free solutions at a voltage of –80 mV. I_{Na-Ca} was maximally activated by switching to **Fig.**

rabbit, guinea pig, and human ventricles *(2,15,19–33)*. Our principal aim in this chapter is to review the extent to which repolarization characteristics differ in ventricular myocardium, to evaluate the ionic and molecular basis for this heterogeneity and to examine the pharmacological implications.

TRANSMURAL AND INTERVENTRICULAR DIFFERENCES IN THE CHARACTERISTICS OF ACTION POTENTIAL REPOLARIZATION IN VENTRICULAR MYOCARDIUM

The ventricles of the heart are comprised of two principal cell types: Specialized conducting cells forming the His-Purkinje system and ventricular working muscle cells making up the ventricular myocardium. The ventricular myocardium, once believed to be largely homogeneous with respect to electrical properties, is today recognized as being comprised of at least three electrophysiologically and functionally distinct cell types: Epicardial, M, and endocardial. These three ventricular myocardial cell types differ principally with respect to phase 1 and phase 3 repolarization characteristics (Fig. 1A). Ventricular epicardial and M, but not endocardial, cells typically display a conspicuous phase 1, due to a prominent 4-aminopyridine (4-AP) sensitive transient outward current (I_{to}), giving the action potential a spike and dome or notched configuration. These regional differences in I_{to}, first suggested on the basis of action potential data *(10)*, have now been demonstrated using whole cell patch clamp techniques in canine *(15)*, feline *(34)*, rabbit *(12)*, rat *(35)*, and human *(36,37)* ventricular myocytes. No information is available about differences in I_{to2}, a calcium-activated component of the transient outward current, among the three ventricular myocardial cell types *(38)*. I_{to2}, initially ascribed to a K^+ current, is now thought to be primarily due to the calcium-activated chloride current ($I_{Cl(Ca)}$) *(38)*. Myocytes isolated from the epicardial region of the left ventricular wall of the rabbit show a higher density of cAMP-activated chloride current (24.9 +/– 12.1 uS/uF) when compared to endocardial myocytes (12.3 +/– 8.5 uS/uF) *(39)*. Major differences in the magnitude of the action potential notch and corresponding differences in I_{to} have also been described between right and left ventricular epicardial *(40)* and M cells *(41)*.

The transmural and interventricular differences in the manifestation of I_{to} have a number of interesting consequences *(1,3,18,40,42–45)* (Table 1).

M cells are distinguished by the ability of their action potentials to prolong more than those of epicardial or endocardial in response to a slowing of rate and/or agents that prolong action potential duration (APD)-(Fig. 2) *(1,19,29)*. The ionic basis for these features of the M cell include the presence of a smaller slowly activating delayed rectifier current (I_{Ks}) *(24)*, a larger late sodium (late I_{Na}) *(46)* and electrogenic sodium-calcium exchange current (I_{Na-Ca}) currents *(47)* (Fig. 1). Some M cells are largely devoid of

---

(Fig. 1. *Continued*) sodium-free external solution at the time indicated by the arrow. **(H)** Midmyocardial sodium-calcium exchanger density is 30% greater than endo density, calculated as the peak outward I_{Na-Ca} normalized by cell capacitance. Endocardial and epi densities were not significantly different. **(I)** TTX-sensitive late sodium current. Cells were held at –80 mV and briefly pulsed to –45 mV to inactivate fast sodium current before stepping to –10 mV. **(J)** Normalized late sodium current measured 300 ms into the test pulse was plotted as a function of test pulse potential. Modified from *(47)* with permission.

Table 1
Consequences of a Prominent I_{to}-mediated Action Potential Notch
in Epicardium but not Endocardium

- J wave (Osborne wave) *(1,18,18)*
- Differential sensitivity to ischemia and components of ischemia *(1,14,17,195)*
- Differential sensitivity to drugs *(1,11,13,14,18,167,170,195)*
  - Neurohormones (Acetylcholine and Isoproterenol)
  - Transient Outward Current Blockers
  - Calcium Channel Blockers
  - Sodium Channel Blockers
  - Potassium Channel Openers

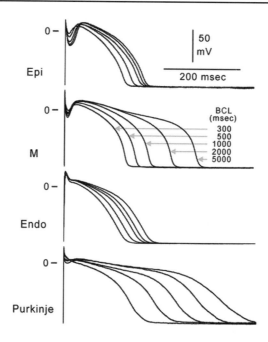

Fig. 2. Transmembrane activity recorded from PF and tissues isolated from the Epi, M and Endo regions of the canine LV at basic cycle lengths (BCL) of 300 to 5000 ms (steady-state conditions).

I_{Ks}. The rapidly activating delayed rectifier (I_{Kr}) and inward rectifier (I_{K1}) currents are similar in the three transmural cell types. It is noteworthy that transmural and apico-basal differences in the density of I_{Kr} channels have been described in the ferret heart; I_{Kr} and channel protein were shown to be much larger in the epicardium *(48)*.

Histologically, M cells are similar to epicardial and endocardial cells. Electrophysiologically and pharmacologically, they appear to be a hybrid between Purkinje and ventricular cells (Table 2). The position of M cells within the ventricular wall has been investigated in greatest detail in the left ventricle (LV) of the canine heart. Although transitional cells are found throughout the wall in the canine LV, M cells displaying the longest action potentials (at BCLs $\geq$ 2000 ms) are often localized in the deep subendocardium to midmyocardium in the anterior wall *(49)*, deep subepicardium to

Table 2
Electrophysiologic Distinctions among Epicardial, Endocardial, M Cells,
and Purkinje Fibers Isolated from the Canine Heart

	Purkinje	M	Epicardial	Endocardial
Long APD, steep APD-rate	Yes	Yes	No	No
Develop EADs in response to agents with class III actions	Yes	Yes	No	No
Develop DADs in response to digitalis, high Ca^{2+}, catecholamines	Yes	Yes	No	No
Display marked increase in APD in response to IK_r blockers	Yes	Yes	No	No
Display marked increase in APD in response to I_{Ks} blockers	No	Yes	Yes	Yes
α1 Agonist-induced change in APD	↑	↓	↔	↔
V_{max}	High	Intermediate	Low in surface tissues	
Phase 4 depolarization	Yes	No	No	No
Depolarize in $[K^+]_o < 2.5$ mM	Yes	No	No	No
Acceleration-induced EADs and APD, prolongation in presence of I_{Kr} block	No	Yes	No	No
EADs sensitive to $[Ca^{2+}]_I$	No	Yes	–	–
Develop DADs with Bay K 8644	No	Yes	No	No
Found in bundles	Yes	No	No	No

APD = action potential duration; EAD = early afterdepolarization; DAD = delayed afterdepolarization

midmyocardium in the lateral wall (19) and throughout the wall in the region of the right ventricular (RV) outflow tracts (6). M cells are also present in the deep layers of endocardial structures, including papillary muscles, trabeculae and the interventricular septum (22). Unlike Purkinje fibers, they are not found in discrete bundles (21,22). The first description of cells with an unusually long APD and rapid V_{max} was made in a papillary muscle preparation (50).

Figure 3 graphically illustrates the transmural distribution of APD_{90} and tissue resistivity in the canine LV. M cells with the longest action potentials are found in the deep subendocardium and transitions in action potential duration are relatively gradual across the ventricular wall, except in the deep subepicardial region (49). A sharp increase in tissue resistivity measured in the deep subepicardium leads to reduced electrotonic interaction, thus permitting cells in this region to exhibit more of their intrinsic properties. The extent to which electrical heterogeneity is manifest across the intact ventricular wall depends on:

1. The magnitude of differences in intrinsic action potential characteristics of cells spanning the wall.
2. The extent to which the cells are electrically coupled in the syncytium (51). When coupling resistance is low, intrinsic differences in APD are highly damped, but are usually perceptible over the full width of the left ventricular wall. As coupling resistance increases, so does the ability to manifest differences of APD and other action potential

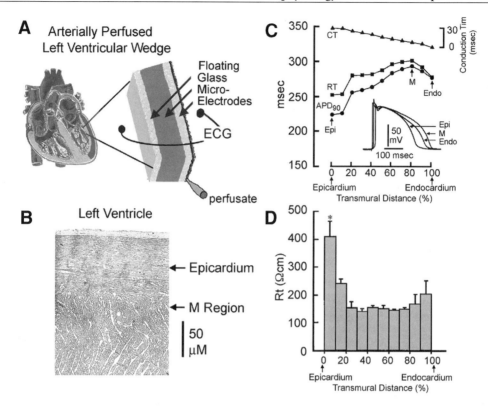

Fig. 3. Transmural distribution of action potential duration and tissue resistivity in the intact ventricular wall. **(A)** Schematic diagram of the arterially perfused canine LV wedge preparation. The wedge is perfused with Tyrode's solution via a small native branch of the left descending coronary artery and stimulated from the endocardial surface. Transmembrane action potentials are recorded simultaneously from epicardial (Epi), M region (M) and endocardial (Endo) sites using three floating microelectrodes. A transmural ECG is recorded along the same transmural axis across the bath, registering the entire field of the wedge. **(B)** Histology of a transmural slice of the LV wall near the epicardial border. The region of sharp transition of cell orientation coincides with the region of high tissue resistivity depicted in panel D and the region of sharp transition of action potential duration illustrated in panel C. **(C)** Distribution of conduction time (CT), APD_{90} and repolarization time (RT = APD_{90} + CT) in a canine LV wall wedge preparation paced at BCL of 2000 ms. A sharp transition of APD_{90} is present between epicardium and subepicardium. Epi: epicardium; M: M Cell; Endo: endocardium. RT: repolarization time; CT: conduction time. **(D)** Distribution of total tissue resistivity (R_t) across the canine left ventricular wall. Transmural distances at 0% and 100% represent epicardium and endocardium, respectively. * $p < 0.01$ compared with R_t at mid-wall. Tissue resistivity increases most dramatically between deep subepicardium and epicardium. Error bars represent SEM (n=5). From *(49)* with permission.

parameters across the wall. In the canine ventricle, transmural heterogeneity is because of differences in intrinsic action potential characteristics as well as differences in tissue resistivity among the various transmural layers *(49)*. A sharp increase in tissue resistivity between the M region and epicardium is responsible for the sharp increase in APD in this region of the wall. This resistive barrier may be still more important in the lateral free wall of the LV where M cells with the longest APD are often found in the deep subepicardial to midmyocardial layers *(19)*. Despite the relatively large increase in tissue resistivity in the deep subepicardium, conduction in this region slows only slightly, consistent with cable theory predictions. Although the basis for the abrupt rise in tissue resistivity is not fully understood, a sudden shift in the orientation of the myocardial cells in this part of the wall is thought to contribute importantly (Fig. 3B) *(49)*. An abrupt shift in cell orientation in the deep subepicardium has been documented throughout the canine heart. A sharp transition in the orientation of cells is also observed in the deep subepicardium of the human LV, where prolonged M cell action potentials are first encountered *(23)*.

The shift in the location of the M cells from the deep subepicardium to the deep subendocardium appears to follow the transmural shift in the muscular layers that envelop the heart, as described by Streeter *(52,53)* and more recently by Lukenheimer and coworkers *(54)*.

Cells with the characteristics of M cells have been described in the canine, guinea pig, rabbit, pig, and human ventricles *(2,15,19–24,26–33,49,55–61)*. Several studies have failed to discern M cells in the ventricles of the human, pig, guinea pig, and rat *(30, 62–64)*. Other studies although clearly demonstrating the presence of M cells in the ventricles of the canine heart in vitro, failed to delineate the unique cell type in vivo *(7,29)*. Methodological considerations thought to be responsible for these differences have been discussed at great length *(6,8,65,66)*. Chief among these is the anesthetic employed. Most anesthetics are thought to importantly reduce transmural dispersion of repolarization owing to their action to block late I_{Na}. Block of this current preferentially abbreviates the action potential of the M cell and dramatically flattens its APD-rate relationship *(57)*. Agents such as pentobarbital are particularly effective in reducing transmural heterogeneities because of the anesthetic's potent effect to block the late sodium current (late I_{Na}) as well as the slowly activating delayed rectifier current (I_{Ks})(unpublished observations). The effect of this dual ion channel inhibition is to prolong the epicardial and endocardial action potential, but abbreviate that of the M cell in the canine heart. A relatively small transmural dispersion of repolarization is generally reported in in vivo studies using pentobarbital or α chloralose for anesthesia *(7,26,29)* vs studies that have used other agents including isoflurane *(32,67,68)* or halothane *(26)*. A recent study by Yamamoto et al. *(69)*, demonstrates the effect of both pentobarbital and isoflurane to suppress quinidine and astemizole-induced torsade de pointes (TdP), suggesting that both reduce transmural heterogeneities. It is noteworthy that Takei and coworkers *(70)* were able to distinguish M cell activity in the midmyocardium of the in vivo dog heart despite the use of pentobarbital anesthesia.

CHARACTERISTICS OF REPOLARIZATION IN HIS-PURKINJE SYSTEM

Purkinje fibers isolated from dog, cow, sheep, and rabbit exhibit a rapid phase 1 repolarization caused by a transient outward current consisting of a large 4AP-sensitive voltage-dependent potassium current I_{to} and a smaller ryanodine-sensitive calcium-dependent chloride current $I_{Cl(Ca)}$ *(71–75)*. Inhibition of I_{to} and $I_{Cl(Ca)}$ slows phase 1 repolarization and elevates the plateau, confirming the important role of these two outward currents during the earliest phases of the action potential. Low concentrations of 4-AP, which selectively inhibit I_{to}, abbreviate APD, whereas higher concentrations, which also inhibit I_{K1}, prolong APD *(71,76)*.

I_{Ks} is undetectable *(77)* or very small *(78)* in voltage clamped Purkinje cells, and action potentials in these cells show virtually no response to inhibition of I_{Ks} using chromanol

293B under basal conditions *(78,79)*. Interestingly, β-adrenergic agonists increase I_{Ks} during the action potential by augmenting maximal conductance, accelerating activation, and causing a negative shift of the activation-voltage toward plateau potentials *(78)*. This coupled with a more positive action potential plateau, secondary to an increase in I_{Ca}, makes possible the activation of I_{Ks} during the Purkinje action potential. I_{Ks} in Purkinje cells may function to prevent disproportionate APD prolongation in the face of β-adrenergic stimulation of I_{Ca}.

I_{Kr} and I_{K1} are the most important repolarizing currents during phase 3 in Purkinje cells. I_{Kr} inhibitors almokalant and sotalol significantly prolong Purkinje APD *(80,81)*, and this prolongation is more pronounced at long cycle lengths *(82)*. I_{Kr} is a small current throughout the plateau, but its amplitude increases during phase 3 repolarization. I_{Kr} density in Purkinje cells is similar to that found in ventricular myocytes *(83)*. Because of strong inward rectification, I_{K1} is undetectable during the plateau, but dramatically increases during final repolarization. I_{K1} density in canine Purkinje cells is four times the density of I_{Kr} *(83)*. In rabbits, the density of Purkinje I_{K1} is half that of ventricular myocytes *(77)*. Concentrations of 4-AP shown to inhibit I_{K1} also slow final repolarization and prolong Purkinje APD *(76)*.

A late component of the sodium current (Late I_{Na}) contributes significantly to the plateau phase of the action potential in both Purkinje and M cells. Late I_{Na} is comprised of:

1. A window current representing the overlap of steady-state activation and inactivation relations *(84)*,
2. Slowly inactivating sodium channels *(85)*,
3. Late re-openings of the sodium channel, and
4. A mode shift that results in bursting behavior of the channel *(86–88)*.

Late I_{Na} maintains the action potential plateau and opposes potassium currents during final repolarization. A majority of studies find that a single population of sodium channels underlies both the fast sodium conductance and Late I_{Na} *(89,90)*. Patlak and Ortiz *(86)* concluded that a single population of sodium channels can function in different modes, each with a different inactivation rate. Low concentrations of sodium channel blockers, which do not significantly affect phase zero upstroke velocity, dramatically reduce both Purkinje and M cell APD, suggesting that the density of late sodium current is similar in the two cell types *(91–94)*.

DEVELOPMENTAL ASPECTS

Ventricular myocardium of the canine neonate is largely homogeneous with respect to electrical properties. Action potential characteristics of midmyocardial cells are no different from those of epicardial or endocardial cells. The spike and dome morphology of the epicardial action potential is generally absent in neonates and appears over the first few months of life, reaching a plateau or quasi-steady-state between 10- and 20-wk-of-age in the dog *(1,95,96)* (Fig. 4). The progressive development of the notch parallels the appearance of I_{to}. Age-related changes in the manifestation of the spike and dome have also been described in human atrial *(97)* and canine Purkinje *(98)* tissues and rat ventricular *(99)* cells. Preliminary studies indicate that distinct M cell behavior is not observed until 2 to 3 mo-of-age in the dog *(100)* and possibly also in the pig *(6,30,100)*. Rodriguez-Sinova and coworkers have shown the absence of a distinct M cell in the LV of the young

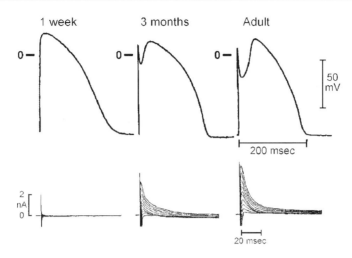

Fig. 4. Age-related spike and dome morphology and changes in I_{to} in canine ventricular epicardium. Each panel depicts transmembrane activity recorded from RV epicardial tissues (upper trace) and transient outward current (lower trace) recorded from LV epicardial cells isolated from a neonate (5 days of age; **(A)**, a young dog (3 months old; **(B)**, and an adult dog **(C)**. BCL = 2000 ms; [K$^+$]o = 4 mM. The spike and dome configuration of the epicardial action potential and I_{to} density are absent in the neonate, relatively small in the young dog, and most prominent in the adult.

pig (1 to 2 mo-of-age) *(30)*. More recent studies have described the presence of M cells in the heart of the 4–6-mo-old pig *(6,55)*.

Thus in the neonate, there are no M cells, epicardial cells or endocardial cells. The changes in ionic current density responsible for the transformation of neonatal cells into distinct adult cell types occurs over the first few weeks and months of life in the dog. Studies are underway to assess whether these developmental changes in ion channel current play a role in sudden infant death syndrome (SIDS) in infants with the congenital long QT or Brugada syndromes. Recent clinical data provide support for this hypothesis *(101,102)*.

MOLECULAR BASIS FOR TRANSMURAL AND INTERVENTRICULAR DIFFERENCES IN REPOLARIZATION

Major breakthroughs in genetics, molecular biology, and immunology over the past two decades have elevated our knowledge from the descriptive Mendelian laws of heredity and the Watson and Crick model of the DNA to practical applications involving identification and engineering of genes. Knowledge of the human brain advanced first in studies of the genome of Drosophila Melanogaster. It soon became evident that many of the genes found in the human brain are also expressed in the heart. The identification and heterologous expression of cardiac genes linked to ion channels, pumps, exchangers, and gap junction proteins involved in the activation and propagation of the cardiac action potential soon led to a better understanding of rhythm disturbances long considered idiopathic in nature. In this section we review key findings dealing with heterogeneous distribution of messenger RNA and/or gene products and assess the extent to which these may be responsible for the electrophysiological heterogeneities discussed throughout the remainder of the chapter. Our principal focus will be on the distribution of messenger ribonucleic acid (mRNA) and gene products in different regions of ventricular myocardium of the normal heart.

Potassium Channels

Potassium channels are the most numerous and diverse family of ion channels expressed in the heart. Their propensity to pair with members of the same and/or different phylogenic branch makes their genetic linkage to cardiac current a daunting task.

OVERVIEW OF SHAKER TYPE CHANNELS

The first voltage-gated potassium channel subunit was cloned from the Shaker locus in Drosophila *(103)* and it was soon discovered that Shaker K$^+$ channels are oligomeric proteins comprised of four units *(104)*. This family consists of four subfamily members of voltage-gated K$^+$ channel genes originally named Shaker, Shab, Shaw, Shal *(105)*, now referred to as Kv1.x, Kv2.x, Kv3.x, and Kv4.x respectively, based on the nomenclature proposed by Chandy *(106)*. We will use this terminology in the remainder of the chapter. Within the Shaker family, 11 genes have been identified at the transcriptional level in the heart: Kv1.1, Kv1.2, Kv1.3, Kv1.4, Kv1.5, Kv1.6, Kv2.1, Kv2.2, Kv3.4, Kv4.2, Kv4.3. Northern blot analysis of rat heart tissues initially revealed the presence of Kv1.1, Kv1.2, Kv1.4, Kv1.5, Kv4.2, and Kv2.1 mRNA *(107)*. Dixon and McKinnon *(108)* subsequently reported the presence of only the Kv1.2, Kv1.4, Kv1.5, and Kv4.2 transcripts in the ventricles using a ribonuclease (RNase) protection assay (RPA). Kv1.2 and Kv4.2 proteins are strongly expressed in rat atrium and ventricles, with Kv4.2 being more abundant in ventricular cells *(109)*. The Kv1.4 proteins are poorly expressed in rat hearts *(109)*.

Kv2.1 is twice as abundant as Kv2.2 and both show a uniform distribution in all regions of the heart. Kv3.4 is threefold more abundant in ventricles than in atria and all members of the Kv4 family are expressed, with Kv4.2 being the most abundant. The link of some members of the Kv1 and Kv2 family to ionic current in the heart remains unclear. In the remainder of this section, we will limit our discussion to genes definitively linked to known ion channels in the heart.

THE ELUSIVE ROLE OF KV1.5 IN THE VENTRICLES (I$_{KUR}$)

Kv1.5 has been linked to I$_{Kur}$, the ultra rapid delayed rectifier current *(110,111)* found in dog atria. A similar current has yet to be found in the ventricles of the dog. Brahmajothi et al. *(112)* described an even distribution of the Kv1.5 mRNA in ferret atria and ventricles. Kv1.5 mRNA is also found in rat ventricles *(108)*, where the protein product is reportedly weakly expressed *(109,113)*. In dog, Kv1.5 proteins are localized at the level of the intercalated disk junctions *(114,115)*. Interestingly, the protein diffuses from the intercalated disk to the sarcolemma of ventricular myocytes during ischemia or in the cells lining the border of an infarct *(114,115)*. The migration of the channels is accompanied by a parallel downregulation of mRNA and proteins, suggesting transcriptional regulation of expression *(116)*.

THE TRANSIENT OUTWARD CURRENT (I$_{TO}$)

The distribution of I$_{to}$ across the ventricular wall is perhaps the most striking example of electrical heterogeneity in the heart. Based on inactivation kinetics and sensitivity to 4-AP of members of the Kv1 and Kv4 families, several attempts have been made to correlate the anatomical location of these genes with the distribution of I$_{to}$. Dixon and

McKinnon *(108)* first showed that the distribution of Kv4.2 parallels the gradient for I_{to} in the rat LV with eight times more mRNA in epicardium than endocardium. The same group later reported that Kv4.3 is uniformly distributed between the epicardium and endocardium of the LV in rat and electrophysiological studies on Kv4.3 strengthened the link to I_{to} *(117)*. Dixon et al. detected the message for Kv4.3 in canine and human LV, but not for Kv4.2 *(118)*. The distribution of Kv4.2 and Kv4.3 in rat preparations suggest that a complex formed by Kv4.2 and Kv4.3 may be responsible for I_{to}. Barry et al. *(109)* further confirmed the expression of Kv4.2 proteins in the sarcolemma of rat ventricular myocytes. In dog and human however, their results suggested that KV4.3 co-assembles with another member of the Shaker or other family to form I_{to}.

In a study conducted in the ferret heart, Brahmajothi et al. *(119)* combined electro-physiological and co-localization techniques to show that Kv4.2 and Kv4.3 are more abundant in the epicardium than in the endocardium, whereas Kv1.4 is observed mostly in endocardium and absent in epicardium. On the apico-basal axis, they found that the Kv4.3 transcript was more abundant at the base of the heart in the RV and LV epicardium. In the same study they report that Kv1.4 is more abundant in the apical LV and septum, whereas Kv4.2 is more abundant in the epicardial region of the LV. Kv4.2 is more diffuse throughout in the RV free wall and septum. The same group also reported the presence of Kv3.x subfamily members in the ferret ventricles *(120)*. The results support the hypothesis that an heteromultimer composed of Kv4.3 and Kv4.2 forms part of I_{to} in the ferret epicardium and that Kv1.4 may contribute to formation of I_{to} in the endocardium. Interestingly, strong signal for Kv1.4 and Kv3.4 were also observed in canine hearts *(118)* but their contribution to I_{to} considered unlikely on the basis of the lack of sensitivity of the current inactivation to oxidizing agents *(118)* and to the channel blocker TEA. Immunoprecipitation studies may help to resolve this issue. One must also be mindful of the fact that co-assembly of different subunits can result in large fluctuations in drug sensitivity, as seen with KCNQ1 and KCNE1 *(121)*.

In a recent elegant study, Rosati et al. *(122)* showed that the transcript of the potassium channel subunit KChIP2 was 25 times more abundant in the epicardium than in endocardium of dog and human heart ventricles. This steep gradient in the mRNA distribution of KChIP2 paralleled the transmural distribution of I_{to} in the LV, leading the authors to conclude that transcriptional regulation of this beta subunit, rather than Kv4.3, was responsible for the expression of the transient outward current. Kuo et al. *(123)* have shown that KChIP2 also plays a determining role in the expression of I_{to} in the mouse heart. Mice deficient in KChIP2 lack I_{to} and as a consequence display prolonged repolarization and ventricular tachycardia. KChIP2 appears to modulate I_{to} levels both by controlling the expression of the channel so as to affect channel density and regulating the function of the channel once expressed *(123–127)*.

The Slowly Activating Delayed Rectifier Current (I_{Ks})

I_{Ks} is formed by co-assembly of the KCNE1 and KCNQ1 gene products *(128,129)*. In acutely dissociated cells from the ferret ventricles, KCNQ1 and KCNE1 mRNA are 34% and 70% more abundant, respectively, in RV vs LV. Our group recently reported a similar interventricular distribution for KCNQ1 mRNA in the canine RV but a 50% more abundant KCNE1 transcript in the LV; protein expression paralleled the transcript distribution *(130)* suggesting important regulation at the transcriptional level. Transmurally, KCNQ1 mRNA was found to be less abundant in the midmyocardium than in epicardium and endocardium of the canine LV *(131)*, consistent with the transmural distribution of I_{Ks}.

The 70 and 50 kD bands seen in canine ventricular cells likely represent the glycosylated protein expressed at the sarcolemmal surface and the unglycosylated protein trapped in the Golgi or ER, respectively. This suggests that the expression of KCNQ1 is regulated at the transcriptional and possibly posttranscriptional levels. Another likely possibility is that the polyclonal antibody also recognizes an alternative splice variant of KCNQ1 of smaller size. Such a splice variant has been identified in human *(132)* and shown to result in an N-terminal truncated isoform which has a dominant negative effect on the expression of normal KCNQ1 channels. Both interpretations of the results predict smaller amplitude of I_{Ks} in the LV, consistent with the electrophysiological data *(41)*. Thus far, our group has been unable to detect the presence of mRNA or cDNA corresponding to truncated form of KCNQ1 in canine heart tissues using reverse transcriptase-polymerase chain reaction (RT-PCR) and 5' RACE, respectively.

Unlike KCNQ1, the distribution of KCNE1 follows an uphill gradient from epicardium to endocardium. These results, suggest that KCNQ1 is the primary determinant of the transmural distribution of I_{Ks} in the canine LV and that KCNE1 act as a modulator of its kinetics and possibly its pharmacology. Because KCNE1 also increases the number of functional channels encoded by the human ether-a-gogo-related gene (HERG), its distribution in the canine ventricle may influence the distribution of HERG channels as well.

THE RAPIDLY ACTIVATING DELAYED RECTIFIER CURRENT (I_{Kr})

The ERG transcript encoding for the α-subunit of I_{Kr} channels *(133–135)* is 20% more abundant in the RV vs LV in the ferret heart. ERG protein is found throughout the myocardium but is more abundant in the epicardium, except near the base of the heart where it is evenly distributed across the ventricular wall *(48)*. Concordance between protein and mRNA distribution indicate transcriptional regulation of the expression of I_{Kr}. Recent data indicate that KCNE1 is a member of a multigene family including KCNE2 (Mirp1) *(136)*. Both genes are known to modulate the function and the gating *(48)* of HERG. It remains to be determined if the distribution of these ancillary subunits share a similar pattern of expression with HERG and to what extent they may modulate the properties of I_{Kr}.

Sodium Channels

The SCN5A (hH1) gene encodes for the α-subunit of the sodium channel, which conducts the tetrodotorin TTX-sensitive *(137,138)* fast sodium current responsible for the upstroke of the cardiac action potential. The protein is homogeneously distributed on the surface of rat atria and ventricular free wall; no transmural differences have been reported in the rat *(139)*. Although the transmural distribution of I_{Na} is not known in the rat heart, in the canine heart I_{Na} is considerably greater in the midmyocardium vs epicardium or endocardium *(21,46)*. Data relative to transmural distribution of channel protein in the dog ventricle are not available. At the cellular level, sodium channel protein is generally more strongly expressed at the level of the T tubules, along the Z bands, with a major concentration at the intercalated disks. This distribution of the cardiac sodium channel within the cell appears to be designed to facilitate conduction via an amplification process akin to neuronal saltatory conduction *(139)*. Recent studies suggest that in addition to $Na_v1.5$ (SCN5A), the heart also contains the brain sodium channel $Na_v1.1$ *(140)*. The extent to which differential expression of these distinct sodium channel species may regulate the transmural expression of early and late I_{Na} is not known.

Gap Junctions

Intercellular communication and impulse conduction depend on the presence of gap junctions, which are comprised of proteins known as connexins (Cx). Each Cx family displays a unique pharmacological and electrophysiological profile as well as anatomical distribution, conferring specific properties to the conductive and muscle tissues of the heart. In rabbits, Cx43 and Cx45 are abundant in atrium and ventricles. Cx40 is also present in the atrium (141,142) and Cx37 and Cx40 are preferentially localized in rabbit ventricular endocardial cells (141).

In dog, Cx40 is threefold more abundant in Purkinje fibers (PF) vs ventricular myocardium with mRNA levels proportional to protein expression (143). Similar levels of Cx43 and Cx44 are found in the ventricles and PF (143) although Cx43 appears to be absent from the AV bundle and possibly the bundle branch. Cx40 has a greater conductance than Cx43. The greater contribution of Cx40 in PF may account for the more rapid impulse propagation of PF.

Chloride Conductances

An increasing endocardial to epicardial gradient of mRNA for an alternatively spliced variant of CFTR has been demonstrated in rabbit and guinea pig ventricles (144,145). This cAMP-activated chloride conductance is activated during adrenergic stimulation (39) and is thought to contribute to the abbreviation of the ventricular action potential. The transmural distribution of cAMP-activated I_{Cl} density in the rabbit is similar to the distribution of the alternative splice variant. Myocytes isolated from the epicardial region of the rabbit LV wall show a cAMP-activated chloride current density twice that of endocardial myocytes (39).

Calcium Channels

Two types of calcium channels are found in the heart. A slowly inactivating, high threshold, and "long lasting" current generated by L-type channels and a more rapid, lower threshold current transient "T" type current. Six genes encode for the α1 subunit, the principal subunit of the Ca^+ channel (146,147). The L-type channel is believed to be encoded by the α1C, α1D, and α1S genes owing to the sensitivity of their protein products to dihydropyridines (DHPs) (148,149). In contrast, the α1A, α1B, and α1E encode for non-DHP sensitive channels (150,151). The α1C gene together with an α2, β, and δ genes encode for the cardiac L-type channel (148). In isolated adult rabbit cardiac myocytes both, the beta2 and the full-length α1C proteins co-localize along T-tubule membranes (152). In guinea pig, the sarcolemmal L-type calcium channels have been shown to be organized in clusters in the transverse tubules (153). In adult rabbit ventricular cells the L-type calcium channel, the Ryanodine receptor (RyR) and the SR triadin overlap along the T-tubules. In atrial cells, the L-type channels are also found in clusters overlapping with RyR and triadin (154). In rat, the α1D mRNA is found in lung, aorta and atria, but not in the ventricles of the heart (155).

The calcium channels are generally found to localize adjacent to junctional sarcoplasmic reticulum, permitting a close coupling of calcium influx to triggers of release of calcium from the intracellular stores. No studies to our knowledge have specifically probed for transmural, apico-basal or interventricular differences in the distribution of the calcium subunits.

Exchangers

Na/Ca Exchanger

Three primary isoforms, NCX1, NCX2, and NCX3, of the sodium-calcium exchanger have been cloned *(156–158)*. NCX1 protein predominates in the rat heart, with little expression of NCX2 and NCX3. Despite several studies showing upregulation of sodium-calcium exchanger expression in response to cardio pathologies that attend or result from increases in intracellular calcium, it is surprising that little is known about the anatomical localization of the three subunits in the normal heart. In all cell types studied, NCXs appear more abundant in the T-tubules *(159–164)*. During development, NCX proteins are homogenously and maximally expressed during embryogenesis and decline to adult levels after birth *(165)*. Regulation is transcriptional and modulated by hormonal levels. In human heart, Prestle et al. *(162)* found no transmural differences in the mRNA level of NCX1 across the LV wall. As previously discussed, in the canine heart, reverse mode $I_{Na\text{-}Ca}$ is nearly 30% larger in midmyocardial cells than in epicardial or endocardial cells (Fig. 1) *(47)*. No data are as yet available relative to the transmural distribution of NCX protein or message in the canine ventricles.

TRANSMURAL AND INTERVENTRICULAR PHARMACOLOGICAL DISTINCTIONS

Epicardium vs Endocardium

One of the consequences of a prominent I_{to}-mediated spike and dome morphology in epicardium but not endocardium is that the two tissues show different, in some cases opposite, responses to a wide variety of pharmacological agents and neurohormones (Table 1).

Epicardium and endocardium respond differently to agents that block I_{to}. In relatively low concentrations (0.5–1.0 mM) 4-AP is a fairly selective blocker of I_{to}; higher concentrations also block I_K and I_{K1} *(76,166)*. Low concentrations of 4-AP are effective in restoring electrical homogeneity and in abolishing arrhythmias induced by ischemia or drugs and neurohormones that cause dispersion of repolarization and phase 2 reentry (i.e., sodium channel blockers and ACh) *(1,14,16,17,167)*. Inhibition of I_{to} by quinidine may contribute to the antiarrhythmic actions of the drug *(168,169)*.

Epicardium and endocardium also show a differential response to both parasympathetic and sympathetic agonists. In the absence of catecholamines (accentuated antagonism), Acetylcholine (ACh, 10^{-5} M) exerts essentially no effect on the action potential of canine ventricular endocardium. In contrast, ACh either prolongs or markedly abbreviates the epicardial action potential under these same conditions *(170)*, providing support for claims of a direct effect of ACh in the feline and human heart in vivo *(171,172)*. Low concentrations (10^{-7}–10^{-6} M) cause a slowing of the second upstroke giving rise to a delay in the achievement of peak plateau. The attending accentuation of the notch of the epicardial action potential results in a prolongation of action potential duration. Interestingly, higher concentrations cause all-or-none repolarization and marked abbreviation of the action potential. These effects of ACh on epicardium are readily reversed with atropine, fail to appear when epicardium is pretreated with the transient outward current blocker 4-AP, are accentuated in the presence of isoproterenol (10^{-7} to 5×10^{-6} M; accentuated antagonism), persist in the presence of propranolol and arc likcly duc to inhibition of I_{Ca} and/or activation of $I_{K\text{-}ACh}$ *(170)*. ACh does not influence I_{to} *(173)*.

Isoproterenol also produces different effects on epicardium and endocardium. Catecholamines diminish the epicardial action potential notch secondary to their effects to augment I_{Ca}. As a consequence, the epicardial action potential abbreviates more than that of endocardium. β adrenergic agonists influence all of the major currents that contribute to phase 1 and phase 3 repolarization, including I_{to}, I_{Ca}, I_K, and calcium- and cAMP-activated I_{Cl} (38,39,174–179).

Calcium channel blockers also exert dissimilar effects on endocardium and epicardium. Organic Ca^{2+} channel blockers such as verapamil (180) and nifedipine (181) and inorganic inhibitors such as $MnCl_2$ (182) are capable of causing loss of the action potential dome in canine ventricular epicardium but not endocardium. Exposure to Ca^{2+}-free Tyrode's solution yields similar results (182). In endocardium, calcium channel blockers cause only a slight abbreviation of the action potential (9,183).

Sodium channel blockers exert different, and in some cases opposite, effects on canine ventricular epicardium and endocardium (11,13). Concentrations of tetrodotoxin, propranolol, and flecainide sufficient to reduce the rate of rise of the action potential (V_{max}) by approx 40–50% abbreviate the action potential in endocardium but prolong it in epicardium. More intense inhibition of I_{Na} leads to a marked abbreviation of the epicardial response secondary to loss of the action potential dome, although producing only a slight abbreviation of the action potential in endocardium. The paradoxical prolongation of the epicardial action potential is due largely to an accentuation and widening of the action potential notch. With greater inhibition of I_{Na}, termination of phase 1 shifts to more negative potentials at which the availability of I_{Ca} is diminished to a level at which the outward currents overwhelm the inward currents active at the end of phase 1. This results is an all-or-none repolarization at the end of phase 1, causing loss of the action potential dome and marked abbreviation of the action potential. These actions of ACh and sodium channel blockers, particularly on RV epicardium, facilitate the development of phase 2 reentry, which is thought to serve as the trigger for sudden death in patients with the Brugada syndrome.

Chronic exposure to amiodarone produces very different electrophysiologic effects in canine ventricular epicardium and endocardium (3,184). Endocardial tissues excised from the ventricles of dogs receiving chronic amiodarone (20–25 mg\kg\day over a 5–6 wk period) show strong rate dependence of V_{max} (30±5.2% decrease with acceleration from a BCL of 2000 to 300 ms) and an action potential duration 16% longer than control. Unlike endocardium, epicardial tissues isolated from amiodarone treated dogs are markedly depressed (inexcitable) immediately after isolation and recover over a period of several hours. As discussed in the next subheading, chronic amiodarone treatment also leads to a reduction in transmural dispersion, because of its differential effects on M cells vs epicardial/endocardial cells.

M Cells vs Epicardium and Endocardium

One of the hallmarks of the M cell is the ability of its action potential to prolong more in response to agents with Class III actions or APD prolonging effects (Table 2). I_{Kr} blockers, including d-sotalol, dofetilide, almokalant, E-4031, and erythromycin, produce a much greater prolongation of APD in M cells than in epicardium or endocardium (Fig. 5, Table 3). In contrast, surface epicardial and endocardial tissues isolated from the canine LV show little response. A similar preferential prolongation of the M cell APD is seen with agents that increase calcium current, I_{Ca}, such as Bay K 8644 as well as with

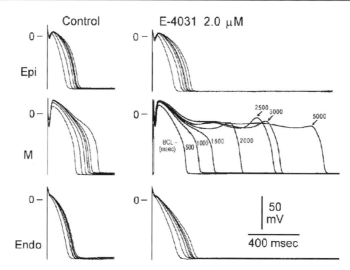

Fig. 5. Effect of the E-4031, a specific I_{Kr} blocker, on transmembrane activity recorded from epicardial (Epi), endocardial (Endo) and deep subepicardial (M cell) sites in a transmural strip of canine LV. **(A)** Each panel shows superimposed action potentials recorded at basic cycle lengths (BCL) of 500 to 5000 ms, before and after E-4031 (2 µM).

Table 3
Early Afterdepolarization (EAD)-induced Triggered Activity and/or Prominent Action Potential Prolongation

	Epicardium	*Endocardium*	*M cells*
Quinidine (3.3 µM)	–	–	+++
4-Aminopyridine (2.5–5 m*M*)	–	–	+++
Amiloride (1–10 µM)	–	–	++
Clofilium (1 µM)	–	–	+++
Bay K 8644 (1 µM)	–	–	++
Cesium (5–10 m*M*)	–	–	++
Sotalol (100 µM)	–	–	+++
Erythromycin (10–100 µg/mL)	–	–	++++
E-4031 (1–5 µM)	–	–	+++
Chronic Amiodarone	+	–	++
ATX–II (10–20 n*M*)	+	++	++++
Azimilide (5–20 µM)	+	++	+++
Chromanol 293B (10–100 µM)	+++	+++	+++

+/– Little to no response; +++++ largest response.

agents that increase late I_{Na} such as ATX-II and anthopleurin-A. An exception to this rule applies to agents that block I_{Ks}, including azimilide, quinidine, pentobarbital, amiodarone, and chromanol 293B. Chromanol 293B is one of the most specific I_{Ks} blockers. In isolated tissues, chromanol 293B produces a similar percentage prolongation of APD in the three transmural cell types. The situation is more complex for drugs affecting two or more ion channels, such as quinidine, pentobarbital, amiodarone, and azimilide. In the case of quinidine, relatively low therapeutic levels of the drug (3–5 µM; 1.14–1.89 µg/mL), produce a marked prolongation of the M cell APD but not of epicardium and endocar-

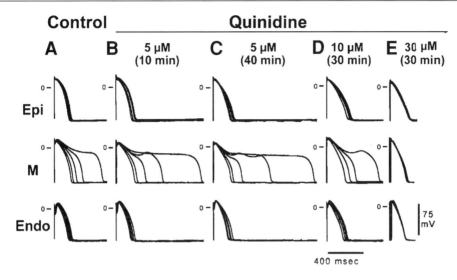

Fig. 6. Effect of 5, 10, and 30 µM quinidine on action potential activity in tissue slices isolated from the endocardial, M, and endocardial regions of the canine ventricular free wall. Preparations were field stimulated at BCLs of 300, 500, 1000, 2000, 5000, and 8000 ms. (**A**) Control, (**B**) Recorded 10 min after addition of 5 µM quinidine; the M cell APD is preferentially prolonged. (**C**) After 40 min of 5 µM, Epi, M, and Endo APD further prolonged. (**D**) 30 min of 10 µM quinidine caused an abbreviation of the M cell action potential but further prolongation of Epi and Endo. (**E**) Recorded after 30 min of 30 µM. Reproduced from *(6)* with permission.

dium, consistent with a predominant effect of quinidine to block I_{Kr} at this concentration (Fig. 6) *(184,185)*. At higher concentrations (10–30 µM; 3.78–11.37 µg/mL), quinidine produces a further prolongation of the epicardial and endocardial action potential, consistent with an effect of the drug to block I_{Ks}, and abbreviate the APD of the M cell, owing to its action to suppress late I_{Na} *(186)*. Voltage clamp studies have shown that low concentration of quinidine (10 µM) potently block I_{Kr}, but not I_{Ks} (15.0±4.6%), whereas higher concentration (25 µM) potently block both I_{Kr} and I_{Ks} (79.8±11%) *(187)*. It is noteworthy that the dose-response relationship in these voltage clamp experiments is markedly shifted to higher concentrations owing to the short exposure (5 min) of the myocytes to the drug. Quinidine exerts its actions to prolong APD with a bi-exponential time-course comprised of two components with time constants of 25 and 435 min, reflecting the time-course of intracellular uptake of the drug *(188–190)*. Thus, over a long exposure period, low concentrations of quinidine produces a preferential prolongation of the M cell APD leading to an increase in transmural dispersion of repolarization. At higher concentrations, the I_{Ks} and I_{Na} blocking effects of the drug cause a greater prolongation of epicardial and endocardial APD, but limit the prolongation of the M cell action potential, thus leading to a more homogeneous prolongation of repolarization across the ventricular wall. These multiple actions of quinidine have been suggested to underlie the ability of the drug to induce TdP at low therapeutic levels, but not at high therapeutic or toxic levels *(187)*.

Like high concentrations of quinidine, chronic amiodarone prolongs the QT interval without increasing transmural dispersion of repolarization. Amiodarone is a potent antiarrhythmic agent used in the management of both atrial and ventricular arrhythmias.

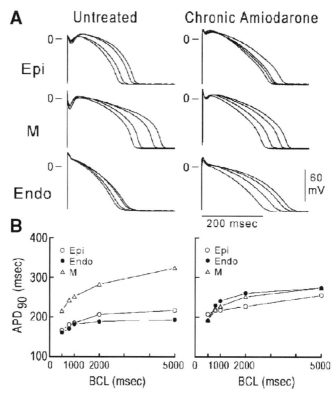

Fig. 7. Effects of chronic amiodarone on the rate dependence of action potential characteristics in Epi, M, and Endo tissues isolated from the hearts of untreated dogs (left) as well as those receiving chronic amiodarone therapy (right). **(A)** Transmembrane activity recorded simultaneously from Epi, M, and Endo preparations at basic cycle lengths (BCL) of 500, 800, 2000, and 5000 ms (steady-state conditions). **(B)** Composite data from 12 untreated and 5 amiodarone treated dogs. The graphs plot APD-rate relations for Epi (open circles), Endo (closed circles), and M (open triangles) of untreated (left) and amiodarone treated animals (right). Each point represents mean ± S.D. * $p<0.01$ amiodarone vs control. [K+]o = 4 mM. Chronic amiodarone treatment leads to much more uniform APD-rate relations in the three cell types.

In addition to its β-blocking properties, amiodarone is known to block the sodium, potassium, and calcium channels in the heart. The high efficacy of the drug as well as its low incidence of proarrhythmia relative to other agents with Class III actions are because of this complex pharmacology. When administered chronically (30–40 mg/kg/day orally for 30–45 d), amiodarone produces a greater prolongation of action potential duration in epicardium and endocardium, but less of an increase, or even a decrease at slow rates, in the M region, thereby reducing transmural dispersion of repolarization (Fig. 7) *(184)*. Chronic amiodarone therapy also suppresses the ability of the I_{Kr} blocker, d-sotalol, to induce a marked dispersion of repolarization or early afterdepolarization activity. Thus, chronic amiodarone treatment differentially alters the cellular electrophysiology of ventricular myocardium so as to produce an important decrease in transmural dispersion of repolarization, especially under conditions in which dispersion is exaggerated. These observations have advanced our understanding of the effectiveness of amiodarone for the treatment of life-threatening arrhythmias as well as our understanding of the relatively low incidence of proarrhythmia *(191)*.

M Cells vs Purkinje Cells

Several distinctions are observed between the response of Purkinje and M cells to pharmacologic agents, and to interventions that elevate internal calcium or manipulate external ion concentration. Purkinje and M cells react differently to α adrenergic agonists resulting from predominance of α_{1a}-adrenoceptors in the former and α_{1b} adrenoceptors in the latter (Table 2) *(192)*. α Agonists, including methoxamine and phenylephrine, produce a prolongation of Purkinje APD, but an abbreviation of the APD of the M cell. Another distinction is the strikingly different mechanisms governing the development of acceleration-induced early afterdepolarizations (EADs) in the two cell types. EADs induced in the M cell are exquisitely sensitive to changes in intracellular calcium levels, whereas EADs elicited in Purkinje are not *(56)*. M cells develop delayed after-depolarizations in response to the calcium channel agonist BAY K 8644 whereas Purkinje cells do not, suggesting differences in calcium handling in the two cell types *(193)*.

Both cell types display an increase in APD as external potassium is lowered, but the response of resting membrane voltage to low external potassium is dissimilar. Possibly owing to a smaller I_{K1} in Purkinje cells, a decline in potassium from 3 mM to 1 mM causes depolarization in Purkinje cells whereas M cell resting potential continues to hyperpolarize *(22)*. M cells do not exhibit phase 4 depolarization in response to low external potassium or isoproterenol because they lack a hyperpolarizing-activated sodium current found in Purkinje cells.

The response to isoproterenol is dependent upon recording conditions. Isoproterenol (0.2 μM) abbreviates APD in both cell types. However, addition of the I_{Ks} inhibitor chromanol 293B in the presence of isoproterenol causes dramatic APD prolongation in the M cell that does not occur in Purkinje cells *(79)*. Addition of a higher concentration of chromanol (50 μM) in the presence of isoproterenol results in prolongation of Purkinje APD *(78)*.

Not all interventions cause dissimilar reactions in the two cell types. TTX inhibits late I_{Na} and significantly shortens Purkinje and M cell APD *(91,92,94)*. Rabbit ventricular myocytes and Purkinje cells also show similar responses to activation of ATP-sensitive potassium current. The ATP-sensitive potassium channel opener levcromakalim results in significant reduction of APD in both cell types, and this response is reversed by the ATP-sensitive potassium channel blocker glibenclamide *(194)*. Both cell types respond in parallel to inhibition of I_{to}, I_{Kr}, and I_{Ca}.

REFERENCES

1. Antzelevitch C, Sicouri S, Litovsky SH, et al. Heterogeneity within the ventricular wall: Electrophysiology and pharmacology of epicardial, endocardial and M cells. Circ Res 1991;69:1427–1449.
2. Antzelevitch C, Sicouri S. Clinical relevance of cardiac arrhythmias generated by afterdepolarizations: The role of M cells in the generation of U waves, triggered activity and torsade de pointes. J Am Coll Cardiol 1994;23:259–277.
3. Antzelevitch C, Sicouri S, Lukas A, et al. Clinical implications of electrical heterogeneity in the heart: The electrophysiology and pharmacology of epicardial, M and endocardial cells. In: Podrid PJ, Kowey PR, eds. Cardiac Arrhythmia: Mechanism, Diagnosis and Management. Baltimore, MD: William & Wilkins, 1995:88–107.
4. Antzelevitch C. The M cell. Invited Editorial Comment. Journal of Cardiovascular Pharmacology and Therapeutics 1997;2:73–76.
5. Antzelevitch C, Yan GX, Shimizu W, Burashnikov A. Electrical heterogeneity, the ECG, and cardiac arrhythmias. In: Zipes DP, Jalife J, eds. Cardiac Electrophysiology: From Cell to Bedside. Philadelphia: W.B. Saunders Co., 1999:222–238.

 6. Antzelevitch C, Shimizu W, Yan GX, et al. The M cell. Its contribution to the ECG and to normal and abnormal electrical function of the heart. J Cardiovasc Electrophysiol 1999;10:1124–1152.
 7. Anyukhovsky EP, Sosunov EA, Gainullin RZ, Rosen MR. The controversial M cell. J Cardiovasc Electrophysiol 1999;10:244–260.
 8. Antzelevitch C, Dumaine R. Electrical heterogeneity in the heart: Physiological, pharmacological and clinical implications. In: Page E, Fozzard HA, Solaro RJ, eds. Handbook of Physiology. The Heart. New York: Oxford University Press, 2002:654–692.
 9. Gilmour RF, Jr., Zipes DP. Different electrophysiological responses of canine endocardium and epicardium to combined hyperkalemia, hypoxia, and acidosis. Circ Res 1980;46:814–825.
10. Litovsky SH, Antzelevitch C. Transient outward current prominent in canine ventricular epicardium but not endocardium. Circ Res 1988;62:116–126.
11. Krishnan SC, Antzelevitch C. Sodium channel blockade produces opposite electrophysiologic effects in canine ventricular epicardium and endocardium. Circ Res 1991;69:277–291.
12. Fedida D, Giles WR. Regional variations in action potentials and transient outward current in myocytes isolated from rabbit left ventricle. J Physiol (Lond) 1991;442:191–209.
13. Krishnan SC, Antzelevitch C. Flecainide-induced arrhythmia in canine ventricular epicardium: Phase 2 Reentry? Circulation 1993;87:562–572.
14. Di Diego JM, Antzelevitch C. Pinacidil-induced electrical heterogeneity and extrasystolic activity in canine ventricular tissues: Does activation of ATP-regulated potassium current promote phase 2 reentry? Circulation 1993;88:1177–1189.
15. Liu DW, Gintant GA, Antzelevitch C. Ionic bases for electrophysiological distinctions among epicardial, midmyocardial, and endocardial myocytes from the free wall of the canine left ventricle. Circ Res 1993;72:671–687.
16. Lukas A, Antzelevitch C. Differences in the electrophysiological response of canine ventricular epicardium and endocardium to ischemia: Role of the transient outward current. Circulation 1993; 88:2903–2915.
17. Di Diego JM, Antzelevitch C. High [Ca^{2+}]-induced electrical heterogeneity and extrasystolic activity in isolated canine ventricular epicardium: Phase 2 reentry. Circulation 1994;89:1839–1850.
18. Yan GX, Antzelevitch C. Cellular basis for the electrocardiographic J wave. Circulation 1996;93: 372–379.
19. Sicouri S, Antzelevitch C. A subpopulation of cells with unique electrophysiological properties in the deep subepicardium of the canine ventricle: The M cell. Circ Res 1991;68:1729–1741.
20. Sicouri S, Antzelevitch C. Drug-induced afterdepolarizations and triggered activity occur in a discrete subpopulation of ventricular muscle cell (M cells) in the canine heart: Quinidine and Digitalis. J Cardiovasc Electrophysiol 1993;4:48–58.
21. Sicouri S, Fish J, Antzelevitch C. Distribution of M cells in the canine ventricle. J Cardiovasc Electrophysiol 1994;5:824–837.
22. Sicouri S, Antzelevitch C. Electrophysiologic characteristics of M cells in the canine left ventricular free wall. J Cardiovasc Electrophysiol 1995;6:591–603.
23. Drouin E, Charpentier F, Gauthier C, Laurent K, Le Marec H. Electrophysiological characteristics of cells spanning the left ventricular wall of human heart: Evidence for the presence of M cells. J Am Coll Cardiol 1995;26:185–192.
24. Liu DW, Antzelevitch C. Characteristics of the delayed rectifier current (I_{Kr} and I_{Ks}) in canine ventricular epicardial, midmyocardial and endocardial myocytes: A weaker I_{Ks} contributes to the longer action potential of the M cell. Circ Res 1995;76:351–365.
25. Antzelevitch C, Nesterenko VV, Yan GX. The role of M cells in acquired long QT syndrome, U waves and torsade de pointes. J Electrocardiol 1996;28(suppl.):131–138.
26. Weissenburger J, Nesterenko VV, Antzelevitch C. Transmural heterogeneity of ventricular repolarization under baseline and long QT conditions in the canine heart in vivo. Torsades de pointes develops with halothane but not pentobarbital anesthesia. J Cardiovasc Electrophysiol 2000;11:290–304.
27. Sicouri S, Quist M, Antzelevitch C. Evidence for the presence of M cells in the guinea pig ventricle. J Cardiovasc Electrophysiol 1996;7:503–511.
28. Li GR, Feng J, Yue L, Carrier M. Transmural heterogeneity of action potentials and Ito1 in myocytes isolated from the human right ventricle. Am J Physiol 1998;275:H369–H377.
29. Anyukhovsky EP, Sosunov EA, Rosen MR. Regional differences in electrophysiologic properties of epicardium, midmyocardium and endocardium: In vitro and in vivo correlations. Circulation 1996;94:1981–1988.

30. Rodriguez-Sinovas A, Cinca J, Tapias A, Armadans L, Tresanchez M, Soler-Soler J. Lack of evidence of M-cells in porcine left ventricular myocardium. Cardiovasc Res 1997;33:307–313.

31. Shimizu W, Antzelevitch C. Sodium channel block with mexiletine is effective in reducing dispersion of repolarization and preventing torsade de pointes in LQT2 and LQT3 models of the long-QT syndrome. Circulation 1997;96:2038–2047.

32. El-Sherif N, Caref EB, Yin H, Restivo M. The electrophysiological mechanism of ventricular arrhythmias in the long QT syndrome: Tridimensional mapping of activation and recovery patterns. Circ Res 1996;79:474–492.

33. Weirich J, Bernhardt R, Loewen N, Wenzel W, Antoni H. Regional- and species-dependent effects of K^+-channel blocking agents on subendocardium and mid-wall slices of human, rabbit, and guinea pig myocardium. [abstr]. Pflugers Arch 1996;431:R130.

34. Furukawa T, Myerburg RJ, Furukawa N, Bassett AL, Kimura S. Differences in transient outward currents of feline endocardial and epicardial myocytes. Circ Res 1990;67:1287–1291.

35. Clark RB, Bouchard RA, Salinas-Stefanon E, Sanchez-Chapula J, Giles WR. Heterogeneity of action potential waveforms and potassium currents in rat ventricle. Cardiovasc Res 1993;27:1795–1799.

36. Wettwer E, Amos GJ, Posival H, Ravens U. Transient outward current in human ventricular myocytes of subepicardial and subendocardial origin. Circ Res 1994;75:473–482.

37. Nabauer M, Beuckelmann DJ, Uberfuhr P, Steinbeck G. Regional differences in current density and rate-dependent properties of the transient outward current in subepicardial and subendocardial myocytes of human left ventricle. Circulation 1996;93:168–177.

38. Zygmunt AC. Intracellular calcium activates chloride current in canine ventricular myocytes. Am J Physiol 1994;267:H1984–H1995.

39. Takano M, Noma A. Distribution of the isoprenaline-induced chloride current in rabbit heart. Pflugers Arch 1992;420:223–226.

40. Di Diego JM, Sun ZQ, Antzelevitch C. I_{to} and action potential notch are smaller in left vs. right canine ventricular epicardium. Am J Physiol 1996;271:H548–H561.

41. Volders PG, Sipido KR, Carmeliet E, Spatjens RL, Wellens HJ, Vos MA. Repolarizing K^+ currents ITO1 and I_{Ks} are larger in right than left canine ventricular midmyocardium. Circulation 1999;99: 206–210.

42. Antzelevitch C, Sicouri S, Lukas A, Nesterenko VV, Liu DW, Di Diego JM. Regional differences in the electrophysiology of ventricular cells: Physiological and clinical implications. In: Zipes DP, Jalife J, eds. Cardiac Electrophysiology: From Cell to Bedside. Philadelphia: W.B. Saunders Co., 1995: 228–245.

43. Lukas A, Antzelevitch C. Phase 2 reentry as a mechanism of initiation of circus movement reentry in canine epicardium exposed to simulated ischemia. The antiarrhythmic effects of 4-aminopyridine. Cardiovasc Res 1996;32:593–603.

44. Antzelevitch C, Di Diego JM, Sicouri S, Lukas A. Selective pharmacological modification of repolarizing currents. Antiarrhythmic and proarrhythmic actions of agents that influence repolarization in the heart. In: Breithardt J, ed. Antiarrhythmic Drugs: Mechanisms of Antiarrhythmic and Proarrhythmic Actions. Berlin: Springer-Verlag, 1995:57–80.

45. Lukas A, Antzelevitch C. The contribution of K^+ currents to electrical heterogeneity across the canine ventricular wall under normal and ischemic conditions. In: Dhalla NS, Pierce GN, Panagia V, eds. Pathophysiology of Heart Failure. Boston: Academic Publishers, 1996:440–456.

46. Eddlestone GT, Zygmunt AC, Antzelevitch C. Larger Late Sodium Current Contributes to the Longer Action Potential of the M Cell in Canine Ventricular Myocardium. [abstr]. PACE 1996;19:4 (Pt 2):569.

47. Zygmunt AC, Goodrow RJ, Antzelevitch C. I_{Na-Ca} contributes to electrical heterogeneity within the canine ventricle. Am J Physiol 2000;278:H1671–H1678.

48. Brahmajothi MV, Morales MJ, Reimer KA, Strauss HC. Regional localization of ERG, the channel protein responsible for the rapid component of the delayed rectifier, K^+ current in the ferret heart. Circ Res 1997;81:128–135.

49. Yan GX, Shimizu W, Antzelevitch C. Characteristics and distribution of M cells in arterially-perfused canine left ventricular wedge preparations. Circulation 1998;98:1921–1927.

50. Solberg LE, Singer DH, Ten Eick RE, Duffin EG. Glass microelectrode studies on intramural papillary muscle cells. Circ Res 1974;34:783–797.

51. Viswanathan PC, Shaw RM, Rudy Y. Effects of I_{Kr} and I_{Ks} heterogeneity on action potential duration and its rate-dependence: A simulation study. Circulation 1999;99:2466–2474.

52. Streeter DD, Spotnitz HM, Patel DP, Ross J, Sonnenblick EH. Fiber orientation in the canine left ventricle during diastole and systole. Circ Res 1969;24:339–347.

53. Streeter DD. Gross morphology and fiber geometry of the heart. In: Berne RM, ed. Handbook of Physiology. Section 2: The Cardiovascular System. Baltimore: Waverly Press, Inc., 1979:61–112.

54. Lunkenheimer PP, Redmann K, Scheld HH, et al. The heart muscle's putative "secondary structure." Functional implications of a band-like anisotropy. Technol Health Care 1997;5:53–64.

55. Stankovicova T, Szilard M, De Scheerder I, Sipido KR. M cells and transmural heterogeneity of action potential configuration in myocytes from the left ventricular wall of the pig heart. Cardiovasc Res 2000;45:952–960.

56. Burashnikov A, Antzelevitch C. Acceleration-induced action potential prolongation and early afterdepolarizations. J Cardiovasc Electrophysiol 1998;9:934–948.

57. Shimizu W, McMahon B, Antzelevitch C. Sodium pentobarbital reduces transmural dispersion of repolarization and prevents torsade de pointes in models of acquired and congenital long QT syndromes. J Cardiovasc Electrophysiol 1999;10:156–164.

58. Shimizu W, Antzelevitch C. Cellular basis for the electrocardiographic features of the LQT1 form of the long QT syndrome: Effects of b-adrenergic agonists, antagonists and sodium channel blockers on transmural dispersion of repolarization and torsade de pointes. Circulation 1998;98:2314–2322.

59. Shimizu W, Antzelevitch C. Cellular and ionic basis for T-wave alternans under Long QT-conditions. Circulation 1999;99:1499–1507.

60. Yan GX, Antzelevitch C. Cellular basis for the normal T wave and the electrocardiographic manifestations of the long QT syndrome. Circulation 1998;98:1928–1936.

61. Balati B, Varro A, Papp JG. Comparison of the cellular electrophysiological characteristics of canine left ventricular epicardium, M cells, endocardium and Purkinje fibres. Acta Physiol Scand 1998;164:181–190.

62. Bryant SM, Wan X, Shipsey SJ, Hart G. Regional differences in the delayed rectifier current (I_{Kr} and I_{Ks}) contribute to the differences in action potential duration in basal left ventricular myocytes in guinea-pig. Cardiovasc Res 1998;40:322–331.

63. Shipsey SJ, Bryant SM, Hart G. Effects of hypertrophy on regional action potential characteristics in the rat left ventricle: a cellular basis for T-wave inversion? Circulation 1997;96:2061–2068.

64. Taggart P, Sutton PM, Opthof T, Coronel R, Trimlett R, Pugsley W, Kallis P. Inhomogeneous transmural conduction during early ischaemia in patients with coronary artery disease. J Mol Cell Cardiol 2000;32:621–630.

65. Antzelevitch C. Transmural dispersion of repolarization and the T wave. Cardiovasc Res 2001;50: 426–431.

66. Vos MA, Jungschleger JG. Transmural repolarization gradients in vivo: the flukes and falls of the endocardium. Cardiovasc Res 2001;50:423–425.

67. El-Sherif N, Chinushi M, Caref EB, Restivo M. Electrophysiological mechanism of the characteristic electrocardiographic morphology of torsade de pointes tachyarrhythmias in the long-QT syndrome. Detailed analysis of ventricular tridimensional activation patterns. Circulation 1997;96:4392–4399.

68. Bauer A, Becker R, Freigang KD, et al. Rate- and site-dependent effects of propafenone, dofetilide, and the new I(Ks)-blocking agent chromanol 293b on individual muscle layers of the intact canine heart. Circulation 1999;100:2184–2190.

69. Yamamoto K, Tamura T, Imai R, Yamamoto M. Acute canine model for drug-induced torsades de pointes in drug safety evaluation-influences of anesthesia and validation with quinidine and astemizole. Toxicol Sci 2001;60:165–176.

70. Takei M, Sasaki Y, Yonezawa T, Lakhe M, Aruga M, Kiyosawa K. The autonomic control of the transmural dispersion of ventricular repolarization in anesthetized dogs. J Cardiovasc Electrophysiol 1999;10:981–989.

71. Kenyon JL, Gibbons WR. 4-Aminopyridine and the early outward current of sheep Purkinje fibers. J Gen Physiol 1979;73:139–157.

72. Kenyon JL, Gibbons WR. Influence of chloride, potassium, and tetraethylammonium on the early outward current of sheep cardiac Purkinje fibers. J Gen Physiol 1979;73:117–138.

73. Kenyon JL, Sutko JL. Ryanodine and aminopyridine sensitive currents of cardiac Purkinje fibers. [abstr]. Biophys J 1985;47:498a.

74. Sipido KR, Callewaert G, Vereecke J, Carmeliet E. [Ca]i-Dependence of a transient outward current in isolated rabbit Purkinje cells [abstr]. Biophys J 1992;61:A509.

75. Sipido KR, Callewaert G, Carmeliet E. [Ca2+]i transients and [Ca2+]i-dependent chloride current in single Purkinje cells from rabbit heart. J Physiol (Lond) 1993;468:641–667.

76. Van Bogaert PP, Snyders DS. Effects of 4-aminopyridine on inward rectifing and pacemaker currents of cardiac purkinje fibers. Pflugers Arch 1982;394:230–238.

77. Cordeiro JM, Spitzer KW, Giles WR. Repolarizing K^+ currents in rabbit heart Purkinje cells. J Physiol 1998;508 (Pt 3):811–823.

78. Han W, Wang Z, Nattel S. Slow delayed rectifier current and repolarization in canine cardiac Purkinje cells. Am J Physiol Heart Circ Physiol 2001;280:H1075–H1080.

79. Burashnikov A, Antzelevitch C. Block of I_{Ks} does not induce early afterdepolarization activity but promotes β-adrenergic agonist-induced delayed afterdepolarization activity in canine ventricular myocardium. J Cardiovasc Electrophysiol 2000;11:458–465.

80. Patterson E, Scherlag BJ, Lazzara R. Early afterdepolarizations produced by d,l-sotalol and clofilium. J Cardiovasc Electrophysiol 1997;8:667–678.

81. Abrahamsson C, Carlsson L, Duker G. Lidocaine and nisoldipine attenuate almokalant-induced dispersion of repolarization and early afterdepolarizations in vitro. J Cardiovasc Electrophysiol 1996;7:1074–1081.

82. Varro A, Nakaya Y, Elharrar V, Surawicz B. Effect of antiarrhythmic drugs on the cycle length-dependent action potential duration in dog Purkinje and ventricular muscle fibers. J Cardiovasc Pharmacol 1986;8:178–185.

83. Gintant GA. Characterization and functional consequences of delayed rectifier current transient in ventricular repolarization. Am J Physiol Heart Circ Physiol 2000;278:H806–H817.

84. Attwell D, Cohen IS, Eisner DA, Ohba M, Ojeda C. The steady-state tetrodotoxin-sensitive ("window") sodium current in cardiac Purkinje fibers. Pflugers Arch 1979;379:137–142.

85. Gintant GA, Daytner NB, Cohen IS. Slow inactivation of a tetrodotoxin-sensitive current in canine cardiac Purkinje fibers. Biophys J 1984;45:509–512.

86. Patlak JB, Ortiz M. Slow currents through single sodium channels of the adult rat heart. J Gen Physiol 1985;86:89–104.

87. Wang DW, Yazawa K, George AL, Jr., Bennett PB. Characterization of human cardiac Na^+ channel mutations in the congenital long QT syndrome. Proc Natl Acad Sci USA 1996;93:13200–13205.

88. Dumaine R, Hartmann HA. Two conformational states involved in the use-dependent TTX blockade of human cardiac Na^+ channel. Am J Physiol 1996;270:H2029–H2037.

89. Kiyosue T, Arita M. Late sodium current and its contribution to action potential configuration in guinea pig ventricular myocytes. Circ Res 1989;64:389–397.

90. Liu Y, DeFelice LJ, Mazzanti M. Na channels that remain open throughout the cardiac action potential plateau. Biophys J 1992;63:654–662.

91. Zygmunt AC, Eddlestone GT, Thomas GP, Nesterenko VV, Antzelevitch C. Larger late sodium conductance in M cells contributes to electrical heterogeneity in canine ventricle. Am J Physiol 2001;281:H689–H697.

92. Coraboeuf E, Deroubaix E, Coulombe A. Effect of tetrodotoxin on action potentials of the conducting system in the dog heart. Am J Physiol 1979;236:H561–H567.

93. Colatsky TJ. Mechanisms of action of lidocaine and quinidine on action potential duration in rabbit cardiac Purkinje fibers: An effect on steady-state sodium current? Circ Res 1982;50:17–27.

94. Aomine M. Tetrodotoxin-sensitive component in action potential plateau of guinea pig Purkinje fibers: comparison with the papillary muscle. Gen Pharmacol 1989;20:791–797.

95. Jeck CD, Boyden PA. Age-related appearance of outward currents may contribute to developmental differences in ventricular repolarization. Circ Res 1992;71:1390–1403.

96. Pacioretty LM, Gilmour RF, Jr. Developmental changes in the transient outward potassium current in canine epicardium. Am J Physiol 1995;268:H2513–H2521.

97. Escande D, Loisance D, Planche C, Coraboeuf E. Age-related changes of action potential plateau shape in isolated human atrial fibers. Am J Physiol 1985;249:H843–H850.

98. Reder RF, Miura DS, Danilo P, Rosen MR. The electrophysiological properties of normal neonatal and adult canine cardiac Purkinje fibers. Circ Res 1981;48:658–668.

99. Kilborn MJ, Fedida D. A study of the developmental changes in outward currents of rat ventricular myocytes. J Physiol (Lond) 1990;430:37–60.

100. Antzelevitch C. Are M cells present in the ventricular myocardium of the pig? A question of maturity. Cardiovasc Res 1997;36:127–128.

101. Schwartz PJ, Stramba-Badiale M, Segantini A, et al. Prolongation of the QT interval and the sudden infant death syndrome. N Engl J Med 1998;338:1709–1714.

102. Priori SG, Napolitano C, Glordano U, Collisani G, Memml M. Brugada syndrome and sudden cardiac death in children. Lancet 2000;355:808–809.

103. Kaplan WD, Trout WE, III. The behavior of four neurological mutants of Drosophila. Genetics 1969;61:399–409.

104. MacKinnon R. Determination of the subunit stoichiometry of a voltage-activated potassium channel. Nature 1991;350:232–235.

105. Butler A, Wei AG, Baker K, Salkoff L. A family of putative potassium channel genes in Drosophila. Science 1989;243:943–947.

106. Chandy KG. Simplified gene nomenclature [letter]. Nature 1991;352:26.

107. Roberds SL, Tamkun MM. Cloning and tissue-specific expression of five voltage-gated potassium channel cDNAs expressed in the heart. Proc Natl Acad Sci USA 1991;88:1798–1802.

108. Dixon EJ, McKinnon D. Quantitative analysis of potassium channel mRNA in atrial and ventricular muscle of rats. Circ Res 1994;75:252–260.

109. Barry DM, Trimmer JS, Merlie JP, Nerbonne JM. Differential expression of voltage-gated K+ channel subunits in adult rat heart. Relation to functional K+ channels? Circ Res 1995;77(2):361–369.

110. Wang ZG, Fermini B, Nattel S. Sustained depolarization-induced outward current in human atrial myocytes: Evidence for a novel delayed rectifier K+ current similar to Kv1.5 cloned channel currents. Circ Res 1993;73:1061–1076.

111. Feng J, Wible BA, Li GR, Wang ZG, Nattel S. Antisence oligodeoxynucleotides directed against Kv1.5 mRNA specifically inhibit ultrarepid delayed rectifier K+ current in cultured adult human atrial myocytes. Circ Res 1997;80:572–579.

112. Brahmajothi MV, Morales MJ, Liu R, Rasmusson RL, Campbell DL, Strauss HC. In situ hybridization reveals extensive diversity of K+ channel mRNA in isolated ferret cardiac myocytes. Circ Res 1996;78:1083–1089.

113. Barry DM, Nerbonne JM. Myocardial potassium channels: Electrophysiological and molecular diversity. Annu Rev Physiol 1996;58:363–394.

114. Mays DJ, Tamkun MM, Boyden PA. Redistribution of the Kv1.5 K+ channel protein on the surface of myocytes from the epicardial border zone of infarcted canine ventricle. Cardiovascular Pathobiology 2000;2 (2):79–87.

115. Mays DJ, Foose JM, Philipson LH, Tamkun MM. Localization of the Kv1.5 K+ channel protein in explanted cardiac tissue. J Clin Invest 1995;96:282–292.

116. Gidh-Jain M, Huang B, Jain P, el Sherif N. Differential expression of voltage-gated K+ channel genes in left ventricular remodeled myocardium after experimental myocardial infarction. Circ Res 1996;79:669–675.

117. Kong W, Po S, Yamagishi T, Ashen MD, Stetten G, Tomaselli GF. Isolation and characterization of the human gene encoding I_{to}: further diversity by alternative mRNA splicing. Am J Physiol 1998;275:H1963–H1970.

118. Dixon EJ, Shi W, Wang H-S, et al. Role of the Kv4.3 K+ channel in ventricular muscle. A molecular correlate for the transient outward current. Circ Res 1996;79:659–668.

119. Brahmajothi MV, Campbell DL, Rasmusson RL, et al. Distinct transient outward potassium current (I_{to}) phenotypes and distribution of fast-inactivating potassium channel alpha subunits in ferret left ventricular myocytes. J Gen Physiol 1999;113:581–600.

120. Brahmajothi MV, Morales MJ, Rasmusson RL, Campbell DL, Strauss HC. Heterogeneity in K+ channel transcript expression detected in isolated ferret cardiac myocytes. PACE 1997;20:388–396.

121. Salata JJ, Jurkiewicz NK, Wang JJ, Orme HT. A novel benzodiazepine that activates cardiac slow delayed rectifier K+ currents. Mol Pharmacol 1998;54:220–230.

122. Rosati B, Pan Z, Lypen S, et al. Regulation of KChIP2 potassium channel beta subunit gene expression underlies the gradient of transient outward current in canine and human ventricle. J Physiol 2001;533:119–125.

123. Kuo HC, Cheng CF, Clark RB, et al. A defect in the Kv channel-interacting protein 2 (KChIP2) gene leads to a complete loss of I(to) and confers susceptibility to ventricular tachycardia. Cell 2001;107: 801–813.

124. An WF, Bowlby MR, Betty M, et al. Modulation of A-type potassium channels by a family of calcium sensors. Nature 2000;403:553–556.

125. Bahring R, Dannenberg J, Peters HC, Leicher T, Pongs O, Isbrandt D. Conserved Kv4 N-terminal domain critical for effects of Kv channel-interacting protein 2.2 on channel expression and gating. J Biol Chem 2001;276:23888–23894.

126. Ohya S, Morohashi Y, Muraki K, et al. Molecular cloning and expression of the novel splice variants of K(+) channel-interacting protein 2. Biochem Biophys Res Commun 2001;282:96–102.

127. Antzelevitch C. Molecular basis for the transmural distribution of the transient outward current. J Physiol 2001;533:1.

128. Sanguinetti MC, Curran ME, Zou AR, et al. Coassembly of KvLQT1 and minK (IsK) proteins to form cardiac I_{Ks} potassium channel. Nature 1996;384:80–83.

129. Barhanin J, Lesage F, Guillemare E, Fink M, Lazdunski M, Romey G. KvLQT1 and IsK (minK) proteins associate to form the I_{Ks} cardiac potassium current. Nature 1996;384:78–80.

130. Ramakers C, Doevendans PA, Vos MA, Antzelevitch C, Dumaine R. KCNQ1 and KCNE1 expression is reduced in dogs with chronic AV block [abstr]. Biophys J 2000;78:220A.

131. Dumaine R, Wu YS, Antzelevitch C. Distribution of KvLQT1 but not mink parallels the distribution of I_{Ks} in the mid-myocardium of canine heart [abstr]. Biophys J 2000;76:A366.

132. Delombe S, Baró I, Péréon Y, et al. A dominant negative isoform of the long QT syndrome 1 gene product. J Biol Chem 1998;273 (12):6837–6843.

133. Trudeau MC, Warmke JW, Ganetzky B, Robertson GA. HERG, a human inward rectifier in the voltage-gated potassium channel family. Science 1995;269:92–95.

134. Sanguinetti MC, Jiang C, Curran ME, Keating MT. A mechanistic link between an inherited and an acquired cardiac arrhythmia: HERG encodes the I_{Kr} potassium channel. Cell 1995;81:299–307.

135. Sanguinetti MC, Curran ME, Spector PS, Keating MT. Spectrum of HERG K^+-channel dysfunction in an inherited cardiac arrhythmia. Proc Natl Acad Sci USA 1996;93:2208–2212.

136. Abbott GW, Sesti F, Splawski I, et al. MiRP1 forms I_{Kr} potassium channels with HERG and is associated with cardiac arrhythmia. Cell 1999;97:175–187.

137. Fozzard HA, Hanck DA. Structure and function of voltage-dependent sodium channels: comparison of brain II and cardiac isoforms. Physiol Rev 1996;76:887–926.

138. Fozzard HA, Lipkind G. The guanidinium toxin binding site on the sodium channel. Jpn Heart J 1996;37:683–692.

139. Cohen SA. Immunocytochemical localization of rH1 sodium channel in adult rat heart atria and ventricle. Presence in terminal intercalated disks. Circulation 1996;94:3083–3086.

140. Dhar MJ, Chen C, Rivolta I, et al. Characterization of sodium channel alpha- and beta-subunits in rat and mouse cardiac myocytes. Circulation 2001;103:1303–1310.

141. Verheule S, van Kempen MJ, te Welscher PH, Kwak BR, Jongsma HJ. Characterization of gap junction channels in adult rabbit atrial and ventricular myocardium. Circ Res 1997;80:673–681.

142. Gros D, Jarry-Guichard T, ten V, et al. Restricted distribution of connexin40, a gap junctional protein, in mammalian heart. Circ Res 1994;74:839–851.

143. Kanter HL, Laing JG, Beau SL, Beyer EC, Saffitz JE. Distinct patterns of connexin expression in canine Purkinje fibers and ventricular muscle. Circ Res 1993;72:1124–1131.

144. Wong KR, Trezise AE, Bryant S, Hart G, Vandenberg JI. Molecular and functional distributions of chloride conductances in rabbit ventricle. Am J Physiol 1999;277:H1403–H1409.

145. James AF, Tominaga T, Okada Y, Tominaga M. Distribution of cAMP-activated chloride current and CFTR mRNA in the guinea pig heart. Circ Res 1996;79:201–207.

146. Hofmann F, Biel M, Flockerzi V. Molecular basis for Ca^{2+} channel diversity. Annu Rev Neurosci 1994;17:399–418.

147. Catterall WA. Structure and function of voltage-gated ion channels. Trends Neurosci 1993;16:500–506.

148. Hu H, Marban E. Isoform-specific inhibition of L-type calcium channels by dihydropyridines is independent of isoform-specific gating properties. Mol Pharmacol 1998;53:902–907.

149. Kamp TJ, Mitas M, Fields KL, et al. Transcriptional regulation of the neuronal L-type calcium channel alpha 1D subunit gene. Cell Mol Neurobiol 1995;15:307–326.

150. Mori Y, Mikala G, Varadi G, et al. Molecular pharmacology of voltage-dependent calcium channels. Jpn J Pharmacol 1996;72:83–109.

151. Zhang JF, Randall AD, Ellinor PT, et al. Distinctive pharmacology and kinetics of cloned neuronal Ca^{2+} channels and their possible counterparts in mammalian CNS neurons. Neuropharmacology 1993;32:1075–1088.

152. Gao T, Puri TS, Gerhardstein BL, Chien AJ, Green RD, Hosey MM. Identification and subcellular localization of the subunits of L-type calcium channels and adenylyl cyclase in cardiac myocytes. J Biol Chem 1997;272:19401–19407.

153. Takahashi Y, Rothery S, Issberner J, Levi AJ, Severs NJ. Spatial distribution of dihydropyridine receptors in the plasma membrane of guinea pig cardiac myocytes investigated by correlative confocal microscopy and label-fracture electron microscopy. J Electron Microsc (Tokyo) 2000;46(2):165–170.

154. Carl SL, Felix K, Caswell AH, et al. Immunolocalization of sarcolemmal dihydropyridine receptor and sarcoplasmic reticular triadin and ryanodine receptor in rabbit ventricle and atrium. J Cell Biol 1995;129:672–682.

155. Takimoto K, Li D, Nerbonne JM, Levitan ES. Distribution, splicing and glucocorticoid-induced expression of cardiac alpha 1C and alpha 1D voltage-gated Ca^{2+} channel mRNAs. J Mol Cell Cardiol 1997;29:3035–3042.

156. Nicoll DA, Longoni S, Philipson KD. Molecular cloning and functional expression of the cardiac sarcolemmal Na(+)-Ca^{2+} exchanger. Science 1990;250:562–565.

157. Li Z, Matsuoka S, Hryshko LV, et al. Cloning of the NCX2 isoform of the plasma membrane Na(+)-Ca^{2+} exchanger. J Biol Chem 1994;269:17434–17439.

158. Nicoll DA, Quednau BD, Qui Z, Xia YR, Lusis AJ, Philipson KD. Cloning of a third mammalian Na^+-Ca^{2+} exchanger, NCX3. J Biol Chem 1996;271:24914–24921.

159. Chen F, Mottino G, Klitzner TS, Philipson KD, Frank JS. Distribution of the Na^+/Ca^{2+} exchange protein in developing rabbit myocytes. Am J Physiol 1995;268:C1126–C1132.

160. Kieval RS, Bloch RJ, Lindenmayer GE, Ambesi A, Lederer WJ. Immunofluorescence localization of the Na-Ca exchanger in heart cells. Am J Physiol 1992;263:C545–C550.

161. Studer R, Reinecke H, Bilger J, et al. Gene expression of the cardiac Na(+)-Ca^{2+} exchanger in end-stage human heart failure. Circ Res 1994;75:443–453.

162. Prestle J, Dieterich S, Preuss M, Bieligk U, Hasenfuss G. Heterogeneous transmural gene expression of calcium-handling proteins and natriuretic peptides in the failing human heart. Cardiovasc Res 1999;43:323–331.

163. Frank JS, Mottino G, Reid D, Molday RS, Philipson KD. Distribution of the Na(+)-Ca^{2+} exchange protein in mammalian cardiac myocytes: an immunofluorescence and immunocolloidal gold-labeling study. J Cell Biol 1992;117:337–345.

164. Porzig H, Li Z, Nicoll DA, Philipson KD. Mapping of the cardiac sodium-calcium exchanger with monoclonal antibodies. Am J Physiol 1993;265:C748–C756.

165. Koban MU, Moorman AF, Holtz J, Yacoub MH, Boheler KR. Expressional analysis of the cardiac Na-Ca exchanger in rat development and senescence. Cardiovasc Res 1998;37:405–423.

166. Toshe N, Haruaki N, Kanno M. a1-adrenoceptor stimulation enhances the delayed rectifier K^+ current of guinea pig ventricular cells through the activation of protein kinase C. Circ Res 1992;71:1441–1446.

167. Antzelevitch C, Di Diego JM. The role of K^+ channel activators in cardiac electrophysiology and arrhythmias. Circulation 1992;85:1627–1629.

168. Imaizumi Y, Giles WR. Quinidine-induced inhibition of transient outward current in cardiac muscle. Am J Physiol 1987;253:H704–H708.

169. Yan GX, Antzelevitch C. Cellular basis for the Brugada Syndrome and other mechanisms of arrhythmogenesis associated with ST segment elevation. Circulation 1999;100:1660–1666.

170. Litovsky SH, Antzelevitch C. Differences in the electrophysiological response of canine ventricular subendocardium and subepicardium to acetylcholine and isoproterenol. A direct effect of acetylcholine in ventricular myocardium. Circ Res 1990;67:615–627.

171. Blair RW, Shimizu T, Bishop VS. The role of vagal afferents in the reflex control of the left ventricular refractory period in the cat. Circ Res 1980;46:378–386.

172. Prystowsky EN, Jackman WM, Rinkenberger RL, et al. Effect of autonomic blockade on ventricular refractoriness and atrioventricular nodal conduction in man. Evidence supporting a direct cholinergic action on ventricular muscle refractoriness. Circ Res 1981;49:511–518.

173. Mubagwa K, Carmeliet E. Effects of acetylcholine on electrophysiological properties of rabbit cardiac Purkinje fibers. Circ Res 1983;53:740–751.

174. Trautwein W, Kameyama M. Intracellular control of calcium and potassium currents in cardiac cells. Jpn Heart J 1986;27 Suppl 1:31–50.

175. Nakayama T, Fozzard HA. Adrenergic modulation of the transient outward current in isolated canine Purkinje cells. Circ Res 1988;62:162–172.

176. Harvey RD, Hume JR. Isoproterenol activates a chloride current, not the transient outward current, in rabbit ventricular myocytes. Am J Physiol 1989;257:C1177–C1181.

177. Zygmunt AC, Gibbons WR. Calcium-activated chloride current in rabbit ventricular myocytes. Circ Res 1991;68:424–437.

178. Zygmunt AC, Gibbons WR. Properties of the calcium-activated chloride current in heart. J Gen Physiol 1992;99:391–414.

179. Hume JR, Harvey RD. Chloride conductance pathways in heart. Am J Physiol 1991;261:C399–C412.

180. Saeki Y, Kamiyama A. Possible mechanism of rate-dependent change of contraction in dog ventricular muscle: Relation to calcium movements. In: Kobayashi T, Sano R, Dhalla NS, eds. Recent Advances in Studies on Cardiac Structure and Metabolism, Vol. II. Baltimore, MD: University Park Press, 1978:131–135.

181. Kimura S, Nakaya H, Kanno M. Electrophysiological effects of diltiazem, nifedipine and Ni^{2+} on the subepicardial muscle cells of canine heart under the condition of combined hypoxia, hyperkalemia and acidosis. Naunyn Schmiedebergs Arch Pharmacol 1983;324:228–232.

182. Kamiyama A, Saeki Y. Myocardial action potentials of right- and left-subepicardial muscles in the canine ventricle and effects of manganese ions. Proc Jap Acad 1974;50:771–774.

183. Kimura S, Bassett AL, Kohya T, Kozlovskis PL, Myerburg RJ. Regional effects of verapamil on recovery of excitability and conduction time in experimental ischemia. Circulation 1987;76: 1146–1154.

184. Sicouri S, Moro S, Litovsky SH, Elizari MV, Antzelevitch C. Chronic amiodarone reduces transmural dispersion of repolarization in the canine heart. J Cardiovasc Electrophysiol 1997;8:1269–1279.

185. Sun ZQ, Eddlestone GT, Antzelevitch C. Ionic mechanisms underlying the effects of sodium pento-barbital to diminish transmural dispersion of repolarization. [abstr]. PACE 1997;20:11–1116.

186. Balser JR, Bennett PB, Hondeghem LM, Roden DM. Suppression of time-dependent outward current in guinea-pig ventricular myocytes. Actions of quinidine and amiodarone. Circ Res 1991;69:519–529.

187. Antzelevitch C, Shimizu W, Yan GX, et al. The M cell: its contribution to the ECG and to normal and abnormal electrical function of the heart. J Cardiovasc Electrophysiol 1999;10:1124–1152.

188. Antzelevitch C, Davidenko JM, Sicouri S, et al. Electrophysiologic effects of quinidine in canine Purkinje fibers and ventricular myocardium. Slow development of the antiarrhythmic and arrhythmo-genic effects of the drug. In: Velasco M, Israel A, Romero E, Silva H, eds. Recent Advances in Pharmacology and Therapeutics. New York: Excerpta Medica, 1989:259–263.

189. Antzelevitch C, Davidenko JM, Sicouri S, et al. Quinidine-induced early afterdepolarizations and triggered activity. J Electrophysiol 1989;5:323–338.

190. Davidenko JM, Cohen L, Goodrow RJ, Antzelevitch C. Quinidine-induced action potential prolonga-tion, early afterdepolarizations, and triggered activity in canine Purkinje fibers. Effects of stimulation rate, potassium, and magnesium. Circulation 1989;79:674–686.

191. van Opstal JM, Schoenmakers M, Verduyn SC, et al. Chronic amiodarone evokes no torsade de pointes arrhythmias despite QT lengthening in an animal model of acquired long-QT syndrome. Circulation 2001;104:2722–2727.

192. Burashnikov A, Antzelevitch C. Differences in the electrophysiologic response of four canine ven-tricular cell types to a_1_adrenergic agonists. Cardiovasc Res 1999;43:901–908.

193. Sicouri S, Antzelevitch C. Afterdepolarizations and triggered activity develop in a select population of cells (M cells) in canine ventricular myocardium: The effects of acetylstrophanthidin and Bay K 8644. PACE 1991;14:1714–1720.

194. Light PE, Cordeiro JM, French RJ. Identification and properties of ATP-sensitive potassium channels in myocytes from rabbit Purkinje fibres. Cardiovasc Res 1999;44:356–369.

195. Antzelevitch C, Litovsky SH, Lukas A. Epicardium vs. endocardium. Electrophysiology and pharma-cology. In: Zipes DP, Jalife J, eds. Cardiac Electrophysiology, From Cell to Bedside. New York: W.B. Saunders, 1990:386–395.

5

How Do We Measure Repolarization Inside the Heart?

Charles Antzelevitch, PhD,
Andrew C. Zygmunt, PhD,
Jeffrey Fish, DVM, Guillermo Perez, PhD,
and Fabiana Scornik, PhD

CONTENTS

INTRODUCTION

Cardiac repolarization can be measured using a variety of electrophysiologic methodologies. Most studies make use of intracellular, extracellular, or optical recording techniques to record action potentials, monophasic action potentials or activation recovery intervals (ARI) from the epicardial or endocardial surfaces of the heart. Electrocardiographic techniques, including body surface mapping, delineate cardiac repolarization characteristics noninvasively, but the extent to which these can be used to assess local heterogeneities of repolarization remains an issue of debate. More recent studies have endeavored to quantitate repolarization characteristics beyond the surfaces of the heart, peering inside the walls of the heart. This chapter will focus on the latter. Our primary goal is to catalog, evaluate, and illustrate the capabilities of methodologies available for the quantitation of transmural heterogeneities of repolarization and probe the ionic basis for these distinctions.

From: *Contemporary Cardiology: Cardiac Repolarization: Bridging Basic and Clinical Science*
Edited by: I. Gussak et al. © Humana Press Inc., Totowa, NJ

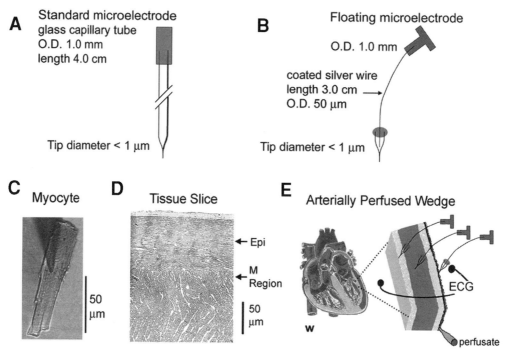

Fig. 1. (A) Standard microelectrode used for recording action potentials, commonly filled with 3 M KCl solution. **(B)** Floating microelectrode; the tip of a standard microelectrode is broken off and a Teflon coated silver wire is inserted into it; the wire is held in place with wax. Standard microelectrodes can be used to record transmembrane activity from isolated myocytes **(C)** and tissue slices **(D)** while floating microelectrodes are used to record transmembrane activity from arterially perfused ventricular wedge preparations **(E)**.

METHODS FOR QUANTITATING REPOLARIZATION AND ITS IONIC BASIS

Experimental Recording Techniques

INTRACELLULAR ACTION POTENTIAL

The gold standard for the measurement of local repolarization is via recording of intracellular transmembrane action potentials using glass microelectrodes filled with 3M KCl. This technique can be applied to enzymatically dissociated single myocytes, tissue slices, or wedge preparations isolated from the heart, or from the intact heart *in situ* or in vivo. In the case of vigorously contracting preparations, floating glass microelectrodes are employed. These are formed by separating the tip of the standard microelectrode and attaching it to a thin strand of silver wire (Fig. 1).

Transmembrane action potentials recorded from cells enzymatically dissociated from different transmural regions of the ventricular myocardium exhibit the greatest range of action potential duration *(1–3)*. Myocytes isolated from the M region display action potential durations (APDs) that are 170 ms longer than those recorded from endocardium or epicardium *(4)*. This transmural dispersion of action potential duration is reduced to 105 ms when recorded from tissue slices isolated from the respective regions of the wall, and further reduced to an average of 64–67 ms when recorded from canine arterially-

Voltage-clamp Methodologies

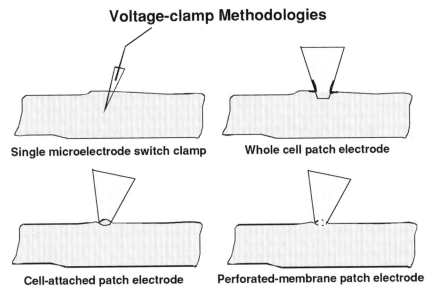

Fig. 2. Voltage/patch clamp techniques.

perfused wedge preparations, in which the three cell types are electrotonically well coupled. In all cases the preparations were paced at a cycle length of 2000 ms.

When these same responses are recorded from transmural tissues or wedge preparations, electrotonic interactions among the three cell types can importantly abbreviate the action potential of the M cell below its intrinsic duration and prolong the APD of epicardial and endocardial cells beyond their intrinsic values, thus reducing transmural dispersion of repolarization *(5)*. The advantages and limitations of each type of preparation will be discussed later in the chapter *(6)*.

ION CHANNEL CURRENT

To elucidate the basis for the intrinsic differences in action potential duration, we can turn to any one of several voltage clamp techniques to quantitate individual ion currents. The use of voltage clamp techniques to study ion channels in acutely dissociated single cardiac myocytes has advanced our understanding of transmural electrical heterogeneity. Each voltage clamp technique has its strengths and limitations (Fig. 2).

Switch Clamp. Discontinuous single-microelectrode voltage clamp, also known as switch clamp technique, is a method in which a high resistance microelectrode serves as both the voltage recording and current passing electrode. Because the high resistance electrode does not dialyze the cell interior, this technique has a minimal impact upon internal calcium buffering and endogenous modulatory pathways. Thus, this technique is preferred when recording ion currents modulated by intracellular calcium or when recording conductances that are dependent upon cytosolic components that can be dialyzed away. Unfortunately, the inability to dialyze the cell is a distinct disadvantage when attempting to separate the many ionic conductances that contribute to electrical activity in the heart. When using this technique, one is left without the ability to make internal ionic substitutions designed to isolate the current of interest. One must resort to measuring currents for which a selective and specific inhibitor is available. This is seldom the case. For example, 5 mM nickel chloride is often applied to characterize the sodium-calcium exchange current. However, nickel also blocks calcium channels and calcium-induced calcium release from the sarcoplasmic reticulum. Inhibition of the calcium transient also blocks the calcium-activated chloride current, and any conductance modulated by internal calcium.

Whole Cell Patch Clamp. The whole cell patch clamp technique uses low resistance patch electrodes that permit substitution of internal ions and better separation of ionic conductances. After sealing the patch electrode to the cell membrane, the membrane beneath the electrode is ruptured by the application of negative pressure, thus permitting rapid dialysis of the cell. This technique is most advantageous when there is an absolute need to isolate a single current for which there is no specific blocker. The limitation of the technique is that cell dialysis disrupts internal calcium levels and eliminates small, soluble modulatory proteins that may be critical for normal channel function. Cell dialysis is known to cause "rundown" of ionic currents, in which the amplitude of the current decreases with the length of the whole cell recording.

Whole Cell Perforated-Patch. Whole cell perforated-patch technique allows substitution of internal monovalent ions without dialysis of larger cellular constituents such as divalent ions and modulatory proteins. Rather than disrupt the membrane beneath the patch electrode, this method uses either amphotericin or nystatin. These antibiotics perforate the membrane and permeabilize it to small ions, thus establishing an electrical connection with the cell interior. Endogenous calcium buffers are maintained, as are the normal calcium transient and contractile function. This method permits the recording of ion channel currents with minimal disturbance of the intracellular milieu. Use of this technique is limited to relatively slow and small currents, since it is otherwise difficult to maintain voltage control.

Cell Attached Patch. The cell attached patch technique is similar to the whole cell patch clamp technique with the exception that the cell membrane is not ruptured. A tight seal between the patch pipet and the cell membrane makes possible the recording of single channel conductances, capable of providing important information about the gating of the channel and the interaction of drugs with the channel.

These techniques may be applied to native cells isolated from the heart of animals or from any one of a number of heterologous expression systems to which the channel of interest is transfected. The pros and cons of these expression systems will be discussed in the next section. Heterologous expression systems are particularly valuable in screening for specific ion channel blocking effects of drugs that may exaggerate dispersion of repolarization within the heart.

Voltage clamp experiments conducted in canine ventricular myocytes have yielded valuable information about the differential contribution of a variety of currents and exchangers to the action potential of epicardial, M, and endocardial cells (Table 1) (*see* Chapter 2 for further details).

MONOPHASIC ACTION POTENTIAL AND UNIPOLAR EXTRACELLULAR ELECTRODES

Unipolar monophasic action potential (MAP) and activation recovery interval (ARI) measurements provide a reasonable approximation of action potential duration at local transmural sites when microelectrode recordings are not possible *(7,8)*. Both recording techniques reasonably approximate local repolarization at transmural sites, thus providing a reasonable estimate of transmural dispersion of repolarization in wedge prepara-

Table 1

Relative Density of Currents that Contribute to Repolarization Among the Four Ventricular Cells Types Found in the Canine Heart

	Epicardial	M	Endocardial	Purkinje
I_{Na}, Late I_{Na}	++	++++	++	++++
I_{Ks}	++++	+	++++	+/−
I_{Kr}	++++	++++	++++	++++
I_{K1}	++++	++++	++++	++
I_{Na-Ca}	++	++++	++	++++
I_{to1}	++++	+++	+	++++

++++, Largest current density; +, Smallest current density; −, No current

Table 2

Transmural Dispersion of APD_{90}, ARI, or MAP Values Measured in Enzymatically Dissociated Myocytes, Tissue Slices, Arterially Perfused LV Wedge Preparations and In Vivo Studies

	Control	I_{Kr} Block (d-Sotalol, 100 μM)	ATX-II (10–30 nM)
Myocytes (BCL=2000 ms)	170 ± 51	–	–
Tissues (BCL=2000 ms)	105 ± 45	286 ± 129	481 ± 155
Perfused Wedge (BCL=2000 ms)	67 ± 15	87 ± 16	178 ± 44
In vivo (BCL=1400–1500 ms)	31 ± 5	88 ± 17	151 ± 29 (7,8)

Mean ± SD (in ms). APD_{90} = action potential duration measured at 90% repolarization measured using floating microelectrodes in the wedge and regular microelectrodes in tissues and cells. MAP = monophasic action potential. ARI = activation-recovery interval. BCL = basic cycle length. Dispersion of APD_{90}: difference between longest APD_{90} (usually M cells) and shortest APD_{90} (generally epicardium). In vivo data were recorded under halothane or isoflurane anesthesia and in some cases from smaller (younger) dogs (7,8).

tions and in the heart in vivo. Drugs with QT prolonging actions, such as d-sotalol, erythromycin, ATX-II, and anthopleurin A, increase transmural dispersion of repolarization to as much as 200 ms in the wedge and in vivo by preferentially prolonging the APD of the M cell (Table 2) (5–7,9). Significant dispersion of repolarization is also observed in the canine heart in vivo with transmural MAP recordings (9) or when unipolar electrodes are used to estimate the ARI (7).

BIPOLAR EXTRACELLULAR ELECTRODES VS UNIPOLAR AND TRANSMEMBRANE RECORDINGS

Unipolar electrograms provide an ARI that can be interpreted on the basis of biophysical theory (10–13) and correlate well with APD under a variety of conditions. In contrast, bipolar electrograms provide a repolarization complex that is not as readily interpretable because it represents the difference in the activity of two sites. Consequently, it is difficult to make a distinction between repolarization times at the two sites, and when differences exist, they are usually obscured. Irrespective of their placement within the wall, ARI values of bipolar electrograms, measured as the interval between the negative peak of the QRS and the *latest* peak of the T wave of the differentiated electrogram *(14)*, can greatly underestimate (by as much as 44%) transmural dispersion of repolarization (Fig. 3) *(15)*.

MULTI-ELECTRODE NEEDLE ELECTRODES VS ULTRA-THIN INDIVIDUAL ELECTRODES

Other factors to consider when selecting a recording method for the measurement of transmural heterogeneities is the degree to which a multiple extracellular electrode needle injures the myocardium, shunts extracellular current, and prevents normal contraction in the region. In previous in vivo and in vitro studies from our laboratory, healing over of the 100–150 μM silver or tungsten electrodes once inserted intramurally is on the order of several minutes (<5 min) *(15,16)*. This is in contrast to the 20 min or more healing over period required for the bulky needle electrodes *(14,17,18)*.

The use of ultra-thin electrodes for the measurement of extracellular potentials is also preferable because the electrodes are flexible, changing shape with the shape of the heart and because they are individually insulated (except at the tip), thus avoiding transmural shunting of extracellular current.

OPTICAL RECORDING TECHNIQUES

Activation and repolarization in the heart follow complex three dimensional pathways that depend on fiber structure, intercellular coupling, and spatial distribution of action potential heterogeneities. Optical recording techniques developed over the past twenty years are capable of mapping these pathways in two dimensions and recent advances are providing information in three dimensions. With the use of voltage dependent fluorescent probes such as di-4-ANEPPS and di-8-ANEPPS, these techniques are used to record action potentials from the surfaces of intact working hearts as well as from arterially perfused wedge preparations. These potentiometric dyes respond to changes in voltage by reducing their emitted fluorescence in the red portion of the light spectrum (above 600 nm) with depolarization. Despite the intrinsically small fractional change (8–15%) of fluorescence during a cardiac action potential, optical recording techniques can provide a high fidelity measurement of the time-course of cardiac action potential *(19)*. Optical mapping with potentiometric dyes provides high-fidelity multisite action potential recordings, the interdependence of temporal, spatial, and voltage resolutions must be considered carefully. For instance, voltage resolution is inversely related to the square of spatial resolution, hence, there exists an inherent trade-off between increased spatial resolution and diminished voltage resolution *(20)*.

A typical recording system consists of a light source, and a lamp or a laser beam of appropriate excitation wavelength for the dye (usually 520 ± 40 nm), that is delivered to the tissue through optic fibers or a lens arrangement. The tissue, loaded with a potentiometric dye, is placed in a recording chamber and illuminated with the excitation light source. Fluorescent light is collected with a high numerical aperture camera lens, long wave-pass filtered (>600 nm), and focused on a detection system consisting of either a CCD camera or a photodiode array, which converts the light signal into an electrical one. The signals are collected and digitized for further analysis. Until recently, this type of optical recording was used almost exclusively to map transmembrane activity from the surface of the heart. Akar et al. *(21,22)*, recently adapted this type of system to record optical maps across the ventricular wall of the canine heart using an arterially perfused

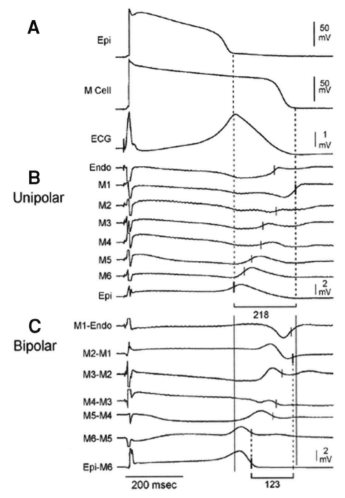

Fig. 3. Accuracy of unipolar vs bipolar extracellular electrode recording techniques. Traces show the correspondence among transmembrane, unipolar, bipolar, and ECG recordings obtained from a canine left ventricular wedge preparation pretreated with ATX-II (20 nmol/L). **(A)** Transmembrane action potentials recorded from M (M2) and epicardial sites together with a transmural ECG at a BCL of 2000 ms; **(B)** Eight intramural unipolar electrograms recorded approx 1.2 mm apart from endocardial (Endo), M (6 sites; M1–M6) and epicardial (Epi) regions (120 µM silver electrodes insulated except at the tip); and **(C)** Bipolar electrograms recorded by differential recording of the unipolar electrodes. Numbers denote the transmural dispersion of repolarization. Dashed vertical lines in the unipolar electrograms mark the time maximum of the first derivative (V_{max}) of the T wave (end of ARI). Dashed vertical lines in each bipolar electrogram show the time of the *latest* peak of the T wave of the differentiated electrogram as defined by Anyukhovsky et al. *(17)*. The data validate unipolar, but invalidate bipolar recordings for the quantitation of repolarization differences in a heterogeneous medium such as the canine left ventricular wall. Modified from *(46)* with permission.

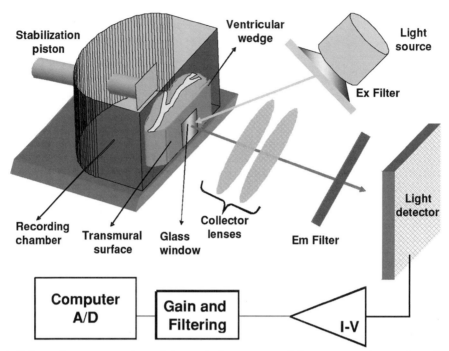

Fig. 4. Schematic representation of the optical system used for transmural mapping of action potentials from an arterially-perfused ventricular wedge preparation. The wedge is placed in a temperature controlled recording chamber and pressed with a stabilization piston against a glass window. The excitation light passes through an excitation filter (Ex filter 540 ± 10 nm) and is directed to the tissue. The fluorescence coming from the di-4-ANEPPS in the preparation is collected by lenses and filtered at 610 nm (Em filter). A 12×12 photodiode array (light detector) can be used to record the changes in light intensity. The photocurrent produced by each of the 144 photodiodes is passed through low noise current to voltage converters (I-V) and then amplified and filtered (gain and filtering). The signals from each photodiode are digitized (A/D) and stored in a computer for further analysis.

wedge preparation. Figure 4 schematically illustrates a typical optical mapping system used to record transmural maps of activation and repolarization.

A major limitation of optical recording techniques is that the preparation studied must, in some cases, be immobilized in order to avoid contraction artifacts. This can impose considerable constraints in the design of the experimental protocol. Contributing to motion artifacts are changes in light transport properties (scattering, absorption, and so on) as well as translational movement of the tissue with heterogeneous distribution of dye among voltage sensing environments and nonspecifically stained regions of the tissue that move with each contraction. Because of the latency of the onset of contraction, motion artifacts do not affect the early phases of the action potential, but may severely distort the repolarization phase. A number of different methods have been used to avoid or compensate for these artifacts. These include mechanical restraints such as a transparent nylon mesh place around the entire heart *(23)* or the use of a vise to immobilize the recording area by pressing the tissue against a glass window (Fig. 4) *(21,24,25)*. However, the pressure applied to the tissue can importantly alter repolarization forces, and if not homogeneously applied, may create artifactual gradients of repolarization. The application of pressure may also accentuate ischemia in preparations that are not well perfused, thus introducing pathophysiological heterogeneities. Another method is to employ agents that uncouple excitation-contraction, such as 2,3-butanedionemonoxime (BDM), diacetyl monoxime (DAM) and cytochalacin D (Cyto D) *(26,27)*. Unfortunately, these agents impose their own electrophysiological effects; BDM and DAM have been shown to affect transmembrane currents (I_{Ca}, I_{to}) *(28,29)* and alter the electrophysiology of the heart *(26)*. Although Cyto D has been reported to be less problematic *(27)*, recent preliminary reports suggest that it too exerts an effect on the action potential.

In recent years, investigators have taken advantage of the dual emission properties of potentiometric dyes *(30,31)*. As discussed previously, these dyes reduce fluorescence in the red portion of the emission spectrum during depolarization. If the dye is excited at shorter wavelengths (470–490 nm), it is possible to obtain dual emission properties in which fluorescence in the green portion of the spectrum (510–576 nm) increases with depolarization whereas fluorescence in the red portion continues to decrease. Assuming that motion artifacts affect both emission wavelengths equally, these artifacts may be cancelled by taking the ratio of the signal recorded in the green portion over that recorded in the red portion of the spectrum. The emitted light is divided in two channels (i.e., green and red) and simultaneously detected in two separate detectors. Rorh and Kucera *(32)* developed a fiber optic detection system for cultured cardiac myocytes in which motion artifacts are completely compensated by the ratiometric approach. Similarly, Knisley et al. *(33)* were able to accurately obtain action potential recordings from epicardial surfaces free of motion artifacts using this dual emission approach. However, the arrangement of light detectors in this study precludes any mapping capabilities of this optical system, and it can only detect changes at the surface of the heart.

A new methodology recently developed involves use of a bundle of fiber optics loaded into a glass micropipet. This device, named an optrode, is inserted into the ventricular wall of a beating heart to record action potentials intramurally *(34)*. The optrode is used to both deliver excitation light from a laser source, and collect emitted light at several radially distributed points inside the heart wall. This system also uses a dual emission ratio-metric technique to process the green and red signals coming from the di-4-ANEPPS present dye. The optrode has brought us a step closer to measuring transmembrane activity in three dimensions, however motion induced artifacts persist.

Other attempts to record intramural activity involve transillumination of a slab of ventricular tissue *(35)*. In this case, a slab of ventricular tissue loaded with di-4-ANEPPS is illuminated from the opposite side of the recording CCD camera. This system also combines recording of optical activity at the surface of the epi-illuminated side. Thus, in transillumination recordings, both the excitation light and the emitted light have to travel across the width of the tissue slab (~8 mm) which results in light scattering and blurring and a reduction in the signal to noise ratio. Despite the light attenuation present in this thick preparation, these investigators were still able to detect intramural reentrant activity that could not be detected in the surface recordings of the same ventricular slab. Thus, transillumination recordings when combined with endocardial and epicardial surface recordings can provide information about three-dimensional propagation of the impulse within the myocardium.

In conclusion, the relatively new optical recording techniques constitute a promising approach for the study of fundamental questions in cardiac electrophysiology that cannot be answered by conventional methods. With progressive improvement of three-dimensional mapping capabilities, this methodological approach should become increasingly more valuable.

Experimental Preparations

ISOLATED TISSUE SLICES

The most direct means to assess dispersion of repolarization in the heart is by recording transmembrane action potentials from tissue slices isolated from different regions. These slices must be kept at a thickness of under 1 mm (semitransparent) to ensure proper oxygenation of the preparation during superfusion. Dissection of the slice is best achieved using a dermatome. Thin slices of isolated tissue generally require two or more hours to recover from the trauma of dissection. Because transmural and trans-septal heterogeneities vary as a function of apico-basal and posterior-anterior position (4,36–39) identification of regional heterogeneities requires that each group of experiments be conducted on tissues from the same region of the heart.

ISOLATED MYOCYTES

Intrinsic differences in the characteristics of repolarization can also be studied in myocytes enzymatically dissociated from different regions of the heart, although this methodology must be applied with great caution. An important limitation of this method is that successful separation of epicardial, M, and endocardial cells requires dissection of very thin layers of the partially digested ventricle. Although it is reasonable that a 1–2 mm thick segment of the ventricle can be acquired under these conditions, this thickness represents an inordinately large fraction of the ventricular wall in species like the rat, guinea pig, and rabbit. In the dog, the thickness of the epicardial layer in the left ventricle is on the order of 500–800 uM (40); thus, when cells are enzymatically dissociated from a 1 mm slice of epicardium, one can expect the fraction to be contaminated with transitional cells and possibly M cells to the extent of 20–50% (1,2). In species with smaller hearts and correspondingly thinner ventricular walls, the problem is greatly compounded in that transitional cells and M cells, if present, will vastly outnumber the epicardial or endocardial cells. Thus, the predominant characteristics of cells in the three layers will be those of the transitional and M cells. This limitation may help to explain why M cells have been reported when guinea pig tissues are studied, but not in isolated ventricular myocytes (41–43). The single cell studies employed myocytes enzymatically dissociated from the epicardial, endocardial, and midmyocardial regions of the guinea pig left ventricular wall (42). Of note, both the electrophysiological and pharmacological profiles of the three cell types isolated fit the profile of an M cell as previously described in guinea pig ventricular tissues. However, the conclusion of the study was that there are no M cells in the guinea pig heart because of the apparent lack of marked heterogeneity of repolarization. Rather than lacking M cells, the myocyte fractions appear to be deficient in epicardial and endocardial cells. These studies highlight the difficulty of using dissociated cells to demonstrate or rule out the absence of M cells in the heart.

Whenever possible, single cell studies should be coupled with experiments designed to examine the electrophysiologic and pharmacologic characteristics of tissues isolated from the respective regions of the ventricular wall as well as with studies of transmural slices of the wall. In dealing with dissociated myocytes, it is also very helpful to use scattergrams or plots of individual experiments to visualize the full range of characteristics of cells isolated from the different transmural regions (1,2,44).

It follows that differences in ionic currents and other parameters measured in isolated epicardial, M, and endocardial myocytes are expected to be underestimated. One can reduce the variability caused by a mixed population of cell types by correlating the ionic current measurements (voltage clamp) with action potential characteristics typically recorded from epicardial, M, and endocardial cells in the same cell (current clamp). These action potential characteristics include spike and dome morphology (when present), APD at a BCL of 2000 ms, and APD-rate relations. This approach was shown to yield a much greater difference in the density of the delayed rectifier current among the three cell types than did measurements made in randomly selected cells from the epicardial, M, and endocardial fractions (2). However, such correlation is often difficult if not impossible because the internal and external solutions needed to isolate the various ionic currents do not permit the development of action potentials.

Studies designed to identify apico-basal and antero-postero differences in action potential and ion channel characteristics using dissociated myocytes from these regions are plagued with similar problems. Selection of a particular transmural population of cells in different parts of the heart as a result of the dissociation and other procedures could generate regional differences where none exist. By the same token, when important intrinsic heterogeneities exist, cell selection may underestimate them. Tissue experiments are extremely helpful in establishing the extent to which action potential heterogeneities exist within these distinct regions.

Electrical heterogeneities of repolarization measured in isolated myocytes are best studied using intracellular microelectrode, switch clamp, or perforated patch clamp techniques in which the intracellular milieu is minimally altered. Whole cell patch clamp techniques are useful in the delineation of ion channel distinctions, but may be problematic for the assessment of APD differences because of the alteration of the intracellular environment. Intracellular calcium is usually highly buffered with EGTA or other chelators under these conditions, resulting in a marked prolongation of the action potential in current clamp mode. It is noteworthy that whole cell and perforated patch clamp techniques are amenable for use both in voltage clamp and current clamp experiments, the latter providing a measurement of action potential activity.

HETEROLOGOUS EXPRESSION SYSTEMS

Heterologous expression systems have proven to be of particular value in studying the individual characteristics of the α and β subunit of ion channel molecules that form the channels that generate the currents responsible for repolarization. They have also proven valuable in screening for specific ion channel blocking effects of drugs capable of amplifying dispersion of repolarization in the heart. Voltage clamp techniques can be applied to any one of a number of heterologous expression systems to which the channel of interest is introduced by viral transfection or microinjected of cDNA (45).

In Xenopus oocytes, ionic currents generally appear 1 to 3 d after injection and can be measured with conventional two-microelectrode voltage clamp recordings (Fig. 5). Whereas this technique is relatively quick and economical, the large size and membrane capacitance of the oocytes limit current measurement to slowly activating voltage-gated channels. The relatively large volume of lipophylic material in the oocyte may influence the response to many drugs. Another major limitation of oocytes is that they cannot be studied at physiological temperatures of the mammal (37°C).

These limitations of Xenopus oocytes have resulted in increasing use of mammalian systems. Most studies use human embryonic kidney cells (HEK293), mouse fibroblasts

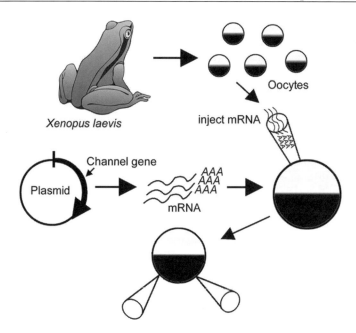

Fig. 5. Expression studies using Xenopus Oocytes.

(C cells), or Chinese hamster ovary (CHO) cells, since these cells have relatively little endogenous voltage activated channel activity. It is noteworthy that differences in IC_{50} of 1–2 orders of magnitude have been reported for the effect of drugs to inhibit ion channel current in different heterologous expressions systems and native cells. In addition to the limitations already discussed, it is important to keep in mind that α subunits expressed in the absence of their β counterparts may exhibit a pharmacological response very different from that of the native channel.

ARTERIALLY PERFUSED VENTRICULAR WEDGE PREPARATION

Data obtained from isolated tissues and cells provide a measure of *intrinsic* regional differences of repolarization, but do not reveal the extent to which dispersion may be present when these cells and tissues are electrotonically well coupled as they are in the intact ventricular wall. This issue can be addressed by studying transmural repolarization in the intact heart *in situ* or in vivo. In the arterially-perfused ventricular wedge preparation, the tissue surrounding a single branch of a coronary artery is isolated, allowing for the recording of transmembrane actions potentials from the interior of the wall using floating microelectrodes. The ability to record a pseudo-ECG across the bath along the same axis permits correlation of transmembrane action potential activity with the electrocardiographic activity of the preparation. This technique has proved to be extremely valuable in the elucidation of the cellular basis of the ECG as well as delineation of mechanisms responsible for the development of cardiac arrhythmias under pathophysiologic conditions *(46,47)*.

Dissection of the wedge is generally done in cardioplegic solution consisting of cold (4°C) or room temperature Tyrode's solution containing 8.5 mmol/L $[K^+]_o$. A native arterial branch of the coronary vasculature is then cannulated and perfused with cardioplegic solution. Unperfused tissue, readily identified by its maintained red appearance (erythrocytes not washed away) is removed using a razor blade. The preparation is then placed in a small tissue bath and arterially perfused with Tyrode's solution bubbled with 95% O_2 and 5% CO_2 and warmed to 35–37°C. The perfusate is delivered to the coronary artery by a roller pump (Cole Parmer Instrument Co., Niles, IL) and perfusion pressure monitored with a pressure transducer (World Precision Instruments, Inc., Sarasota, FL) and maintained between 40 and 50 mm Hg by adjustment of the perfusion flow rate. The preparations remain immersed in the arterial perfusate, which is allowed to rise to a level 2 to 3 mm above the tissue surface when possible. To facilitate impalement with floating microelectrodes, the bath solution is lowered to a level just shy of the top of the wedge and the chamber is covered with coverslips to the extent possible so as to avoid a temperature gradient between the top and lower segments of the wedge. Preparations displaying significant ST segment elevation or depression or in which temperature gradients are evident along the length of the preparation are excluded. There are a number of advantages to using the perfused wedge preparation to define repolarization heterogeneities and their contribution to the ECG and to arrhythmogenesis. Prominent among these is:

1. The ability to record transmembrane action potentials from multiple transmural as well as surface sites.
2. The ability to simultaneously record and correlate transmembrane and electrocardiographic activity.
3. The ability to induce arrhythmias under long QT and other conditions; and most importantly.
4. The absence of anesthesia or other drugs which may be necessary in in vivo studies.

In Vivo Studies

In vivo experiments permit recording of repolarization characteristics under more physiological conditions, but the accuracy of the data is limited in part by the use of anesthetics. Recent studies have shown that transmural dispersion of repolarization observed in vivo can vary dramatically as a function of the anesthetic used. Dispersion of repolarization measured across the anterior canine left ventricular wall (transmural MAP recordings) is smaller with sodium pentobarbital anesthesia than with halothane. The effect of pentobarbital to dissipate transmural heterogeneity under control conditions is still more evident in the presence of agents that prolong the action potential (16,48). d-sotalol produces a prominent increase in transmural dispersion of repolarization under halothane, but a much smaller increase under sodium pentobarbital anesthesia (16). As a consequence, d-sotalol-induced torsade de pointes (TdP) is not observed under sodium pentobarbital anesthesia, but readily develops under halothane anesthesia.

Clinically relevant concentrations of sodium pentobarbital dramatically reduce transmural dispersion of repolarization in the arterially-perfused canine left ventricular wedge preparation under control conditions (Fig. 6) and following exposure of the preparation to d-sotalol and ATX-II (46,48). Pentobarbital totally suppresses d-sotalol- and ATX-II-induced TdP. Pentobarbital-induced abbreviation or diminished prolongation of the M cell APD (owing to block of late I_{Na}) but prominent prolongation of the APD of epicardium and endocardium (secondary to block of I_{Ks}) contribute to these effects of the anesthetic (49). The data demonstrate the effect of sodium pentobarbital to differentially alter the electrophysiology of the three principal ventricular cell types so as to importantly diminish transmural dispersion of repolarization across the ventricular wall. As a

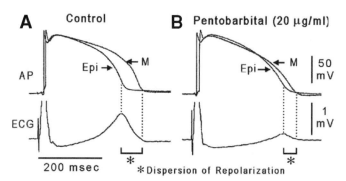

Fig. 6. Effect of sodium pentobarbital (20 µg/mL) on transmembrane and ECG activity in an arterially-perfused canine left ventricular wedge preparation. All traces depict action potentials simultaneously recorded from M and epicardial (Epi) sites together with a transmural ECG. BCL = 2000 ms. Pentobarbital slows phase 3 repolarization, flattens the T wave and reduces transmural dispersion of repolarization from 51 to 37 ms. Reproduced from *(48)*, with permission.

consequence, the development of TdP is under conditions mimicking the LQT2 and LQT3 forms of the congenital LQTS *(48)*. These findings indicate the need to exercise caution in the interpretation of the results of in vivo studies performed under pentobarbital anesthesia.

The cellular and ionic basis for the effects of sodium pentobarbital have been studied in great detail, however data regarding other anesthetics are just emerging. α Chloralose, another commonly used anesthetic, has also been shown to importantly reduce transmural dispersion of repolarization via abbreviation of the APD of the M cell with little or no change in the APD of epicardium and endocardium *(46)*. This may be because of an effect of the anesthetic to block late I_{Na}. Use of α chloralose may be especially problematic in studies of drugs that block I_{Na}.

Use of pentobarbital or α chloralose can contribute to the failure of studies to discern significant repolarization gradients across the canine left ventricular wall in vivo *(14, 16–18,50)*. A relatively small transmural dispersion of repolarization has been reported (at slow rates) in in vivo studies using pentobarbital or α chloralose for anesthesia *(9,14,18,50)* vs studies using other agents including isoflurane *(7,8)* or halothane *(16)*. It is noteworthy that the development of in vivo models of TdP has met with failure when sodium pentobarbital was used for anesthesia *(9,51)*, whereas TdP readily develops when halothane or isoflurane are employed *(7–9,52)* or when no anesthesia is used *(53,54)*. In the case of α chloralose anesthesia, TdP may develop when I_{Kr} block is combined with α adrenergic agonists and/or hypokalemia *(55,56)*. It is noteworthy that a recent study by Yamamoto et al. *(57)* demonstrated the effect of pentobarbital and isoflurane to suppress quinidine and astemizole-induced TdP, suggesting that both reduce transmural dispersion of repolarization *(56)*.

ELECTROCARDIOGRAPHIC MEASURE OF DISPERSION OF REPOLARIZATION

$T_{peak}-T_{end}$

Differences in the time-course of repolarization of the predominant ventricular myocardial cell types are thought to be largely responsible for the inscription of the electro-

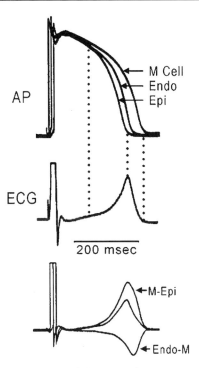

Fig. 7. Voltage gradients on either side of the M region are responsible for inscription of the electrocardiographic T wave. Top: Action potentials simultaneously recorded from endocardial (Endo), epicardial (Epi) and M region sites of an arterially-perfused canine left ventricular wedge preparation. Middle: ECG recorded across the wedge. Bottom: Computed voltage differences between the epicardium and M region action potentials ($\Delta V_{M\text{-}Epi}$) and between the M region and endocardium responses ($\Delta V_{Endo\text{-}M}$).

cardiographic T wave *(58)* (*see* Chapter 4 for further details). Currents flowing down voltage gradients on either side of the M region contribute prominently to inscription of the T wave (Fig. 7) *(58)*. The interplay between these opposing transmural forces determines the height and width of the T wave and the extent to which the T wave may be interrupted, resulting in a bifid or notched appearance.

The T wave starts when the plateau of the epicardial action potential diverges from that of the M cell. As epicardium repolarizes, the voltage gradient between epicardium and the M region continues to grow giving rise to the ascending limb of the T wave. The voltage gradient between the M region and epicardium ($\Delta V_{M\text{-}Epi}$) reaches a peak when the epicardium is fully repolarized—this marks the peak of the T wave. On the other end of the ventricular wall, the endocardial plateau deviates from that of the M cell, generating an opposing voltage gradient ($\Delta V_{Endo\text{-}M}$) and corresponding current that limits the amplitude of the T wave and contributes to the initial part of the descending limb of the T wave. The voltage gradient between endocardium and the M region reaches a peak when the endocardium is fully repolarized. The gradient continues to decline as the M cells repolarize. All voltage gradients are extinguished when the longest M cells are fully repolarized.

When the T wave is upright, the epicardial response is the earliest to repolarize and the M cell action potential is the latest. Full repolarization of the epicardial action potential

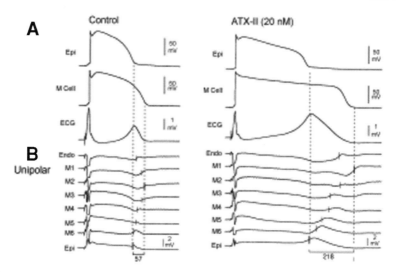

Fig. 8. T_{peak}-T_{end} as a measure of transmural dispersion of repolarization. The traces show the correspondence between the peak of the T wave and repolarization of epicardium and between the end of the T wave and repolarization of the M region in transmembrane, unipolar, and ECG traces simultaneously recorded form a canine left ventricular wedge preparation in the absence (left) and the presence (right) of ATX-II (20 nmol/L). Each panel shows: **(A)** Transmembrane action potentials recorded from M (M2) and epicardial (Epi) sites of a canine left ventricular wedge preparation together with a transmural ECG recorded across the bath (BCL of 2000 ms); **(B)** Eight intramural unipolar electrograms recorded approximately 1.2 mm apart from endocardial (Endo), M (6 sites; M1–M6) and epicardial (Epi) regions (120 µM silver electrodes insulated except at the tip) inserted midway into the wedge preparation. Dashed vertical lines in the unipolar electrograms denote the time maximum of the first derivative (V_{max}) of the T wave (end of ARI). Note the correspondence between the repolarization time of the cells deep within the wedge and those at the cut surface, attesting to the uniformity of the electrical activity in the respective transmural layers. Modified from *(46)*, with permission.

coincides with the peak of the T wave and repolarization of the M cells is coincident with the end of the T wave. Thus, the duration of the M cell action potential determines the QT interval, whereas that of the epicardial action potential determines the QTpeak interval. In addition, these studies suggested that the T_{peak}–T_{end} interval may provide an index of transmural dispersion of repolarization *(46,58)*. Figure 8 illustrates these relationships under baseline and long QT conditions. ATX-II, a sea anemone toxin, mimics the LQT3 form of the long QT syndrome by augmenting the late sodium current, which helps to sustain the plateau of the action potential. ATX-II, like most agents that prolong the action potential, causes a preferential prolongation of the M cell response, thus producing a dramatic accentuation of the transmural dispersion of repolarization, which is reflected on the ECG as a prolongation of the T_{peak}-T_{end} interval. An increase in transmural dispersion of repolarization is a common feature of all LQTS models and has been shown to provide the substrate for the development of TdP under long QT conditions *(6,46,59)*.

The available data suggest that T_{peak}-T_{end} measurements should be limited to precordial leads since these leads may more accurately reflect *transmural* dispersion of repolarization. Recent studies have also provided guidelines for the estimation of transmural dispersion of repolarization in the case of more complex T waves, including negative, biphasic, and triphasic T waves *(60)*. In these cases, the interval from the nadir of the first component of the T wave to the end of the T wave provides an accurate electrocardiographic approximation of transmural dispersion of repolarization.

The T_{peak}-T_{end} index remains to be fully validated in vivo, and the clinical applicability of these concepts remains to be rigorously tested. An important initial step toward validation of the T_{peak}-T_{end} interval as an index of transmural dispersion was provided in a report by Lubinski et al. *(61)*, which showed an increase of this interval in patients with congenital long QT syndrome. Recent studies provide further validation, suggesting that the T_{peak}-T_{end} interval may be useful as an index of transmural dispersion and thus prognostic of arrhythmic risk under a variety of conditions *(62,63)*.

Wolk and coworkers *(64)* recently reported that the results of a study designed to investigate changes in T_{peak}-T_{end} and other traditional indices of electrical dispersion in patients with hypertensive left ventricular hypertrophy (LVH). The main effect of LVH was to increase in QT_{peak} dispersion in the 12 lead ECG. QT dispersion was unaffected, as was T_{peak}-T_{end}, with the exception of lead V2, which showed a significant increase. The authors suggest that these data point to a nonuniform prolongation of action potential duration within ventricular epicardium, leading to a dispersion of transepicardial repolarization, which may underlie the higher level of arrhythmogenesis associated with LVH. This is an interesting observation that merits further consideration.

It seems clear that a great deal of work remains to be done to establish the value of these noninvasive indices of electrical heterogeneity and to assess their prognostic value in the assignment of arrhythmic risk.

REFERENCES

1. Liu DW, Gintant GA, Antzelevitch C. Ionic bases for electrophysiological distinctions among epicardial, midmyocardial, and endocardial myocytes from the free wall of the canine left ventricle. Circ Res 1993;72:671–687.
2. Liu DW, Antzelevitch C. Characteristics of the delayed rectifier current (I_{Kr} and I_{Ks}) in canine ventricular epicardial, midmyocardial and endocardial myocytes: A weaker I_{Ks} contributes to the longer action potential of the M cell. Circ Res 1995;76:351–365.
3. Lukas A, Antzelevitch C. Differences in the electrophysiological response of canine ventricular epicardium and endocardium to ischemia: Role of the transient outward current. Circulation 1993;88:2903–2915.
4. Sicouri S, Antzelevitch C. A subpopulation of cells with unique electrophysiological properties in the deep subepicardium of the canine ventricle: The M cell. Circ Res 1991;68:1729–1741.
5. Antzelevitch C, Sun ZQ, Zhang ZQ, Yan GX. Cellular and ionic mechanisms underlying erythromycin-induced long QT and torsade de pointes. J Am Coll Cardiol 1996;28:1836–1848.
6. Shimizu W, Antzelevitch C. Sodium channel block with mexiletine is effective in reducing dispersion of repolarization and preventing torsade de pointes in LQT2 and LQT3 models of the long-QT syndrome. Circulation 1997;96:2038–2047.
7. El-Sherif N, Caref EB, Yin H, Restivo M. The electrophysiological mechanism of ventricular arrhythmias in the long QT syndrome: Tridimensional mapping of activation and recovery patterns. Circ Res 1996;79:474–492.
8. El-Sherif N, Chinushi M, Caref EB, Restivo M. Electrophysiological mechanism of the characteristic electrocardiographic morphology of torsade de pointes tachyarrhythmias in the long-QT syndrome. Detailed analysis of ventricular tridimensional activation patterns. Circulation 1997;96:4392–4399.
9. Weissenburger J, Nesterenko VV, Antzelevitch C. M Cells contribute to transmural dispersion of repolarization and to the development of torsade de pointes in the canine heart in vivo. [abstr]. PACE 1996;19:II-707.
10. Plonsey R. Action potential sources and their volume conductor fields. Proc IEEE 1977;65:601–611.
11. Spach MS, Barr RC, Serwer GA, Kootsey JM, Johnson EA. Extracellular potentials related to intracellular action potentials in the dog Purkinje system. Circ Res 1972;30:505–519.

12. Haws CW, Lux RL. Correlation between in vivo transmembrane action potential durations and action-recovery intervals from electrograms. Effects of interventions that alter repolarization time. Circulation 1990;81:281–288.

13. Steinhaus BM. Estimating cardiac transmembrane activation and recovery times from unipolar and bipolar extracellular electrograms: a simulation study. Circ Res 1989;64:449–462.

14. Anyukhovsky EP, Sosunov EA, Rosen MR. Regional differences in electrophysiologic properties of epicardium, midmyocardium and endocardium: In vitro and in vivo correlations. Circulation 1996;94:1981–1988.

15. Antzelevitch C, Shimizu W, Yan GX, et al. The M cell: its contribution to the ECG and to normal and abnormal electrical function of the heart. J Cardiovasc Electrophysiol 1999;10:1124–1152.

16. Weissenburger J, Nesterenko VV, Antzelevitch C. Transmural heterogeneity of ventricular repolarization under baseline and long QT conditions in the canine heart in vivo. Torsades de pointes develops with halothane but not pentobarbital anesthesia. J Cardiovasc Electrophysiol 2000;11:290–304.

17. Anyukhovsky EP, Sosunov EA, Feinmark SJ, Rosen MR. Effects of quinidine on repolarization in canine epicardium, midmyocardium, and endocardium. II. In vivo study. Circulation 1997;96: 4019–4026.

18. Anyukhovsky EP, Sosunov EA, Gainullin RZ, Rosen MR. The controversial M cell. J Cardiovasc Electrophysiol 1999;10:244–260.

19. Shimizu A, Nozaki A, Rudy Y, Waldo AL. Onset of induced atrial flutter in the canine pericarditis model. J Am Coll Cardiol 1991;17:1223–1234.

20. Girouard SD, Laurita KR, Rosenbaum DS. Unique properties of cardiac action potentials recorded with voltage-sensitive dyes. J Cardiovasc Electrophysiol 1996;7:1024–1038.

21. Akar FG, Laurita KR, Rosenbaum DS. Cellular basis for dispersion of repolarization underlying reentrant arrhythmias. J Electrocardiol 2000;33 Suppl:23–31.

22. Akar FG, Yan GX, Antzelevitch C, Rosenbaum DS. Use {7178} [abstr]. Submitted 2002;96(8):I-355.

23. Samie FH, Berenfeld O, Anumonwo J, et al. Rectification of the background potassium current: a determinant of rotor dynamics in ventricular fibrillation. Circ Res 2001;89:1216–1223.

24. Chen J, Mandapati R, Berenfeld O, Skanes AC, Jalife J. High-frequency periodic sources underlie ventricular fibrillation in the isolated rabbit heart. Circ Res 2000;86:86–93.

25. Samie FH, Mandapati R, Gray RA, et al. A mechanism of transition from ventricular fibrillation to tachycardia: effect of calcium channel blockade on the dynamics of rotating waves. Circ Res 2000;86:684–691.

26. Wu J, Biermann M, Rubart M, Zipes DP. Cytochalasin D as excitation-contraction uncoupler for optically mapping action potentials in wedges of ventricular myocardium [see comments]. J Cardiovasc Electrophysiol 1998;9:1336–1347.

27. Lee MH, Lin SF, Ohara T, et al. Effects of diacetyl monoxime and cytochalasin D on ventricular fibrillation in swine right ventricles. Am J Physiol Heart Circ Physiol 2001;280:H2689–H2696.

28. Coulombe A, Lefevre IA, Deroubaix E, Thuringer D, Coraboeuf E. Effect of 2,3-butanedione 2-monoxime on slow inward and transient outward currents in rat ventricular myocytes. J Mol Cell Cardiol 1990;22:921–932.

29. Chapman RA. The effect of oximes on the dihydropyridine-sensitive Ca current of isolated guinea-pig ventricular myocytes. Pflugers Arch 1993;422:325–331.

30. Bullen A, Saggau P. High-speed, random-access fluorescence microscopy: II. Fast quantitative measurements with voltage-sensitive dyes. Biophys J 1999;76:2272–2287.

31. Beach JM, McGahren ED, Xia J, Duling BR. Ratiometric measurement of endothelial depolarization in arterioles with a potential-sensitive dye. Am J Physiol 1996;270:H2216–H2227.

32. Rohr S, Kucera JP. Optical recording system based on a fiber optic image conduit: assessment of microscopic activation patterns in cardiac tissue. Biophys J 1998;75:1062–1075.

33. Knisley SB, Justice RK, Kong W, Johnson PL. Ratiometry of transmembrane voltage-sensitive fluorescent dye emission in hearts. Am J Physiol Heart Circ Physiol 2000;279:H1421–H1433.

34. Hooks DA, LeGrice IJ, Harvey JD, Smaill BH. Intramural multisite recording of transmembrane potential in the heart. Biophys J 2001;81:2671–2680.

35. Baxter WT, Mironov SF, Zaitsev AV, Jalife J, Pertsov AM. Visualizing excitation waves inside cardiac muscle using transillumination. Biophys J 2001;80:516–530.

36. Sicouri S, Fish J, Antzelevitch C. Distribution of M cells in the canine ventricle. J Cardiovasc Electrophysiol 1994;5:824–837.

37. Antzelevitch C, Sicouri S, Litovsky SH, Lukas A, Krishnan SC, Di Diego JM, Gintant GA, Liu DW. Heterogeneity within the ventricular wall: Electrophysiology and pharmacology of epicardial, endocardial and M cells. Circ Res 1991;69:1427–1449.

38. Balati B, Varro A, Papp JG. Comparison of the cellular electrophysiological characteristics of canine left ventricular epicardium, M cells, endocardium and Purkinje fibres. Acta Physiol Scand 1998;164: 181–190.

39. Sicouri S, Antzelevitch C. Electrophysiologic characteristics of M cells in the canine left ventricular free wall. J Cardiovasc Electrophysiol 1995;6:591–603.

40. Yan GX, Shimizu W, Antzelevitch C. Characteristics and distribution of M cells in arterially-perfused canine left ventricular wedge preparations. Circulation 1998;98:1921–1927.

41. Sicouri S, Quist M, Antzelevitch C. Evidence for the presence of M cells in the guinea pig ventricle. J Cardiovasc Electrophysiol 1996;7:503–511.

42. Bryant SM, Wan X, Shipsey SJ, Hart G. Regional differences in the delayed rectifier current (I_{Kr} and I_{Ks}) contribute to the differences in action potential duration in basal left ventricular myocytes in guinea-pig. Cardiovasc Res 1998;40:322–331.

43. Shipsey SJ, Bryant SM, Hart G. Effects of hypertrophy on regional action potential characteristics in the rat left ventricle: a cellular basis for T-wave inversion? Circulation 1997;96:2061–2068.

44. Di Diego JM, Sun ZQ, Antzelevitch C. I_{to} and action potential notch are smaller in left vs. right canine ventricular epicardium. Am J Physiol 1996;271:H548–H561.

45. Dascal N. The use of Xenopus oocytes for the study of ion channels. CRC Crit Rev Biochem 1987;22: 317–387.

46. Antzelevitch C, Shimizu W, Yan GX, et al. The M cell. Its contribution to the ECG and to normal and abnormal electrical function of the heart. J Cardiovasc Electrophysiol 1999;10:1124–1152.

47. Antzelevitch C, Dumaine R. Electrical heterogeneity in the heart: Physiological, pharmacological and clinical implications. In: Page E, Fozzard HA, Solaro RJ, eds. Handbook of Physiology. The Heart. New York: Oxford University Press, 2002:654–692.

48. Shimizu W, McMahon B, Antzelevitch C. Sodium pentobarbital reduces transmural dispersion of repolarization and prevents torsade de pointes in models of acquired and congenital long QT syndromes. J Cardiovasc Electrophysiol 1999;10:156–164.

49. Sun ZQ, Eddlestone GT, Antzelevitch C. Ionic mechanisms underlying the effects of sodium pentobarbital to diminish transmural dispersion of repolarization. [abstr]. PACE 1997;20:11–1116.

50. Freigang KD, Becker R, Bauer A, Voss F, Senges J, Brachmann J. Electrophysiological properties of individual muscle layers in the in vivo canine heart [abstr]. J Am Coll Cardiol 1996;27(supplA):124A.

51. Duker GD, Linhardt GS, Rahmberg M. An animal model for studying class III-induced proarrhythmias in the halothane-anesthetized dog. [abstr]. J Am Coll Cardiol 1994;23:326A.

52. Vos MA, Verduyn SC, Gorgels APM, Lipcsei GC, Wellens HJ. Reproducible induction of early afterdepolarizations and torsade de pointes arrhythmias by d-sotalol and pacing in dogs with chronic atrioventricular block. Circulation 1995;91:864–872.

53. Weissenburger J, Davy JM, Chezalviel F, et al. Arrhythmogenic activities of antiarrhythmic drugs in conscious hypokalemic dogs with atrioventricular block: comparison between quinidine, lidocaine, flecainide, propranolol and sotalol. J Pharmacol Exp Ther 1991;259:871–883.

54. Weissenburger J, Davy JM, Chezalviel F. Experimental models of torsades de pointes. Fundam Clin Pharmacol 1993;7:29–38.

55. Buchanan LV, Kabell GG, Brunden MN, Gibson JK. Comparative assessment of ibutilide, D-sotalol, clofilium, E-4031, and UK-68,798 in a rabbit model of proarrhythmia. J Cardiovasc Pharmacol 1993;22:540–549.

56. Carlsson L, Almgren O, Duker GD. Qtu-prolongation and torsades-de-pointes induced by putative class-III antiarrhythmic agents in the rabbit—etiology and interventions. J Cardiovasc Pharmacol 1990;16:276–285.

57. Yamamoto K, Tamura T, Imai R, Yamamoto M. Acute canine model for drug-induced torsades de pointes in drug safety evaluation-influences of anesthesia and validation with quinidine and astemizole. Toxicol Sci 2001;60:165–176.

58. Yan GX, Antzelevitch C. Cellular basis for the normal T wave and the electrocardiographic manifestations of the long QT syndrome. Circulation 1998;98:1928–1936.

59. Shimizu W, Antzelevitch C. Differential effects of beta-adrenergic agonists and antagonists in LQT1, LQT2 and LQT3 models of the long QT syndrome. J Am Coll Cardiol 2000;35:778–786.

60. Emori T, Antzelevitch C. Cellular basis for complex T waves and extrasystolic activity in a model of combined acquired and congenital long QT syndrome [abstr]. PACE 2000;23:615.

61. Lubinski A, Lewicka-Nowak E, Kempa M, Baczynska AM, Romanowska I, Swiatecka G. New insight into repolarization abnormalities in patients with congenital long QT syndrome: the increased transmural dispersion of repolarization. PACE 1998;21:172–175.

62. Wolk R, Stec S, Kulakowski P. Extrasystolic beats affect transmural electrical dispersion during programmed electrical stimulation. Eur J Clin Invest 2001;31:293–301.

63. Tanabe Y, Inagaki M, Kurita T, et al. Sympathetic stimulation produces a greater increase in both transmural and spatial dispersion of repolarization in LQT1 than LQT2 forms of congenital long QT syndrome. J Am Coll Cardiol 2001;37:911–919.

64. Wolk R, Mazurek T, Lusawa T, Wasek W, Rezler J. Left ventricular hypertrophy increases transepicardial dispersion of repolarisation in hypertensive patients: a differential effect on QT_{peak} and QT_{end} dispersion. Eur J Clin Invest 2001;31:563–569.

6

Contribution of Electrical Heterogeneity of Repolarization to the ECG

*Charles Antzelevitch, PhD
and Vladislav V. Nesterenko, PhD*

Contents

INTRODUCTION

Willem Einthoven first recorded the electrocardiogram (ECG) near the turn of the last century, initially using a capillary electrometer and then a string galvanometer *(1,2)*. Today, nearly a century later, physicians and scientists are still learning how to extract valuable information from the ECG and still debating the cellular basis for the various waves of the ECG. In this chapter, our focus will be on the cellular basis for the J, T, and U waves of the ECG. These three waves represent repolarization forces within the ventricles of the heart. The J wave and T wave are thought to arise as a consequence of voltage gradients that develop as a result of the electrical heterogeneity that exists within the ventricular myocardium. The basis for the U wave has long been a matter of debate. One theory attributes the U wave to mechano-electrical feedback. A second theory ascribes it to voltage gradients within ventricular myocardium and a third to voltage gradients between the ventricular myocardium and the His-Purkinje system. An understanding of the ECG clearly requires that we have an understanding of the electrical heterogeneity that exists within the heart, which we review briefly below and discuss in much more detail in Chapter 2.

ELECTRICAL HETEROGENEITY

As early as 15 yr ago, ventricular myocardium was thought to be largely homogeneous with respect to its electrical properties and responsiveness to drugs. Studies from a

From: *Contemporary Cardiology: Cardiac Repolarization: Bridging Basic and Clinical Science*
Edited by: I. Gussak et al. © Humana Press Inc., Totowa, NJ

number of laboratories have demonstrated ventricular myocardium to be comprised of three electrophysiologically distinct cell types: epicardial, M, and endocardial (3–5). These three ventricular myocardial cell types differ principally with respect to phase 1 and phase 3 repolarization characteristics. Ventricular epicardial and M, but not endocardial, action potentials display a prominent phase 1, owing to a prominent 4-aminopyridine (4-AP) sensitive transient outward current (I_{to}), giving rise to a spike and dome or notched configuration. These regional differences in I_{to} have been demonstrated in canine (6,7), feline (8), rabbit (9), rat (10), and human (11,12) ventricular myocytes. Important differences also exist in the magnitude of I_{to} and action potential notch between right and left ventricular epicardial and M cells with right ventricular cells displaying a much greater I_{to} (13,14). The transmural and interventricular differences in the manifestation of I_{to} have a number of interesting consequences (13,15–21), including the creation of a transmural voltage gradient responsible for the inscription of the electrocardiographic J wave.

M cells are distinguished by the ability of their action potential to prolong more than other ventricular myocardial cell types in response to a slowing of rate and/or in response to agents with Class III actions (15,22,23). These features of the M cell are owing to the presence of a smaller slowly activating delayed rectifier current (I_{Ks}) (24), a larger late sodium current (late I_{Na}) (25), and a larger electrogenic sodium-calcium exchange current (I_{Na-Ca}) (26). Electrophysiologically and pharmacologically, M cells appear to be a hybrid between Purkinje and ventricular cells (3–5). M cells displaying the longest action potentials are often localized in the deep subendocardium to midmyocardium in the anterior wall (27), deep subepicardium to midmyocardium in the lateral wall (22), and throughout the wall in the region of the right ventricular (RV) outflow tracts (5). Unlike Purkinje fibers, they are not found in discrete bundles (28). M cells are also present in the deep layers of endocardial structures, including papillary muscles, trabeculae, and the interventricular septum (29). Cells with the characteristics of M cells have been described in the canine (7,22,23,30–33) guinea pig (34), rabbit (35), pig (36), and human (37,38) ventricles.

CONTRIBUTION OF TRANSMURAL HETEROGENEITY TO THE ECG

Transmural Distribution of I_{to} as the Basis for the J Wave

The presence of a prominent action potential notch in epicardium but not endocardium leads to the development of a transmural voltage gradient during ventricular activation that manifests as a late delta wave following the QRS or what is more commonly referred to as a J wave (18) or Osborn wave. The J wave and elevated J point have been described in the ECG of animals and humans for over forty years (39), since Osborn's observation in the early 1950s (40). A distinct J wave is commonly observed in the ECG of some animal species including dogs and baboons, under baseline conditions and is considerably amplified under hypothermic conditions (41–43). An elevated J point is commonly encountered in humans and some animal species under normal conditions. In humans, a prominent J wave in the ECG is considered pathognomonic of hypothermia (44–47) or hypercalcemia (48,49).

A transmural gradient in the distribution of I_{to} is responsible for the transmural gradient in the magnitude of phase 1 and action potential notch, which gives rise to a voltage gradient across the ventricular wall responsible for the inscription of the J wave or J point elevation in the ECG (6,7,16,17). Direct evidence in support of the hypothesis that the J

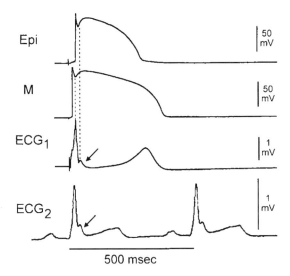

Fig. 1. Relationship between the spike-and-dome morphology of the epicardial action potential and the appearance of the J wave. ECG_2 is a lead V_5 ECG recorded from the dog in vivo. ECG_1 is a transmural ECG recorded across the arterially perfused left ventricular wedge isolated from the heart of the same dog. Both display a prominent J wave at the R-ST junction (arrows). The two upper traces are transmembrane action potentials simultaneously recorded from the epicardial (Epi) and M regions with floating microelectrodes. The preparation was paced at a basic cycle length of 4000 ms. The sinus cycle length at the time ECG_2 was recorded was 500 ms. The J wave is temporally coincident with the notch of the epicardial action potential. Although the M cell action potential also exhibits a prominent notch, it occurs too early to exert an important influence on the manifestation of the J wave. (From *[18]*, with permission.)

wave is caused by a transmural gradient in the magnitude of the I_{to}-mediated action potential notch derives from experiments conducted in the arterially-perfused right ventricular wedge preparation (Fig. 1) *(18)*. The data derived from the wedge preparations indicated a highly significant correlation between the amplitude of the epicardial action potential notch and that of the J wave recorded during interventions that alter the appearance of the electrocardiographic J wave, including hypothermia, premature stimulation (restitution), and block of I_{to} by 4-AP (Figs. 2–4).

Ventricular activation from endocardium to epicardium, with epicardium activated last, is an important prerequisite for the appearance of the J wave. This sequence permits the establishment of a voltage gradient of the early phases of the action potential after activation of the preparation is completed (i.e., after the QRS). Stimulation of the preparation from an epicardial site does not produce a J wave despite the maintenance of cellular differences in the morphology of the action potential; the J wave is buried in the QRS.

Conduction time across the wall is another determining factor. Because the right ventricular wall is relatively thin, transmural activation may be so rapid as to bury the J wave inside the QRS. Thus, although the action potential notch is most prominent in right ventricular epicardium, right ventricular myocardium would be expected to contribute very little to the manifestation of the J wave. These observations are consistent with the manifestation of the J wave in ECG leads in which the mean vector axis is transmurally oriented across the left ventricle and septum. Accordingly, the J wave in the dog is most

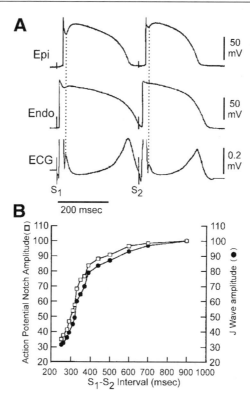

Fig. 2. Relation between restitution of epicardial action potential notch amplitude and J wave amplitude. (**A**) Simultaneous recording of a transmural ECG and transmembrane action potentials from the epicardial (Epi) and endocardial (Endo) regions of an isolated arterially perfused right ventricular wedge. A significant action potential notch in epicardium is associated with a prominent J wave (arrow) during basic stimulation (S_1–S_1: 4000 ms). Premature stimulation (S_1–S_2: 300 ms) causes a parallel decrease in the amplitude of the epicardial action potential notch and that of the J wave (arrow). (**B**) Plot of the amplitudes of the epicardial action potential notch (□) and J wave (O) as a function of the S_1–S_2 interval. The amplitude of the epicardial action potential notch and that of the J wave are normalized to the value recorded at an S_1–S_2 interval of 900 ms. (From *[18]*, with permission.)

prominent in leads II, III, aVR, aVF, and mid to left precordial leads V_3 through V_6. A similar picture is seen in the human ECG *(44,47,49)*. In addition, vectorcardiography indicates that the J wave forms an extra loop that occurs at the junction of the QRS and T loops *(50)*. It is directed leftward and anteriorly, which explains its prominence in leads associated with the left ventricle.

The J wave was first noted in animal experiments involving hypercalcemia conducted in the 1920s *(48)*. The first extensive description and characterization appeared 30 yr later in a study by Osborn involving experimental hypothermia in dogs *(40)*. As a consequence, this wave, which appears at the R-ST junction, is often referred to as either a J wave or an Osborn wave.

The spike-and-dome morphology of the epicardial action potential is absent in canine neonates, gradually appearing over the first few months of life *(16)*. The progressive development of the notch is paralleled by the appearance of I_{to} *(16,52,53)*. It is therefore not surprising that a J wave is not observed in neonatal dogs *(18,83)*.

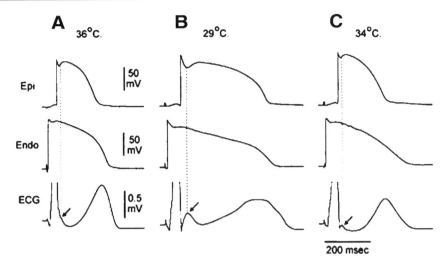

Fig. 3. Effect of hypothermia on action potential and ECG morphology. Each panel shows transmembrane recordings obtained from the epicardial (Epi) and endocardial (Endo) regions of an isolated arterially perfused canine left ventricular wedge and a transmural ECG recorded simultaneously. **(A)** A small but distinct action potential notch in epicardium but not in endocardium is associated with an elevated J-point at the R-ST junction (arrow) under normothermic conditions (36°C). **(B)** A decrease in the temperature of the perfusate and bath to 29°C results in an increase in the amplitude and width of the action potential notch in epicardium but not in endocardium, leading to a prominent J wave on the transmural ECG (arrow). **(C)** Rewarming to a temperature of 34°C is attended by a parallel reduction in the amplitude and width of the J wave and epicardial action potential notch. (From [18], with permission.)

The appearance of a prominent J wave in the clinic is typically associated with pathophysiological conditions such as hypothermia (44,47) and hypercalcemia (48,49). A modest J wave is observed in some patients who have completely recovered from hypothermia (54,55). The prominent J wave induced by hypothermia is the result of a marked accentuation of the spike-and-dome morphology of the action potential of M and epicardial cells (i.e., an increase in both width and magnitude of the notch) as illustrated in Fig. 3. This may be the result of slowing of the kinetics of activation of I_{to} less than the kinetics of the calcium current, I_{Ca}. In addition to inducing a more prominent notch, hypothermia produces a slowing of conduction which allow the epicardial notch to clear the QRS so as to manifest a distinct J wave. Thus, the additional conduction delay from endocardium to epicardium together with the widening of the epicardial action potential notch serve to unmask a latent J wave by moving it out of the QRS complex (Fig. 3).

Association of hypercalcemia with the appearance of the J wave (48,49,56) may also be explained on the basis of an accentuation of the epicardial action potential notch, possibly as a result of an augmentation of the calcium-activated chloride current and a decrease in I_{Ca} (57).

As discussed in Chapter 9, the presence of a prominent action potential notch predisposes canine ventricular epicardium to all-or-none repolarization and phase 2 reentry. Under ischemic conditions and in response to sodium channel blockers, parasympathetic agonists, potassium channel blockers and a variety of other drugs, canine ventricular epicardium exhibits an all-or-none repolarization at the end of phase 1 of the action

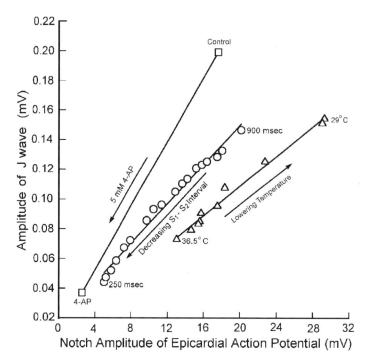

Fig. 4. Graph showing correlation between amplitude of J wave of transmural ECG and amplitude of epicardial action potential notch recorded at different S_1–S_2 intervals (O) and temperatures (29°C to 36.5°C, Δ) and in the absence and presence of 5 mmol/L 4-AP (□). Three separate preparations. Basic cycle length was 4000 ms. In the case of the hypothermia and restitution plots, the solid lines were obtained by linear regression (r^2=.99 for both). (From *[18]*, with permission.)

potential. Failure of the dome to develop results in a marked (40% to 70%) abbreviation of the action potential. Under these conditions, the action potential dome is usually abolished at some epicardial sites but not others, causing a marked dispersion of repolarization. Propagation of the action potential dome from sites at which it is maintained to sites at which it is abolished can cause local reexcitation of the preparation. This mechanism, called phase 2 reentry, produces extrasystolic activity, which can then initiate one or more cycles of circus movement reentry *(3)*. Because the J wave provides an index of the prominence of the spike-and-dome morphology of the epicardial response, it can be of diagnostic and prognostic value in identifying subjects predisposed to phase 2 reentry or individuals who may be inclined to develop life-threatening arrhythmias such as the Brugada syndrome *(58,59)*.

Transmural Dispersion of Repolarization as the Basis for the T Wave

M cells have been shown to play a determining role in the inscription of the electrocardiographic T wave. Data from the arterially-perfused wedge have provided new insights into the cellular basis of the T wave showing that currents flowing down voltage gradients on either side of the M region are in large part responsible for the T wave (Fig. 5) *(60)*. The interplay between these opposing currents establishes the height and width of the T wave as well as the degree to which either the ascending or descending limb of the T wave is interrupted, leading to a bifurcated or notched appearance. The voltage

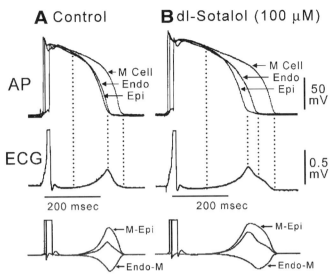

Fig. 5. Voltage gradients on either side of the M region are responsible for inscription of the electrocardiographic T wave. Top: Action potentials simultaneously recorded from endocardial, epicardial and M region sites of an arterially-perfused canine left ventricular wedge preparation. Middle: ECG recorded across the wedge. Bottom: Computed voltage differences between the epicardium and M region action potentials ($\Delta V_{M\text{-}Epi}$) and between the M region and endocardium responses ($\Delta V_{Endo\text{-}M}$). If these traces are representative of the opposing voltage gradients on either side of the M region, responsible for inscription of the T wave, then the weighted sum of the two traces should yield a trace (middle trace in bottom grouping) resembling the ECG, which it does. The voltage gradients are weighted to account for differences in tissue resistivity between M and Epi and Endo and M regions, thus yielding the opposing currents flowing on either side of the M region. **(A)** Under control conditions the T wave begins when the plateau of epicardial action potential separates from that of the M cell. As epicardium repolarizes, the voltage gradient between epicardium and the M region continues to grow giving rise to the ascending limb of the T wave. The voltage gradient between the M region and epicardium ($\Delta V_{M\text{-}Epi}$) reaches a peak when the epicardium is fully repolarized—this marks the peak of the T wave. On the other end of the ventricular wall, the endocardial plateau deviates from that of the M cell, generating an opposing voltage gradient ($\Delta V_{Endo\text{-}M}$) and corresponding current that limits the amplitude of the T wave and contributes to the initial part of the descending limb of the T wave. The voltage gradient between the endocardium and the M region reaches a peak when the endocardium is fully repolarized. The gradient continues to decline as the M cells repolarize. All gradients are extinguished when the longest M cells are fully repolarized. **(B)** DL-sotalol (100 μM) prolongs the action potential of the M cell more than those of the epicardial and endocardial cells, thus widening the T wave and prolonging the QT interval. The greater separation of epicardial and endocardial repolarization times also gives rise to a notch in the descending limb of the T wave. Once again, the T wave begins when the plateau of epicardial action potential diverges from that of the M cell. The same relationships as described for panel A are observed during the remainder of the T wave. The sotalol-induced increase in dispersion of repolarization across the wall is accompanied by a corresponding increase in the T_{peak}-T_{end} interval in the pseudo-ECG. Modified from *(60)* with permission.

gradients result from more positive plateau potentials in the M region than in epicardium or endocardium and from differences in the time-course of phase 3 of the action potential of the three predominant ventricular cell types. Under baseline and long QT conditions, the epicardial response is the earliest to repolarize and the M cell action potential is the last. Full repolarization of the epicardial action potential is coincident with peak of the

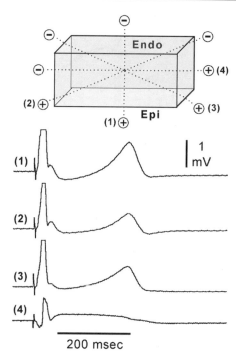

Fig. 6. Contribution of transmural vs apico-basal and anterior-posterior gradients to the registration of the T wave. The four ECG traces were simultaneously recorded at 0°, 45°, –45°, and 90° (apico-basal) angles relative to the transmural axis of an arterially-perfused left ventricular wedge preparation. Inscription of the T wave is largely the result of voltage gradients along the transmural axis. Modified from *(60)* with permission.

T wave and repolarization of the M cells coincides with the end of the T wave. The duration of the M cell action potential determines the duration of the QT interval under a wide variety of conditions in which the QT interval can be altered, including changes in pacing rate, prematurity, alterations in $[K^+]_o$ and exposure to APD-prolonging drugs. Under these conditions, the T_{peak}–T_{end} interval provides an index of transmural dispersion of repolarization, which may prove to be a valuable prognostic tool *(60,61)*, as recently reported by Lubinski et al. *(62)*.

Previous studies have suggested apico-basal repolarization gradients measured along the epicardial surface may play a role in the registration of the T wave *(63)*. In contrast, more recent studies involving the perfused wedge suggest little or no contribution, owing to the fact that the ECG recorded along the apico-basal axis fails to display a T wave (Fig. 6) *(60,64)*. These findings suggest that in this part of the canine left ventricular wall (anterior, mid apico-basal) the inscription of the T wave is largely the result of voltage gradients along the transmural axis.

Role of Transmural Heterogeneity in Inscription of the U Wave

A number of interesting theories have been advanced to explain the cellular basis for the U wave. Since the original description of this wave by Einthoven, who hypothesized that the U wave is the representation of the late repolarization of certain regions of myocardium *(2)*, the following theories have been proposed to explain the physiologic mechanisms responsible for its genesis. Several myocardial sources of the U wave have been considered:

1. Ventricular septum *(65)*
2. Papillary muscles *(66)*
3. Negative afterpotentials *(67,68)*
4. Purkinje system *(69,70)*
5. Early or delayed afterdepolarizations *(68)*
6. "Mechano-electrical feedback" *(71,72)*

The major idea behind these concepts was to find some electrical processes in myocardium that last far beyond repolarization of endocardial and epicardial surfaces of the heart.

The most popular hypothesis ascribes the U wave to delayed repolarization of the His-Purkinje system *(69,70)*. The small mass of the specialized conduction system is difficult to reconcile with the sometimes very large U wave deflections reported in the literature, especially in cases of acquired and congenital long QT syndrome. It has previously been suggested that the M cells, more abundant in mass and possessing delayed repolarization characteristics similar to those of Purkinje fibers, may be responsible for the inscription of the pathophysiologic U wave *(73)*. However, the original simulations *(74)* failed to reproduce U waves of width comparable to those observed clinically *(75)* even when myocardial resistivity was assumed much higher than normal. More recent findings derived from the wedge clearly indicate that what many clinicians refer to as an accentuated or inverted U wave is not a U wave, but rather a component of the T wave whose descending or ascending limb (especially during hypokalemia) is interrupted (Fig. 7) *(60,76)*. A transient reversal in current flow across the wall owing to shifting voltage gradients between epicardium and the M region and endocardium and the M region appear to underlie these phenomena. The data suggest that the "pathophysiologic U wave" that develops under conditions of acquired or congenital LQTS is part of the T wave and that the various hump morphologies represent different levels of interruption of the ascending limb of the T wave, arguing for use of the term T2 in place of U to describe these events, as previously suggested by Lehmann et al. *(60,77)*.

What then is responsible for the normal U wave, the very small distinct deflection following the T wave? The repolarization of the His–Purkinje system as previously suggested by Hoffman, Crenfield and Lepeshkin *(69)* and by Watanabe and coworkers *(70)* remains a most plausible hypothesis. Repolarization of the Purkinje system is temporally aligned with the expected appearance of the U wave in the perfused wedge preparation (Fig. 8) *(60)*. The lack of a U wave in the wedge is likely related to a low density of the Purkinje system in the dog. A test of this hypothesis awaits the availability of an experimental model displaying a prominent U wave.

Indirect support for the hypothesis derives from the recent finding that isoproterenol-induced changes in the repolarization of Purkinje fibers parallel those of the U wave *(78)*. In healthy humans, isoproterenol abbreviates both QT and QU intervals, whereas in LQT1 patients (defective I_{Ks}) isoproterenol remarkably prolongs the QT interval but apparently abbreviates the QU interval *(79)*. Experimental studies involving canine left ventricular M cell preparations and Purkinje fibers demonstrate that isoproterenol abbreviates the action potential of both cell types under normal conditions, but that under

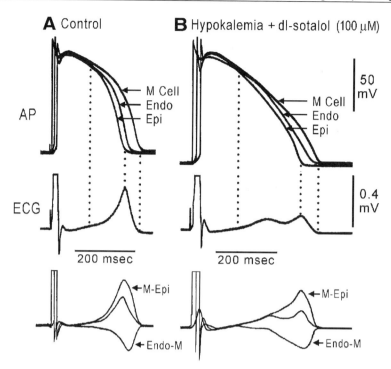

Fig. 7. Transient shift of voltage gradients on either side of the M region results in T wave bifurcation. The format is the same as in Fig. 5. All traces were simultaneously recorded from an arterially perfused left ventricular wedge preparation. **(A)** Control. **(B)** In the presence of hypokalemia ($[K^+]_o = 1.5$ mM), the I_{Kr} blocker dl-sotalol (100 μM) prolongs the QT interval and produces a bifurcation of the T wave, a morphology some authors refer to as T-U complex. The rate of repolarization of phase 3 of the action potential is slowed giving rise to smaller opposing transmural currents that cross-over producing a low amplitude bifid T wave. Initially the voltage gradient between the epicardium and M regions (M-Epi) is greater than that between endocardium and M region (Endo-M). When endocardium pulls away from the M cell, the opposing gradient (Endo-M) increases, interrupting the ascending limb of the T wave. Predominance of the M-Epi gradient is restored as the epicardial response continues to repolarize and the Epi-M gradients increases, thus resuming the ascending limb of the T wave. Full repolarization of epicardium marks the peak of the T wave. Repolarization of both endocardium and the M region contribute importantly to the descending limb. BCL = 1000 ms. Modified from *(60)* with permission.

conditions mimicking LQT1 (use of chromanol 293B to block I_{Ks}) isoproterenol abbreviates the Purkinje fiber action potential, but markedly prolongs that of the M cell *(78)*. The isoproterenol-induced changes in the action potential duration (APD) of Purkinje parallel those of the QU interval, thus providing indirect support for the hypothesis that repolarization of the Purkinje system is responsible for the inscription of the U wave.

Another hypothesis that endures despite a lack of direct experimental and clinical evidence is that the normal U wave is associated with the mechanical activity of the heart (mechano-electrical feedback). This concept in essence combines the four remaining hypotheses 1., 2., 5., and 6. listed previously into one. Lepeshkin *(68)* was the first to propose that U wave may be associated with late afterdepolarizations. Around the same time Furbetta et al. *(66)* reported that the U wave correlates temporally with the mechanical activity of papillary muscles, substantiating the well-known fact that the beginning

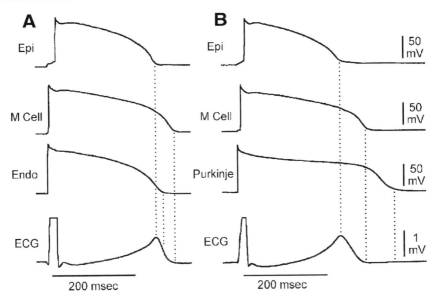

Fig. 8. Correlation of transmembrane and electrocardiographic activity. Transmembrane potentials and a transmural ECG recorded from two different arterially-perfused canine left ventricular wedge preparations. **(A)** Action potentials from epicardial (Epi), midmyocardial (M) and endocardial (Endo) sites were simultaneously recorded using floating glass microelectrodes. A transmural ECG was recorded concurrently across the bath. **(B)** Action potentials from epicardium (Epi), midmyocardium (M) and subendocardial Purkinje were recorded simultaneously together with a transmural ECG. In both cases, repolarization of epicardium is coincident with the peak of the T wave of the ECG, whereas repolarization of the M cells is coincident with the end of the T wave. The endocardial APD is intermediate (panel A). Note that although repolarization of the Purkinje fiber occurs after that of the M cell (panel B), it does not register on the ECG. BCL = 2000 ms. Modified from *(60)* with permission.

of the U wave coincides with the second heart sound. A few years earlier, it was shown that the tip of papillary muscles and the upper part of the ventricular septum have enhanced sensitivity to the mechanical "injury" (pressure or touching by a catheter) giving rise to ectopic beats *(80,81)*. These observations contributed to the hypothesis put forth by Lepeshkin *(82)* that the sudden release of tension on the papillary muscles secondary to opening of the mitral and tricuspid valves in early diastole may generate a delayed afterdepolarization in this mechano-sensitive area. This hypothesis received further support from data obtained in pig hearts *in situ* using monophasic action potentials *(71)*. In a series of elegant experiments, Max Lab *(71)* showed that sudden myocardial stretch (or release) results in APD prolongation that can be ascribed to triggering of Ca efflux from the sarcoplasmic reticulum which in turn is capable of generating an inward Na-Ca exchange current-induced depolarization. A possible contribution from another "sensitive" area—the upper part of the intraventricular septum—could not be excluded. This area at the base of the ventricles is thinner than the wall of the apex and it experiences rapid distention during early diastole. The region of the outflow tracts have recently been shown to have a disproportionately large fraction of M cells, which have been shown to develop delayed afterdepolarization more readily than other ventricular myocytes under a variety of conditions *(51)*. Also of note is the fact that this region of the ventricular

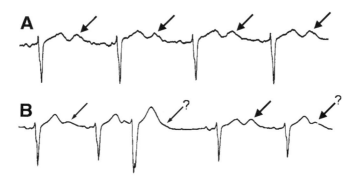

Fig. 9. Spectrum of T-U transitions in lead II recorded in the 71 year-old-male on amiodarone (for atrial fibrillation). **(A)** The U wave (thick arrows) is completely separated from the T wave and may be erroneously excluded in measurement of the QT interval. The QTc (without the U) is 400 ms, too short for a patient on amiodarone, whereas the QTc (with the U) is 600 ms, very long even for a patient on amiodarone. In this case, the U wave is pathologic (T2) and the QT is abnormally prolonged. **(B)** ECG recorded the next day in the same patient. The U waves are greatly diminished (thin arrows) but appear to become much more prominent (thick arrows) following a post-extrasystolic compensatory pause. The post-pause T2 augmentation suggests that, regardless of their origin, these pathophysiologic waves reflect early afterdepolarizations (EADs), increased dispersion of repolarization or both. Question marks indicate intermediate T-U configurations that are very difficult to classify as either T2 or U.

myocardium is densely innervated with sympathetic nerves. M cells are also found in the deep layers of papillary muscles.

Several well-established facts provide support, albeit indirect, for the mechano-electrical hypothesis. For example, conditions that increase ventricular filling (slow heart rate) produce a greater mechanical influence due to a greater ventricular and papillary muscle extension. Delayed depolarizations are facilitated by cardiac hypertrophy, a condition known to be associated with larger U waves. Mild hypertrophy may also increase mechanical stress due to the larger size of the heart. Hypokalemia, which potentiates the appearance of U wave, reduces resting outward currents, thus facilitating the development of delayed afterdepolarizations (DADs). It is noteworthy that the differential effect of isoproterenol on the T wave and U wave in LQT1 patients *(79)* could be explained by this hypothesis if there is preferential shortening of mechanical systole relative to the electrical systole in the presence of catecholamines.

The need to understand the U wave is not purely academic. High amplitude U waves have been implicated in the generation of "triggered" extrasystoles capable of precipitating life-threatening arrhythmias, including torsade de pointes. The question however that we must ask at this juncture is whether many of these examples in the literature represent cases in which T2 is confused for a U wave. A continuous spectrum of TU transitions can make distinction of the two difficult at times. Such distinction however becomes paramount when studying the effects of agents with Class III antiarrhythmic actions. QTc may be grossly underestimated if a T2 is judged to be a U wave and excluded from the measurement of the QT interval. Figure 9 shows a clinical example in a patient receiving amiodarone, illustrating how such confusion can arise. The prominent apparent U waves are actually T2 waves. If excluded from the measurement of QT, a value of 400 ms would be obtained, far shorter than the actual QT interval of 600 ms.

Table 1
Consequences of a Prominent I_{to}-mediated Action Potential Notch
in Epicardium but not Endocardium

J wave (Osborne wave) *(15,18)*
Differential sensitivity to ischemia & components of ischemia *(15,57,84,85)*
Differential sensitivity to drugs *(15,18,84–89)*
      Neurohormones (Acetylcholine and Isoproterenol)
      Transient Outward Current Blockers
      Calcium Channel Blockers
      Sodium Channel Blockers
      Potassium Channel Openers

ACKNOWLEDGMENT

Supported by grants from the National Institutes of Health (HL 47678), the American Heart Association, New York State Affiliate, and the Masons of New York State and Florida. We are grateful to Dr. Sami Viskin for providing the clinical trace shown in Fig. 8.

REFERENCES

1. Einthoven W. The galvanometric registration of the human electrocardiogram, likewise a review of the use of the capillary electrometer in physiology. Pflugers Arch 1903;99:472–480.
2. Einthoven W. Uber die Deutung des Electrokardiogramms. Pflugers Arch 1912;149:65–86.
3. Antzelevitch C, Dumaine R. Electrical heterogeneity in the heart: Physiological, pharmacological and clinical implications. In: Page E, Fozzard HA, Solaro RJ, eds. Handbook of Physiology. The Heart. New York: Oxford University Press, 2002:654–692.
4. Antzelevitch C. Heterogeneity of cellular repolarization in LQTS. The role of M cells. Eur Heart J 2001;Suppl 3:K-2–K-16.
5. Antzelevitch C, Shimizu W, Yan GX, et al. The M cell. Its contribution to the ECG and to normal and abnormal electrical function of the heart. J Cardiovasc Electrophysiol 1999;10:1124–1152.
6. Litovsky SH, Antzelevitch C. Transient outward current prominent in canine ventricular epicardium but not endocardium. Circ Res 1988;62:116–126.
7. Liu DW, Gintant GA, Antzelevitch C. Ionic bases for electrophysiological distinctions among epicardial, midmyocardial, and endocardial myocytes from the free wall of the canine left ventricle. Circ Res 1993;72:671–687.
8. Furukawa T, Myerburg RJ, Furukawa N, Bassett AL, Kimura S. Differences in transient outward currents of feline endocardial and epicardial myocytes. Circ Res 1990;67:1287–1291.
9. Fedida D, Giles WR. Regional variations in action potentials and transient outward current in myocytes isolated from rabbit left ventricle. J Physiol (Lond) 1991;442:191–209.
10. Clark RB, Bouchard RA, Salinas-Stefanon E, Sanchez-Chapula J, Giles WR. Heterogeneity of action potential waveforms and potassium currents in rat ventricle. Cardiovasc Res 1993;27:1795–1799.
11. Wettwer E, Amos GJ, Posival H, Ravens U. Transient outward current in human ventricular myocytes of subepicardial and subendocardial origin. Circ Res 1994;75:473–482.
12. Nabauer M, Beuckelmann DJ, Uberfuhr P, Steinbeck G. Regional differences in current density and rate-dependent properties of the transient outward current in subepicardial and subendocardial myocytes of human left ventricle. Circulation 1996;93:168–177.
13. Di Diego JM, Sun ZQ, Antzelevitch C. I_{to} and action potential notch are smaller in left vs. right canine ventricular epicardium. Am J Physiol 1996;271:H548–H561.
14. Volders PG, Sipido KR, Carmeliet E, Spatjens RL, Wellens HJ, Vos MA. Repolarizing K+ currents ITO1 and IKs are larger in right than left canine ventricular midmyocardium. Circulation 1999;99:206–210.

15. Antzelevitch C, Sicouri S, Litovsky SH, et al. Heterogeneity within the ventricular wall: Electrophysiology and pharmacology of epicardial, endocardial and M cells. Circ Res 1991;69:1427–1449.

16. Antzelevitch C, Sicouri S, Lukas A, Nesterenko VV, Liu DW, Di Diego JM. Regional differences in the electrophysiology of ventricular cells: Physiological and clinical implications. In: Zipes DP, Jalife J, eds. Cardiac Electrophysiology: From Cell to Bedside. Philadelphia: W.B. Saunders Co., 1995:228–245.

17. Antzelevitch C, Sicouri S, Lukas A, et al. Clinical implications of electrical heterogeneity in the heart: The electrophysiology and pharmacology of epicardial, M and endocardial cells. In: Podrid PJ, Kowey PR, eds. Cardiac Arrhythmia: Mechanism, Diagnosis and Management. Baltimore, MD: William & Wilkins, 1995:88–107.

18. Yan GX, Antzelevitch C. Cellular basis for the electrocardiographic J wave. Circulation 1996;93: 372–379.

19. Lukas A, Antzelevitch C. Phase 2 reentry as a mechanism of initiation of circus movement reentry in canine epicardium exposed to simulated ischemia. The antiarrhythmic effects of 4–aminopyridine. Cardiovasc Res 1996;32:593–603.

20. Antzelevitch C, Di Diego JM, Sicouri S, Lukas A. Selective pharmacological modification of repolarizing currents. Antiarrhythmic and proarrhythmic actions of agents that influence repolarization in the heart. In: Breithardt J, ed. Antiarrhythmic Drugs: Mechanisms of Antiarrhythmic and Proarrhythmic Actions. Berlin: Springer-Verlag, 1995:57–80.

21. Lukas A, Antzelevitch C. The contribution of K^+ currents to electrical heterogeneity across the canine ventricular wall under normal and ischemic conditions. In: Dhalla NS, Pierce GN, Panagia V, eds. Pathophysiology of Heart Failure. Boston: Academic Publishers, 1996:440–456.

22. Sicouri S, Antzelevitch C. A subpopulation of cells with unique electrophysiological properties in the deep subepicardium of the canine ventricle: The M cell. Circ Res 1991;68:1729–1741.

23. Anyukhovsky EP, Sosunov EA, Rosen MR. Regional differences in electrophysiologic properties of epicardium, midmyocardium and endocardium: In vitro and in vivo correlations. Circulation 1996;94:1981–1988.

24. Liu DW, Antzelevitch C. Characteristics of the delayed rectifier current (I_{Kr} and I_{Ks}) in canine ventricular epicardial, midmyocardial and endocardial myocytes: A weaker I_{Ks} contributes to the longer action potential of the M cell. Circ Res 1995;76:351–365.

25. Eddlestone GT, Zygmunt AC, Antzelevitch C. Larger late sodium current contributes to the longer action potential of the M cell in canine ventricular myocardium. [abstr]. PACE 1996;19:4, Pt 2:569.

26. Zygmunt AC, Goodrow RJ, Antzelevitch C. I_{Na-Ca} contributes to electrical heterogeneity within the canine ventricle. Am J Physiol 2000;278:H1671–H1678.

27. Yan GX, Shimizu W, Antzelevitch C. Characteristics and distribution of M cells in arterially-perfused canine left ventricular wedge preparations. Circulation 1998;98:1921–1927.

28. Sicouri S, Fish J, Antzelevitch C. Distribution of M cells in the canine ventricle. J Cardiovasc Electrophysiol 1994;5:824–837.

29. Sicouri S, Antzelevitch C. Electrophysiologic characteristics of M cells in the canine left ventricular free wall. J Cardiovasc Electrophysiol 1995;6:591–603.

30. Weissenburger J, Nesterenko VV, Antzelevitch C. Transmural heterogeneity of ventricular repolarization under baseline and long QT conditions in the canine heart in vivo. Torsades de pointes develops with halothane but not pentobarbital anesthesia. J Cardiovasc Electrophysiol 2000;11:290–304.

31. Rodriguez-Sinovas A, Cinca J, Tapias A, Armadans L, Tresanchez M, Soler-Soler J. Lack of evidence of M-cells in porcine left ventricular myocardium. Cardiovasc Res 1997;33:307–313.

32. El-Sherif N, Caref EB, Yin H, Restivo M. The electrophysiological mechanism of ventricular arrhythmias in the long QT syndrome: Tridimensional mapping of activation and recovery patterns. Circ Res 1996;79:474–492.

33. Balati B, Varro A, Papp JG. Comparison of the cellular electrophysiological characteristics of canine left ventricular epicardium, M cells, endocardium and Purkinje fibres. Acta Physiol Scand 1998;164: 181–190.

34. Sicouri S, Quist M, Antzelevitch C. Evidence for the presence of M cells in the guinea pig ventricle. J Cardiovasc Electrophysiol 1996;7:503–511.

35. McIntosh MA, Cobbe SM, Smith GL. Heterogeneous changes in action potential and intracellular Ca^{2+} in left ventricular myocyte sub-types from rabbits with heart failure. Cardiovasc Res 2000;45:397–409.

36. Stankovicova T, Szilard M, De Scheerder I, Sipido KR. M cells and transmural heterogeneity of action potential configuration in myocytes from the left ventricular wall of the pig heart. Cardiovasc Res 2000;45:952–960.

37. Drouin E, Charpentier F, Gauthier C, Laurent K, Le Marec H. Electrophysiological characteristics of cells spanning the left ventricular wall of human heart: Evidence for the presence of M cells. J Am Coll Cardiol 1995;26:185–192.

38. Li GR, Feng J, Yue L, Carrier M. Transmural heterogeneity of action potentials and Ito1 in myocytes isolated from the human right ventricle. Am J Physiol 1998;275:H369–H377.

39. Gussak I, Bjerregaard P, Egan TM, Chaitman BR. ECG phenomenon called the J wave. History, pathophysiology, and clinical significance. J Electrocardiol 1995;28:49–58.

40. Osborn JJ. Experimental hypothermia: respiratory and blood pH changes in relation to cardiac function. Am J Physiol 1953;175:389–398.

41. Hugo N, Dormehl IC, Van Gelder AL. A positive wave at the J-point of electrocardiograms of anaesthetized baboons. J Med Primatol 1988;17:347–352.

42. West TC, Frederickson EL, Amory DW. Single fiber recording of the ventricular response to induced hypothermia in the anesthetized dog. Correlation with multicellular parameters. Circ Res 1959;7: 880–888.

43. Santos EM, Frederick KC. Electrocardiographic changes in the dog during hypothermia. Am Heart J 1957;55:415–420.

44. Clements SD, Hurst JW. Diagnostic value of ECG abnormalities observed in subjects accidentally exposed to cold. Am J Cardiol 1972;29:729–734.

45. Thompson R, Rich J, Chmelik F, Nelson WL. Evolutionary changes in the electrocardiogram of severe progressive hypothermia. J Electrocardiol 1977;10:67–70.

46. Dillon SM, Allessie MA, Ursell PC, Wit AL. Influences of anisotropic tissue structure on reentrant circuits in the epicardial border zone of subacute canine infarcts. Circ Res 1988;63:182–206.

47. Eagle K. Images in clinical medicine. Osborn waves of hypothermia. N Engl J Med 1994;10:680.

48. Kraus F. Ueber die wirkung des kalziums auf den kreislauf. Dtsch Med Wochenschr 1920;46:201–203.

49. Sridharan MR, Horan LG. Electrocardiographic J wave of hypercalcemia. Am J Cardiol 1984;54: 672–673.

50. Emslie-Smith D, Sladden GE, Stirling GR. The significance of changes in the electrocardiogram in hypothermia. Br Heart J 1959;21:343–351.

51. Antzelevitch C, Sicouri S. Clinical relevance of cardiac arrhythmias generated by afterdepolarizations: The role of M cells in the generation of U waves, triggered activity and torsade de pointes. J Am Coll Cardiol 1994;23:259–277.

52. Jeck CD, Boyden PA. Age-related appearance of outward currents may contribute to developmental differences in ventricular repolarization. Circ Res 1992;71:1390–1403.

53. Pacioretty LM, Gilmour RF, Jr. Developmental changes in the transient outward potassium current in canine epicardium. Am J Physiol 1995;268:H2513–H2521.

54. Phillipson EA, Herbert FA. Accidental exposure to freezing: clinical and laboratory observations during convalescence from near-fatal hypothermia. Can Med Assoc J 1967;97:786–792.

55. Okada M, Nishimura F, Yoshino H, Kimura M, Ogino T. The J wave in accidental hypothermia. J Electrocardiol 1983;16:23–28.

56. Sridharan MR, Johnson JC, Horan LG, Sohl GS, Flowers NC. Monophasic action potentials in hypercalcemic and hypothermic "J" waves—a comparative study. Am Fed Clin Res 1983;31:219.

57. Di Diego JM, Antzelevitch C. High [Ca^{2+}]-induced electrical heterogeneity and extrasystolic activity in isolated canine ventricular epicardium: Phase 2 reentry. Circulation 1994;89:1839–1850.

58. Yan GX, Antzelevitch C. Cellular basis for the Brugada Syndrome and other mechanisms of arrhythmogenesis associated with ST segment elevation. Circulation 1999;100:1660–1666.

59. Antzelevitch C. The Brugada syndrome: Ionic basis and arrhythmia mechanisms. J Cardiovasc Electrophysiol 2001;12:268–272.

60. Yan GX, Antzelevitch C. Cellular basis for the normal T wave and the electrocardiographic manifestations of the long QT syndrome. Circulation 1998;98:1928–1936.

61. Antzelevitch C. The M cell. Invited Editorial Comment. Journal of Cardiovascular Pharmacology and Therapeutics 1997;2:73–76.

62. Lubinski A, Lewicka-Nowak E, Kempa M, Baczynska AM, Romanowska I, Swiatecka G. New insight into repolarization abnormalities in patients with congenital long QT syndrome: the increased transmural dispersion of repolarization. PACE 1998;21:172–175.

63. Cohen IS, Giles WR, Noble D. Cellular basis for the T wave of the electrocardiogram. Nature 1976;262:657–661.

64. Noble D, Cohen IS. The interpretation of the T wave of the electrocardiogram. Cardiovasc Res 1978;12:13–27.

65. Zuckerman R, Cabrera-Cosio E. La ondu U. Arch Inst Cardiol Mex 1947;17:521–532.
66. Furbetta D, Bufalari A, Santucci F, Solinas P. Abnormality of the U wave and the T-U segment of the electrocardiogram: The syndrome of the papillary muscles. Circulation 1956;14:1129–1137.
67. Nahum LH, Hoff HE. The interpretation of the U wave of the electrocardiogram. Am Heart J 1939;17:585–598.
68. Lepeschkin E. Genesis of the U wave. Circulation 1957;15:77–81.
69. Hoffman BF, Cranefield PF. Electrophysiology of the Heart. New York: McGraw-Hill, 1960:202.
70. Watanabe Y. Purkinje repolarization as a possible cause of the U wave in the electrocardiogram. Circulation 1975;51:1030–1037.
71. Lab MJ. Contraction-excitation feedback in myocardium: Physiologic basis and clinical revelance. Circ Res 1982;50:757–766.
72. Choo MH, Gibson DG. U waves in ventricular hypertrophy: possible demonstration of mechano-electrical feedback. Br Heart J 1986;55:428–433.
73. Antzelevitch C, Nesterenko VV, Yan GX. The role of M cells in acquired long QT syndrome, U waves and torsade de pointes. J Electrocardiol 1996;28(suppl.):131–138.
74. Nesterenko VV, Antzelevitch C. Simulation of the electrocardiographic U wave in heterogeneous myocardium: effect of the local junctional resistance. Proc "Computers in Cardiology," IEEE Computer Society Press, Los Alamitos, CA 1992:43–46.
75. Surawicz B. U wave: facts, hypotheses, misconceptions, and misnomers. J Cardiovasc Electrophysiol 1998;9:1117–1128.
76. Shimizu W, Antzelevitch C. Sodium channel block with mexiletine is effective in reducing dispersion of repolarization and preventing torsade de pointes in LQT2 and LQT3 models of the long-QT syndrome. Circulation 1997;96:2038–2047.
77. Lehmann MH, Suzuki F, Fromm BS, Frankovich D, Elko P, Steinman RT, Fresard J, Baga JJ, Taggart RT. T-wave "humps" as a potential electrocardiographic marker of the long QT syndrome. J Am Coll Cardiol 1994;24:746–754.
78. Burashnikov A, Antzelevitch C. Is the Purkinje system the source of the electrocardiographic U wave? [abstr]. Circulation 1999;100:II-386.
79. Zhang L, Compton SJ, Antzelevitch C, Timothy KW, Vincent GM, Mason JW. Differential response of QT and QU intervals to adrenergic stimulation in long QT patients with I_{Ks} defects [abstr]. J Am Coll Cardiol 1999;33:138A.
80. Hellerstein HK, Katz LN. The electrical effects of injury at various myocardial locations. Am Heart J 1948;36:184–220.
81. Zimmerman HA, Hellerstein HK. Cavity potentials of the human ventricle. Circulation 1951;3:95–104.
82. Lepeschkin E. Physiologic basis of the U wave. In: Schlant RC, Hurst JW, eds. Advances in Electrocardiography. New York: Grune & Stratton, 1971:431–437.
83. Yan GX, Antzelevitch C. Cellular basis for the electrocardiographic J wave. [abstr]. Circulation 1995;92:I-71.
84. Antzelevitch C, Litovsky SH, Lukas A. Epicardium vs. endocardium. Electrophysiology and pharmacology. In: Zipes DP, Jalife J, eds. Cardiac Electrophysiology, from Cell to Bedside. New York: W.B. Saunders, 1990:386–395.
85. Di Diego JM, Antzelevitch C. Pinacidil-induced electrical heterogeneity and extrasystolic activity in canine ventricular tissues: Does activation of ATP-regulated potassium current promote phase 2 reentry? Circulation 1993;88:1177–1189.
86. Antzelevitch C, Di Diego JM. The role of K^+ channel activators in cardiac electrophysiology and arrhythmias. Circulation 1992;85:1627–1629.
87. Krishnan SC, Antzelevitch C. Flecainide-induced arrhythmia in canine ventricular epicardium: Phase 2 reentry? Circulation 1993;87:562–572.
88. Krishnan SC, Antzelevitch C. Sodium channel blockade produces opposite electrophysiologic effects in canine ventricular epicardium and endocardium. Circ Res 1991;69:277–291.
89. Litovsky SH, Antzelevitch C. Differences in the electrophysiological response of canine ventricular subendocardium and subepicardium to acetylcholine and isoproterenol. A direct effect of acetylcholine in ventricular myocardium. Circ Res 1990;67:615–627.

7

Electrical and Structural Remodeling of the Ventricular Myocardium in Disease

Antonis A. Armoundas, PhD
and Gordon F. Tomaselli, MD

CONTENTS

INTRODUCTION

Abnormalities of ventricular repolarization are a reoccurring feature of structural heart disease and likely contributors to the increased incidence of sudden death in patients with cardiac hypertrophy and heart failure (HF). Several clinical observations support this contention. Over two million Americans suffer from heart failure and more than 200,000 die annually. The incidence is estimated to be 400,000 per year with a prevalence of over 4.5 million, numbers that will increase with the aging of the US population *(1)*. The majority of patients with heart failure have coronary artery disease as the cause of heart failure or concomitant with myocardial failure. Despite remarkable improvements in medical therapy the prognosis of patients with myocardial failure remains poor with over 15% of patients dying within one year of initial diagnosis and up to an 80% six-year mortality *(2)*. Of the deaths in patients with heart failure, 50% are sudden and unexpected.

The distinction between true mechanisms and mere markers of disease has been particularly difficult in heart failure, because the cascade of physiological, neurohumoral,

From: *Contemporary Cardiology: Cardiac Repolarization: Bridging Basic and Clinical Science*
Edited by: I. Gussak et al. © Humana Press Inc., Totowa, NJ

and biochemical abnormalities observed in heart failure is the result of a complex interaction of a number of environmental and genetic factors. Yet making the distinction between mechanisms and markers of disease may have far-reaching therapeutic implications.

ELECTRICAL AND STRUCTURAL REMODELING OF THE DISEASED VENTRICLE

The hypertrophic and failing heart undergoes a complex series of changes in both myocyte and nonmyocyte elements. In an attempt to compensate for the reduction in cardiac function the sympathetic nervous (SNS), renin-angiotensin-aldosterone (RAAS) systems and other neurohumoral mechanisms are activated but ultimately prove to be maladaptive. Neurohumoral activation predisposes to myocyte loss, ventricular chamber remodeling including interstitial fibrosis, resulting in a progressive reduction in force development and impairment of ventricular relaxation. The precise pathways involved in left ventricular (LV) remodeling are still unclear, however the following molecular scenario has been proposed. As myocytes stretch, local norepinephrine, angiotensin, and endothelin are increased. These changes induce qualitative and quantitive changes in protein expression in the interstitium and myocyte hypertrophy. In addition, increased activation of aldosterone and cytokines may also stimulate collagen synthesis, thus leading to fibrosis and remodeling of the extracellular matrix. The remodeling that is most relevant to changes in repolarization is that occurring in active membrane properties of the cardiac myocyte.

Intrinsic cardiac and neurohumoral responses to myocardial hypertrophy and failure adversely alter the electrophysiology of the heart predisposing patients with heart failure to an increased risk of arrhythmic death. With progression of heart failure there is an increase in the frequency and complexity of ventricular ectopy (3,4). Total mortality in heart failure patients correlates with LV function and the presence of complex ventricular ectopy (5–7). However, there is no clear correlation between sudden cardiac death (SCD) and ventricular function or ventricular ectopy. Moreover, death can be disproportionately sudden in patients with hypertrophy or more modest myocardial dysfunction (8). A major caveat is that the mechanism of sudden death is highly heterogeneous.

This chapter will review the major changes that have been observed in the electrophysiology of ventricular myocytes isolated from hypertrophic or failing hearts and uninvolved regions of infarcted ventricles with an emphasis on altered ventricular repolarization.

CHANGES IN THE ACTION POTENTIAL PROFILE AND DURATION

An elementary and distinctive signature of any excitable tissue is its action potential profile. Cardiac myocytes possess a characteristically long action potential (Fig. 1): After an initial rapid upstroke, there is a plateau of maintained depolarization before repolarization. The duration of the action potential is primarily responsible for the time course of repolarization of the heart; prolongation of the action potential produces delays in cardiac repolarization.

Changes in action potential duration and profile result from alterations in the functional expression of depolarizing and repolarizing currents. Prolongation of the action potential is characteristic of cells and tissues isolated from the ventricles of animals with

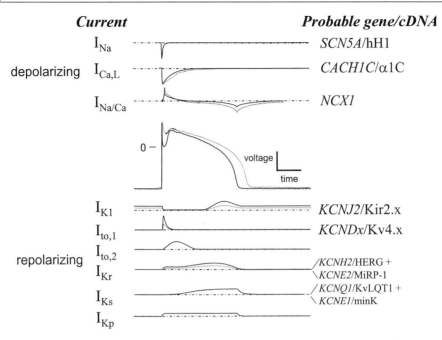

Fig. 1. Schematic of the depolarizing and repolarizing currents that shape the action potential in the mammalian ventricle. A schematic of the time course of each of the currents is shown as well as the gene product that underlies the current. The dotted line represents the trajectory in the failing heart.

hypertrophy or heart failure independent of the mechanism (Fig. 1), including pressure and/or volume overload *(9–24)*, genetic *(25–27)*, metabolic *(28)*, ischemia/infarction *(29–32)*, and chronic pacing tachycardia models *(33–35)*. Similarly tissues *(36–38)* and cells *(39–41)* from failing human ventricles exhibit action potential prolongation.

The pathophysiological significance of action potential prolongation in myocytes isolated from hypertrophied and failing hearts has been debated on several grounds. First, most action potential recordings from ventricular myocytes are made at unphysiologically slow rates and indeed the difference in duration between cells from failing and control ventricles converges at high stimulation frequency *(38,42)*. However, slow heart rates and pauses after premature contractions are common in heart failure, and the post-pause prolongation of the action potential duration may be highly significant. Second, isolated myocytes are no longer electrically coupled to other cells in the cardiac synctium; however, intact muscle preparations from failing hearts *(37)*, monophasic action potential recordings in whole hearts *(43)* and optical mapping from transmural sections of failing hearts *(44)* also exhibit action potential prolongation. Finally, the duration of the action potential is quite sensitive to mechanical load and increasing the load has been reported to shorten action potential duration and refractoriness more in failing than in normal hearts *(45)*, however cellular studies suggest that mechanical stretch prolongs action potential duration (APD) *(46)*.

An important and understudied question is the effect of hypertrophy and failure on regional differences in APD. APDs vary across the myocardial wall *(47–50)* and in different regions *(51)* of the mammalian heart. Data from a limited number of experimental animal models of hypertrophy *(13,16)* and heart failure *(44,52)* suggest exaggerated regional inhomogeneity in APD. The finding of enhanced spatial and temporal dispersion of monophasic APD, refractoriness, and electrocardiographic QT intervals in humans (53,54), and animals with heart failure (43,44) is consistent with an exaggerated dispersion of APD that may predispose to ventricular arrhythmias.

ALTERATIONS IN CA²⁺ HOMEOSTASIS

Although altered myocyte calcium handling is characteristic of HF in both human (55,56) and animal models, the basic mechanisms involved in myocardial remodeling of excitation-contraction coupling remain controversial. Different forms of remodeling are associated with distinct patterns of gene expression, and hence with different molecular phenotypes (57).

The density of Ca current has been studied in a number of animal models of ventricular hypertrophy and failure (58). The severity of hypertrophy or failure appears to be inversely correlated with the density of the L-type current (12,14,21,59–63) or number of diydropyridine (DHP) binding sites (64–69). The L-type current is generally increased in mild-moderate hypertrophy and unchanged or decreased in severe hypertrophy and heart failure.

The changes in L-type current in cells isolated from failing human hearts parallel those obtained from animal models with severe hypertrophy or failure; human cells exhibit either no change (39,70–72) or a decrease in the current density (73) or DHP binding sites (35,74,75). A recent study showed a decrease of L-type current with increased stimulation frequency in failing human myocytes (76). In most studies of Ca currents in cells isolated from failing hearts, there are no changes in either kinetics or voltage dependence. However, a slowing of the decay of the whole-cell current has been observed in some models, a change that could alter excitation-contraction coupling and would tend to prolong the action potential duration (Fig. 2) (9,12,77–79). It should be noted that most measurements of L-type currents have been performed under highly unphysiologic conditions; notably the conventional use of high affinity intracellular Ca^{2+} buffers, such as EGTA, will suppress the Ca^{2+}-mediated component of L-type channel inactivation and thus may potentially lead to an underestimation of kinetic differences between normal and failing myocytes (80).

The molecular basis of changes in the density of the L-type current is unknown. A reduction in the number of DHP binding sites has been reported in various animal models (66–69,81,82), whereas in failing human hearts the steady-state level of α_{1c} mRNA has been reported to be decreased by Northern blot (74,83), but was unchanged by ribonuclease protection assay (84). Two reports of changes in human Ca channel β subunit mRNA are conflicting. Northern blots of samples from the left ventricle of failing hearts revealed no change in β subunit mRNA (83). In contrast, samples from right ventricular endomyocardial biopsies revealed an inverse relationship between β subunit mRNA levels measured by PCR and LV end-diastolic pressure in explanted hearts (85). No data are available yet on possible changes in the level of immunoreactive β subunit protein in human cardiac hypertrophy or failure.

Measurements of intracellular Ca^{2+} have revealed a reduction in the amplitude of the calcium transient and its rate of decay in intact muscles (37) and cells isolated from failing ventricles compared with normal controls (39,42,71,86–91).

Despite agreement that Ca sequestration by the SR is defective in the failing myocardium (Fig. 2), there is controversy regarding the molecular mechanisms. SERCA2a

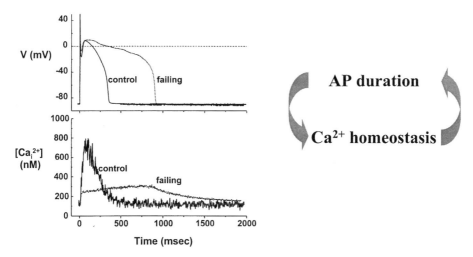

Fig. 2. (Left) Action potential and Ca^{2+} transients recorded in canine ventricular myocytes isolated from a normal heart and failing heart. The action potentials and transients are prolonged and the transient amplitude is decreased. (Right) Action potential duration and Ca^{2+} handling are intimately linked by several mechanisms (*see* text for details).

mRNA is decreased in many studies *(55,74,92–100)*, but fewer studies have shown a reduction in the immunoreactive protein *(42,99–103)*. In human heart failure, some studies have shown a reduction in SERCA2a mRNA (Mercadier et al.) and protein levels *(91,92,94,95,104–106)*, although others have shown no change of the SERCA2a mRNA and protein *(94,107,108)*.

SERCA2a function may be indirectly altered in hypertrophy and heart failure, by changes in the functional expression of the regulatory protein phospholamban (PLB). PLB mRNA is generally reduced in failing human hearts *(55,94–96,109)*, but changes in the level of immunoreactive PLB protein have not been as consistent *(94–96,108,110)*. Data regarding the level of phosphorylation of PLB in the failing human heart are contradictory *(108,111,112)*. The combination of a reduction in the level of phosphorylation of PLB, and a decrease in the level of immunoreactive SERCA and PLB would be expected to reduce the rate of uptake of Ca^{2+} by the SR. Indeed a decrease in the SERCA2a to PLB ratio has been associated with defective Ca^{2+} handling and contraction *(113–116)*.

The level of ryanodine receptor (RyR) mRNA in the left ventricle is decreased in some studies of terminal human heart failure *(117,118)*, but no change in RyR immunoreactive protein has been demonstrated by others *(106)*. Hyperphosphorylation of RyR by PKA in the failing heart has been associated with dissociation of the macromolecular complex FKBP12.6 from the RyR, which has been argued to reduce the EC coupling gain *(119–121)*. Nevertheless, a reported decrease in the EC coupling gain *(90)* has not been confirmed in large animal *(122)* or in human *(123)* heart failure studies. Furthermore, a decrease in EC coupling gain would not adequately explain the fact that Ca^{2+} transients are generally similar in normal and failing myocytes at slow pacing rates.

The sodium-calcium exchanger (NCX) importantly contributes to the control of intracellular $[Ca^{2+}]$, extruding Ca^{2+} from the cell by electrogenically exchanging it for extracellular $[Na^+]$. Most studies from human and animal hypertrophied and failing hearts have demonstrated an increase in both NCX mRNA *(93,124–127)* and/or protein *(93,116,124, 125,127,128)*, suggesting that enhanced NCX function compensates for defective SR removal of Ca^{2+} from the cytoplasm in the failing heart. A prominent increase in NCX function has been demonstrated in both animal models and human heart failure *(9,124,128–130)*. Na^+-dependent Ca^{2+} flux into the cell (reverse mode Na/Ca exchange) has been shown to be increased in human sarcolemmal preparations *(128)*. Thus, in the context of a prolonged calcium transient, the NCX is likely to play a significant role in reshaping the action potential profile. Forward-mode exchanger function (Na^+ in and Ca^{2+} out) compensates for defective SR Ca^{2+} removal at the expense of depletion of the releasable pool of Ca^{2+} *(131–133)*, increasing depolarizing current. Reverse mode exchange (Na^+ out and Ca^{2+} in) has been suggested to provide inotropic support to the failing heart *(124,134)* and contribute to the slow decay of the calcium transient in failing human myocytes *(41)*. Computer simulations based on the canine pacing tachycardia model suggest that augmentation of reverse mode exchanger function during the early plateau will tend to shorten the action potential duration. However, with exaggerated forward mode function and changes in the decay rate of the L-type Ca current, the net effect is prolongation of the action potential *(80)*.

DOWNREGULATION OF POTASSIUM CURRENTS

Functional downregulation of K currents is a recurring theme in hypertrophied and failing ventricular myocardium. A reduction in the current density of I_{to} is the most consistent ionic current change in cardiac hypertrophy and failure. Several notable exceptions are studies of compensated pressure overload hypertrophy which were associated with either no change *(12,135)* or an increase in I_{to} density *(18,136)*. Downregulation of I_{to}, without a significant change in the voltage dependence or kinetics of the current has also been observed in cells isolated from terminally failing human hearts *(40,137,138)*.

The density of I_{to} and other K currents, notably the delayed rectifiers (I_{Kr} and I_{Ks}) vary regionally and transmurally in the heart, and there is some evidence that I_{to} may be reduced differentially in heart failure *(137,138)*. The regional differences in current expression are further complicated by presence of inhomogenous structural heart disease such as myocardial infarction. In the rabbit pacing-induced heart failure model, there has been a reduction in the I_{to} density in myocytes isolated from the apex of the left ventricle *(35)*. The mechanisms underlying regional and transmural differences in I_{to} density in the heart are not clear. Some data suggest that there are differences in the level of expression of the gene encoding Kv4.x channel or its accessory subunit KChIP2 *(139)*; alternatively, distinct gene products may underlie I_{to} in different regions of the heart (e.g., Kv4.x vs Kv1.4) and at various stages of development *(140,141)*.

Changes in I_{to} density have been observed in different regions and cell types in the infarcted heart. In the early postinfarction period in the canine heart Purkinje myocytes in the infarcted region exhibit a 50% reduction in I_{to} density without changes in the voltage dependence of gating but an alteration of kinetics consisting of a hastening of current decay and slowing of recovery from inactivation *(142)*. Thus the reduction in I_{to} would be exaggerated at high heart rates. Ventricular myocytes isolated from the epicardial border zone five days after infarction in the dog expressed little or no I_{to} *(29)*. Other studies of remodeling after healed myocardial infarction have focused on regions remote from the infarction that undergo hypertrophy in response to the loss of muscle mass in the infarct region. These studies generally reveal a reduction in I_{to} density *(29,30,143,144)*.

In humans, it has been hypothesized that Kv1.4 is the predominant gene that encodes endocardial I_{to}, whereas Kv4.3 underlies mid-myocardial and epicardial I_{to} (*145*). Interestingly, these two K channels (Kv1.4 and [Kv4.3 or Kv4.2]) exhibit distinct kinetic behaviors when heterologously expressed, with Kv1.4 having much slower inactivation recovery kinetics than Kv4.x (*146–149*). Preferential expression of Kv1.4 in the endocardium may underlie the different electrophysiological behavior of I_{to} in human cells isolated from the subendocardium and subepicardium (*137,138*).

The molecular mechanism of I_{to} downregulation in structural heart disease is likely to be multifactorial. I_{to} is regulated by neurohumoral mechanisms, specifically α_1 adrenergic stimulation which reduces the current size (*150–152*). In animal models (*32*) and human heart failure (*84*), a reduction in the steady-state level of Kv4 mRNA has been associated with downregulation of I_{to}. In the rat, reduction in the steady-state level of mRNA is associated with a commensurate decrease in the level of immunoreactive Kv4 protein (*32*). The reduction in mRNA level results from a change in the balance between transcription and mRNA degradation, but the precise molecular mechanism is unknown. It is interesting to note that regulated expression of I_{to} and Kv4 mRNA and protein occurs during development (*140*) and exposure to thyroid hormone (*141,153*).

I_{to} profoundly influences rapid early repolarization (phase 1) and the level of the plateau thereby affecting all of the currents that are active later in the action potential. Because I_{to} is brief, its role in setting the action potential duration in larger animals and humans remains controversial. Most of the studies examining I_{to} in heart failure have used Ca^{2+}-buffered internal solutions, thus distorting any possible role of calcium-dependent processes. Under these conditions, several lines of evidence suggest that reduced I_{to} density prolongs the overall action potential duration (*33,34,40,154*). Nevertheless, it is not clear whether this conclusion would also apply under more physiological conditions. In fact, computer simulations of the canine ventricular AP suggest that reductions in I_{to} decrease the APD when Ca^{2+} cycling is intact (*155*).

Changes in other K currents in hypertrophy and heart failure have been reported, but not with the consistency of downregulation of I_{to}. In ventricular hypertrophy, I_{K1} has been reported to be increased (*17*), decreased (*12*), or unchanged (*9,12,14,21,135*). Similar inconsistencies have been observed in pacing tachycardia models: reduced I_{K1} density has been seen in the dog (*33*), although unchanged current density was found in the rabbit (*34,35,156*). In human heart failure, ventricular myocytes exhibit significantly reduced current density at negative voltages. The underlying basis of the downregulation of I_{K1} in human heart failure is uncertain. Kääb et al. reported no change in the steady-state level of Kir2.1 mRNA in failing compared to control hearts (*84*). In studies of human ventricular I_{K1}, a differential reduction in the current was noted between cells isolated from failing hearts with dilated vs ischemic cardiomyopathy. The whole-cell slope conductance near the reversal potential for K^+ was significantly smaller in cells from hearts with dilated cardiomyopathy; these cells also had longer action potentials with slower terminal (phase 3) repolarization (*157*). Ventricular myocytes isolated from controls and hearts with ischemic cardiomyopathy exhibited voltage dependence of the open probability of I_{K1}, a response that was absent in cells from hearts of patients with dilated cardiomyopathy (*157*).

Studies of the delayed rectifier K currents in hypertrophic and failing hearts are more limited. Myocytes isolated from hypertrophied right (*17*) and left ventricles (*59,158*) of the cat have reduced I_K density with slowed activation and faster deactivation. The reduction in the outward current over the plateau phase of the action potential, in cells from the hypertrophied feline left ventricle, exhibit a greater predisposition to developing potentially arrhythmogenic early afterdepolarizations (EADs) *(158)*. In contrast, studies of cells isolated from pressure-overload guinea pig *(9,21)* or spontaneously hypertensive rat *(12)* ventricles demonstrate no change in I_K. Recently, in the pacing-induced heart failure model in the rabbit, both E-4031-sensitive and -resistant components were found to be significantly smaller than those in control hearts, without a significant change in the voltage dependence or kinetics of the currents *(35)*. The chronic atrioventricular block dog is a well-characterized model of arrhythmogenic cardiac hypertrophy *(159)*. These animals exhibit increased monophasic APD, exaggerated dispersion of the APD, and enhanced susceptibility to pacing and class III antiarrhythmic drug induced torsades de pointes *(159,160)*. A significant downregulation of the slow component of the delayed rectifier, I_{Ks}, has been identified *(135)* and preliminary data suggest a downregulation of steady-state mRNA and protein levels of the transcripts and gene products of KCNQ1 and KCNE1 (personal communication M. Vos). In the rabbit both E4031-sensitive and resistant components of I_K were decreased in the pacing tachycardia-induced heart failure *(35)*.

In experimental myocardial infarction reduction of sustained K currents has been described. In a five–day canine myocardial infarction model, ventricular myocytes isolated from the ischemic zone (IZ, a thin layer of subepicardial tissue overlying the infarction) exhibited significantly reduced I_{Kr} and I_{Ks} densities compared with myocytes isolated from the noninfarcted zone (NZ) *(161)*. The changes in delayed rectifier current density were associated with a reduction in KvLQT1, ERG, and minK mRNA levels two days after coronary occlusion, at five days postinfarction the level of KvLQT1 mRNA had normalized while the others remained depressed compared to the NZ *(161)*. In a chronic feline myocardial infarction model, ventricular myocytes from the border zone of the infarct exhibited depressed I_K with a shift in the voltage-dependence of activation in the positive direction compared to cells isolated from noninfarcted hearts. When quinidine was applied to ventricular myocytes isolated from the infarcted hearts, action potential prolongation was blunted compared with cells isolated from normal ventricles *(162)* consistent with reduced repolarizing reserve in cells isolated from the diseased hearts. No change was found in the steady-state level of HERG mRNA in human HF *(84)*, although others have reported a decrease in failing compared to control hearts *(163)*.

The ATP-gated potassium channel (I_{K-ATP}) is the principal mediator of action potential shortening in response to ischemia in the heart. Differences in the behavior of I_{K-ATP} in hypertrophied or failing hearts may have profound implications for susceptibility to arrhythmias induced by myocardial ischemia. Human ventricular I_{K-ATP} in cells isolated from failing ventricles is functionally similar to that observed in myocytes from control ventricles, but less sensitive to ATP inhibition *(164)*. Action potential shortening that occurs in response to ischemia or metabolic inhibition is exaggerated in cells from hypertrophied compared to normal ventricles *(59)*. The differential sensitivity of the action potential duration to ischemic stress may be a result of altered I_{K-ATP} sensitivity to intracellular (ATP); however, the L-type Ca current in myocytes from hypertrophied hearts is also more profoundly suppressed by metabolic inhibition than it is in cells from control hearts *(59)*.

Na^+-K^+-ATPase

The Na^+-K^+ adenosine triphosphatase (ATPase), or Na pump, is responsible for the establishment and maintenance of the major ionic gradients across the cardiac cell membrane. The Na pump belongs to the widely distributed class of P-type ATPases that are responsible for transporting a number of cations. The P-type designation of this family of enzymes refers to the formation of a phosphorylated aspartyl intermediate during the catalytic cycle. The Na^+-K^+ ATPase hydrolyzes a molecule of ATP to transport K^+ into the cell and Na^+ out with a stoichiometry of 2:3 therefore generating a time-independent outward current.

The majority of experimental data suggests that the expression and function of the Na^+-K^+-ATPase are reduced in failing compared with control hearts (165–169). The density of the Na^+-K^+ ATPase decreases in heart failure as assessed by ^{3}[H]-ouabain binding. The decrease occurs without a significant impact on the inotropic effect of digitalis glycosides in human ventricular myocardium (170). Decreased Na pump function in heart failure has several consequences that might be relevant to production of arrhythmias. First, the reduction in the outward repolarizing current that would tend to prolong action potential duration. Second, reduced pump function would lead to an increase in intracellular [Na^+] and enhanced reverse-mode NCX, increasing depolarizing current. Finally, cells with less Na^+-K^+-ATPase activity have greater difficulty handling changes in extracellular [K^+]. Low [K^+]$_o$ itself tends to inhibit the ATPase, while increases in [K^+]$_o$ would tend to be cleared less rapidly in the setting of relative pump inhibition.

Pacemaker Current, I_f

I_f is a current that contributes to diastolic depolarization in pacemaking cells in the heart. The current is found in many cell types, but its features are variable; for example, I_f is present in ventricular myocytes, but its activation voltage is so negative that it is not likely to be of physiological significance in the ventricle (171). I_f activates slowly on hyperpolarization and deactivates rapidly with depolarization, supporting a mixed monovalent cation (Na^+ and K^+) current with a reversal potential of –20 to –30 mV; β-adrenergic stimulation increases I_f and hastens diastolic depolarization. Support for I_f as the pacemaker current in the heart comes from a genetic model of bradycardia in zebrafish with a dramatically reduced I_f current (172); nevertheless, in other species the linkage is not certain.

In the rat I_f density increases with the severity of cardiac hypertrophy (173). In contrast, although I_f is found in higher density in ventricular myocytes from failing human hearts, the difference from controls did not reach statistical significance. Furthermore, no differences in the voltage dependence, kinetics or isoproterenol-induced gating shift were noted in cells from failing compared to control hearts (174). Nonetheless, the trend toward an increase in I_f in the setting of reduced I_{K1} density may predispose ventricular myocytes isolated from failing hearts to enhanced automaticity.

Gap Junctions

Although alteration in ionic currents represent a central feature of electrical remodeling, ultimately the way myocytes function in the cardiac synctium is the final arbitor of the effect of remodeling on the electrical and contractile function of the heart. The most fundamental level of integration of myocytes is via their contact through gap junctions. Gap junctions are specialized membrane structures that contain multiple intercellular ion channels that facilitate electrical and chemical communication between cells. Mammalian gap junction channels or connexons are built by the oligomerization of a family of closely related genes encoding connexins. Connexins are transmembrane proteins consisting of four highly conserved membrane-spanning α-helices, two extracellular and one intracellular loop. Three different connexins have been detected in mammalian heart: connexin-40, connexin-43 and connexin-45 named for their molecular masses.

In virtually all structural heart disease studied to date, there are changes in the number and distribution of gap junctions. The changes in expression of gap junction channels are associated with changes in cellular coupling and an increased risk of malignant arrhythmias. Significant changes in the density and distribution of the major cardiac connexins have been demonstrated in ischemic *(175)*, hypertrophic *(176)*, and dilated cardiomyopathies *(177)* and acute cardiac rejection *(178)* in humans. Connexin-43, the major gap junction protein in ventricular myocardium is uniformly decreased and exhibits major changes in spatial localization including immunostaining extensively over the surface of the myocyte (lateralization) compared with more restricted expression at intercalated disks in normal tissue *(see [179])*. Total connexin-43 content is down-regulated in failing human LV myocardium of both ischemic and nonischemic etiologies with a reduction in steady-state mRNA levels *(177)*. In a canine myocardial infarction model abnormally distributed connexin-43 was spatially coincident with central common pathways of figure-of-eight reentry circuits *(180)*.

The regulation of expression of connexin-43 is remarkably dynamic with protein half-lives as short as 1.3 h *(181)*, such rapid turnover times suggests that one of many mechanisms for controlling cellular coupling in the heart is regulation of the number of gap junction channels. Posttranslational modification of gap junction proteins also plays a significant role in regulating cell-to-cell communication in normal and diseased hearts. Acute ischemia is associated with a rise in intracellular $[Ca^{2+}]$ and $[H^+]$ that can reduce gap junction channel activity, however dephosphorylation of Cx-43 also occurs with a time course that mimics electrical uncoupling *(182)*. In cardiomyopathic hamsters, progressive mechanical dysfunction is associated with reduced gap junctional communication via c-Src-mediated tyrosine phosphorylation of connexin-43 *(183)*. Alterations in beta-adrenergic and RAAS signaling in the failing heart is associated with depressed junctional conductance *(184,185)*. However, in vitro experiments in rat neonatal ventricular myocytes revealed a significant increase in connexin-43 expression upon exposure to angiotensin II, an effect which could be blocked by losartan *(186)*.

Transgenic mouse models have further reinforced the role of abnormalities of gap junctions in arrhythmia production. Cardiac restricted knock-out of connexin-43 is associated with sudden death due to ventricular arrhythmias at an early age in these animals in the presence of significant decrements in both longitudinal and transverse epicardial conduction velocities with augmented anisotropy *(187)*. Although the mechanism of initiation of lethal ventricular arrhythmias in this model is unknown, the absence of connexin-43 is a key molecular feature of arrhythmia susceptibility.

Altered Autonomic Signaling

In the face of impaired LV pump function, the body attempts to maintain circulatory homeostasis (cardiac output) through a complex series of neurohumoral changes. Prominently, the SNS and RAAS are activated. Activation of the SNS increases heart rate and contractility and redistributes blood flow centrally by peripheral vasoconstriction. The RAAS similarly causes vasoconstriction and increases circulatory volume, allowing individuals to respond appropriately to physiological stress or exercise. However, these powerful compensatory mechanisms are also utilized to deal with hemodynamic overload, and they are activated when myocardial contractile function is compromised for any reason. Chronic β-adrenergic receptor stimulation by catecholamines can be cardiotoxic, and multiple regulatory adjustments produce desensitization of downstream effector responses in the failing heart. Although these neurohumoral changes are initially adaptive, maintaining systolic function and vital organ perfusion, ultimately progression of the heart failure phenotype ensues. The combination of neurohumoral activation and mechanical stress activates signal transduction cascades that produce myocyte hypertrophy and result in the elaboration of trophic factors that increase the interstitial content of collagen. Activation of these cascades have profound effects on the electrophysiology of the failing heart.

Since the initial observations of Bristow et al. *(188)*, adrenergic signaling in human heart failure has been the subject of extensive study *(189,190)*. The β_1-, β_2-, and α_1-adrenergic receptors mediate the effects of increased catecholamines, both circulating epinephrine and norepinephrine, released from cardiac nerve terminals in the heart *(191)*. These receptor subtypes are coupled to different signaling systems. The β_1- and β_2-receptors are coupled by stimulatory G proteins to adenylyl cyclase; activation results in increased cellular levels of cAMP, which may be quite local in the case of β_2-receptors *(192)*. The α_1-receptor is coupled through a G protein to phospholipase C (PLC) which hydrolyzes inositol phospholipids increasing cellular inositol 1,4,5-trisphosphate (IP3) and diacylglycerol (DAG). Activation of the α-adrenergic pathway initiates a cascade of events that trigger cell growth and alter the intracellular Ca^{2+} load. The possible adverse consequences of increased Ca^{2+} load include activation of phospholipases, proteases, and endonucleases, culminating in cell necrosis or apoptosis and perhaps progression of the failing phenotype.

In human and animal models of chronic HF the cardiac response to β-adrenergic stimulation is blunted and there is a positive correlation between increased plasma catecholamine levels and the degree of the diminution of the β-adrenergic response *(188,193–195)*. In most studies of end-stage human heart failure *(188,193,196)* and some failing animal models *(195)*, the β_1–adrenergic receptor undergoes subtype-selective downregulation such that the proportions of β_1–:β_2–adrenergic receptors are nearly equal in abundance compared to the 70–80% dominance of the β_1–subtype in normal hearts. In addition, the remaining β-adrenergic receptors are significantly desensitized due to uncoupling of the receptors from their respective signaling pathways *(197,198)*.

The β-adrenergic receptor subtype signaling pathways may have markedly different chronic effects on cardiac hypertrophic response, as manifested by the distinct phenotypes of transgenic mice overexpressing cardiac β_1– vs β_2–adrenergic receptors *(199)*. Recent evidence suggests that the β-adrenergic receptor subtypes even have opposing effects on apoptosis in cultured rat cardiomyocytes: β_1–stimulation induces apoptosis whereas β_2–stimulation inhibits apoptosis *(200,201)*.

In chronic heart failure in both humans *(202–204)* and animal models *(195)*, a marked increase in G_i mRNA levels has been reported. Studies in rat and guinea pig have shown that chronic infusion of catecholamines increases the expression of G_i *(202,205)*, whereas, when the human β_2–adrenergic receptor was overexpressed in transgenic mice, G_i protein abundance was significantly enhanced *(199)*.

Protein phosphorylation mediated by β-adrenergic activation is decreased in the failing human heart *(206,207)*. The PKA signaling pathway appears to be downregulated at several levels beyond the β-receptor, with the functional implication of limiting PKA signaling in important subcellular locations such as the sarcolemma and the SR in the failing cardiac myocytes *(208)*. There is now increasing evidence for local regulation of PKA activity by binding of PKA to A-kinase anchoring proteins (AKAP) *(209,210)*. Such compartmentalization of PKA in the human heart may be disrupted in heart failure as yet another mechanism of abnormal autonomic signaling in the failing heart *(211)*.

The β- and α-adrenergic signaling pathways affect the function of a number of ion channels and transporters. The net effect of β-adrenergic stimulation is to shorten the ventricular action potential duration owing to an increase of I_K current density *(212)*, despite β_1 receptor stimulation of depolarizing current through the L-type Ca channel. α_1-adrenergic receptor stimulation inhibits several K currents in the mammalian heart, including I_{to}, I_{K1} and I_K, with the net effect of prolonging action potential duration *(213)*. Alterations in β-receptor number and the increased of G_i will impact all down stream effectors including ion channels and transporters. A well-documented example is the blunted β-adrenergic agonist-mediated stimulation of I_{Ca} in the failing heart *(39)*. The depressed stimulatory (β-receptor downregulation and desensitization) and enhanced inhibitory responses to beta adrenergic receptor stimulation are consistent with the overall electrical profile in failing ventricular myocardium.

STRUCTURAL REMODELING IN THE FAILING VENTRICLE

Myocytes and nonmyocytes in the heart are interconnected by connective tissue and extracellular matrix. Nonmyocyte cardiac cells include fibroblasts responsible for turnover of the extracellular matrix that consists predominantly of fibrillar type I and III collagens. The fibrillar collagen matrix contributes to the maintenance of ventricular geometry, the structural alignment of adjoining myocytes and coordinated transmission of contractile force to the ventricular chamber. Components of the extracellular matrix include collagens, proteoglycans, glycoproteins, peptide growth factors, and proteases. The extracellular matrix is an important determinant of the structural characteristics of the myocardium.

Pathologic myocardial hypertrophy is associated with interstitial fibrosis, which may alter the electrical and mechanical properties of the myocardium. On the other hand, a reduction or alteration of certain structural proteins could compromise the integrity of the extracellular matrix and lead to chamber dilation. Alterations in collagen structure and composition have been reported to occur within the left ventricle in structural heart disease, which in turn may influence ventricular geometry and result in discontinuity of the fibrillar collagen network *(214–217)*.

Following a myocardial infarction, a fraction of cardiac myocytes is replaced by scar tissue. The scar tissue at the border zone of the infarction consists of type I and III collagens and atrophied surrounding myocytes, whereas remaining viable myocytes may hypertrophy. Another prominent feature of the structural remodeling of myocardium in ischemic cardiomyopathy is an accumulation of fibrillar collagen that is not related to myocyte necrosis. This reactive interstitial fibrosis is generally remote from the infarct site and involves both right and left ventricles, including the interventricular septum *(218–221)*.

Metalloproteinases (MMPs) are a family of enzymes with high affinity for extracellular matrix components. Recent evidence has shown an increased abundance and activity of MMPs in experimental models of HF and in end-stage human cardiomyopathy of both ischemic and nonischemic etiologies *(222–224)*. Enhanced MMP activity in the LV may contribute to the remodeling processes. Although it is likely that different extracellular stimuli will induce different profiles of MMP expression, increased left ventricular MMP activity almost certainly contributes to structural remodeling in both ischemic and nonischemic cardiomyopathies.

In the infarcted heart collagen turnover at sites of tissue repair is governed by myofibroblasts, a phenotypically transformed fibroblast that expresses α-smooth muscle actin. Actin microfilaments confer myofibroblasts with contractile behavior that contributes to scar tissue remodeling and whose tonic contraction could alter myocardial stiffness. Fibroblast-like cells regulate matrix remodeling. Myofibroblast collagen turnover is mediated by signaling molecules found in the interstitial space. Transforming growth factor-β1 (TGF-β1), a cytokine derived from inflammatory cells, is released into the tissue fluid where it serves to regulate myofibroblast collagen synthesis. TGF-β1 is derived from cells entering the infarct zone and by resident myofibroblasts. Myofibroblast TGF-β1 expression is regulated in an autocrine manner by angiotensin II (ATII) generated at sites of repair *(225)*.

Chronic elevations of ATII are associated with myocardial fibrosis *(226,227)*. The same holds true for chronic elevations of aldosterone, the other effector hormone of the circulating RAAS. The existence of other pathways for upregulation of the RAAS in heart failure has been suggested. In a recent study activation of p53 with ventricular pacing upregulates the myocyte RAAS with the generation and secretion of ATII that may promote myocyte growth and death *(228)*. In any case, chronic activation of the RAAS in heart failure is pathological and contributes to the progressive structural remodeling of cardiac tissue *(217)* with profound implications for electrical conduction in the heart.

MECHANISMS OF VENTRICULAR ARRHYTHMIAS SECONDARY TO ELECTRICAL AND STRUCTURAL REMODELING

Ventricular arrhythmias are multifactorial in patients with heart failure. The variability in the reported electrophysiological changes are certainly in part methodological, but also reflect a high degree of heterogeneity in the pathophysiology of hypertrophy and heart failure in animal models and human disease. The stage of disease is crucial in determining the degree and character of electrical remodeling and arrhythmic risk. The changes in risk of sudden death with progression of heart disease are likely to be a reflection of changes in electrophysiological substrate. The great challenge remains to understand the mechanisms of ventricular arrhythmias in terms of cellular and tissue electrophysiology and the molecular changes in hypertrophy and heart failure that alter the electrophysiology of the cells, tissues and intact hearts of patients.

Altered Automaticity

Abnormal automaticity may arise in hypertrophied and failing hearts in the setting of a reduction in resting membrane potential or acceleration of phase 4 diastolic depolarization such that the threshold for activation of the Na current is rapidly achieved. A number of changes in the failing heart that may alter automaticity in the ventricles including: Reexpression of I_{Ca-T}; changes in the voltage dependence, β-adrenergic sensitivity, or an increased density of I_f; and reduced I_{K1} density. Additionally, the augmentation of time-independent depolarizing currents may hasten diastolic depolarization and/or reduce the maximal diastolic potential.

Triggered automaticity arising from afterdepolarizations could be enhanced by several electrophysiological changes described in the failing and hypertrophied heart. Cells isolated from failing animal and human hearts consistently reveal a significant prolongation of action potentials compared to those in normal hearts, independent of the mechanism of HF. The plateau phase of the action potential is known to be quite labile. The longer the action potential, the more labile is the repolarization process *(229)*. Action potential lability may be manifested as variability in duration and/or secondary depolarizations that interrupt action potential repolarization, such as early afterdepolarizations (EADs) that can initiate triggered arrhythmias including torsades de pointes ventricular tachycardia. Indeed, enhanced susceptibility to afterdepolarization-mediated ventricular arrhythmias has been demonstrated experimentally as summarized below.

Prolongation of repolarization *(230–232)*, enhanced dispersion of repolarization and susceptibility to cesium-induced action potential prolongation have been demonstrated in the canine pacing-tachycardia heart failure model, an animal model with a high incidence of sudden death *(43)*. Ventricular myocytes isolated from the failing canine heart exhibit more spontaneous EADs than cells from control hearts and have an exaggerated response (more frequent and complex EADs) to reduction of the bath K^+ concentration and the addition of the nonspecific K channel blocker CsCl *(233)*. Complex afterdepolarizations and triggered arrhthythmias are more common in hypertrophied rat ventricular myocardium exposed to K channel blockers *(234)* and dogs with LVH exposed to the Ca channel agonist BayK 8644 *(235)* or antiarrhythmic drugs with class III action *(159)*. Alterations in Ca current density or kinetics can predispose to EAD- or DAD-mediated arrhythmias *(229)*. Changes in the cellular environment such as hypokalemia, hypomagnesemia, and elevated levels of catecholamines may further increase the susceptibility to afterdepolarization-mediated triggered arrhythmias *(38)*.

The changes in Ca^{2+} handling in the hypertrophic and failing heart may also contribute to electrical instability. The characteristic slow decay of the calcium transients and increased diastolic Ca^{2+} can predispose to oscillatory release of Ca^{2+} from the SR and DAD-mediated triggered arrhythmias. The slow decay of the Ca^{2+} transient will influence ion flux through the NCX and may also predispose to late phase 3 EAD-mediated triggered arrhythmias. Recently, NCX current has been implicated as the major underlying mechanism of delayed afterdepolarizations in hypertrophied and failing ventricular myocardium *(127,236,237)*.

Reentry in the Failing Heart

The vast majority of patients with heart failure because of coronary artery disease have suffered a myocardial infarction. The resulting scar and its border zone contain surviving myocyte fiber bundles in which conduction is slowed, thus facilitating reentry and giving rise to ventricular tachycardia. In addition to the presence of scar, reorganization of intercellular connections in infarct border zones may contribute to conduction slowing that is critical for maintenance of reentry.

Patients with idiopathic, nonischemic, dilated cardiomyopathy are likely to experience ventricular arrhythmias that are mechanistically distinct from those in patients with prior myocardial infarction. Several electrophysiological abnormalities have been identified in the hypertrophied and failing noninfarcted heart that may predispose to reentry. Altered conduction through the myocardium and exaggerated dispersion of recovery or repolarization may predispose to functional or nonexcitable gap reentry in the hypertrophied or failing ventricle. Increased excitation threshold, decreased resting membrane potential and resultant depression of the action potential upstroke may contribute to slowing conduction velocity *(230,238,239)*. Alterations in intracellular [Ca^{2+}] *(240,241)*, redistribution of gap junctions *(242,243)* and changes in cell size will affect cell-to-cell coupling *(244)*. Modified cellular coupling and fibrosis will alter anisotropic conduction leading to spatial nonuniformities of electrical loading resulting in conduction block and reentry *(245)*.

Defective repolarization the result of action potential prolongation is a prominent feature of the hypertrophied and failing heart that has been also associated with lethal ventricular arrhythmias *(229,230,246,247)*. Prolonged and labile action potentials may predispose to arrhythmic afterdepolarizations, as importantly exaggerated dispersion of repolarization may predispose to conduction block and reentry.

Mechanical load is an important modulator of excitability in the heart. The effect of altered hemodynamic load may be exaggerated in the failing compared with the normal ventricle. Furthermore, the effect of load is not likely to be distributed uniformly across the ventricular wall or throughout the myocardium, and thus has the potential to increase dispersion in action potential duration with arrhythmogenic consequences.

Autonomic Nervous System and Cardiac Arrhythmias in Heart Failure

Heart failure is characterized by sympathetic activation and parasympathetic withdrawal *(248,249)*. Resting plasma and whole body norepinephrine levels are increased and heart rate variability is reduced, indicative of parasympathetic withdrawal. The autonomic disturbances in heart failure may promote ventricular arrhythmias in many ways. Increased sympathetic tone, reduced vagal tone, and diminished baroreceptor responsiveness increase the likelihood of ventricular fibrillation during acute ischemia. β-adrenergic stimulation increases intracellular calcium and promotes delayed afterdepolarizations. α-adrenergic stimulation can prolong action potential duration, promoting early afterdepolarizations. Sympathetic stimulation may increase heterogeneity of recovery times within the heart, facilitating reentry.

CONCLUSIONS

There is little doubt that myocardial remodeling in structural heart disease is multifactorial with changes in myocytes, intercellular coupling, and the interstitium. The alterations in the ventricular myocardium will vary depending upon the nature of the underlying heart disease and exhibits regional heterogeneity that may be particularly pronounced in the case of coronary artery disease and prior myocardial infarction. The changes that attend the remodeled ventricle include myocyte hypertrophy and apoptosis, altered expression of ion channel genes and transporters that modify the electrical and contractile phenotype and quantitative and qualitative changes in the extracellular matrix.

It is necessary that information garnered from cellular and molecular models together with data obtained from clinical trials, be used to generate strategies designed to optimize symptom control, prevent sudden death and disease progression.

ACKNOWLEDGMENTS

Support provided by an AHA Fellowship #0020257U (AAA). Support for the study of heart failure and associated sudden death was provided by a Specialized Center of Research from the NHLBI, NIH (P50 HL 52307).

REFERENCES

1. Changes in mortality from heart failure—United States, 1980–1995. MMWR Morb Mortal Wkly Rep 1998;47:633–637.
2. Konstam MA, Remme WJ. Treatment guidelines in heart failure. Prog Cardiovasc Dis 1998;48:65–72.
3. Kjekshus J. Arrhythmias and mortality in congestive heart failure. Am J Cardiol 1990;65:421–481.
4. Chakko CS, Gheorghiade M. Ventricular arrhythmias in severe heart failure: incidence, significance, and effectiveness of antiarrhythmic therapy. Am Heart J 1985;109:497–504.
5. Wilson JR, Schwartz JS, Sutton MS, et al. Prognosis in severe heart failure: relation to hemodynamic measurements and ventricular ectopic activity. J Am Coll Cardiol 1983;2:403–410.
6. von Olshausen K, Schafer A, Mehmel HC, Schwarz F, Senges J, Kubler W. Ventricular arrhythmias in idiopathic dilated cardiomyopathy. Br Heart J 1984;51:195–201.
7. Califf RM, McKinnis RA, Burks J, et al. Prognostic implications of ventricular arrhythmias during 24 hour ambulatory monitoring in patients undergoing cardiac catheterization for coronary artery disease. Am J Cardiol 1982;50:23–31.
8. Cohn JN, Archibald DG, Ziesche S, et al. Effect of vasodilator therapy on mortality in chronic congestive heart failure. Results of a Veterans Administration Cooperative Study. N Engl J Med 1986;314:1547–1552.
9. Ahmmed GU, Dong PH, Song G, et al. Changes in Ca(2+) cycling proteins underlie cardiac action potential prolongation in a pressure-overloaded guinea pig model with cardiac hypertrophy and failure. Circ Res 2000;86:558–570.
10. Bassett AL, Gelband H. Chronic partial occlusion of the pulmonary artery in cats. Change in ventricular action potential configuration during early hypertrophy. Circ Res 1973;32:15–26.
11. Benitah JP, Gomez AM, Bailly P, et al. Heterogeneity of the early outward current in ventricular cells isolated from normal and hypertrophied rat hearts. J Physiol (Lond) 1993;469:111–138.
12. Brooksby P, Levi AJ, Jones JV. The electrophysiological characteristics of hypertrophied ventricular myocytes from the spontaneously hypertensive rat. J Hyperten 1993;11:611–622.
13. Bryant SM, Shipsey SJ, Hart G. Regional differences in electrical and mechanical properties of myocytes from guinea-pig hearts with mild left ventricular hypertrophy. Cardiovasc Res 1997;35:315–323.
14. Cerbai E, Barbieri M, Li Q, Mugelli A. Ionic basis of action potential prolongation of hypertrophied cardiac myocytes isolated from hypertensive rats of different ages. Cardiovasc Res 1994; 28:1180–1187.
15. Coulombe A, Momtaz A, Richer P, Swynghedauw B, Coraboeuf E. Reduction of calcium-independent transient outward potassium current density in DOCA salt hypertrophied rat ventricular myocytes. Pflugers Archiv European J Physiol 1994;427:47–55.
16. Keung EC, Aronson RS. Non-uniform electrophysiological properties and electrotonic interaction in hypertrophied rat myocardium. Circ Res 1981;49:150–158.
17. Kleiman RB, Houser SR. Outward currents in normal and hypertrophied feline ventricular myocytes. Am J Physiol 1989;256:H1450–H1461.
18. Li Q, Keung EC. Effects of myocardial hypertrophy on transient outward current. Am J Physiol 1994;266:H1738–H1745.

19. Gulch RW. Alterations in excitation of mammalian myocardium as a function of chronic loading and their implications in the mechanical events. Basic Res Cardiol 1980;75:73–80.
20. Nordin C, Siri F, Aronson RS. Electrophysiologic characteristics of single myocytes isolated from hypertrophied guinea-pig hearts. J Molec & Cell Cardiol 1989;21:729–739.
21. Ryder KO, Bryant SM, Hart G. Membrane current changes in left ventricular myocytes isolated from guinea pigs after abdominal aortic coarctation. Cardiovasc Res 1993;27:1278–1287.
22. Tomita F, Bassett AL, Myerburg RJ, Kimura S. Diminished transient outward currents in rat hypertrophied ventricular myocytes. Circ Res 1994;75:296–303.
23. Potreau D, Gomez JP, Fares N. Depressed transient outward current in single hypertrophied cardiomyocytes isolated from the right ventricle of ferret heart. Cardiovasc Res 1995;30:440–448.
24. Takimoto K, Li D, Hershman KM, Li P, Jackson EK, Levitan ES. Decreased expression of Kv4.2 and novel Kv4.3 K+ channel subunit mRNAs in ventricles of renovascular hypertensive rats. Circ Res 1997;81:533–539.
25. Li GR, Ferrier GR, Howlett SE. Calcium currents in ventricular myocytes of prehypertrophic cardiomyopathic hamsters. Am J Physiol 1995;268:H999–H1005.
26. Thuringer D, Coulombe A, Deroubaix E, Coraboeuf E, Mercadier JJ. Depressed transient outward current density in ventricular myocytes from cardiomyopathic Syrian hamsters of different ages. J Mol Cell Cardiol 1996;28:387–401.
27. Thuringer D, Deroubaix E, Coulombe A, Coraboeuf E, Mercadier JJ. Ionic basis of the action potential prolongation in ventricular myocytes from Syrian hamsters with dilated cardiomyopathy. Cardiovasc Res 1996;31:747–757.
28. Xu XP, Best PM. Decreased transient outward K+ current in ventricular myocytes from acromegalic rats. Am J Physiol 1991;260:H935–H942.
29. Lue WM, Boyden PA. Abnormal electrical properties of myocytes from chronically infarcted canine heart. Alterations in Vmax and the transient outward current. Circulation 1992;85:1175–1188.
30. Qin D, Zhang ZH, Caref EB, Boutjdir M, Jain P, el-Sherif N. Cellular and ionic basis of arrhythmias in postinfarction remodeled ventricular myocardium. Circ Res 1996;79:461–473.
31. Bril A, Forest MC, Gout B. Ischemia and reperfusion-induced arrhythmias in rabbits with chronic heart failure. Am J Physiol 1991;261:H301–H307.
32. Gidh-Jain M, Huang B, Jain P, el-Sherif N. Differential expression of voltage-gated K+ channel genes in left ventricular remodeled myocardium after experimental myocardial infarction. Circ Res 1996;79:669–675.
33. Kääb S, Nuss HB, Chiamvimonvat N, et al. Ionic mechanism of action potential prolongation in ventricular myocytes from dogs with pacing-induced heart failure. Circ Res 1996;78:262–273.
34. Rozanski GJ, Xu Z, Whitney RT, Murakami H, Zucker IH. Electrophysiology of rabbit ventricular myocytes following sustained rapid ventricular pacing. J Mol Cell Cardiol 1997;29:721–732.
35. Tsuji Y, Opthof T, Kamiya K, et al. Pacing-induced heart failure causes a reduction of delayed rectifier potassium currents along with decreases in calcium and transient outward currents in rabbit ventricle. Cardiovasc Res 2000;48:300–309.
36. Coltart DJ, Meldrum SJ. Intracellular action potential in hypertrophic obstructive cardiomyopathy. British Heart Journal 1972;34:7112–7497.
37. Gwathmey JK, Copelas L, MacKinnon R, et al. Abnormal intracellular calcium handling in myocardium from patients with end-stage heart failure. Circ Res 1987;61:70–76.
38. Vermeulen JT, McGuire MA, Opthof T, et al. Triggered activity and automaticity in ventricular trabeculae of failing human and rabbit hearts. Cardiovasc Res 1994;28:1547–1554.
39. Beuckelmann DJ, Nabauer M, Erdmann E. Intracellular calcium handling in isolated ventricular myocytes from patients with terminal heart failure. Circulation 1992;85:1046–1055.
40. Beuckelmann DJ, Nabauer M, Erdmann E. Alterations of K+ currents in isolated human ventricular myocytes from patients with terminal heart failure. Circ Res 1993;73:379–385.
41. Dipla K, Mattiello JA, Margulies KB, Jeevanandam V, Houser SR. The sarcoplasmic reticulum and the Na+/Ca2+ exchanger both contribute to the Ca2+ transient of failing human ventricular myocytes. Circ Res 1999;84:435–444.
42. O'Rourke B, Kass DA, Tomaselli GF, Kääb S, Tunin R, Marbán E. Mechanisms of altered excitation-contraction coupling in canine tachycardia-induced heart failure, I: experimental studies. Circ Res 1999;84:562–570.
43. Pak PH, Nuss HB, Tunin RS, et al. Repolarization abnormalities, arrhythmia and sudden death in canine tachycardia-induced cardiomyopathy. J Am Coll Cardiol 1997;30:576–584.

44. Akar FG, Rosenbaum DS. Transmural heterogeneities of cellular repolarization underlie polymorphic ventricular tachycardia in failing myocardium. Circulation 2001;104:25.

45. Pye MP, Cobbe SM. Arrhythmogenesis in experimental models of heart failure: the role of increased load. Cardiovasc Res 1996;32:248–257.

46. Kamkin A, Kiseleva I, Isenberg G. Stretch-activated currents in ventricular myocytes: amplitude and arrhythmogenic effects increase with hypertrophy. Cardiovasc Res 2000;48:409–420.

47. Litovsky SH, Antzelevitch C. Rate dependence of action potential duration and refractoriness in canine ventricular endocardium differs from that of epicardium: role of the transient outward current. J Am Coll Cardiol 1989;14:1053–1066.

48. Fedida D, Giles WR. Regional variations in action potentials and transient outward current in myocytes isolated from rabbit left ventricle. J Physiol 1991;442:191–209.

49. Lukas A, Antzelevitch C. Differences in the electrophysiological response of canine ventricular epicardium and endocardium to ischemia. Role of the transient outward current. Circulation 1993;88:2903–2915.

50. Drouin E, Charpentier F, Gauthier C, Laurent K, Le Marec H. Electrophysiologic characteristics of cells spanning the left ventricular wall of human heart: evidence for presence of M cells [see comments]. J Am Coll Cardiol 1995;26:185–192.

51. Di Diego JM, Sun ZQ, Antzelevitch C. I(to) and action potential notch are smaller in left vs. right canine ventricular epicardium. Am J Physiol 1996;271:H548–H561.

52. McIntosh MA, Cobbe SM, Smith GL. Heterogeneous changes in action potential and intracellular Ca2+ in left ventricular myocyte sub-types from rabbits with heart failure. Cardiovasc Res 2000;45:397–409.

53. Barr CS, Naas A, Freeman M, Lang CC, Struthers AD. QT dispersion and sudden unexpected death in chronic heart failure. Lancet 1994;343:327–329.

54. Berger RD, Kasper EK, Baughman KL, Marban E, Calkins H, Tomaselli GF. Beat-to-beat QT interval variability: novel evidence for repolarization lability in ischemic and nonischemic dilated cardiomyopathy. Circulation 1997;96:1557–1565.

55. Arai M, Alpert NR, MacLennan DH, Barton P, Periasamy M. Alterations in sarcoplasmic reticulum gene expression in human heart failure. A possible mechanism for alterations in systolic and diastolic properties of the failing myocardium. Circ Res 1993;72:463–469.

56. Morgan JP, Erny RE, Allen PD, Grossman W, Gwathmey JK. Abnormal intracellular calcium handling, a major cause of systolic and diastolic dysfunction in ventricular myocardium from patients with heart failure. Circulation 1990;81.

57. Calderone A, Takahashi N, Izzo NJ, Thaik CM, Colucci WS. Pressure- and volume-induced left ventricular hypertrophies are associated with distinct myocyte phenotypes and differential induction of peptide growth factor mRNAs. Circulation 1995;92:2385–2390.

58. Hart G. Cellular electrophysiology in cardiac hypertrophy and failure. Cardiovasc Res 1994;28: 933–946.

59. Furukawa T, Myerburg RJ, Furukawa N, Kimura S, Bassett AL. Metabolic inhibition of ICa,L and IK differs in feline left ventricular hypertrophy. Am J Physiol 1994;266:H1121–H1131.

60. Gomez AM, Benitah JP, Henzel D, Vinet A, Lorente P, Delgado C. Modulation of electrical heterogeneity by compensated hypertrophy in rat left ventricle. Am J Physiol 1997;272.

61. Xiao YF, McArdle JJ. Elevated density and altered pharmacologic properties of myocardial calcium current of the spontaneously hypertensive rat. J Hypertens 1994;12:783–790.

62. Mukherjee R, Hewett KW, Walker JD, Basler CG, Spinale FG. Changes in L-type calcium channel abundance and function during the transition to pacing-induced congestive heart failure. Cardiovasc Res 1998;37:432–444.

63. Gidh-Jain M, Huang B, Jain P, Battula V, el-Sherif N. Reemergence of the fetal pattern of L-type calcium channel gene expression in non infarcted myocardium during left ventricular remodeling. Biochemical & Biophysical Research Communications 1995;216:892–897.

64. Creazzo TL. Reduced L-type calcium current in the embryonic chick heart with persistent truncus arteriosus. Circ Res 1990;66:1491–1498.

65. Mayoux E, Callens F, Swynghedauw B, Charlemagne D. Adaptational process of the cardiac Ca2+ channels to pressure overload: biochemical and physiological properties of the dihydropyridine receptors in normal and hypertrophied rat hearts. J Cardiovasc Pharmacol 1988;12:390–396.

66. Wagner JA, Weisman HF, Snowman AM, Reynolds IJ, Weisfeldt ML, Snyder SH. Alterations in calcium antagonist receptors and sodium-calcium exchange in cardiomyopathic hamster tissues. Circ Res 1989;65:205–214.

67. Dixon IM, Lee SL, Dhalla NS. Nitrendipine binding in congestive heart failure due to myocardial infarction. Circ Res 1990;66:782–788.
68. Vatner DE, Sato N, Kiuchi K, Shannon RP, Vatner SF. Decrease in myocardial ryanodine receptors and altered excitation-contraction coupling early in the development of heart failure. Circulation 1994;90:1423–1430.
69. Gengo PJ, Sabbah HN, Steffen RP, et al. Myocardial beta adrenoceptor and voltage sensitive calcium channel changes in a canine model of chronic heart failure. J Mol Cell Cardiol 1992;24:1361–1369.
70. Rasmussen RP, Minobe W, Bristow MR. Calcium antagonist binding sites in failing and nonfailing human ventricular myocardium. Biochem Pharmacol 1990;39:691–696.
71. Beuckelmann DJ, Erdmann E. Ca(2+)-currents and intracellular [Ca2+]i-transients in single ventricular myocytes isolated from terminally failing human myocardium. Basic Res Cardiol 1992;87: 235–243.
72. Mewes T, Ravens U. L-type calcium currents of human myocytes from ventricle of non-failing and failing hearts and from atrium. J Mol Cell Cardiol 1994;26:1307–1320.
73. Ouadid H, Albat B, Nargeot J. Calcium currents in diseased human cardiac cells. J Cardiovasc Pharmacol 1995;25:282–291.
74. Takahashi T, Allen PD, Lacro RV, et al. Expression of dihydropyridine receptor (Ca2+ channel) and calsequestrin genes in the myocardium of patients with end-stage heart failure. J Clin Invest 1992;90:927–935.
75. Gruver EJ, Morgan JP, Stambler BS, Gwathmey JK. Uniformity of calcium channel number and isometric contraction in human right and left ventricular myocardium. Basic Research in Cardiology 1994;89:139–148.
76. Sipido KR, Stankovicova T, Flameng W, Vanhaecke J, Verdonck F. Frequency dependence of Ca2+ release from the sarcoplasmic reticulum in human ventricular myocytes from end-stage heart failure. Cardiovasc Res 1998;37:478–488.
77. Ryder KO, Bryant SM, Hart G. Changes in cell length consequent on depolarization in single left ventricular myocytes from guinea-pigs with pressure-overload left ventricular hypertrophy. Proceedings of the Royal Society of London Series B: Biological Sciences 1993;253:35–42.
78. Keung EC. Calcium current is increased in isolated adult myocytes from hypertrophied rat myocardium. Circ Res 1989;64:753–763.
79. Kleiman RB, Houser SR. Calcium currents in normal and hypertrophied isolated feline ventricular myocytes. Am J Physiol 1988;255:H1434–H1442.
80. Winslow RL, Rice J, Jafri S, Marbán E, O'Rourke B. Mechanisms of altered excitation-contraction coupling in canine tachycardia-induced heart failure, II: model studies. Circ Res 1999;84:571–586.
81. Finkel MS, Marks ES, Patterson RE, Speir EH, Steadman KA, Keiser HR. Correlation of changes in cardiac calcium channels with hemodynamics in Syrian hamster cardiomyopathy and heart failure. Life Sci 1987;41:153–159.
82. Colston JT, Kumar P, Chambers JP, Freeman GL. Altered sarcolemmal calcium channel density and Ca(2+)-pump ATPase activity in tachycardia heart failure. Cell Calcium 1994;16:349–356.
83. Schroeder F, Handrock R, Beuckelmann DJ, et al. Increased availability and open probability of single L-type calcium channels from failing compared with nonfailing human ventricle. Circulation 1998;98:969–976.
84. Kääb S, Dixon J, Duc J, et al. Molecular basis of transient outward potassium current downregulation in human heart failure: A decrease in Kv4.3 mRNA correlates with a reduction in current density. Circulation 1998;98:1383–1393.
85. Hullin RA, Asmus F, Berger HJ, Boekstegers P. Differential expression of the subunits of the cardiac L-type calcium channel in diastolic failure of the transplanted heart. Circulation 1997;96:1–55.
86. Siri FM, Krueger J, Nordin C, Ming Z, Aronson RS. Depressed intracellular calcium transients and contraction in myocytes from hypertrophied and failing guinea pig hearts. Am J Physiol 1991; 261:H514–H530.
87. Bailey BA, Houser SR. Calcium transients in feline left ventricular myocytes with hypertrophy induced by slow progressive pressure overload. J Mol Cell Cardiol 1992;24:365–373.
88. Bailey BA, Dipla K, Li S, Houser SR. Cellular basis of contractile derangements of hypertrophied feline ventricular myocytes. J Mol Cell Cardiol 1997;29:1823–1835.
89. Wang J, Flemal K, Qiu Z, Ablin L, Grossman W, Morgan JP. Ca2+ handling and myofibrillar Ca2+ sensitivity in ferret cardiac myocytes with pressure-overload hypertrophy. Am J Physiol 1994;267.
90. Gomez AM, Valdivia HH, Cheng H, et al. Defective excitation-contraction coupling in experimental cardiac hypertrophy and heart failure. Science 1997;276:800–806.

91. Beuckelmann DJ, Nabauer M, Kruger C, Erdmann E. Altered diastolic [Ca2+]i handling in human ventricular myocytes from patients with terminal heart failure. Am Heart J 1995;129:684–689.

92. Mercadier JJ, Lompre AM, Duc P, et al. Altered sarcoplasmic reticulum Ca2(+)-ATPase gene expression in the human ventricle during end-stage heart failure. J Clin Investig 1990;85:305–309.

93. Studer R, Reinecke H, Bilger J, et al. Gene expression of the cardiac Na(+)-Ca2+ exchanger in end-stage human heart failure. Circ Res 1994;75:443–453.

94. Schwinger RH, Bohm M, Schmidt U, et al. Unchanged protein levels of SERCA II and phospholamban but reduced Ca2+ uptake and Ca(2+)-ATPase activity of cardiac sarcoplasmic reticulum from dilated cardiomyopathy patients compared with patients with nonfailing hearts. Circulation 1995;92: 3220–3228.

95. Flesch M, Schwinger RH, Schnabel P, et al. Sarcoplasmic reticulum Ca2+ATPase and phospholamban mRNA and protein levels in end-stage heart failure due to ischemic or dilated cardiomyopathy. J Molec Med 1996;74:321–332.

96. Linck B, Boknik P, Eschenhagen T, et al. Messenger RNA expression and immunological quantification of phospholamban and SR-Ca(2+)-ATPase in failing and nonfailing human hearts. Cardiovasc Res 1996;31:625–632.

97. Kuo TH, Tsang W, Wang KK, Carlock L. Simultaneous reduction of the sarcolemmal and SR calcium ATPase activities and gene expression in cardiomyopathic hamster. Biochim Biophys Acta 1992;1138:343–349.

98. Feldman AM, Weinberg EO, Ray PE, Lorell BH. Selective changes in cardiac gene expression during compensated hypertrophy and the transition to cardiac decompensation in rats with chronic aortic banding. Circ Res 1993;73:184–192.

99. Zarain-Herzberg A, Afzal N, Elimban V, Dhalla NS. Decreased expression of cardiac sarcoplasmic reticulum Ca(2+)-pump ATPase in congestive heart failure due to myocardial infarction. Molecular & Cellular Biochemistry 1996;164:285–290.

100. Gupta RC, Mishra S, Mishima T, Goldstein S, Sabbah HN. Reduced sarcoplasmic reticulum Ca(2+)-uptake and expression of phospholamban in left ventricular myocardium of dogs with heart failure. J Mol Cell Cardiol 1999;31:1381–1389.

101. Kiss E, Ball NA, Kranias EG, Walsh RA. Differential changes in cardiac phospholamban and sarcoplasmic reticular Ca(2+)-ATPase protein levels. Effects on Ca2+ transport and mechanics in compensated pressure-overload hypertrophy and congestive heart failure. Circ Res 1995;77:759–764.

102. Hasenfuss G, Reinecke H, Studer R, et al. Relation between myocardial function and expression of sarcoplasmic reticulum Ca(2+)-ATPase in failing and nonfailing human myocardium. Circ Res 1994;75:434–442.

103. Currie S, Smith GL. Enhanced phosphorylation of phospholamban and downregulation of sarco/endoplasmic reticulum Ca2+ ATPase type 2 (SERCA 2) in cardiac sarcoplasmic reticulum from rabbits with heart failure. Cardiovasc Res 1999;41:135–146.

104. Pieske B, Kretschmann B, Meyer M, et al. Alterations in intracellular calcium handling associated with the inverse force-frequency relation in human dilated cardiomyopathy. Circulation 1995;92: 1169–1178.

105. Hasenfuss G, Mulieri LA, Leavitt BJ, Allen PD, Haeberle JR, Alpert NR. Alteration of contractile function and excitation-contraction coupling in dilated cardiomyopathy. Circ Res 1992;70: 1225–1232.

106. Meyer M, Schillinger W, Pieske B, et al. Alterations of sarcoplasmic reticulum proteins in failing human dilated cardiomyopathy. Circulation 1995;92:778–784.

107. Movsesian MA, Bristow MR, Krall J. Ca2+ uptake by cardiac sarcoplasmic reticulum from patients with idiopathic dilated cardiomyopathy. Circ Res 1989;65:1141–1144.

108. Schwinger RH, Munch G, Bolck B, Karczewski P, Krause EG, Erdmann E. Reduced Ca(2+)-sensitivity of SERCA 2a in failing human myocardium due to reduced serin-16 phospholamban phosphorylation. J Mol Cell Cardiol 1999;31:479–491.

109. Feldman AM, Ray PE, Silan CM, Mercer JA, Minobe W, Bristow MR. Selective gene expression in failing human heart. Quantification of steady-state levels of messenger RNA in endomyocardial biopsies using the polymerase chain reaction. Circulation 1991;83:1866–1872.

110. Movsesian MA, Karimi M, Green K, Jones LR. Ca(2+)-transporting ATPase, phospholamban, and calsequestrin levels in nonfailing and failing human myocardium. Circulation 1994;90:653–657.

111. Bohm M, Reiger B, Schwinger RH, Erdmann E. cAMP concentrations, cAMP dependent protein kinase activity, and phospholamban in non-failing and failing myocardium. Cardiovasc Res 1994;28:1713–1719.

112. Schmidt U, Hajjar RJ, Kim CS, Lebeche D, Doye AA, Gwathmey JK. Human heart failure: cAMP stimulation of SR Ca(2+)-ATPase activity and phosphorylation level of phospholamban. Am J Physiol 1999;277:H474–H480.
113. Hajjar RJ, Schmidt U, Kang JX, Matsui T, Rosenzweig A. Adenoviral gene transfer of phospholamban in isolated rat cardiomyocytes. Rescue effects by concomitant gene transfer of sarcoplasmic reticulum Ca(2+)-ATPase. Circ Res 1997;81:145–153.
114. Hajjar RJ, Kang JX, Gwathmey JK, Rosenzweig A. Physiological effects of adenoviral gene transfer of sarcoplasmic reticulum calcium ATPase in isolated rat myocytes. Circulation 1997;95:423–429.
115. Meyer M, Bluhm WF, He H, et al. Phospholamban-to-SERCA2 ratio controls the force-frequency relationship. Am J Physiol 1999;276:H779–H785.
116. Ito K, Yan X, Tajima M, Su Z, Barry WH, Lorell BH. Contractile reserve and intracellular calcium regulation in mouse myocytes from normal and hypertrophied failing hearts. Circ Res 2000;87: 588–595.
117. Brillantes AM, Allen P, Takahashi T, Izumo S, Marks AR. Differences in cardiac calcium release channel (ryanodine receptor) expression in myocardium from patients with end-stage heart failure caused by ischemic versus dilated cardiomyopathy [published erratum appears in Circ Res 1992; 71(6):1538]. Circ Res 1992;71:18–26.
118. Go LO, Moschella MC, Watras J, Handa KK, Fyfe BS, Marks AR. Differential regulation of two types of intracellular calcium release channels during end-stage heart failure. J Clin Invest 1995;95:888–894.
119. Marx SO, Reiken S, Hisamatsu Y, et al. PKA phosphorylation dissociates FKBP12.6 from the calcium release channel (ryanodine receptor): defective regulation in failing hearts. Cell 2000;101:365–376.
120. Ono K, Yano M, Ohkusa T, et al. Altered interaction of FKBP12.6 with ryanodine receptor as a cause of abnormal Ca(2+) release in heart failure. Cardiovasc Res 2000;48:323–331.
121. Yano M, Ono K, Ohkusa T, et al. Altered stoichiometry of FKBP12.6 versus ryanodine receptor as a cause of abnormal Ca(2+) leak through ryanodine receptor in heart failure. Circulation 2000;102: 2131–2136.
122. Hobai IA, O'Rourke B. Decreased sarcoplasmic reticulum calcium content is responsible for defective excitation-contraction coupling in canine heart failure. Circulation 2001;103:1577–1584.
123. Li S, Margulies KB, Cheng H, Houser SR. Calcium current and calcium transients are depressed in failing human ventricular myocytes and recover in patients supported with left ventricular assist devices. (Abstract). Circulation 1999;100:I60.
124. Flesch M, Schwinger RH, Schiffer F, et al. Evidence for functional relevance of an enhanced expression of the Na(+)-Ca2+ exchanger in failing human myocardium. Circulation 1996;94:992–1002.
125. Studer R, Reinecke H, Vetter R, Holtz J, Drexler H. Expression and function of the cardiac Na+/Ca2+ exchanger in postnatal development of the rat, in experimental-induced cardiac hypertrophy and in the failing human heart. Basic Res Cardiol 1997;92:53–58.
126. Yoshiyama M, Takeuchi K, Hanatani A, et al. Differences in expression of sarcoplasmic reticulum Ca2+-ATPase and Na+-Ca2+ exchanger genes between adjacent and remote noninfarcted myocardium after myocardial infarction. J Mol Cell Cardiol 1997;29:255–264.
127. Pogwizd SM, Qi M, Yuan W, Samarel AM, Bers DM. Upregulation of Na(+)/Ca(2+) exchanger expression and function in an arrhythmogenic rabbit model of heart failure [see comments]. Circ Res 1999;85:1009–1019.
128. Reinecke H, Studer R, Vetter R, Holtz J, Drexler H. Cardiac Na+/Ca2+ exchange activity in patients with end-stage heart failure. Cardiovasc Res 1996;31:48–54.
129. Hobai IA, O'Rourke B. Enhanced Ca(2+)-activated Na(+)-Ca(2+) exchange activity in canine pacing-induced heart failure. Circ Res 2000;87:690–698.
130. O'Rourke B, Kääb S, Kass DA, Tomaselli GF, Marbán E. Role of Ca2+-activated Cl-current in shaping the action potential of canine ventricular myocytes from normal and failing hearts. Biophysical J 1996;70:A373.
131. Gwathmey JK, Slawsky MT, Hajjar RJ, Briggs GM, Morgan JP. Role of intracellular calcium handling in force-interval relationships of human ventricular myocardium. J Clin Invest 1990;85:1599–1613.
132. Hasenfuss G, Reinecke H, Studer R, et al. Calcium cycling proteins and force-frequency relationship in heart failure. Basic Res Cardiol 1996;91:17–22.
133. Pieske B, Sutterlin M, Schmidt-Schweda S, et al. Diminished post-rest potentiation of contractile force in human dilated cardiomyopathy. Functional evidence for alterations in intracellular Ca2+ handling. J Clin Invest 1996;98:764–776.
134. Mattiello JA, Margulies KB, Jeevanandam V, Houser SR. Contribution of reverse-mode sodium-calcium exchange to contractions in failing human left ventricular myocytes. Cardiovasc Res 1998;37:424–431.

135. Volders PG, Sipido KR, Vos MA, et al. Downregulation of delayed rectifier K(+) currents in dogs with chronic complete atrioventricular block and acquired torsades de pointes. Circulation 1999;100: 2455–2461.

136. Ten Eick RE, Zhang K, Harvey RD, Bassett AL. Enhanced functional expression of transient outward current in hypertrophied feline myocytes. Cardiovascular Drugs & Therapy 1993;3:611–619.

137. Wettwer E, Amos GJ, Posival H, Ravens U. Transient outward current in human ventricular myocytes of subepicardial and subendocardial origin. Circ Res 1994;75:473–482.

138. Nabauer M, Beuckelmann DJ, Uberfuhr P, Steinbeck G. Regional differences in current density and rate-dependent properties of the transient outward current in subepicardial and subendocardial myocytes of human left ventricle. Circulation 1996;93:168–177.

139. Rosati B, Pan Z, Lypen S, et al. Regulation of KChIP2 potassium channel. J Physiol 2001;533: 119–125.

140. Xu H, Dixon JE, Barry DM, et al. Developmental analysis reveals mismatches in the expression of K+ channel alpha subunits and voltage-gated K+ channel currents in rat ventricular myocytes. J Gen Physiol 1996;108:405–419.

141. Wickenden AD, Kaprielian R, Parker TG, Jones OT, Backx PH. Effects of development and thyroid hormone on K+ currents and K+ channel gene expression in rat ventricle. J Physiol (Lond) 1997;504:271–286.

142. Jeck C, Pinto J, Boyden P. Transient outward currents in subendocardial Purkinje myocytes surviving in the infarcted heart. Circulation 1995;92:465–473.

143. Rozanski GJ, Xu Z, Zhang K, Patel KP. Altered K+ current of ventricular myocytes in rats with chronic myocardial infarction. Am J Physiol 1998;274:H259–H265.

144. Aimond F, Alvarez JL, Rauzier JM, Lorente P, Vassort G. Ionic basis of ventricular arrhythmias in remodeled rat heart during long-term myocardial infarction. Cardiovasc Res 1999;42:402–415.

145. Nabauer M, Barth A, Kääb S. A second calcium-independent transient outward current present in human left ventricular myocardium. Circulation 1998;98:1–231.

146. Blair TA, Roberds SL, Tamkun MM, Hartshorne RP. Functional characterization of RK5, a voltage-gated K+ channel cloned from the rat cardiovascular system. FEBS Lett 1991;295:211–213.

147. Po S, Snyders DJ, Baker R, Tamkun MM, Bennett PB. Functional expression of an inactivating potassium channel cloned from human heart. Circ Res 1992;71:732 736.

148. Dixon JE, Shi W, Wang HS, et al. Role of the Kv4.3 K+ channel in ventricular muscle. A molecular correlate for the transient outward current [published erratum appears in Circ Res 1997;80(1):147]. Circ Res 1996;79:659–668.

149. Kong W, Po S, Yamagishi T, Ashen MD, Stetten G, Tomaselli GF. Isolation and characterization of the human gene encoding the transient outward potassium current: further diversity by alternative mRNA splicing. Am J Physiol 1998;275:H1963–H1970.

150. Apkon M, Nerbonne JM. Alpha 1-adrenergic agonists selectively suppress voltage-dependent K+ current in rat ventricular myocytes. Proc Natl Acad Sci USA 1988;85:8756–8760.

151. Fedida D, Shimoni Y, Giles WR. A novel effect of norepinephrine on cardiac cells is mediated by alpha 1-adrenoceptors. Am J Physiol 1989;256:H1500–H1504.

152. Braun AP, Fedida D, Clark RB, Giles WR. Intracellular mechanisms for alpha 1-adrenergic regulation of the transient outward current in rabbit atrial myocytes. J Physiol (Lond) 1990;431:689–712.

153. Shimoni Y, Fiset C, Clark RB, Dixon JE, McKinnon D, Giles WR. Thyroid hormone regulates post-natal expression of transient K+ channel isoforms in rat ventricle. J Physiol (Lond) 1997;500:65–73.

154. Hoppe UC, Johns DC, Marban E, O'Rourke B. Manipulation of cellular excitability by cell fusion: effects of rapid introduction of transient outward K+ current on the guinea pig action potential. Circ Res 1999;84:964–972.

155. Greenstein JL, Wu R, Po S, Tomaselli GF, Winslow RL. Role of the calcium-independent transient outward current i(to1) in shaping action potential morphology and duration [In Process Citation]. Circ Res 2000;87:1026–1033.

156. Pogwizd SM, Schlotthauer K, Li L, Yuan W, Bers DM. Arrhythmogenesis and contractile dysfunction in heart failure: Roles of sodium-calcium exchange, inward rectifier potassium current, and residual beta-adrenergic responsiveness. Circ Res 2001;88:1159–1167.

157. Koumi S, Backer CL, Arentzen CE. Characterization of inwardly rectifying K+ channel in human cardiac myocytes. Alterations in channel behavior in myocytes isolated from patients with idiopathic dilated cardiomyopathy. Circulation 1995;92:164–174.

158. Furukawa T, Bassett AL, Furukawa N, Kimura S, Myerburg RJ. The ionic mechanism of reperfusion-induced early afterdepolarizations in feline left ventricular hypertrophy. J Clin Invest 1993;91: 1521–1531.
159. Vos MA, Verduyn SC, Gorgels AP, Lipcsei GC, Wellens HJ. Reproducible induction of early afterdepolarizations and torsade de pointes arrhythmias by d-sotalol and pacing in dogs with chronic atrioventricular block. Circulation 1995;91:864–872.
160. Vos MA, de Groot SH, Verduyn SC, et al. Enhanced susceptibility for acquired torsade de pointes arrhythmias in the dog with chronic, complete AV block is related to cardiac hypertrophy and electrical remodeling. Circulation 1998;98:1125–1135.
161. Jiang M, Cabo C, Yao J, Boyden PA, Tseng G. Delayed rectifier K currents have reduced amplitudes and altered kinetics in myocytes from infarcted canine ventricle. Cardiovasc Res 2000;48:34–43.
162. Yuan F, Pinto JM, Li Q, et al. Characteristics of I(K) and its response to quinidine in experimental healed myocardial infarction. J Cardiovasc Electrophysiol 1999;10:844–854.
163. Choy A-M, Kuperschmidt S, Lang CC, Pierson RN, Roden DM. Regional expression of HERG and KvLQT1 in heart failure. Circulation 1996;94:164.
164. Koumi SI, Martin RL, Sato R. Alterations in ATP-sensitive potassium channel sensitivity to ATP in failing human hearts. Am J Physiol 1997;272:H1656–H1665.
165. Dhalla NS, Dixon IM, Rupp H, Barwinsky J. Experimental congestive heart failure due to myocardial infarction: sarcolemmal receptors and cation transporters. Basic Res Cardiol 1991;86:13–23.
166. Houser SR, Freeman AR, Jaeger JM, et al. Resting potential changes associated with Na-K pump in failing heart muscle. Am J Physiol 1981;240:H168–H176.
167. Kjeldsen K, Bjerregaard P, Richter EA, Thomsen PE, Norgaard A. Na+,K+-ATPase concentration in rodent and human heart and skeletal muscle: apparent relation to muscle performance. Cardiovasc Res 1988;22:95–100.
168. Spinale FG, Clayton C, Tanaka R, et al. Myocardial Na+,K(+)-ATPase in tachycardia induced cardiomyopathy. J Mol Cell Cardiol 1992;24:277–294.
169. Zahler R, Gilmore-Hebert M, Sun W, Benz EJ. Na, K-ATPase isoform gene expression in normal and hypertrophied dog heart. Basic Res Cardiol 1996;91:256–266.
170. Schwinger RH, Bohm M, Erdmann E. Effectiveness of cardiac glycosides in human myocardium with and without "downregulated" beta-adrenoceptors. J Cardiovasc Pharmacol 1990;15:692–697.
171. Ranjan R, Chiamvimonvat N, Thakor NV, Tomaselli GF, Marban E. Mechanism of anode break stimulation in the heart. Biophys J 1998;74:1850–1863.
172. Baker K, Warren KS, Yellen G, Fishman MC. Defective "pacemaker" current (Ih) in a zebrafish mutant with a slow heart rate. Proc Natl Acad Sci USA 1997;94:4554–4559.
173. Cerbai E, Barbieri M, Mugelli A. Occurrence and properties of the hyperpolarization-activated current If in ventricular myocytes from normotensive and hypertensive rats during aging. Circulation 1996;94:1674–1681.
174. Hoppe UC, Jansen E, Sudkamp M, Beuckelmann DJ. Hyperpolarization-activated inward current in ventricular myocytes from normal and failing human hearts. Circulation 1998;97:55–65.
175. Smith JH, Green CR, Peters NS, Rothery S, Severs NJ. Altered patterns of gap junction distribution in ischemic heart disease. An immunohistochemical study of human myocardium using laser scanning confocal microscopy. Am J Pathol 1991;139:801–821.
176. Peters NS, Green CR, Poole-Wilson PA, Severs NJ. Reduced content of connexin43 gap junctions in ventricular myocardium from hypertrophied and ischemic human hearts. Circulation 1993;88: 864–875.
177. Dupont E, Matsushita T, Kaba RA, et al. Altered connexin expression in human congestive heart failure. J Mol Cell Cardiol 2001;33:359–371.
178. Lerner DL, Chapman Q, Green KG, Saffitz JE. Reversible down-regulation of connexin43 expression in acute cardiac allograft rejection. J Heart Lung Transplant 2001;20:93–97.
179. Jongsma HJ, Wilders R. Gap junctions in cardiovascular disease. Circ Res 2000;86:1193–1197.
180. Peters NS, Coromilas J, Severs NJ, Wit AL. Disturbed connexin-43 gap junction distribution correlates with the location of reentrant circuits in the epicardial border zone of healing canine infarcts that cause ventricular tachycardia. Circulation 1997;95:988–996.
181. Saffitz JE, Laing JG, Yamada KA. Connexin expression and turnover: implications for cardiac excitability. Circ Res 2000;86:723–728.
182. Beardslee MA, Lerner DL, Tadros PN, et al. Dephosphorylation and intracellular redistribution of ventricular connexin43 during electrical uncoupling induced by ischemia. Circ Res 2000;87:656–662.

183. Toyofuku T, Yabuki M, Otsu K, Kuzuya T, Tada M, Hori M. Functional role of c-Src in gap junctions of the cardiomyopathic heart. Circ Res 1999;85:672–681.
184. De Mello WC. Renin-angiotensin system and cell communication in the failing heart. Hypertension 1996;27:1267–1272.
185. De Mello WC. Impaired regulation of cell communication by beta-adrenergic receptor activation in the failing heart. Hypertension 1996;27:265–268.
186. Dodge SM, Beardslee MA, Darrow BJ, Green KG, Beyer EC, Saffitz JE. Effects of angiotensin II on expression of the gap junction channel protein connexin43 in neonatal rat ventricular myocytes. J Am Coll Cardiol 1998;32:800–807.
187. Gutstein DE, Morley GE, Tamaddon H, et al. Conduction slowing and sudden arrhythmic death in mice with cardiac-restricted inactivation of connexin43. Circ Res 2001;88:333–339.
188. Bristow MR, Ginsburg R, Minobe W, et al. Decreased catecholamine sensitivity and beta-adrenergic-receptor density in failing human hearts. N Engl J Med 1982;307:205–211.
189. Bristow MR. Changes in myocardial and vascular receptors in heart failure. J Am Coll Cardiol 1993;22:61A–71A.
190. Bohm M, Flesch M, Schnabel P. Beta-adrenergic signal transduction in the failing and hypertrophied myocardium. J Mol Med 1997;75:842–848.
191. Dash R, Kadambi VJ, Schmidt AG, et al. Interactions between phospholamban and beta-adrenergic drive may lead to cardiomyopathy and early mortality. Circulation 2001;103:889–896.
192. Zhou YY, Cheng H, Bogdanov KY, et al. Localized cAMP-dependent signaling mediates beta 2–adrenergic modulation of cardiac excitation-contraction coupling. Am J Physiol 1997;273: H1611–H1618.
193. Bristow MR, Ginsburg R, Umans V, et al. Beta 1- and beta 2-adrenergic-receptor subpopulations in nonfailing and failing human ventricular myocardium: coupling of both receptor subtypes to muscle contraction and selective beta 1-receptor down-regulation in heart failure. Circ Res 1986;59:297–309.
194. Bristow MR, Hershberger RE, Port JD, et al. Beta-adrenergic pathways in nonfailing and failing human ventricular myocardium. Circulation 1990;82:112–125.
195. Kiuchi K, Shannon RP, Komamura K, et al. Myocardial beta-adrenergic receptor function during the development of pacing-induced heart failure. J Clin Invest 1993;91:907–914.
196. Brodde OE. Beta 1- and beta 2-adrenoceptors in the human heart: properties, function, and alterations in chronic heart failure. Pharmacol Rev 1991;43:203–242.
197. Bristow MR, Hershberger RE, Port JD, Minobe W, Rasmussen R. Beta 1- and beta 2-adrenergic receptor-mediated adenylate cyclase stimulation in nonfailing and failing human ventricular myocardium. Mol Pharmacol 1989;35:295–303.
198. Bristow MR, Anderson FL, Port JD, et al. Differences in beta-adrenergic neuroeffector mechanisms in ischemic versus idiopathic dilated cardiomyopathy. Circulation 1991;84:1024–1039.
199. Xiao RP, Avdonin P, Zhou YY, et al. Coupling of beta2-adrenoceptor to Gi proteins and its physiological relevance in murine cardiac myocytes. Circ Res 1999;84:43–52.
200. Communal C, Singh K, Pimentel DR, Colucci WS. Norepinephrine stimulates apoptosis in adult rat ventricular myocytes by activation of the beta-adrenergic pathway. Circulation 1998;98:1329–1334.
201. Chesley A, Lundberg MS, Asai T, et al. The beta(2)-adrenergic receptor delivers an antiapoptotic signal to cardiac myocytes through G(i)-dependent coupling to phosphatidylinositol 3'-kinase. Circ Res 2000;87:1172–1179.
202. Eschenhagen T, Mende U, Nose M, et al. Increased messenger RNA level of the inhibitory G-protein alpha subunit Gialpha-2 in human end-stage heart failure. Circ Res 1992;70:688–696.
203. Bohm M, Eschenhagen T, Gierschik P, et al. Radioimmunochemical quantification of Gi alpha in right and left ventricles from patients with ischaemic and dilated cardiomyopathy and predominant left ventricular failure. J Mol Cell Cardiol 1994;26:133–149.
204. Feldman AM, Cates AE, Veazey WB, et al. Increase of the 40,000-mol wt pertussis toxin substrate (G protein) in the failing human heart. J Clin Invest 1988;82:189–197.
205. Mende U, Eschenhagen T, Geertz B, et al. Isoprenaline-induced increase in the 40/41 kDa pertussis toxin substrates and functional consequences on contractile response in rat heart. Naunyn Schmiedebergs Arch Pharmacol 1992;345:44–50.
206. Bodor GS, Oakeley AE, Allen PD, Crimmins DL, Ladenson JH, Anderson PA. Troponin I phosphorylation in the normal and failing adult human heart. Circulation 1997;96:1495–1500.
207. Zakhary DR, Moravec CS, Stewart RW, Bond M. Protein kinase A (PKA)-dependent troponin-I phosphorylation and PKA regulatory subunits are decreased in human dilated cardiomyopathy. Circulation 1999;99:505–510.

208. Zakhary DR, Fink MA, Ruehr MA, Bond M. Selectivity and regulation of A-kinase anchoring proteins in the heart: the role of autophosphorylation of the Type-II regulatory subunit of cAMP-dependent protein kinase. J Biol Chem 2000;275:41389–41395.

209. Dell'Acqua ML, Scott JD. Protein kinase A anchoring. J Biol Chem 1997;272:12881–12884.

210. Huang LJ, Durick K, Weiner JA, Chun J, Taylor SS. Identification of a novel protein kinase A anchoring protein that binds both type I and type II regulatory subunits. J Biol Chem 1997;272:8057–8064.

211. Zakhary DR, Moravec CS, Bond M. Regulation of PKA binding to AKAPs in the heart: alterations in human heart failure. Circulation 2000;101:1459–1464.

212. Hartzell HC, Duchatelle-Gourdon I. Regulation of the cardiac delayed rectifier K current by neurotransmitters and magnesium. Cardiovasc Drugs Ther 1993;7 Suppl 3:547–554.

213. Fedida D, Braun AP, Giles WR. Alpha 1-adrenoceptors in myocardium: functional aspects and transmembrane signaling mechanisms. Physiol Rev 1993;73:469–487.

214. Spinale FG, Holzgrefe HH, Mukherjee R, et al. Angiotensin-converting enzyme inhibition and the progression of congestive cardiomyopathy. Effects on left ventricular and myocyte structure and function. Circulation 1995;92:562–578.

215. Spinale FG, Coker ML, Thomas CV, Walker JD, Mukherjee R, Hebbar L. Time-dependent changes in matrix metalloproteinase activity and expression during the progression of congestive heart failure: relation to ventricular and myocyte function. Circ Res 1998;82:482–495.

216. Dollery CM, McEwan JR, Henney AM. Matrix metalloproteinases and cardiovascular disease. Circ Res 1995;77:863–868.

217. Weber KT, Brilla CG. Pathological hypertrophy and cardiac interstitium. Fibrosis and renin-angiotensin-aldosterone system. Circulation 1991;83:1849–1865.

218. Volders PG, Willems IE, Cleutjens JP, Arends JW, Havenith MG, Daemen MJ. Interstitial collagen is increased in the non-infarcted human myocardium after myocardial infarction. J Mol Cell Cardiol 1993;25:1317–1323.

219. van Krimpen C, Schoemaker RG, Cleutjens JP, et al. Angiotensin I converting enzyme inhibitors and cardiac remodeling. Basic Res Cardiol 1991;86:149–155.

220. Smits JF, van Krimpen C, Schoemaker RG, Cleutjens JP, Daemen MJ. Angiotensin II receptor blockade after myocardial infarction in rats: effects on hemodynamics, myocardial DNA synthesis, and interstitial collagen content. J Cardiovasc Pharmacol 1992;20:772–778.

221. Beltrami CA, Finato N, Rocco M, et al. Structural basis of end-stage failure in ischemic cardiomyopathy in humans. Circulation 1994;89:151–163.

222. Spinale FG, Coker ML, Krombach SR, et al. Matrix metalloproteinase inhibition during the development of congestive heart failure: effects on left ventricular dimensions and function. Circ Res 1999; 85:364–376.

223. Thomas CV, Coker ML, Zellner JL, Handy JR, Crumbley AJ, Spinale FG. Increased matrix metalloproteinase activity and selective upregulation in LV myocardium from patients with end-stage dilated cardiomyopathy. Circulation 1998;97:1708–1715.

224. Li YY, Feldman AM, Sun Y, McTiernan CF. Differential expression of tissue inhibitors of metalloproteinases in the failing human heart. Circulation 1998;98:1728–1734.

225. Weber KT. Extracellular matrix remodeling in heart failure: a role for de novo angiotensin II generation. Circulation 1997;96:4065–4082.

226. Everett AD, Tufro-McReddie A, Fisher A, Gomez RA. Angiotensin receptor regulates cardiac hypertrophy and transforming growth factor-beta 1 expression. Hypertension 1994;23:587–592.

227. Reiss K, Capasso JM, Huang HE, Meggs LG, Li P, Anversa P. ANG II receptors, c-myc, and c-jun in myocytes after myocardial infarction and ventricular failure. Am J Physiol 1993;264:H760–H769.

228. Barlucchi L, Leri A, Dostal DE, et al. Canine ventricular myocytes possess a renin-angiotensin system that is upregulated with heart failure. Circ Res 2001;88:298–304.

229. Aronson RS, Ming Z. Cellular mechanisms of arrhythmias in hypertrophied and failing myocardium. Circulation 1993;87:76–83.

230. Li HG, Jones DL, Yee R, Klein GJ. Electrophysiologic substrate associated with pacing-induced heart failure in dogs: potential value of programmed stimulation in predicting sudden death. J Am Coll Cardiol 1992;19:444–449.

231. Li HG, Jones DL, Yee R, Klein GJ. Arrhythmogenic effects of catecholamines are decreased in heart failure induced by rapid pacing in dogs. Am J Physiol 1993;265:H1654–H1662.

232. Wang Z, Taylor LK, Denney WD, Hansen DE. Initiation of ventricular extrasystoles by myocardial stretch in chronically dilated and failing canine left ventricle. Circulation 1994;90:2022–2031.

233. Nuss HB, Kääb S, Kass DA, Tomaselli GF, Marbán E. Increased susceptibility to arrhythmogenic early after depolarization and oscillatory prepotentials in failing canine ventricular myocytes. Circulation 1995;92:434.

234. Aronson RS. Afterpotentials and triggered activity in hypertrophied myocardium from rats with renal hypertension. Circ Res 1981;48:720–727.

235. Ben-David J, Zipes DP, Ayers GM, Pride HP. Canine left ventricular hypertrophy predisposes to ventricular tachycardia induction by phase 2 early afterdepolarizations after administration of BAY K 8644. Journal of the American College of Cardiology 1992;20:1576–1584.

236. Koster OF, Szigeti GP, Beuckelmann DJ. Characterization of a [Ca2+]i-dependent current in human atrial and ventricular cardiomyocytes in the absence of Na+ and K+. Cardiovasc Res 1999;41:175–187.

237. Sipido KR, Volders PG, de Groot SH, et al. Enhanced Ca(2+) release and Na/Ca exchange activity in hypertrophied canine ventricular myocytes: potential link between contractile adaptation and arrhythmogenesis. Circulation 2000;102:2137–2144.

238. Shechter JA, O'Connor KM, Friehling TD, Mark R, Uboh C, Kowey PR. Electrophysiologic effects of left ventricular hypertrophy in the intact cat. Am J Hypertens 1989;2:81–85.

239. Gelband H, Bassett AL. Depressed transmembrane potentials during experimentally induced ventricular failure in cats. Circ Res 1973;32:625–634.

240. Noma A, Tsuboi N. Dependence of junctional conductance on proton, calcium and magnesium ions in cardiac paired cells of guinea-pig. J Physiol (Lond) 1987;382:193–211.

241. Maurer P, Weingart R. Cell pairs isolated from adult guinea pig and rat hearts: effects of [Ca2+]i on nexal membrane resistance. Pflugers Arch 1987;409:394–402.

242. Peters NS. New insights into myocardial arrhythmogenesis: distribution of gap-junctional coupling in normal, ischaemic and hypertrophied human hearts. Clin Sci (Colch) 1996;90:447–452.

243. Severs NJ. Gap junction alterations in the failing heart. Eur Heart J 1994;15 Suppl D:53–57.

244. Spach MS, Heidlage JF, Dolber PC, Barr RC. Electrophysiological effects of remodeling cardiac gap junctions and cell size: experimental and model studies of normal cardiac growth. Circ Res 2000;86:302–311.

245. Spach MS, Boineau JP. Microfibrosis produces electrical load variations due to loss of side-to-side cell connections: a major mechanism of structural heart disease arrhythmias. Pacing Clin Electrophysiol 1997;20:397–413.

246. Marbán E. Heart failure: the electrophysiologic connection. J Cardiovasc Electrophysiol 1999;10:1425–1428.

247. Tomaselli GF, Marbán E. Electrophysiological remodeling in hypertrophy and heart failure. Cardiovascular Research 1999: in press.

248. Porter TR, Eckberg DL, Fritsch JM, et al. Autonomic pathophysiology in heart failure patients. Sympathetic-cholinergic interrelations. J Clin Invest 1990;85:1362–1371.

249. Cohn JN, Levine TB, Olivari MT, et al. Plasma norepinephrine as a guide to prognosis in patients with chronic congestive heart failure. N Engl J Med 1984;311:819–823.

8

Ischemia-Related Changes in Repolarization

André G. Kléber, MD
and Michiel J. Janse, MD, PhD

CONTENTS

INTRODUCTION
CHANGES IN THE TRANSMEMBRANE ACTION POTENTIAL AND UNDERLYING MECHANISMS
SUBACUTE AND CHRONIC INFARCTION
REPERFUSION
CONSEQUENCES OF CHANGED REPOLARIZATION FOR IMPULSE CONDUCTION AND ARRHYTHMOGENESIS
REFERENCES

INTRODUCTION

Myocardial ischemia and infarction are among the most common disorders in the western world and are, and will remain, the leading cause of mortality and morbidity *(1)*. A large part of mortality is related to the occurrence of ventricular arrhythmias leading to sudden cardiac death *(2)*. Acute myocardial ischemia caused by coronary thrombosis results in changes of myocardial electrical function that occur within minutes after cessation or reduction of coronary flow. If the individual survives the acute phase of myocardial ischemia, further electrophysiological changes occur over a period of several days in surviving myocardial layers and in Purkinje fibers. In the course of several months, the electrophysiological properties of surviving cells return close to normal *(3)*. In this stage of a healed infarct, it is the architecture of the surviving myocardial strands that forms the substrate for reentrant arrhythmias *(4)*.

Over the past decades, a variety of experimental models have been used to define the basic characteristics of ischemic arrhythmias *(5)*. Although a large number of variables may contribute to arrhythmogenesis in a patient with coronary artery disease (genetic predisposition, extent of collateral circulation, activity of the sympathetic nervous system, antiarrhythmic or other drugs, remodeling by preexisting heart disease or general disease *[6]*), a distinction of different stages of myocardial ischemia using classical animal models has proven to be useful *(3)*. In this chapter we will concentrate on the

From: *Contemporary Cardiology: Cardiac Repolarization: Bridging Basic and Clinical Science*
Edited by: I. Gussak et al. © Humana Press Inc., Totowa, NJ

153

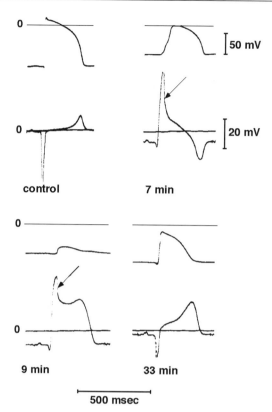

Fig. 1. Transmembrane action potentials (top trace in each panel) and extracellular electrograms (bottom trace) during the early phase of ischemia in an isolated perfused pig heart. The time in minutes after coronary artery occlusion is indicated beneath each panel. Electrical activity virtually disappeared after 9 min (lower left), but improved after 33 min (unpublished observation).

changes in cellular electrophysiology and related mechanisms during the various phases following acute coronary artery occlusion and discuss their relevance for arrhythmogenesis. In some pathologic settings, for example the long QT-syndromes or drug related arrhythmias, specific ion channels involved in repolarization are affected. Accordingly, a discussion about related mechanisms can be very specific *(7,8)*. However, in myocardial ischemia, changes in repolarization often arise indirectly from alterations in resting potential, depolarization, ccll-to-cell coupling, and tissue architecture. This complexity implies that a comprehensive description of changes in repolarization has to include a discussion of all these factors as well.

The first reports on the changes in the transmembrane action potential appeared in the 1970s when it became possible to directly record with microelectrodes from the intact heart *(9)*.

CHANGES IN THE TRANSMEMBRANE ACTION POTENTIAL AND UNDERLYING MECHANISMS

Acute Ischemia

Description of action potential changes: Malignant ventricular arrhythmias are observed within minutes after total occlusion of a coronary artery and divided in 2 phases,

5 min occl.

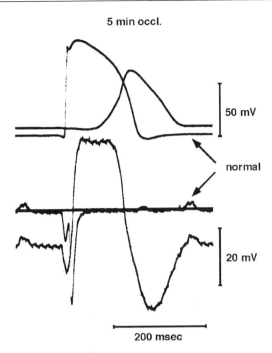

Fig. 2. Transmembrane potentials and local direct current electrograms before (top) and 5 min after coronary occlusion. Note alteration in action potential amplitude and duration (modified from ref *12*).

the so-called type 1A (2–10 min after occlusion) and type 1B (15 to 30 min) arrhythmias *(10)*. It has been shown that the early phase type 1A arrhythmias are entirely due to changes in the transmembrane action potential *(11)*. Figures 1–3 depict the essential changes of the transmembrane action potential after total arrest of coronary flow. A microelectrode recording is shown together with a local DC ("direct-current") extracellular electrogram in Figs. 1–3. Within the first minute resting membrane potential decreases (i.e., it shifts to more positive values) and the action potential amplitude, upstroke velocity and action potential duration decrease *(9,12)*. After approx 8–10 min the ischemic cells become unexcitable at levels of resting membrane potentials of 55–60 mV *(13)*. When the occlusion is maintained, a temporary recovery of the action potential is observed after 20 to 30 min *(11)*. In ischemia, the action potential shortening occurs concomitantly to the changes in resting potential and action potential amplitude. This is in contrast to hypoxia, where a marked shortening of the action potential occurs with only a slight decrease in resting potential and action potential upstroke *(14)*.

As shown in Fig. 2, a period of electrical alternans frequently precedes the period of inexcitability, especially at rapid heart rates *(9,12)*. The electrical alternans in acute ischemia does involve both action amplitude and duration. Several reports have shown that it often precedes the onset of ventricular tachycardia and fibrillation *(9,15–19)*. As discussed below, the phenomenon of electrical alternans may be explained by several ion current systems becoming unstable. Moreover, electrical alternans does not occur uniformly throughout the myocardium but is observed regionally, whereby the various regions may be out of phase *(15)*. Although the changes shown in Figs. 1 and 2 stand for the prototype of the transmembrane potentials during ischemia, several factors affect

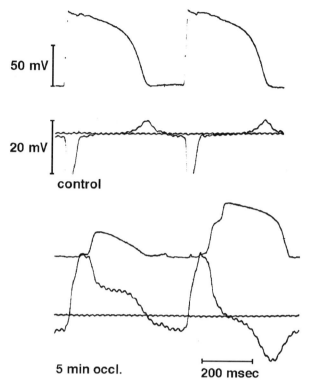

50 mV

20 mV

control

5 min occl.   200 msec

Fig. 3. Transmembrane potentials and local DC current electrograms recorded from an *in situ* dog heart. Potentials before and after 5 min of coronary artery occlusion are superimposed, using as time reference the stimulus artifact on the atrium. Note the extreme delay in activation of the ischemic subepicardial cell, which is depolarized at the time normoxic cells are already repolarized. The negative "T wave" in the local electrogram represents in fact the intrinsic deflection caused by the delayed activity (modified from ref *11).*

repolarization in addition. Already during normal cardiac propagation, the time of normal repolarization is determined by both the conduction time and action potential duration. The effect of conduction time on local repolarization can get extreme during acute ischemia, as shown in Fig. 3. In this example local depolarization in an ischemic region occurs at a time when the normal myocardium is already repolarized, because of conduction slowing in the ischemic myocardium. Thus even in presence of a relatively short action potential, repolarization of the ischemic zone may outlast repolarization of normoxic tissue. This delayed repolarization can produce marked T-wave negativity, and has been associated with arrhythmogenesis *(15).* A further characteristic of regional myocardial ischemia is electrical inhomogeneity. Although the alterations in action potentials shown on Figs. 1–3 are typical for the ischemic center, ischemic cells close to the border with normal myocardium have almost normal resting potentials, normal action potential amplitude and upstroke but show marked action shortening. The mechanisms underlying electrical inhomogeneity are complex and will be discussed below.

Mechanisms: Very important determinants of the cellular electrical changes in myocardial ischemia are anoxia, accumulation of extracellular K^+, and acidification. Although many of the observed changes can be qualitatively mimicked by elevation of extracellular

K^+ alone, addition on anoxia and acidification exert a marked potentiating effect *(14,20)*. As shown by measurements using K^+-sensitive electrodes, extracellular K^+ can rise up 15–20 mmoles/liter within 10 min of ischemia *(21,22)*. This early cellular K^+ loss is fully reversible upon reperfusion, therefore it is not caused by injury of the cell membrane but has been attributed to a regulatory change in cellular ion homeostasis. Although a large number of studies on this subject have been carried out, there is still no unanimity on the underlying mechanisms *(23,24)*. The following mechanisms have been postulated: Partial inhibition of Na^+/K^+ pumping, opening of ATP-sensitive K^+ channels, opening of nonspecific cation channels with concomitant Na^+ overload, compensatory K^+ movement secondary to anion shifts. A major problem in analyzing this mechanism resides in the fact that the overall loss of cellular K^+ is very small in relation to the whole cellular K^+ pool. The large change of K^+ concentration is then a consequence of the small volume of extracellular compartment relative to intracellular space *(25)*. This has made it exceedingly difficult to prove whether the cellular K^+ loss is compensated by a movement of other cations in the opposite direction or a movement of anions in the same direction. However, the observation that the changes in resting membrane potential closely follow the changes in the level of extracellular K^+, speaks against the hypothesis that opening of ATP-sensitive K^+ channels or other K^+ channels are responsible for net K^+ loss. This is because K^+ ion distribution is expected always to be in electro-chemical equilibrium if a large K^+ electrical conductance, for example in presence of opened ATP-sensitive K channels, largely dominates over the other ion conductances. Thus, from the mechanistic point of view, the loss of cellular K^+ in acute ischemia seems to be rather a consequence than a cause of the change in resting potential. However, more accurate methods to determine changes in intracellular ions, such as Na^+, K^+, and Ca^{2+}, need to become available to answer to this question in a fully conclusive way.

Relevant for the discussion of changes in repolarization and arrhythmogenesis is the observation that extracellular K^+ levels are not homogenous within the ischemic zone. In general, they decrease from the center to the ischemic border and gradients in the order of 8 mmoles/liter have been recorded over a distance in the order of 1 cm *(see* Fig. 4) *(26)*. Importantly, these differences occur in "fully ischemic tissue," i.e., at sites were oxygen supply is completely absent. Two mechanisms have been invoked: 1. Convective movement of extracellular K^+ ions toward the normoxic myocardium owing to the mechanical heart action *(26)*. 2. Diffusion of CO_2 trapped in the ischemic myocardium *(27,28)*.

In an experimental system where CO_2 accumulation in the ischemic tissue was completely prevented, no cellular K^+ loss and extracellular accumulation occurred *(27)*.

At the phenomenological level, most of the electrical changes in acute ischemia can be described on the basis of inhomogeneity of extracellular K^+. The shortening of the transmembrane action potential in elevated K^+ is a classical observation in cardiac electrophysiology, and it is mainly because of an increase in conductance of I_{K1} *(29,30)*. In normoxic cells, at normal resting potentials, the recovery of excitability is primarily voltage dependent, and excitability is restored as the cell repolarizes. Consequently, the period of relative refractoriness falls into the repolarization phase of the transmembrane action potential. In partially depolarized fibers, recovery from inactivation of both the fast Na and the slower Ca inward current is markedly delayed, until many milliseconds after completion of repolarization *(31)*. This so-called "postrepolarization refractoriness" has been demonstrated in ischemic myocardium *(9,32)* and is considered as a key change for explaining the electrical behavior of the tissue *(see* Fig. 5). Thus, in the center of the

REGIONAL ISCHEMIA L.A.D.
10 min

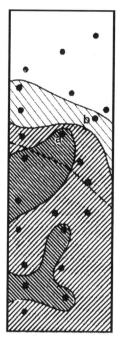 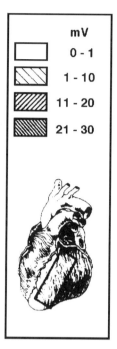

Fig. 4. Map of the distribution of the changes in potassium equilibrium potential (delta E_K in mV), as measured from multiple K^+-sensitive electrodes in and around the ischemic zone, 10 min after occlusion of the left coronary artery (inset depicts the area where the electrodes (black dots in left panel) were inserted). Delta E_K of 0–1 mV corresponds to an extracellular K^+ concentration around 4 mmole/liter, delta E_K of 28 mV corresponds to an extracellular K^+ concentration around 12 mmole/liter (modified from ref *73*).

ischemic zone, at high levels of extracellular K^+ and low levels of resting membrane potentials, refractory periods are actually longer than those in normal myocardium despite action potential shortening *(9)*. In contrast, refractory periods of ischemic cells close to the border where action potentials are short but resting potentials are close to normal, refractory periods are shorter than in normoxic myocardium *(33)*.

If severe hypoxia or anoxia are produced in absence of elevation of extracellular K^+, the refractory period shortens along with the shortening of the action potential *(14)*. Action potential shortening in anoxia can be extreme, and action potential of 30 ms in duration or shorter have been described *(34)*. However, such short action potentials are never observed in ischemic myocardium. Opening of ATP-sensitive K^+ channels is the main cause of action potential shortening in myocardial anoxia and can be reversed by application of ATP-sensitive K channel inhibitors *(35,36)*. Adding anoxia to elevated extracellular K^+ potentiates the changes in transmembrane action potentials observed in presence of elevated K^+ alone and closely mimic the changes observed in ischemia *(14)*. Thus, postrepolarization refractoriness is more marked in combined hypoxia/elevated K^+ conditions vs elevated $[K^+]_o$ alone. Comparison of action potentials recorded from the ischemic border zone with those from the ischemic center suggests that the extracellular K^+ accumulation is the dominating change in the center, while anoxia mostly determines

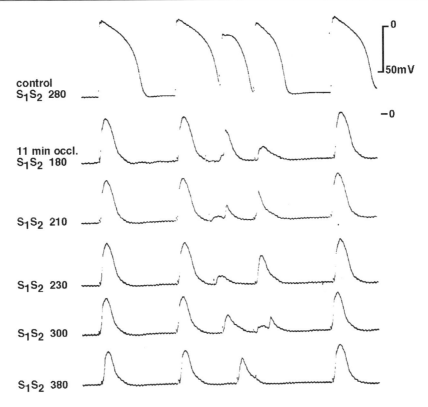

control
$S_1 S_2$ 280

11 min occl.
$S_1 S_2$ 180

$S_1 S_2$ 210

$S_1 S_2$ 230

$S_1 S_2$ 300

$S_1 S_2$ 380

Fig. 5. Postrepolarization refractoriness. Stimuli were delivered within 1 mm from the cell recorded from. In the control situation, recovery of excitability closely follows repolarization. After 11 min of ischemia, the heart responds to a premature test stimulus with a coupling interval that is 100 ms shorter than in the control situation. However the latency between stimulus and response is now more than 100 ms, indicating that the strong stimulus must have excited tissue at a distance with a shorter refractory period. At a coupling interval of 230 ms there is minimal latency but a very small response. Action potential with a significant amplitude and minimal latency occurred only when the coupling interval was increased to 380 ms, well after completion of repolarization (modified from ref *9*).

alterations close to the border. Both the fact that only a very few open ATP-sensitive K^+ channels are necessary to produce marked action potentials shortening and the large variability of ATP-levels reported from ischemic myocardium make it difficult to quantitatively predict the role of ATP-sensitive K^+ channels in acute ischemia. However, it is important to note that in the presence of marked extracellular K^+ elevation, activation of $I_{K,ATP}$ may not only affect action potential duration but exerts an additional depressing effect on propagation spread *(37)*. Activation of $I_{K,ATP}$ is likely to be one factor explaining the observation that conduction block in ischemia occurs at lower levels of extracellular K^+ than during perfusion with elevated K^+ alone *(38)*.

Humoral factors released from arterial thrombi are among further important factors modifying electrical changes and arrhythmogenesis in acute ischemia *(39–41)*. Thus, a thrombotic coronary artery occlusion is more arrhythmogenic than ischemia produced by coronary artery ligation. This is owing to the fact that during the first three minutes of ischemia, the electrophysiological changes occur more rapidly during a thrombotic occlusion than during coronary ligation *(41)*. The precise factors mediating these changes are as yet unknown. It has been suggested that phospholipoglycerides produced in the vascular endothelium, as a consequence of the release of serin proteases from the thrombi, are responsible *(40,42)*. It is well-known that very small amounts of released lysophophoglycerides are highly arrhythmogenic.

SUBACUTE AND CHRONIC INFARCTION

Although most of the myocardial cells subjected to persistent ischemia die within 40 to 60 min, some cells receive enough oxygen, either via collateral vessels (subepicardial cells) or via the cavitary blood (subendocardial Purkinje fibers), and survive. These surviving cells develop changes in ion channel function that alter their transmembrane potentials. This process is referred to as electrical remodeling (for a recent review *see 43*). Most experimental studies have been performed on infarcted canine hearts either 24 to 48 h or 4–5 d after the onset of ischemia. Only a few studies have been published on human hearts with a chronic infarct. Changes after 24 to 48 h in Purkinje fibers differ from those in subepicardial muscle: Purkinje fibers have a reduced resting potential and upstroke velocity and a prolonged action potential duration, whereas subepicardial cells show a shortening and a triangularization of the action potential. Figure 6 shows how the changes of action potential configuration of subepicardial cells overlying the infarct develop over time and return to normal within several months.

The increase in action potential duration of the subendocardial Purkinje fibers that are in close proximity to the infarct is most likely owing to a decrease in the density of both the transient outward current and the inward rectifier I_{K1} *(44,45)*, as well as a reduced density of the L-type Ca^{2+} current *(46)*. In the surviving epicardial cells, maximum upstroke velocity is reduced, because of a decrease in the density in the inward Na^+ current, whereas recovery from inactivation of the Na^+ current is prolonged, which accounts for postrepolarization refractoriness *(47)*. The density of the L-type Ca^{2+} current is reduced to about 2/3 of the control values *(48)*. The loss of the notch in the early repolarization phase is caused by a reduction of the non-Ca-dependent transient outward current *(49)*. In addition, densities of I_{Kr} and I_{Ks} are significantly reduced *(50)*. This alone would retard repolarization, but apparently the reduction in the L-type Ca^{2+} current overrules the changes in the delayed rectifier current accounting for the shortening and the triangularization of the action potential in the epicardial border zone.

There are also changes in cell-to-cell electrical coupling, caused by both a redistribution and reduction of Cx43 proteins *(51)*.

As shown in Fig. 6, the action potential of the epicardial border zone returns to normal over a period of several months. Microelectrode recordings from surviving myocardial bundles in human infarcts, many months after the acute event, have shown that transmembrane potential are close to normal *(52)*. Conduction velocity parallel to fiber orientation in these bundles is normal as well *(4,53)*. These findings suggest that the initial downregulation of ion channels is followed by normalization of ion channel function, but voltage clamp data from late phases of myocardial infarction are lacking.

In addition to the changes in fibers that survive within an infarct, the remote noninfarcted myocardium also undergoes electrical remodeling, because of the development of hypertrophy. The action potential of hypertrophied myocardium is prolonged,

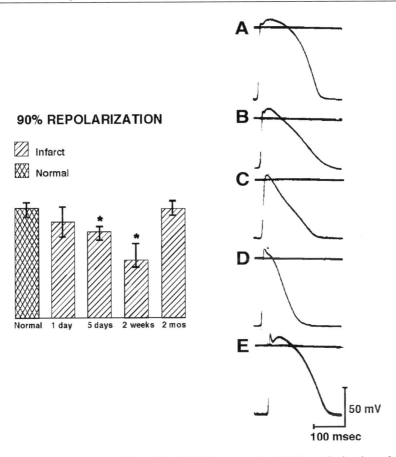

Fig. 6. Changes in action potential duration (APD) measured at 90% repolarization of subepicardial muscle fibers overlying a canine infarct with increasing time after coronary artery occlusion. At the right are shown representative transmembrane potentials: **(A)** is from a noninfarcted heart, **(B)** from a 1-day-old infarct, **(C)** from a 5-day-old infarct, **(D)** from a 2-week-old infarct, and **(E)** from a 2-month-old infarct (modified from ref *74*).

especially at slow heart rates *(54)* and this is mainly caused by a reduction in the density of the delayed rectifier I_K *(55)*.

REPERFUSION

It has been known for more than 150 yr that reperfusion following a relatively brief ischemic episode of 10–20 min frequently results in ventricular fibrillation *(56)*. Microelectrode recordings from the reperfused myocardium have shown that resting membrane potential, action potential amplitude, and upstroke velocity return to normal within seconds following restoration of coronary flow. Resting membrane potentials even hyperpolarize. In addition there is a very marked shortening of the action potential to durations that are shorter than those in normal myocardium *(57)*. The reperfused cells take up K^+ ions at a rapid rate so that extracellular K^+ concentrations become even lower than those in normally perfused myocardium *(57)*. The reasons for the marked action potential shortening have not been conclusively established, but enhanced activity of the sodium potassium pump, stimulated by intracellular Na^+ overload, may be responsible. This activity would also explain depletion of extracellular potassium. The arrhythmias are initiated by a focal mechanism within the reperfused zone, most likely delayed afterdepolarizations caused by intracellular Ca^{2+} overload. Since refractory periods of the reperfused myocardium are shorter than those of the normal myocardium, unidirectional block develops at the border between reperfused and normal myocardium, setting up reentrant excitation in the reperfused zone (57).

CONSEQUENCES OF CHANGED REPOLARIZATION FOR IMPULSE CONDUCTION AND ARRHYTHMOGENESIS

Typically, arrhythmia mechanisms are subdivided in disturbances of impulse generation and impulse conduction. In most types of arrhythmias these mechanisms may coexist. In the setting of myocardial ischemia both circus movement with reentry and focal mechanisms can initiate ventricular tachycardias, although the persistence of tachycardias and the deterioration to ventricular fibrillation is mostly owing to reentry (58–60). A further useful subdivision of arrhythmia mechanisms relates to the underlying anatomical substrate. Although reentry and circus movement in early ischemia are mostly because of functional, reversible changes at the level of the transmembrane action potential and/ or to cell-to-cell uncoupling at the level of the gap junctions, the disappearance of the dense myocardial architecture and the highly discontinuous tissue excitation in scars form the arrhythmogenic substrate in chronic infarction (3,52).

Changes in repolarization of the cardiac action potential are known to be important for both reentry and focal initiation. In reentrant arrhythmias during acute ischemia, which occur in absence of major anatomical obstacles, changes in repolarization are relevant in two respects. First, shortening of the transmembrane action potential in moderately depolarized tissue, especially in the ischemic border zone, is expected to decrease the wavelength of excitation. This decrease reduces the size of reentrant circuits and increases the likelihood for reentry to occur (61). Second, changes in repolarization are nonhomogenous in ischemic tissue. In regions with steep gradients in repolarization propagating waves are deviated in the direction of the excitable sites. At such sites rotating waves develop that may either initiate reentrant arrhythmias or form daughter waves in the case of a transition from ventricular tachycardia to ventricular fibrillation.

As mentioned previously, the interpretation of changes in repolarization for arrhythmogenesis in acute ischemia is not straightforward. This is because the recovery of Na^+ and Ca^{2+} channels from previous inactivation is markedly prolonged (31). It is this prolongation of the recovery time constants rather than the level of membrane potential during repolarization that determines excitability. In this situation, the previous "history" of excitation of a given site in the myocardium determines whether or not and at what velocity the impulse is conducted. Sites with a very long recovery interval, for instance sites which showed conduction block during the previous passage of excitation, conduct the impulse faster than sites with a short recovery interval (11,15). On the basis of theoretical work, the slope of the recovery curve of action potential duration has been postulated as a key parameter determining whether a reentrant tachycardia splits into multiple waves and produces fibrillation (62,63). It needs to be emphasized that in depolarized tissue the recovery of the action potential upstroke (recovery from inactivation of Na^+ channels) and concomitant recovery of propagation rather than action potential duration is the most important change.

Changes in action potential duration reflecting changes in net repolarizing ion current are also involved in the generation of early and late afterdepolarizations (EAD's and DAD's). These oscillations of membrane potential that can initiate arrhythmias are the result of an imbalance between repolarizing and depolarizing currents during the plateau phase of the action potential *(64)* and after repolarization *(65)*. As a consequence, changes in repolarizing currents during ischemia may affect the generation of focal arrhythmias. During acute ischemia, there is evidence that foci which are located in the ischemic border zone do contribute to arrhythmia initiation. However, with exception of the reperfusion arrhythmias, there is no direct evidence that either EAD's or DAD's play a role in acute ischemia. The fact that the overall membrane conductance is increased in depolarized ischemic tissue (probably owing to a substantial part to activation of ATP-sensitive K^+ channels) suggest that the membrane potential is stabilized by strong repolarizing forces which prevent formation of EAD's and DAD's. Accordingly it was not possible to elicit DAD's in simulated ischemia and hypoxia, when extracellular $[K^+]_o$ was elevated *(66)*. This makes the formation of DAD's unlikely in the center of the ischemic zone but does not rule out their generation in the ischemic border zone.

A detailed discussion about the relation between changes in repolarization and arrhythmogenesis in subacute and chronic infarction is difficult because of lack of experimental data. In general, the arrhythmias in the four days healing infarct and in the several months-old healed infarct are determined by structural changes, either involving changes in distribution and number of gap junctions in the epicardial border zone, or the separation of viable muscle bundles by connective tissue in chronic infarcts *(51,67)*. There are both arguments that speak against and in favor of structural changes modulating the role of repolarization in arrhythmogenesis.

In the case of discontinuous conduction (or "zig-zag" conduction) in infarcts scars, propagation along the surviving fiber bundles occurs at a normal rate, although large delays are present if the wave encounters fiber branches or any site with a discontinuity in tissue architecture *(52,53)*. At such sites wavefronts are forced to turn around tissue obstacles and lose speed because of curvature and current-to-load mismatch *(68)*. The result of the changing propagation velocity in reentrant circuits is the formation of a so-called excitable gap between the head of the wavefront and the tail of the previous wavefront *(69,70)*. The more excitable gaps are formed, the less changes in repolarization will affect the behavior of the circulating excitation.

Although one may postulate as a general rule that changes in repolarization are more relevant for functionally than structurally-defined reentry, the degree of cell-to-cell coupling and tissue architecture is likely to affect repolarization *per se*, in addition to the state, the type and the quantity of repolarizing ion channels. Intrinsic differences in repolarization between different groups of cells may be unmasked by partial uncoupling. In normal, well coupled myocardium, electrotonic current flow during repolarization will attenuate the intrinsic differences by lengthening short action potentials and shortening long ones. Thus, in general terms, it may be said that electrical uncoupling will increase the dispersion in repolarization. In the setting of acute ischemia it was shown that the so-called 1B type arrhythmias occur during the onset of cell-to-cell uncoupling *(71)*. It has been shown that a certain degree of coupling between the markedly depolarized, and inexcitable midmyocardium and the less depolarized subepicardium is needed to depress excitability in the surviving subepicardial layers and cause reentry. When uncoupling between mid-myocardium and subepicardium is complete, electrical activity in the subepicardium recovers and reentry no longer occurs *(72)*.

A further mechanism that involves the changes in repolarization in ischemia relates to the excitatory role of injury current. Injury current flows across the border between ischemic and nonischemic tissue consequently to local differences in membrane potential. Usually, injury currents are invoked to explain the changes in the QT- and ST-segments of the electrocardiogram. If the ischemic repolarization is markedly delayed, the currents of injury produce a deep negative T-wave in the ischemic region. The associated flow of injury current is large and exerts a depolarizing effect in the nonischemic region, Thus it may facilitate excitation in the nonischemic border zone and contribute to arrhythmogenesis *(12,13)*.

REFERENCES

1. Murray C, Lopez A. Alternative projections of mortality and disability by cause 1990–2020: Global burden of disease study. The Lancet 1997;349:1498–1504.
2. Myerburg R, Spooner P. Opportunities for sudden death prevention: directions for new clinical and basic research. Cardiovasc Res 2001;50:177–185.
3. Janse MJ, Wit AL. Electrophysiological mechanisms of ventricular arrhythmias resulting from myocardial ischemia and infarction. Physiol Rev 1989;69:1049–1169.
4. de Bakker JM, Coronel R, Tasseron S, et al. Ventricular tachycardia in the infarcted, Langendorff-perfused human heart: role of the arrangement of surviving cardiac fibers. J Am Coll Cardiol 1990;15:1594–1607.
5. Janse MJ, Opthof T, Kléber AG. Animal models of cardiac arrhythmias. Cardiovasc Res 1998;39:165–177.
6. Myerburg RJ, Interian A, Mitrani RM, Kessler KM, Castellanos A. Frequency of sudden cardiac death and profiles of risk. Am J Cardiol 1997;80:10F–19F.
7. Priori SG, Barhanin J, Hauer RN, et al. Genetic and molecular basis of cardiac arrhythmias: impact on clinical management part III. Circulation 1999;99:674–681.
8. Priori SG, Barhanin J, Hauer RN, et al. Genetic and molecular basis of cardiac arrhythmias: impact on clinical management parts I and II. Circulation 1999;99:518–528.
9. Downar E, Janse MJ, Durrer D. The effect of acute coronary artery occlusion on subepicardial transmembrane potentials in the intact porcine heart. Circulation 1977;56:217–224.
10. Kaplinsky E, Ogawa S, Balke CW, Dreifus LS. Two periods of early ventricular arrhythmias in the canine acute myocardial infarction model. Circulation 1979;60:397–403.
11. Janse MJ, Kléber AG. Electrophysiological changes and ventricular arrhythmias in the early phase of regional myocardial ischemia. Circ Res 1981;49:1069–1081.
12. Kléber AG, Janse MJ, van Capelle FJL, Durrer D. Mechanism and time course of S-T and T-Q segment changes during acute regional myocardial ischemia in the pig heart determined by extracellular and intracellular recordings. Circ Res 1978;42:603–613.
13. Kléber AG. Resting membrane potential, extracellular potassium activity, and intracellular sodium activity during acute global ischemia in isolated perfused guinea pig hearts. Circ Res 1983;52:442–450.
14. Kodama I, Wilde AAM, Janse MJ, Durrer D, Yamada K. Combined effects of hypoxia, hyperkalemia and acidosis on membrane action potential and excitability of guinea-pig ventricular muscle. J Mol Cell Cardiol 1984;16:247–259.
15. Janse MJ, van Capelle FJ, Morsink H, et al. Flow of "injury" current and patterns of excitation during early ventricular arrhythmias in acute regional myocardial ischemia in isolated porcine and canine hearts. Evidence for two different arrhythmogenic mechanisms. Circ Res 1980;47:151–165.
16. Nearing BD, Oesterle SN, Verrier RL. Quantification of ischaemia induced vulnerability by precordial T wave alternans analysis in dog and human. Cardiovasc Res 1994;28:1440–1449.
17. Pastore JM, Girouard SD, Laurita KR, Akar FG, Rosenbaum DS. Mechanism linking T-wave alternans to the genesis of cardiac fibrillation. Circulation 1999;99:1385–1394.
18. Rosenbaum DS, Albrecht P, Cohen RJ. Predicting sudden cardiac death from T wave alternans of the surface electrocardiogram: promise and pitfalls. J Cardiovasc Electrophysiol 1996;7:1095–1111.
19. Verrier RL, Nearing BD. Electrophysiologic basis for T wave alternans as an index of vulnerability to ventricular fibrillation. J Cardiovasc Electrophysiol 1994;5:445–461.

20. Moréna H, Janse MJ, Fiolet JWT, Krieger WJG, Crijns H, Durrer D. Comparison of the effects of regional ischemia, hypoxia, hyperkalemia, and acidosis on intracellular and extracellular potentials and metablolism in the isolated porcine heart. Circ Res 1980;46:635–646.
21. Hirche H, Franz C, Bös L, Lang R, Schramm M. Myocardial extracellular K^+ and H^+ increase and noradrenaline release as possible cause of early arrhythmias following acute coronary artery occlusion in pigs. J Mol Cell Cardiol 1980;12:579–593.
22. Hill JL, Gettes LS. Effect of acute coronary artery occlusion on local myocardial extracellular K^+ activty in swine. Circulation 1980;61:768–778.
23. Kléber AG. Extracellular potassium accumulation in acute myocardial ischemia. J Mol Cell Cardiol 1984;16:389–394.
24. Wilde AA, Aksnes G. Myocardial potassium loss and cell depolarisation in ischaemia and hypoxia. Cardiovasc Res 1995;29:1–15.
25. Johnson EA. First electrocardiographic sign of myocardial ischemia: an electrophysiological conjecture. Circulation 1976;53 (Suppl. I):82–84.
26. Coronel R. Distribution of extracellular potassium during myocardial ischemia. Thesis, University of Amsterdam, The Netherlands. 1988.
27. Cascio WE, Yan G-X, Kléber AG. Early changes in extracellular potassium in ischemic rabbit myocardium. The role of extracellular carbon dioxide accumulation and diffusion. Circ Res 1992;70:409–422.
28. Case RB, Felix A, Castellana FS. Rate of rise of myocardial PCO2 during early myocardial ischemia in the dog. Circ Res 1979;45:324–330.
29. Weidmann S. Shortening of the cardiac action potential due to a brief injection of KCl following the onset of activity. J Physiol (Lond) 1956;132:157–163.
30. Carmeliet E, Vereecke J. Electrogenesis of the action potential and automaticity. In: Berne RAPS, ed. Handbook of Physiology, the Cardiovascular System. Maryland: 1979:269–334.
31. Gettes LS, Reuter H. Slow recovery from inactivation of inward currents in mammalian myocardial fibres. J Physiol (Lond) 1974;240:703–724.
32. Scherlag BJ, El-Sherif N, Hope R, Lazzara R. Characterization and localization of ventricular arrhythmias resulting from myocardial ischemia and infarction. Circ Res 1974;35:372–383.
33. Janse MJ, Capucci A, Coronel R, Fabius MA. Variability of recovery of excitability in the normal canine and the ischaemic porcine heart. Eur Heart J 1985;6:41–52.
34. Riegger CB, Alperovich G, Kléber AG. Effect of oxygen withdrawal on active and passive electrical properties of arterially perfused rabbit ventricular muscle. Circ Res 1989;64:532–541.
35. Wilde AAM, Escande D, Schumacher CA, Thuringer D, Mestre M, Fiolet JWT, Janse MJ. Potassium accumulation in the globally ischemic mammalian heart. Circ Res 1990;67:835–843.
36. Gasser RA, Vaughan-Jones RD. Mechanism of potassium efflux and action potential shortening during ischemia in isolated mammalian cardiac muscle. J Physiol (Lond) 1990;431:713–741.
37. Shaw RM, Rudy Y. Electrophysiologic effects of acute myocardial ischemia: a theoretical study of altered cell excitability and action potential duration. Cardiovasc Res 1997;35:256–272.
38. Kléber AG, Janse MJ, Wilms Schopmann FJ, Wilde AA, Coronel R. Changes in conduction velocity during acute ischemia in ventricular myocardium of the isolated porcine heart. Circulation 1986;73: 189–198.
39. Goldstein JA, Butterfield MC, Ohnishi Y, Shelton TJ, Corr PB. Arrhythmogenic influence of intracoronary thrombosis during acute myocardial ischemia. Circulation 1994;90:139–147.
40. McHowat J, Corr PB. Thrombin-induced release of lysophosphatidylcholine from endothelial cells. J Biol Chem 1993;268:15605–15610.
41. Coronel R, Wilms-Schopman FJ, Janse MJ. Profibrillatory effects of intracoronary thrombus in acute regional ischemia of the in situ porcine heart. Circulation 1997;96:3985–3991.
42. Park TH, McHowat J, Wolf RA, Corr PB. Increased lysophosphatidylcholine content induced by thrombin receptor stimulation in adult rabbit cardiac ventricular myocytes. Cardiovasc Res 1994;28:1263–1268.
43. Pinto JM, Boyden PA. Electrical remodeling in ischemia and infarction. Cardiovasc Res 1999;42: 284–297.
44. Boyden PA, Albala A, Dresdner KP. Electrophysiology and ultrastructure of canine subendocardial Purkinje cells isolated from control and 24-hour infarcted hearts. Circ Res 1989;65:955–970.
45. Pinto JM, Boyden PA. Reduced inward rectifying and increased E-4031-sensitive K^+ current density in arrhythmogenic subendocardial purkinje myocytes from the infarcted heart. J Cardiovasc Electrophysiol 1998;9:299–311.

46. Boyden PA, Pinto JM. Reduced calcium currents in subendocardial Purkinje myocytes that survive in the 24- and 48-hour infarcted heart. Circulation 1994;89:2747–2759.

47. Pu J, Boyden PA. Alterations of Na^+ currents in myocytes from epicardial border zone of the infarcted heart. A possible ionic mechanism for reduced excitability and postrepolarization refractoriness. Circ Res 1997;81:110–119.

48. Aggarwal R, Boyden PA. Diminished Ca^{2+} and Ba^{2+} currents in myocytes surviving in the epicardial border zone of the 5-day infarcted canine heart. Circ Res 1995;77:1180–1191.

49. Lue WM, Boyden PA. Abnormal electrical properties of myocytes from chronically infarcted canine heart. Alterations in Vmax and the transient outward current. Circulation 1992;85:1175–1188.

50. Jiang M, Yao J-A, Wymore R, Boyden P, Tseng G-N. Suppressed transcription and function of delayed rectifier K channels in post myocardial infarction canine ventricle. Circulation. 1998;98:I-818 (abstract).

51. Peters NS, Coromilas J, Severs NJ, Wit AL. Disturbed connexin-43 gap junction distribution correlates with the location of reentrant circuits in the epicardial border zone of healing canine infarcts that cause ventricular tachycardia. Circulation 1997;95:988–996.

52. De Bakker JMT, Van Capelle FJL, Janse MJ, et al. Slow conduction in the infarcted human heart–zigzag course of activation. Circulation 1993;88:915–926.

53. de Bakker JM, van Capelle FJ, Janse MJ, et al. Reentry as a cause of ventricular tachycardia in patients with chronic ischemic heart disease: electrophysiologic and anatomic correlation. Circulation 1988;77:589–606.

54. Vermeulen JT, McGuire MA, Opthof T, et al. Triggered activity and automaticity in ventricular trabeculae of failing human and rabbit hearts. Cardiovasc Res 1994;28:1547–1554.

55. Qin D, Zhang ZH, Caref EB, Boutjdir M, Jain P, el-Sherif N. Cellular and ionic basis of arrhythmias in postinfarction remodeled ventricular myocardium. Circ Res 1996;79:461–473.

56. Conheim J, Schulthess–Rechberg A. Ueber die Folgen der Kranzarterienverschliessung für das Herz. Virchows Arch 1881;85:503–537.

57. Coronel R, Wilms-Schopman FJ, Opthof T, Cinca J, Fiolet JW, Janse MJ. Reperfusion arrhythmias in isolated perfused pig hearts. Inhomogeneities in extracellular potassium, ST and TQ potentials, and transmembrane action potentials. Circ Res 1992;71:1131–1142.

58. Janse MJ, Kléber AG, Capucci A, Coronel R, Wilms-Schopmann FJG. Electrophysiological basis for arrhythmias caused by acute ischemia. Role of subendocardium. J Moll Cell Cardiol 1986;18:339–355.

59. Pogwizd SM, Corr PB. Reentrant and nonreentrant mechanisms contribute to arrhythmogenesis during early myocardial ischemia: results using three-dimensional mapping. Circ Res 1987;61: 352–371.

60. Pogwizd SM, Corr PB. Mechanisms underlying the development of ventricular fibrillation during early myocardial ischemia. Circ Res 1990;66:672–695.

61. Allessie MA, Bonke FIM, Schopman FJC. Circus movement in rabbit atrial muscle as a mechanism of tachycardia. III. The "leading circle" concept: a new model of circus movement in cardiac tissue without the involvement of an anatomical obstacle. Circ Res 1977;41:9–18.

62. Qu Z, Weiss JN, Garfinkel A. Cardiac electrical restitution properties and stability of reentrant spiral waves: a simulation study. Am J Physiol 1999;276:H269–H283.

63. Karma A. Spiral breakup in model equations of action potential propagation in cardiac tissue. Phys Rev Lett 1993;71:1103–1106.

64. Zeng J, Rudy Y. Early afterdepolarizations in cardiac myocytes: mechanism and rate dependence. Biophys J 1995;68:949–964.

65. Wit A, Rosen M. Afterdepolarization and triggered activity. In: Fozzard H, Katz, AM, Haber E, Jennings R, Morgan H, eds. The Heart and the Cardiovascular System. New York: Raven Press, 1986:1449–1490.

66. Saman S, Coetzee WA, Opie LH. Inhibition by simulated ischemia or hypoxia of delayed afterdepolarizations provoked by cyclic AMP: significance for ischemic and reperfusion arrhythmias. J Mol Cell Cardiol 1988;20:91–95.

67. Peters NS, Wit AL. Myocardial architecture and ventricular arrhythmogenesis. Circulation 1998; 97:1746–1754.

68. Fast VG, Kléber AG. Role of wavefront curvature in propagation of cardiac impulse. Cardiovasc Res 1997;33:258–271.

69. Schalij MJ. Anisotropic conduction and ventricular tachycardia. In: Maastricht, The Netherlands: Rijksuniversiteit Limburg, 1988.

70. Schalij MJ, Lammers WEJP, Rensma PL, Allessie MA. Anisotropic conduction and reentry in perfused epicardium of rabbit left ventricle. Am J Physiol 1992;263:H1466–H1478.
71. Smith WT, Fleet WF, Johnson TA, Engle CL, Cascio WE. The 1b phase of ventricular arrhythmias in ischemic in situ porcine heart is related to changes in cell-to-cell coupling. Circulation 1995;92: 3051–3060.
72. De Groot J, FJG W-S, Opthof T, Remme C, Coronel R. Late ventricular arrhythmias during acute regional ischemia in the isolated blood perfused pig heart. Cardiovasc Res 2001;50:362–372.
73. Coronel R, Fiolet JW, Wilms-Schopman FJ, et al. Distribution of extracellular potassium and its relation to electrophysiologic changes during acute myocardial ischemia in the isolated perfused porcine heart. Circulation 1988;77:1125–1138.
74. Ursell PC, Gardner PI, Albala A, Fenoglio JJ, Wit AL. Structural and electrophysiological changes in the epicardial border zone of canine myocardial infarcts during infarct healing. Circ Res 1985;56: 436–451.

9

The Long QT Syndrome
Molecular and Genetic Aspects

Carlo Napolitano, MD, PhD
and Silvia G. Priori, MD, PhD

INTRODUCTION

The Long QT syndrome (LQTS) is an inherited arrhythmogenic disease occurring in the structurally normal heart that may cause sudden death and that usually manifests in children and teen-agers *(1)*. The prevalence of this disorder is still undefined, however it is estimated to be between 1:10000–1:5000.

Initially, two LQTS variants were described: An autosomal dominant form (Romano-Ward [RW] syndrome) and an autosomal recessive form (Jervell Lange Nielsen [JLN] syndrome). Both variants share the cardiac phenotype that includes QT interval prolongation and ventricular tachyarrhythmias manifesting as syncope or sudden cardiac death (SCD); the autosomal recessive JLN syndrome is also associated with sensineural deafness *(2)*. Recently it has become evident that other diseases combine repolarization abnormalities and extracardiac phenotypes, namely Andersen Syndrome (AS) and LQTS with syndactyly. These conditions will be reviewed here as they may be considered as novel and rare variants of LQTS.

Since the autosomal dominant RW syndrome *(3,4)* is by far the most common variant, most of the data reported in the following sections of this chapter pertain to this latter group of patients.

MOLECULAR BASIS AND PATHOPHYSIOLOGY

An understanding of the pathophysiological substrate of LQTS dates back only a decade to a period when Keating and coworkers discovered, within few years, five of the

From: *Contemporary Cardiology: Cardiac Repolarization: Bridging Basic and Clinical Science*
Edited by: I. Gussak et al. © Humana Press Inc., Totowa, NJ

genes accounting for the disease. It became clear that the distinguishing cardiac pheno-type of LQTS is caused by dysfunction of cardiac ion channels. Therefore, the typical presentation is that of a "primary electrical disease" in which the development of cardiac arrhythmias is not associated with structural abnormalities.

The Long QT Syndrome Genes

Five genes and six loci have been associated with the LQTS phenotype. Based on this information 50–60% of the clinically affected patients may be successfully genotyped *(5,6)*: In the remaining patients a genetic defect of unknown gene(s) is postulated. The application of molecular genetics to the study of LQTS started in 1991 with the linkage analysis investigation that led to the identification of the first locus (LQT1) on chromo-some 11p15.1 *(7)*. Shortly after, three additional loci were identified on chromosome 7q35–36 (LQT2), 3p21–23 (LQT3) *(8)* and 4q25–27 (LQT4) *(9)*. The gene on chromo-some 11, *KCNQ1* was identified using positional cloning *(10)* whereas candidate gene approach led to the identification of the genes *KCNH2* and *SCN5A* mapping on chromo-some 7 and 3, respectively *(11,12)*. The gene on chromosome 4 (LQT4) is still unknown. More recently, mutations in two genes on chromosome 21p22.1 were also reported: *KCNE1* (LQT5) and *KCNE2* (LQT6) *(13,14)*. The five genes so far identified encode for subunits of ion channels that play a critical role in controlling the excitability of cardiac myocytes.

The application of molecular screening to LQTS patients has led to the identification of large number of mutations thus providing data to define the molecular epidemi-ology of the disease. It is now clear that we should adopt the term "long QT Syn-dromes" to refer to a family of diseases that share common phenotypes (polymorphic VT and prolonged repolarization) but that also present distinguishing features (triggers precipitating cardiac events, morphology of QT interval, lethality of the disease, response to therapy) (Table 1).

In the following paragraphs we will briefly outline some aspects of the functional abnormalities of mutated ion channels and how they influence ventricular repolarization and susceptibility to cardiac arrhythmias. We will then summarize current knowledge on genotype-phenotype correlation trying to highlight their practical implications in the management of LQTS patients.

In Vitro Characterization of LQTS Mutations

The proteins encoded by the LQTS genes constitute transmembrane channels conduct-ing ionic currents that control myocardial cells excitability. Four of the five genes thus far identified encode for subunits of ion channels conducting the delayed rectifier current. The *KCNQ1* and *KCNE1* genes encode respectively the alpha and the beta subunits of the slow component of the cardiac delayed rectifier current (I_{Ks}) *(15,16)*. *KCNH2* and *KCNE2* encode respectively the alpha and for the beta subunits of I_{Kr}, the rapid component of the delayed rectifier *(14,17)*. The fifth gene related to the RW syndrome is *SCN5A* encoding for the cardiac sodium channel protein conducting I_{Na} *(18)*. Most of the probands affected by any of the five genetic variants of LQTS present missense mutations leading to the substitution of a single amino acid. At variance with other genetic diseases in which few mutations account for most clinical cases, in LQTS nearly every family carries a different mutation. As a consequence there are hundreds of DNA mutations that cause the pheno-type of LQTS suggesting that almost any constitutive amino acid is critical to ensure the

Table 1
Clinical and Genetic Variants of LQTS

	Symbol	OMIM ID	Gene(s)	Cardiac Phenotype	Associated Phenotype
Romano-Ward	LQT1	192500	KCNQ1	QT interval prolongation – Polymophic VT – VF – 2:1 AV block (rare)	None
	LQT2	152427	KCNH2	"	None
	LQT3	603830	SCN5A	"	None
	LQT4	600919	Unknown	+ Sinus node dysfunction and atrial fibrillation	None
	LQT5	176261	KCNE1	QT interval prolongation – Polymophic VT – VF	None
	LQT6	603796	KCNE2	"	None
Jervell and Lange-Nielsen	JLN1 JLN2	220400*	KCNQ1 KCNE1	" "	Sensineural deafness
LQTS with syndactyly	LQTsynd	601005	Unknown	QT interval prolongation – Polymophic VT – VF – 2:1 AV block	Syndactyly – congenital heart defect – metabolic disturbances (?)
Andersen Syndrome	LQTAnd	170390	KCNJ2	QT interval prolongation – bidirectional VT – "giant" U waves	Periodic paralysis – dysmorphic features

VT = Ventricular Tachycardia; VF = Ventricular Fibrillation; * = the OMIM database has only one entry for JLN1 and JLN2.

171

appropriate function of a cardiac ion channel. So far little correlation has been found between the position of a mutation and its functional consequence, and mutations localized in distant regions may cause very similar functional abnormalities. Even less evident is the relationship between the severity of the dysfunction assessed in vitro and the clinical phenotype as carriers of "severe" mutations may have a completely silent phenotype (Fig. 1). The only evidence of regional cluster of mutations that share a relatively similar phenotype is represented by the defects in the carboxy-terminus of *KCNQ1* that are often associated with a milder phenotype *(19)*.

In vitro expression studies have demonstrated that the prolongation of QT interval is the counterpart of action potential prolongation caused by either a "reduction" of repolarizing (outward) currents or an increase of "depolarizing" (inward) currents. Accordingly, it has been shown that defects in the potassium channel subunits cause a "loss of function" *(13,20,21)*, whereas mutations in the cardiac sodium channel cause a "gain of function" *(22,23)*.

Functional studies have demonstrated that DNA mutations cause the LQTS phenotype by different mechanisms. Genetic defects that truncate the protein (in heterozygous individuals) lead to a 50% reduction in the number of functional channels (haploinsufficiency). Other mutations may lead to a similar effect by hampering intracellular protein trafficking thus preventing incorporation of ion channels in the cellular membrane *(24,25)*. However, most of the defects exert more subtle actions as they alter the kinetic and the gating properties of the channels *(26–29)* or they alter the interaction with the beta subunits *(15)*: In these instances the functional consequence of a mutation is therefore difficult to predict based on the type of DNA defect and therefore expression of ion channels mutations identified in LQTS patients is a most important tool for the understanding of the disease.

GENOTYPE-PHENOTYPE IN ROMANO-WARD LONG QT SYNDROME

A reliable quantification of the relative prevalence of the LQTS genetic variants is now available based on extensive genotyping experience worldwide. There is a general agreement that mutations in *KCNQ1* and *KCNH2* account for the majority of genotyped individuals. In the report by Splawsky et al. *(5)* LQT2 (*KCNH2* related LQTS variant) was more common than LQT1 (*KCNQ1* related LQTS), although in our experience LQT1 is the most prevalent variant *(6)*. Overall, in any case the LQT1 and LQT2 subtypes account for 70–80% of genotyped patients.

The LQTS variant associated with *SCN5A* mutations, LQT3, is less common, accounting for 10–15% of genotyped patients *(6)*. Mutations in *KCNE1* and *KCNE2* accounting for LQT5 and LQT6 respectively, are rare and include no more than 5% of the genotyped cases *(5,6)*. So far, no additional families have been linked to the chromosome 4 locus (LQT4) after the first identification *(9)*. Most of the genotype-phenotype studies in LQTS have therefore targeted the LQT1, LQT2, and LQT3 forms of the disease.

Morphology of the QT-T Wave

The analysis of electrocardiographic parameters by genotype showed that T wave morphology allows the distinction between LQT1, LQT2, and LQT3 subtypes with an

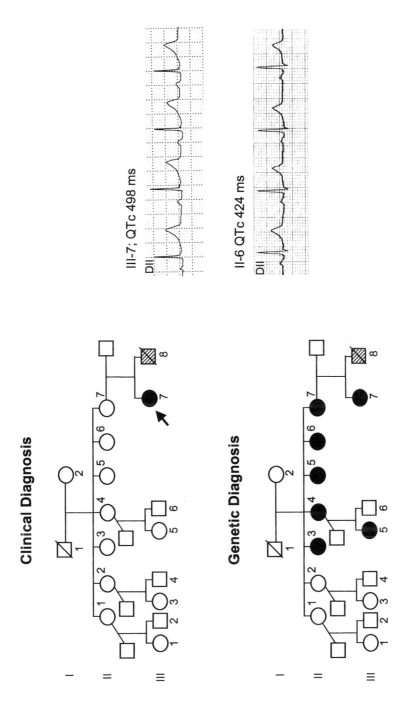

Fig. 1. Incomplete penetrance in LQTS. Comparison between clinical diagnosis (upper left panel) and molecular diagnosis (lower left panel) in a family with low penetrance. Filled symbols represent individuals identified as affected. The right panel depicts two representative ECG tracings from individual II-7 (proband) with prolonged QT interval and II-6 with normal QT interval despite being mutation carrier.

173

acceptable degree of accuracy. Three distinguishing patterns were initially identified by Moss and coworkers *(30)* and other variants have subsequently been identified by Zhang et al. *(31)*. Despite analysis of the ECG is not a substitute for genetic testing, it may be very helpful in directing genetic screening allowing faster and cheaper genotyping of affected individuals.

QT Interval Adaptation to Heart Rate

Following the initial identification of the LQTS genes we developed a cellular model mimicking the electrophysiological consequences of the mutations at cellular level. The results of this study pointed to a differential degree of adaptation of action potential duration to changes in cycle length, thus suggesting possible differences in QT interval behavior in the affected patients. This hypothesis was indeed confirmed by the clinical observations showing that LQT3 patients may present faster and more pronounced adaptation to fast rates than LQT1 patients *(32)*. This distinguishing behavior of QT interval may be used to differentiate among genetic variants of the disease *(33,34)*. Furthermore, an impaired adaptation may increase the diagnostic performance of QT interval measurement in borderline cases *(34)* (Fig. 2).

The ability of LQT3 to shorten their QT interval during tachycardia supports the view that LQT3 patients may benefit from receiving a pacemaker. However, there is no evidence demonstrating that the QT shortening at relatively faster rates is associated with a reduction of the risk of arrhythmias.

Severity of Clinical Manifestations

Analysis of cardiac events by genotype showed that the event rate (number of syncope and cardiac arrests) is higher in LQT1 patients than in other genetic variants. However, although the number of events is lowest in LQT3, mortality is higher suggesting that lethality of cardiac events in also higher in this variant *(35)*.

Triggers for Cardiac Events

The evaluation of the events preceding syncope and or cardiac arrest (defined as "triggers") suggests that there are specific factors that precipitate arrhythmias in the different phenotype. It is widely recognized that the majority of patients with LQTS experience cardiac events during increased sympathetic activation induced either by physical exercise or stress and emotion. However, some patients may experience cardiac events at rest and even during sleep. It is now known that carriers of *KCNQ1* mutations gene have 68% of events during physical or emotional stress and only 9% at rest, whereas LQT3 and LQT2 have a higher probability of developing events at rest or during sleep (64% and 49%) *(36)*. This observation fits the current understanding of the pathophysiology of the different genetic variants of LQTS. Since the defective protein in LQT1 is the I_{Ks} component of I_K, that causes action potential duration (APD) shortening at fast rates and during adrenergic stimulation it is expected that in LQT1 patients repolarization is more vulnerable during physical or emotional stress. Additional novel observations have linked "triggering events" to a specific genetic variant of the disease. For example, auditory stimuli are almost invariably observed in LQT2 patients *(37)* whereas swimming is mainly associated with cardiac events in LQT1 patients *(38,39)*.

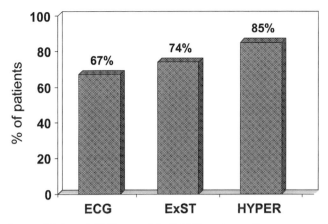

Fig. 2. Diagnostic sensitivity of QT interval in LQT1 patients. Bars represent the percentage of LQT1 showing QTc interval above the normal limits (440 ms in males and 460 ms in females) at baseline ECG or during relative tachycardia obtained at exercise stress test (ExST) or hyperventilation (HYPER).

Clinical Implications of Genotype-Phenotype Correlations

Genotype-phenotype correlation have practical implications for diagnosis and for risk stratification. For example when the genetic defect is known, gene-specific lifestyle modifications may be recommended: Physical activity (especially swimming) is to be more rigorously avoided in LQT1 patients, whereas, given the highest lethality of cardiac events, a more aggressive therapeutic strategy might be considered in LQT3.

Although useful information having emerged from genotype-phenotype studies, several limitations have also been highlighted and should be taken into consideration when managing patients from genotyped families.

Although individuals with a genetic defect on the same gene share some common characteristics, they also present large variability in the severity of clinical manifestations. Data available from genotyped patients demonstrate that the presence of a genetic defect in a gene that causes LQTS should be regarded as a risk factor that "increases the probability of cardiac arrhythmias." However, given the incomplete penetrance of the disease *(40)* (Fig. 1) it is impossible to define the individual risk of events in each subject. Even within the same family, mutation carriers may show large variability of clinical manifestations ranging from being asymptomatic to developing ventricular fibrillation. Extreme examples of low penetrance in LQTS are the demonstration of a recessively inherited RW phenotype *(41)* and by the case of drug-induced torsades de pointes *(42,43)*, where the mutation only constitute a predisposing factor for cardiac events.

Similarly although LQT3 patients may have a more adverse prognosis than patients with other genetic variants of the disease, it is impossible to rank mutations by the degree of "malignancy." Concepts such as "malignant" or "benign" mutations do not exist in LQTS and each mutation may be associated to severe or benign manifestations.

In summary, genotype-phenotype correlation in LQTS provided valuable information for diagnosis and clinical management of the patients. However, the decision making process in each specific patient has to take into account that the variable penetrance may significantly modify the outcome *(44)*.

LONG QT SYNDROME WITH EXTRACARDIAC MANIFESTATIONS

Although the RW syndrome is the most prevalent LQTS variant, in rare instances QT interval prolongation may be associated with abnormal extra-cardiac phenotypes. This occurs in the Jervell and Lange Nielsen (JLN) syndrome, in the LQTS associated with syndactyly (LQT-Synd) and the Andersen Syndrome (LQT-And). Even if epidemiological data on these rare variants is still limited, it seems that the natural history of these diseases significantly diverge from that of RW syndrome.

Jervell and Lange Nielsen Syndrome

Jervell and Lange Nielsen syndrome (JLN) is the autosomal recessive form of LQTS presenting sensineural deafness associated with the cardiac phenotype. Most of the patients present "severe-to-profound" hearing impairment *(2)*, however, more recently, the availability of genetic testing allowed the identification of recessively transmitted mutations associated with mild or absent hearing impairment *(25,41)* (Fig. 3). Two JLN causing genes have been identified so far: *KCNQ1* (JLN1) on chromosome 1p15.5 and *KCNE1* (JLN2) on chromosome 21q22.1–22.2 *(45–48)*. Both genes were previously shown to be linked to the autosomal dominant form of LQTS (*KCNQ1*, LQT1 and *KCNE1*, LQT5).

Although, the functional consequences of JLN mutations have been elucidated in vitro by heterologous expression of the mutated channels and pathophysiologically linked to the cardiac phenotype, the mechanisms leading to hearing impairment are less clearly understood. *KCNQ1* and *KCNE2* are expressed in the inner ear *(49)* where the I_{Ks} current appears to be a major player in endolymph homeostasis. Under normal conditions, the $[K^+]$ of the endolymph, and the K^+ fluxes into hair cells are essential to the transduction of sound into neural signals. Recycling of K^+ from the hair cells back to the endolymph, possibly through I_{Ks}, by maintaining the appropriate high levels of K^+ in that fluid is a crucial step for normal hearing. This view is supported by the studies on *KCNE1* and *KCNQ1* knock-out models *(50,51)* that demonstrated a progressive loss of endolymph in the sensory epithelium and hair-cell degeneration. Interestingly, these animal models also provided evidence of involvement of extra-cardiac structures as a consequence of gene function disruption. *KCNQ1* deficient mice present gastric hyperplasia where this ion channel could be involved in the regulation of acid secretion *(52)*. On the other hand, *KCNE1* knock-out mice show hypokalemia and higher plasma aldosterone concentrations *(50)*. However, so far there is no evidence of such abnormalities in JLN patients.

The low prevalence of JLN syndrome curtails the achievement of detailed knowledge concerning its natural history and clinical features. JLN appears to be more malignant than RW-LQTS *(53)*. We recently reported preliminary data on 136 JLN individuals showing that 90% of them present cardiac events and that on average occur at a younger age than those occurring in RW patients. Furthermore, it seems also that the response to beta-blockers may be less satisfactory in JLN than in the heterozygous *KCNQ1* carriers *(54)*. If confirmed these data would advocate a more aggressive therapeutic approach in JLN patients *(44)*.

LQTS with Syndactyly

In rare instances, QT interval prolongation presents with cutaneous syndactyly (LQT-synd). The prevalence of LQT-synd in the general population is unknown but its occur-

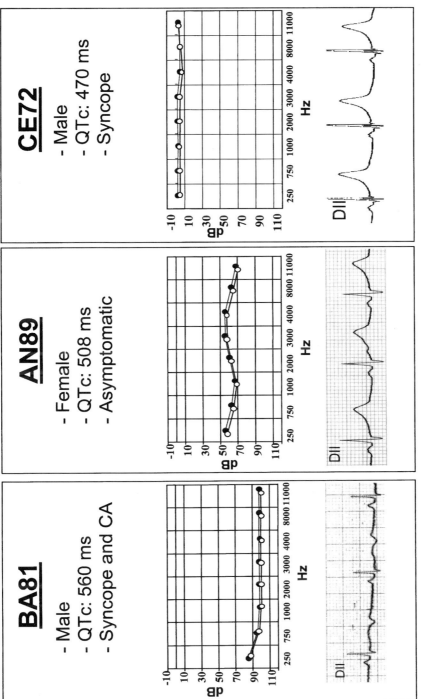

Fig. 3. Examples of variable hearing impairment in recessive Long QT syndrome. Left and middle panels show audiograms and representative ECGs of two genotyped patients (KCNQ1 and KCNE2, respectively), diagnosed as JLN and presenting with profound and moderate hearing loss. The patient CE72 (right panels) presents with normal hearing despite being homozygous carrier of a KCNQ1 mutation. The patient was clinically diagnosed as a Romano-Ward syndrome (*see 41*) and it may also be considered an example of incomplete penetrance of auditory phenotype in JLN.

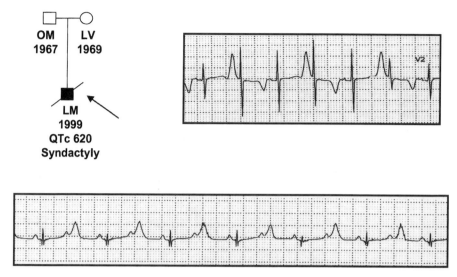

Fig. 4. Pedigree and ECG tracings showing macroscopic T wave alternans (upper panel) and 2:1 functional AV block (lower panel) in a patient with LQTS associated with syndactyly.

rence in the clinical practice is low. Only a few such cases have been described *(55–58)* in the literature and the available data depict a complex and distinctive phenotype.

We have recently reported five cases of LQT-synd, four sporadic and one with familial occurrence *(59)* and we performed a literature search in order to delineate the most relevant clinical features of this disorder and identified seven additional cases. Based on the 12 patients it appears that LQT-synd is usually characterized by a markedly prolonged QT interval with QTc exceeding 550 ms in 67% of cases. Functional 2:1 atrio-ventricular (AV) block (reported in 75% of cases), and macroscopic T wave alternans are distinguishing electrocardiographic features of LQT-synd (Fig. 4) *(55,56,59)*. Interestingly, 42% of patients showed severe bradycardia and AV block during anesthesia with halothane, suggesting an idiosyncratic response to volatile anesthetics of still unknown origin. Moreover, congenital heart defects, consisting mainly in patent ductus arteriosus and patent foramen ovalem that have been reported in 58% of cases.

Syndactyly, typically involving the 3rd to the 5th finger, is invariably cutaneous (i.e., not involving tendons and finger bones) and in the majority of cases it involves both hands and feet. Peculiar extra-cardiac abnormal phenotypes are sometimes evident. Recurrent infections have been reported in 33% of the patients and in our series two out of five cases developed severe hypoglycemia during follow up *(59)*.

Only scanty follow-up information are available to assess the "long-term" prognosis of LQT-synd. Among the ten patients with reported follow-up information (in most cases not exceeding 2.5 yr), six deaths occurred with a mean age of death of 22 mo despite the use of beta blocker in all the reported cases. Therefore, a poor prognosis appears to characterize LQT-synd. The available evidence suggests that sudden death may occur either due to tachyarrhythmias or for bradyarrhythmias. Moreover, LQT-synd patients could also present a predisposition to severe infections and altered glucose metabolism. In this regard, we have recently described *(59)* a case of a 28-mo-old child who, given the extreme QT interval prolongation, the frequent episodes of T wave alternans and 2:1 AV block (not responding to sodium channel blockers administration), received a prophylactic implantable cardioverter defibrillator (ICD) at age 13 mo. At age 24 mo he experienced syncope and the review of ICD stored electrogram showed three appropriately delivered therapies. Four months later another syncopal episode occurred. No arrhythmias were documented but severe hypoglycemia was observed leading to coma. The patient died shortly after because of the irreversible brain damage secondary to the hypoglycemia.

The genetic basis of LQT-synd is still unknown and its identification is complicated by the infrequency of the disease. No chromosomal abnormalities have been demonstrated by standard karyotyping (55,56). Based upon pedigree analysis *de novo* mutations and autosomal recessive transmission constitute the two most likely patterns. However, the lack of parental consanguinity challenges the presence of autosomal recessive transmission, and may point to compound heterozygosity.

In summary LQT-synd appears as a rare but highly malignant condition. When recognized, it is of utmost importance that all the possible preventive measures are undertaken, in order to avoid not only tachy- but also brady-arrhythmias.

Andersen Syndrome (LQT-And)

In 1971 Andersen et al. (60) reported the case of an 8-yr-old with short stature, hypertelorism, broad nasal root, and defect of soft and hard palate. The definition of Andersen syndrome (LQT-And) was used for the first time in 1994 by Tawil et al. (61) to describe a clinical disorder consisting of three major features: Potassium-sensitive periodic paralysis, ventricular arrhythmias, and dysmorphic features (similar to those described by Andersen in 1971). The presence of a variable degree of QT interval prolongation was pointed out in the first systematic description of the disease (61) and subsequently, Sansone et al. strengthened its crucial diagnostic significance (62). Besides QT interval prolongation, LQT-And patients may also present repolarization abnormalities consisting in a late repolarization component resembling a "giant" U wave. Bi-directional ventricular tachycardia has also been reported as a distinguishing pattern of arrhythmias in LQT-And (Fig. 5).

Although sudden death being reported (63), arrhythmias do not appear to be a major cause of death in LQT-And and the disease often has a benign outcome (62,64).

The genetic background of LQT-And has been recently elucidated by genome-wide linkage analysis by Plaster et al. (61) who successfully linked this disorder to the locus 17q23 in a large family. A candidate gene screening was carried out in the critical region and a missense mutation was identified in the *KCNJ2* gene. Additional mutations were subsequently identified in eight unrelated individuals, thus providing the proof that *KCNJ2* is the cause of at least some of the LQT-And cases. *KCNJ2* encodes an inwardly rectifying potassium channel, Kir2.1, highly expressed in the heart where it appears to act as a determinant factor of resting membrane potential. Interestingly, since dysmorphic facial appearance constitutes a distinctive trait of LQT-And, the data provided by Plaster et al. also strongly suggest that Kir2.1 plays a major role in developmental signaling.

CLINICAL MANAGEMENT

Risk Stratification

The central features of all variants of LQTS are an abnormally prolonged QT interval and syncopal episodes owing to the onset of polymorphic, self-terminating ventricular

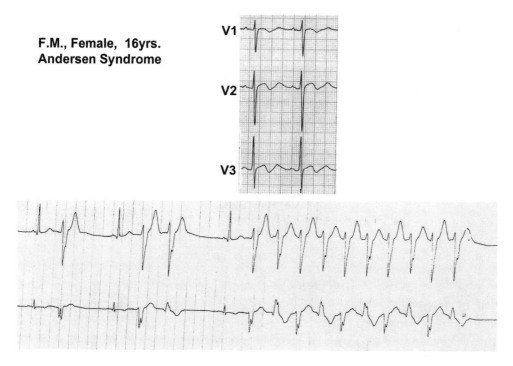

Fig. 5. ECG in the Andersen syndrome. Upper panel: typical ECG with QT interval prolongation and "giant" U waves in the precordial leads. Lower panel; example of ventricular tachycardia with a bi-directional pattern.

tachycardia, generally referred to as torsades de pointes. Ventricular arrhythmias may also degenerate into ventricular fibrillation leading to sudden death. Clinical manifestations of LQTS may be highly variable, ranging from fully blown disease with markedly prolonged QT interval and recurrent syncope, to subclinical forms with borderline QT interval prolongation.

The guidelines for risk stratification and prevention of life-threatening cardiac events have recently been published in the Task Force on SCD of the European Society of Cardiology *(44)* and have been based mainly on the data published over the years by the International Long QT Syndrome Registry (Table 2).

LQTS patients are often not inducible *(65)*, therefore, programmed electrically stimulation is not a valuable risk stratification tool. Despite in clinical practice a clinician will always consider with more concern a patient with a family history of juvenile SCD, quantitative data are not available to support the view that family history of unexplained sudden death should be regarded as a risk factor and mandate aggressive treatment of family members *(44)*.

The amount of QT interval prolongation has been associated with increased risk *(53)* such that the longer the QTc, the greater the risk for cardiac events. However, there have also been observations that 5% of family members with a normal QT interval (QTc < 440 ms) had syncope or cardiac arrest. Thus, mild QT prolongation or even normal QT (in gene carriers) does not always translate into a benign outcome. Increased QT interval dispersion and macroscopic T wave alternans have also been associated with increased

Table 2
Recommendations for Prevention of Sudden Death in Long QT Syndrome
(from ref. *44* with permission)

	Recommendations	*Level of evidence*
Primary Prevention		
Avoidance of QT prolonging agents/K$^+$ lowering agents		
Symptomatic	Class IIa	C
Silent Gene Carriers	Class IIa	C
Asymptomatic	Class IIa	C
Avoidance of competitive sport/strenuous activity		
Symptomatic	Class I	C
Silent Gene Carriers	Class IIa	C
Asymptomatic	Class IIa	C
Beta blockers		
Symptomatic	Class I	B
Asymptomatic	Class IIa	C
Left Cardiac Sympathetic Denervation + Beta blockers		
Symptomatic with recurrences on beta blockers	Class IIb	B
Pace makers (plus beta blockers)		
Symptomatic with pause- or bradycardia-dependent arrhythmias	Class IIb	C
ICD + Beta blockers		
Symptomatic with recurrences on beta blockers	Class IIa	C
Secondary Prevention		
ICD + Beta blockers	Class I	C
Avoidance of competitive sport/strenuous activity*	Class I	C
Avoidance of QT prolonging agents*	Class I	C

*Lifestyle measures to be adopted in conjunction with ICD implant in CA survivors

risk of arrhythmias but no prospective trials quantifying their actual predictive value are so far available *(66)*.

Gender differences in cardiac event rate have been demonstrated in LQTS patients. Events tend to occur earlier in males than in females, and males who are still asymptomatic at age 20 can be considered at low risk for manifesting cardiac events. Females maintain the same risk of becoming symptomatic in adulthood and they are at increased risk in the first year after delivery *(67,68)*.

Prevention of Sudden Death in LQTS

Pharmacological treatment of LQTS is largely based on the use of beta-blockers. Propranolol (2–4 mg/kg/day) or Nadolol (1–2 mg/kg/day) are the most frequently prescribed compounds. No randomized controlled clinical trials have specifically addressed the issue of the effectiveness of beta-blockers in this disease. Nonetheless, this therapeutic approach is generally accepted as the more effective available based on the retrospective analysis reported in the literature. Schwartz and Moss provided the first indication of the effectiveness of antiadrenergic therapy in 1979 *(69)*. Subsequently, a retrospective survival analysis on 233 patients showed 9% mortality for the group treated with antiadrenergic therapy (β-blockers and/or left cardiac sympathetic denervation) and close to 60% for the patients with nonantiadrenergic therapy or left without treatment *(70)*. More recently, a reappraisal of beta-blocker therapy in LQTS has been carried out by the International LQTS Registry investigators *(71)*. Cardiac event rate analysis in matched periods (5 yr) before and after the beginning of therapy confirmed a highly statistically significant reduction of events on therapy. The five-year incidence of cardiac arrest or SCD was below 1% for those asymptomatic at treatment initiation, 3% for those who had suffered syncope, and 13% for those who already had a cardiac arrest. Thus, when considering only patients presenting with an aborted SCD, a significant residual risk a second life threatening event (Hazard Ratio of 12.6) remains despite the use of beta-blockers *(71)*. It is fair to observe that beta-blocker therapy may have differential effectiveness according to genotype being highly effective especially in LQT1 patients *(46)*, who present an impairment of I_{Ks}, a catecholamine-sensitive current.

Based on the previously mentioned findings, the use of ICD has been recommended in survivors of cardiac arrest, in children with syndactyly, and in symptomatic JLN patients *(44)* (Table 2). Finally, sympathetic denervation, may also be indicated for patients who continue to have syncope despite full dose β-blocking therapy or who are not compliant with medical therapy *(44,72)*.

Gene specific therapy has been proposed for the management of patients with LQT3 and LQT2, i.e., those in which beta-blockers may be less effective.

The use of sodium channel blockers in LQT3 individuals has been suggested based on experimental *(73)* and on preliminary clinical data *(32)*. It has been confirmed by other groups that sodium channel blockers shorten QT interval, however no data are available to demonstrate their efficacy in preventing cardiac events. One of our LQT3 patients who survived cardiac arrest and remained asymptomatic for five years, died suddenly while being treated with beta-blockers and mexiletine. Another LQT3 patient who was prophylactically treated with beta-blockers and sodium channel blockers experienced cardiac arrest that represented the first manifestation of the disease in this five-yr-old child. Based on this experience we consider that extreme caution should be used when considering novel treatment strategies in LQT3 patients.

Compton et al. *(74)* suggested that increase in extracellular potassium may represent a gene specific strategy for individuals affected by LQT2. This approach is based on the experimental evidence that in the presence of high extracellular K^+, I_{Kr} current increases, thus "compensating" for the reduced function of the *KCNH2* defective protein. Preliminary clinical data demonstrated a reduction in QT interval duration but also in this case data on large series of patients and data suggesting a reduction of cardiac events is not available.

REFERENCES

1. Priori SG, Napolitano C. Genetic of arrhythmogenic disorders. In: Prodrid PJ, Kowey PR, eds. Cardiac Arrhythmia: Mechanisms, Diagnosis and Management. 2nd Edition. Philadelphia: Lippincott Williams and Wilkins, 2001:81–107.
2. Jervell A, Lange-Nielsen F. Congenital deaf mutism, functional heart disease with prolongation of the QT interval and sudden death. Am Heart J 1957;54:59–61.
3. Romano C, Gemme G, Pongiglione R. Aritmie cardiache rare in eta' pediatrica. Clin Ped 1963;45:656–657.
4. Ward DC. New familial cardiac syndrome in children. J Irish Med Ass 1964;54:103.
5. Splawski I, Shen J, Timothy KW, et al. Spectrum of mutations in long-QT syndrome genes : KVLQT1, HERG, SCN5A, KCNE1, and KCNE2. Circulation 2000;102:1178–1185.
6. Napolitano C, Ronchetti E, Memmi M, et al. Molecular epidemiology of the Long QT Syndrome in a cohort of 267 probands. J Am Coll Cardiol 2001;37(abs.suppl A):87A.

7. Keating MT, Atkinson D, Dunn C, Timothy K, Vincent GM, Leppert M. Linkage of a cardiac arrhythmia, the long QT syndrome, and the Harvey ras-1 gene. Science 1991;252:704–706.

8. Jiang C, Atkinson D, Towbin JA, et al. Two long QT syndrome loci map to chromosomes 3 and 7 with evidence for further heterogeneity. Nat Genet 1994;8:141–147.

9. Schott JJ, Charpentier F, Peltier S, et al. Mapping of a gene for long QT syndrome to chromosome 4q25–27. Am J Hum Genet 1995;57:1114–1122.

10. Wang Q, Curran ME, Splawski I, et al. Positional cloning of a novel potassium channel gene: KVLQT1 mutations cause cardiac arrhythmias. Nat Genet 1996;12:17–23.

11. Curran ME, Splawski I, Timothy KW, Vincent GM, Green ED, Keating MT. A molecular basis for cardiac arrhythmia: HERG mutations cause long QT syndrome. Cell 1995;80:795–803.

12. Wang Q, Shen J, Splawski I, et al. SCN5A mutations associated with an inherited cardiac arrhythmia, long QT syndrome. Cell 1995;80:805–811.

13. Splawski I, Tristani-Firouzi M, Lehmann MH, Sanguinetti MC, Keating MT. Mutations in the hminK gene cause long QT syndrome and suppress I_{Ks} function. Nat Genet 1997;17:338–340.

14. Abbott GW, Sesti F, Splawski I, et al. MiRP1 forms I_{Kr} potassium channels with HERG and is associated with cardiac arrhythmia. Cell 1999;97:175–187.

15. Barhanin J, Lesage F, Guillemare E, Fink M, Lazdunski M, Romey G. K(V)LQT1 and lsK (minK) proteins associate to form the I(Ks) cardiac potassium current. Nature 1996;384:78–80.

16. Sanguinetti MC, Curran ME, Zou A, et al. Coassembly of K(V)LQT1 and minK (IsK) proteins to form cardiac I(Ks) potassium channel. Nature 1996;384:80–83.

17. Sanguinetti MC, Jiang C, Curran ME, Keating MT. A mechanistic link between an inherited and an acquired cardiac arrhythmia: HERG encodes the I_{Kr} potassium channel. Cell 1995;81:299–307.

18. Gellens ME, George AL, Jr., Chen LQ, et al. Primary structure and functional expression of the human cardiac tetrodotoxin-insensitive voltage-dependent sodium channel. Proc Natl Acad Sci USA 1992;89:554–558.

19. Donger C, Denjoy I, Berthet M, et al. KVLQT1 C-terminal missense mutation causes a forme fruste long-QT syndrome. Circulation 1997;96:2778–2781.

20. Sanguinetti MC, Curran ME, Spector PS, Keating MT. Spectrum of HERG K$^+$-channel dysfunction in an inherited cardiac arrhythmia. Proc Natl Acad Sci USA 1996;93:2208–2212.

21. Priori SG, Napolitano C, Brown AM, et al. The loss of function induced by HERG and KVLQT1 mutations does not correlate with the clinical severity of the Long QT Syndrome. Circulation 1998;98(suppl1):I-457.

22. Bennett PB, Yazawa K, Makita N, George AL, Jr. Molecular mechanism for an inherited cardiac arrhythmia. Nature 1995;376:683–685.

23. Dumaine R, Wang Q, Keating MT, et al. Multiple mechanisms of Na$^+$ channel-linked long-QT syndrome. Circ Res 1996;78:916–924.

24. Zhou Z, Gong Q, Epstein ML, January CT. HERG channel dysfunction in human long QT syndrome. Intracellular transport and functional defects. J Biol Chem 1998;273:21061–21066.

25. Bianchi L, Shen Z, Dennis AT, et al. Cellular dysfunction of LQT5-minK mutants: abnormalities of I_{Ks}, I_{Kr} and trafficking in long QT syndrome. Hum Mol Genet 1999;8:1499–1507.

26. Wang DW, Yazawa K, George AL, Jr., Bennett PB. Characterization of human cardiac Na$^+$ channel mutations in the congenital long QT syndrome. Proc Natl Acad Sci USA 1996;93:13200–13205.

27. Bennett PB. Long QT syndrome: biophysical and pharmacologic mechanisms in LQT3. J Cardiovasc Electrophysiol 2000;11:819–822.

28. Sanguinetti MC. Dysfunction of delayed rectifier potassium channels in an inherited cardiac arrhythmia. Ann NY Acad Sci 1999;868:406–413.

29. Zou A, Xu QP, Sanguinetti MC. A mutation in the pore region of HERG K$^+$ channels expressed in Xenopus oocytes reduces rectification by shifting the voltage dependence of inactivation. J Physiol 1998;509 (Pt 1):129–137.

30. Moss AJ, Zareba W, Benhorin J, et al. ECG T-wave patterns in genetically distinct forms of the hereditary long QT syndrome. Circulation 1995;92:2929–2934.

31. Zhang L, Timothy KW, Vincent GM, et al. Spectrum of ST-T-wave patterns and repolarization parameters in congenital long-QT syndrome: ECG findings identify genotypes. Circulation 2000;102:2849–2855.

32. Schwartz PJ, Priori SG, Locati EH, et al. Long QT syndrome patients with mutations of the SCN5A and HERG genes have differential responses to Na$^+$ channel blockade and to increases in heart rate. Implications for gene-specific therapy. Circulation 1995;92:3381–3386.

33. Swan H, Vittasalo M, Piippo K, Laitinen P, Kontula K, Toivonen L. Sinus node function and ventricular repolarization during exercise stress test in long QT syndrome patients with KvLQT1 and HERG potassium channel defects. J Am Coll Cardiol 1999;34:823–829.
34. Moretti P, Calcaterra G, Napolitano C, et al. High prevalence of concealed Long QT Syndrome among carriers of KVLQT1 defects. Circulation 2001;102(abs suppl):II–584.
35. Zareba W, Moss AJ, Schwartz PJ, et al. Influence of genotype on the clinical course of the long-QT syndrome. International Long-QT Syndrome Registry Research Group. N Engl J Med 1998;339: 960–965.
36. Schwartz PJ, Priori SG, Spazzolini C, et al. Genotype-phenotype correlation in the long-QT syndrome: gene-specific triggers for life-threatening arrhythmias. Circulation (Online) 2001;103:89–95.
37. Wilde AM, Jongbloed RJ, Doevendans PA, et al. Auditory stimuli as a trigger for arrhythmic events differentiate HERG-related (LQTS2) patients from KVLQT1-related patients (LQTS1). J Am Coll Cardiol 1999;33:332.
38. Moss AJ, Robinson JL, Gessman L, et al. Comparison of clinical and genetic variables of cardiac events associated with loud noise versus swimming among subjects with the long QT syndrome. Am J Cardiol 1999;84:876–879.
39. Ackerman MJ, Tester DJ, Porter CJ. Swimming, a gene-specific arrhythmogenic trigger for inherited long QT syndrome. Mayo Clin Proc 1999;74:1088–1094.
40. Priori SG, Napolitano C, Schwartz PJ. Low penetrance in the long-QT syndrome: clinical impact. Circulation 1999;99:529–533.
41. Priori SG, Schwartz PJ, Napolitano C, et al. A recessive variant of the Romano-Ward long-QT syndrome? Circulation 1998;97:2420–2425.
42. Napolitano C, Schwartz PJ, Brown AM, et al. Evidence for a cardiac ion channel mutation underlying drug-induced QT prolongation and life-threatening arrhythmias. J Cardiovasc Electrophysiol 2000;11:691–696.
43. Schulze-Bahr E, Haverkamp W, Hordt M. A genetic basis for quinidine-induced (acquired) long QT syndrome. Eur Heart J 1997;18:29.
44. Priori SG, Aliot E, Blomstrom-Lundqvist C, et al. Task force on sudden cardiac death of the European Society of Cardiology. Eur Heart J 2001;22:1374–1450.
45. Chen Q, Zhang D, Gingell RL, et al. Homozygous deletion in KVLQT1 associated with Jervell and Lange-Nielsen syndrome. Circulation 1999;99:1344–1347.
46. Vincent GM, Schwartz PJ, Swan H, Piippo K, Bithell C. Effectiveness of beta-blockers in the LQT1 genotype of long QT syndrome. Circulation 2001;104 (suppl II):463.
47. Duggal P, Vesely MR, Wattanasirichaigoon D, Villafane J, Kaushik V, Beggs AH. Mutation of the gene for IsK associated with both Jervell and Lange-Nielsen and Romano-Ward forms of Long-QT syndrome. Circulation 1998;20;97:142–146.
48. Schulze-Bahr E, Wang Q, Wedekind H, et al. KCNE1 mutations cause Jervell and Lange-Nielsen syndrome. Nat Genet 1997;17:267–268.
49. Nicolas M, Dememes D, Martin A, Kupershmidt S, Barhanin J. KCNQ1/KCNE1 potassium channels in mammalian vestibular dark cells. Hear Res 2001;153:132–145.
50. Arrighi I, Bloch-Faure M, Grahammer F, et al. Altered potassium balance and aldosterone secretion in a mouse model of human congenital long QT syndrome. Proc Natl Acad Sci USA 2001;98:8792–8797.
51. Vetter DE, Mann JR, Wangemann P, et al. Inner ear defects induced by null mutation of the isk gene. Neuron 1996;17:1251–1264.
52. Lee MP, Ravenel JD, Hu RJ, et al. Targeted disruption of the Kvlqt1 gene causes deafness and gastric hyperplasia in mice. J Clin Invest 2000;106:1447–1455.
53. Moss AJ, Schwartz PJ, Crampton RS, et al. The long QT syndrome. Prospective longitudinal study of 328 families. Circulation 1991;84:1136–1144.
54. Cerrone M, Schwartz PJ, Priori SG, et al. Natural history and genetic aspects of the Jervell and Lange-Nielsen syndrome. Circulation 2001;104 (suppl II):463.
55. Marks ML, Whisler SL, Clericuzio C, Keating M. A new form of long QT syndrome associated with syndactyly. J Am Coll Cardiol 1995;25:59–64.
56. Marks ML, Trippel DL, Keating MT. Long QT syndrome associated with syndactyly identified in females. Am J Cardiol 1995;76:744–745.
57. Joseph-Reynolds AM, Auden SM, Sobczyzk WL. Perioperative considerations in a newly described subtype of congenital long QT syndrome. Paediatr Anaesth 1997;7:237–241.
58. Levin SE. Long QT syndrome associated with syndactyly in a female. Am J Cardiol 1996;78:380.

59. Napolitano C, Bloise R, Lunati M, et al. Prolongation of QT interval and Syndactyly: characterization of a Novel Variant of the Long QT Syndrome. Circulation 2001;104(suppl II):365.
60. Andersen ED, Krasilnikoff PA, Overvad H. Intermittent muscular weakness, extrasystoles, and multiple developmental anomalies. A new syndrome? Acta Paediatr Scand 1971;60:559–564.
61. Tawil R, Ptacek LJ, Pavlakis SG, et al. Andersen's syndrome: potassium-sensitive periodic paralysis, ventricular ectopy, and dysmorphic features. Ann Neurol 1994;35:326–330.
62. Sansone V, Griggs RC, Meola G, et al. Andersen's syndrome: a distinct periodic paralysis. Ann Neurol 1997;42:305–312.
63. Levitt LP, Rose LI, Dawson DM. Hypokalemic periodic paralysis with arrhythmia. N Engl J Med 1972;286:253–254.
64. Gutmann L. Periodic paralyses. Neurol Clin 2000;18:195–202.
65. Bhandari AK, Shapiro WA, Morady F, Shen EN, Mason J, Scheinman MM. Electrophysiologic testing in patients with the long QT syndrome. Circulation 1985;71:63–71.
66. Schwartz PJ, Priori SG, Napolitano C. The Long QT Syndrome. In: Zipes DP, Jalife J, eds. Cardiac Electrophysiology. From Cell to Bedside. Philadelphia: WB Saunders Co., 2000:597–615.
67. Locati EH, Zareba W, Moss AJ, et al. Age- and sex-related differences in clinical manifestations in patients with congenital long-QT syndrome: findings from the International LQTS Registry. Circulation 1998;97:2237–2244.
68. Rashba EJ, Zareba W, Moss AJ, et al. Influence of pregnancy on the risk for cardiac events in patients with hereditary long QT syndrome. LQTS Investigators. Circulation 1998;97:451–456.
69. Moss AJ, Schwartz PJ. Sudden death and the idiopathic long QT syndrome. Am J Med 1979;66:6–7.
70. Schwartz PJ, Locati E. The idiopathic long QT syndrome: pathogenetic mechanisms and therapy. Eur Heart J 1985;6 Suppl D:103–14:103–114.
71. Moss AJ, Zareba W, Hall WJ, et al. Effectiveness and limitations of beta-blocker therapy in congenital long-QT syndrome. Circulation 2000;101:616–623.
72. Schwartz PJ, Locati EH, Moss AJ, Crampton RS, Trazzi R, Ruberti U. Left cardiac sympathetic denervation in the therapy of congenital long QT syndrome. A worldwide report. Circulation 1991;84:503–511.
73. Priori SG, Napolitano C, Cantu F, Brown AM, Schwartz PJ. Differential response to Na+ channel blockade, beta-adrenergic stimulation, and rapid pacing in a cellular model mimicking the SCN5A and HERG defects present in the long-QT syndrome. Circ Res 1996;78:1009–1015.
74. Compton SJ, Lux RL, Ramsey MR, et al. Genetically defined therapy of inherited long-QT syndrome. Correction of abnormal repolarization by potassium. Circulation 1996;94:1018–1022.

10 Ion Channel Disease as a Cause of the Brugada Syndrome

Molecular and Genetic Aspects

Connie R. Bezzina, PhD
and Arthur A. M. Wilde, MD, PhD

INTRODUCTION

In recent years, research on the genetic basis of inherited cardiac channelopathies, namely the Long QT syndrome, the Brugada syndrome, and more recently catecholamine-induced polymorphic ventricular tachycardia, has initiated an increased understanding of the molecular blueprints of myocardial electrical function. The electrophysiological analysis of naturally-occurring mutant ion channels associated with these disorders provides insight, not only into mechanisms of disease but also, for instance, into the biophysical properties of the native channel, its pharmacology, its association with other subunits and its contribution to the myocardial action potential. This, in turn, should ultimately enable more specific pharmacological intervention in the management of these syndromes and other related and possibly more common arrhythmias.

The Brugada syndrome *(1,2)*, first presented as a distinct clinical entity by Pedro and Josep Brugada in 1992 *(3)*, is characterized by ventricular fibrillation and sudden cardiac death associated with the electrocardiographic (ECG) pattern of ST-segment elevation in leads V1 through V3 (Fig. 1). This typical ECG pattern might not be consistently present; day-to-day or hour-to-hour variability in the magnitude of the ST-segment elevation has been recognized *(4–9)*. The ST-segment abnormalities have been described as "coved-," originally described in the 1992 paper by Brugada and Brugada *(3)*, and

From: *Contemporary Cardiology: Cardiac Repolarization: Bridging Basic and Clinical Science*
Edited by: I. Gussak et al. © Humana Press Inc., Totowa, NJ

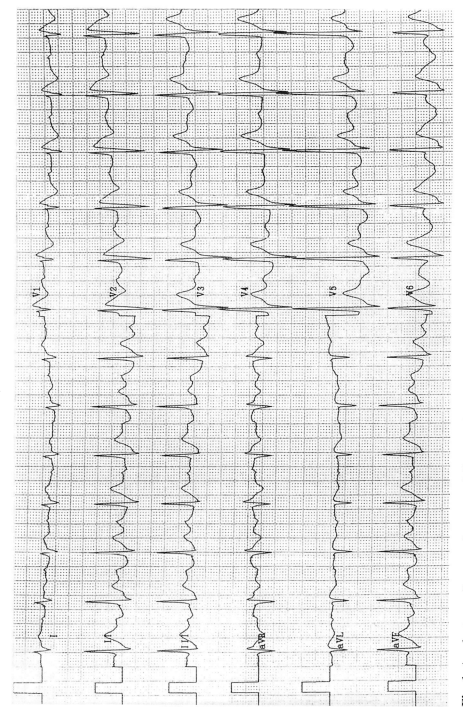

Fig. 1. An electrocardiogram of a successfully resuscitated 41-yr-old male. Note the 5 mm elevated J point in lead V2 followed by a down-sloping T wave terminated by a negative deflection. The axis is slightly deviated to the right, the PQ interval is lengthened (280 ms), and the QRS width is 100 ms. During EPS, 2 extrasystoles (BCL 600) repeatedly induced ventricular fibrillation.

"saddle back-" types. Other characteristic ECG-features include a terminal negative T-wave in the right precordial leads and specific (i.e., left anterior hemiblock) or nonspecific (QRS widening) conduction disorders. The HV-interval was prolonged in the vast majority of patients in whom it has been measured *(1)*. The diagnosis "Brugada syndrome" should be reserved for those cases in which structural heart disease is excluded by means of extensive clinical investigation with particular focus on right ventricular structure and function. Important differential diagnostic considerations include any form of right ventricular cardiomyopathy, ischemia, and intrathoracic pathology. Absence of these abnormalities implies a primary electrical disease.

From a recent survey *(1)*, dealing with 163 patients, several remarkable epidemiological features emerge. Firstly, there is a strong male preponderance (92%). Secondly, the entity seems particularly common in South East-Asian people *(10)* and, thirdly, a suspect familial history is present in 22% of cases (range in the different series 4–40%; ref *1*). The predominant occurrence of events during sleep, reported in 17 out of 21 Southeast-Asian patients *(1)*, was confirmed in a more recent study using ICD data *(11)*. The mean age of arrhythmic events varies between 2 and 77 yr *(3)*, but the vast majority of individual patients become symptomatic in their fourth decade. Extremes are symptomatic twins at the age of 2 in the initial Brugada series, a recently described highly "malignant" family with sudden cardiac death in very young children resembling sudden infant death syndrome *(12)*, and an asymptomatic (for arrhythmias) individual with documented ECG changes over 40 yr at the age of 85 *(13)*.

ELECTROPHYSIOLOGICAL BASIS

Ever since the initial report of Brugada and Brugada *(3)*, wherein it was suggested that a functional cardiac disorder, rather than a subclinical cardiomyopathy underlies the syndrome, electrical heterogeneity, particularly in the right ventricular outflow tract (RVOT), has been postulated to underlie the different electrophysiological aspects of the syndrome *(1,2,14)*. Indeed, experimental data by Antzelevitch and coworkers *(15)* in perfused canine right ventricle wedge preparations favor this explanation. In these studies, pharmacological modulation of currents, including the use of sodium channel blockers, targeted at phase 1 of the action potential, modulate the ECG in a manner that is in agreement with this hypothesis *(15)*.

Sodium channel blockers aggravate the ECG abnormalities and may increase the propensity for ventricular tachycardia/ventricular fibrillation in patients, although they may precipitate the ECG abnormalities in asymptomatic family members. This, taken together with the high prevalence of associated conduction disorders, indicated that reduced sodium channel function could—at least in a subset of patients—underlie the Brugada syndrome.

The postulated mechanism whereby reduced sodium channel function is thought to result in the ECG features of Brugada syndrome involves an interaction of different ion channels active during the upstroke of the cardiac action potential: phase 0, caused by the sodium current, I_{Na}; the early repolarization phase 1, involving the transient outward potassium current, I_{to}; and the phase 2 plateau, involving the L-type calcium current I_{Ca-L} *(1,2,15)*. All of the channels involved are voltage-gated, that is they are activated only at particular voltages. Reduced I_{Na}, secondary to pharmacological sodium channel blockade or mutation in *SCN5A*, the gene encoding the α-subunit of the cardiac sodium channel

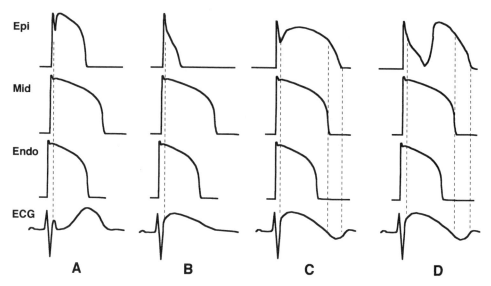

Fig. 2. Putative epicardial and endocardial action potential morphology and surface ECG in normal subjects (**A**) and patients with the Brugada syndrome (**B**). Note the abbreviated epicardial action potential as proposed by Charles Antzelevitch *(14)* as the basis of ST-segment elevation in Brugada syndrome. (**C and D**) Alternative hypotheses proposed for the secondary negative T-wave observed in the right precordial leads in Brugada syndrome: (**C**) prolongation of the action potential of the epicardial layer outlasts that of the midmural layer leading to transmural membrane current flow from epicardium to midmyocardium ensuing in a terminal negative T-wave; or (**D**) a secondary upstroke in the epicardial layer, elicited by local current flow from the plateau-phase of the midmural layer to the (partly) repolarized epicardial cells, will lead to prolonged repolarization in the epicardial layer with the same result.

(see below), leads to a depressed phase 0, thereby lowering conduction velocity and leading to the conduction disturbances often manifested in the Brugada syndrome. More significantly, in Brugada syndrome, reduced I_{Na} would result in a less depolarized voltage at the start of phase 1. Although this reduced voltage may be expected to reduce I_{to}, resulting in less early repolarization during phase 1, computer simulations have shown that I_{to} is only a little depressed *(16)*. The net effect of reduced I_{Na} and (near) normal I_{to} is that phase 1 ends at a more repolarized voltage. This voltage may be so repolarized that I_{Ca-L} may fail to be activated. This could lead to a loss of phase 2 (the action potential goes from phase 1 straight to the final repolarization phase 3) and a marked shortening of action potential duration.

Importantly, this scenario is played out in the epicardium, but not in the endocardium (refer to Fig. 2A, B), since I_{to} density is much larger in epicardium than in endocardium in man (similar to other species), both in the left *(17,18)* and right ventricle *(19)*. Thus, while action potential duration in epicardium is greatly shortened, it is normal in endocardium, resulting in strongly increased dispersion of refractoriness and setting the stage for reentry. The electrotonic current flow during phase 2 from endocardium to epicardium underlies the ST elevation of Brugada syndrome (Fig. 2B) and forms the basis for reentrant tachyarrhythmias during this phase (phase 2 reentry) with the reentry circuit incorporating the different transmural layers *(1,15,20)*. Why the ST elevations are only apparent in the right precordial leads, is not clear. I_{to} may be more abundant in right ventricular epicardium than in left ventricular epicardium in man *(17,19)*, as it is in dog *(21)*. Alternatively, it has been proposed that the contribution of the epicardium to the ECG is larger in the right ventricle than in the left ventricle, because it has a larger relative contribution to the right ventricular mass than to the left ventricular mass *(1,22)*. Finally, regional differences may follow from differences in autonomic innervation as shown with MIBG imaging by some *(23,24)*, but not all *(6)*, since the manifestations of Brugada syndrome are strongly dependent on autonomic tone, as discussed previously. In any case, the hypothesis that (phase 2) reentry is responsible for the tachyarrhythmias of Brugada syndrome is corroborated by a number of clinical and experimental findings.

However, one should realize that clinical data, i.e., monophasic action potential recordings from the epicardial surface, to prove this reasoning are as yet lacking. One study *(22)* demonstrated changes in endocardial monophasic action potentials in the RVOT, but not the right ventricular apex, in a patient with recurrent syncope and transient right precordial ST elevation in whom these ST elevations were precipitated by ajmaline administration. In light of the great number of patients with earlier generation ICDs (with epicardial patches) and their returning need for replacement, it does not seem impossible to obtain epicardial recordings.

An aspect of the repolarization abnormality in the right precordial leads that has not received much attention is the secondary negative T-wave. It has been shown that the action potential initially lengthens upon exposure to flecainide before the action potential dome is lost *(25)*. Whenever the action potential duration of the epicardial layer outlasts those of the midmural layer, transmural membrane current will flow from epicardium to midmyocardium and a terminal negative T-wave will ensue (Fig. 2C). Alternatively, a secondary upstroke in the epicardial layer, elicited by local current flow from the plateau-phase of the midmural layer to the (partly) repolarized epicardial cells, will lead to prolonged repolarization in the epicardial layer with the same result (Fig. 2D). Intuitively, the latter sequence of events seems highly arrhythmogenic to us and because a terminal negative T-wave has not been reported to precede the onset of arrhythmias, less likely.

GENETIC BASIS

The Brugada syndrome displays an autosomal dominant inheritance *(26)* with incomplete penetrance *(27,28)*. Based on the postulated involvement of reduced sodium current, the *SCN5A* gene became an obvious candidate for the disorder, leading to the identification of aberrations in *SCN5A* in several small affected families and in individual cases (Fig. 3; *26,28–33*). In strict terms these findings do not prove causal involvement of *SCN5A* in Brugada syndrome, but compelling evidence, including functional aberrations of identified mutants, continues to emerge *(34)*.

Absence of linkage to *SCN5A* in a large family with the disorder indicates genetic heterogeneity *(35)*. This family linkage was identified to the chromosomal region 3p22–25. Thus, at least one other gene—close to the *SCN5A* locus on 3p21—is involved. Moreover, in three studies, mutation in *SCN5A* was identified only in a relatively small proportion of Brugada syndrome patients: *SCN5A* mutation was found in only 8 (15%) of 52 probands investigated by Priori and coworkers *(36)*; out of 18 Japanese patients studied by Akai et al. *(32)*, *SCN5A* mutation was only found in 1 patient with the disorder; and Schulze-Bahr et al. *(37)* identified *SCN5A* mutation in only 2 out of 20 unrelated

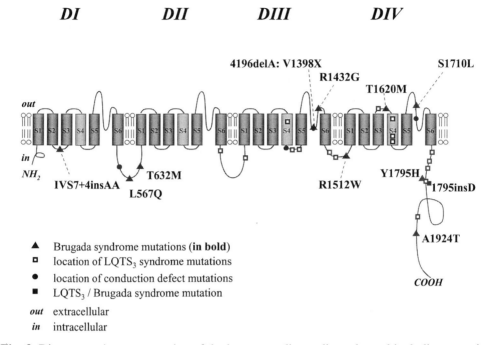

Fig. 3. Diagrammatic representation of the human cardiac sodium channel including mutations reported to date in this channel. Identity of Brugada syndrome mutations is indicated, while in the case of Long QT type 3 and conduction defect mutations, only locations of the mutations are shown.

individuals with Brugada syndrome upon mutation analysis of the *SCN5A* gene (90% of the coding region checked in this latter study).

When other genes are also implicated, mutations affecting the genes encoding the channels for I_{to} are immediate candidates; however, as yet no mutations have been found in the *KCND3* (Kv4.3) gene, the gene thought to encode (or part of) I_{to} in man *(37,38)*.

THE CARDIAC SODIUM CHANNEL

The cardiac Na^+ channel (Fig. 3; *39*) is a member of the voltage-dependent family of Na^+ channels *(40)* that are composed of heteromeric assemblies of an α-subunit, the pore-forming component, the function of which is modulated by association with one or two ancillary β-subunits. The cardiac Na^+ channel α-subunit is a heavily glycosylated protein of ~260 kDa consisting of 2016 amino acid residues *(41)*. It is encoded by the *SCN5A* gene *(42)* located on chromosome 3p21 *(43)*. This channel displays the typical modular architecture (Fig. 3) and the hallmarks of structure-function relation of this family of channels. It consists of four internally homologous domains (DI-DIV) linked by transmembrane segments residing on the cytoplasmic side of the channel. In turn, each domain is made up of six linked transmembrane segments (S1–S6). Ion selectivity and conductance properties *(44)* are determined by the S5–S6 linkers from each domain which line the ion-conducting pore *(45)*. Structures important for gating include the S4 segment from each domain, which act as a voltage sensor bringing about activation gating in response to voltage changes across the membrane *(46)*. The DIII-DIV linker mediates at least in part (fast) inactivation *(46,47)* through occlusion of the pore at the cytoplasmic end. Other structural determinants of (slow) inactivation probably reside within P-loops *(48–50)* and the C-terminal domain of the protein *(31)*.

A role for an interaction between the cardiac sodium channel and the β1–subunit (encoded by the *SCN1B* gene), a 218-amino-acid protein with a single transmembrane segment highly expressed in heart, has been suggested *(reviewed in 51)*. Though a rather consistent finding appears to be an increase in level of expression of the α-subunit, expression studies have produced conflicting results on the effect of this subunit on the kinetics of the cardiac Na-channel α-subunit.

GENOTYPE-PHENOTYPE RELATIONSHIP
IN THE BRUGADA SYNDROME

Theoretically, reduction of whole-cell Na-channel current may result from reduced numbers of functional Na-channels incorporated in the cell membrane or reduction of current through Na-channels (unitary current). Reduced incorporation into the cell membrane may result from defective protein trafficking possibly secondary to protein misfolding. Reduced unitary current may result from mutations that reduce channel pore permeability or those which modulate gating behavior. In general, shifts of the steady-state inactivation curve to more negative voltages (leftward shift) or of the steady-state activation curve to more positive voltages (rightward shift) reduce Na-channel availability. The Na-channel inactivation process seems particularly important, as both the time required for development of inactivation and recovery from it may be affected by mutations. In addition, it must be taken into account that Na-channel inactivation comprises different components (fast inactivation and slow inactivation, which are mediated by different structural features and which can be distinguished by the time required for the development and recovery from inactivation) *(40)* that may be affected in distinct manners. Here, we briefly outline the ways in which the *SCN5A* mutations identified thus far in Brugada syndrome have been shown to reduce Na-current. Notwithstanding, we emphasize caution in attempting to translate the functional changes of the mutations into the clinical phenotype, as the experimental conditions may play a profound role.

One of the initially described mutations (Fig. 3, *26*) putatively results in truncation of the protein: A single nucleotide (A) deletion at codon 1397 leading to the creation of an in-frame stop codon at 1398, resulting in truncation of the protein at the level of the pore region of transmembrane domain III (i.e., elimination of DIIIS6, DIV, and the C-terminal tail). Another mutation reported in the same study was an insertion of two nucleotides (AA) which disrupts the donor splice site of intron 7; the functional consequences of the latter mutation are harder to predict, but the authors speculated that it may also result in truncation of the protein.

Although it is intuitively not hard to envisage that truncated proteins may result in reduced whole-cell Na-current, the exact mechanism has not been elucidated. A reduction, or rather in this case abolishment, of Na-current also applies to the mutation R1432G *(30,33)*, located the extracellular loop between the pore region and the sixth transmembrane segment of domain III. This mutation was reported to result in no measurable current *(30,33)* when expressed in mammalian cells. Localization studies demonstrated that this was owing to a disruption in the localization of the channel to the plasma membrane *(33)*, thereby demonstrating that trafficking defects may indeed play a role in the reduced expression of mutant *SCN5A* channels in Brugada syndrome, as has been demonstrated for Long QT syndrome associated mutant human ether a go-go related gene (HERG)-channels *(52)*. Moreover, for some mutants that do lead to membrane expression of channels (with altered biophysical properties, discussed below), a decreased peak current density was observed (Y1795H, *[31]*; 1795insD, *[53]*).

The biophysical properties of the S1710L Na$^+$ channel (Table 1) include enhanced inactivation, a hyperpolarizing shift of steady-state inactivation, a depolarizing shift of steady-state activation and a delayed recovery from inactivation, all consistent with a decrease in net inward Na$^+$ current *(32)*, expected of *SCN5A* mutations associated with this disorder.

Functional characterization (*54*; Table 1) of the 1795insD mutation (located in the C-terminal tail), responsible for the mixed phenotype of Brugada syndrome and Long QT Syndrome (LQTS$_3$) in a large kindred *(53)*, has provided a satisfactory explanation for the seemingly paradoxical coexistence of the Brugada phenotype (putatively associated with reduced Na-channel function) and LQTS$_3$ phenotype (increased Na-channel function) in the same patients. This explanation revolves around differential effects on the distinct components of inactivation. Although this mutation yields increased slow inactivation, leading to more ST-elevations at fast heart rates (short diastolic intervals do not allow sufficient time for recovery from slow inactivation, thereby reducing the number of Na-channels which are available for activation), it reduces fast inactivation, thereby resulting in the noninactivating Na-current which causes QT prolongation at slow heart rates (at long diastolic intervals, recovery from slow inactivation is complete and the effects of reduced fast inactivation now predominate).

Not unexpectedly, the biophysical properties of two other mutations at the same Tyr-1795 residue, Y1795H *(31)* associated with a Brugada syndrome presentation, and Y1795C *(31)* associated with a LQTS presentation, bear resemblance to those of 1795insD. Like the 1795insD channel, the Y1795C and Y1795H channels display an enhanced entry into a slow (intermediate) inactivation phase compared to wild-type. For the Y1795H mutation, this enhanced development of slow inactivation, together with a negative shift in channel availability and the speeding of the onset of inactivation, is consistent with the loss of channel activity. The Y1795C mutation, on the other hand, prolongs action potential duration and consequently QT interval as a result of a slowed onset of (fast) inactivation and the occurrence of sustained late sodium current. This is most pronounced at slow heart rates since at faster rates sustained Na$^+$ current through this channel is reduced and inactivation becomes faster, which, together with the enhanced entrance into the slowly developing inactivation phase of this channel (which as explained above reduces I_{Na} at faster rates), is expected to reduce peak current (and decrease QT interval) at faster rates. This ties up with observations that LQTS$_3$ patients have prolonged QT-intervals at slower rates and suggestions of a bradycardia-dependent trigger for arrhythmias and mode of death in these patients *(51)*. Taken together this data not only points at the involvement of the C-terminal domain, and possibly the Tyr-1795 residue, in slow (intermediate) inactivation *(31)*, but also provides further evidence of the overlap in pathophysiology of these disorders at the level of the biophysical behavior of the mutant channels (discussed further below).

Patch-clamp studies of the other Brugada syndrome *SCN5A* mutations reported so far have been less consistent in providing evidence for reduced Na-channel function (Table 1). For instance, voltage clamp studies of one of the first reported *SCN5A* mutations

Table 1

Electrophysiological Characteristics of Mutant Cardiac Sodium Channels Associated with the Brugada Syndrome. Changes and/or shifts are relative to the wild-type channel.

Mutation	Domain	Shift in $V_{1/2}$ of activation	Shift in $V_{1/2}$ inactivation	Recovery from inactivation	Time-course of inactivation	Persistent I_{Na}	Ref.
R1512W	DIII-DIV linker	−5.1 mV	−3.8 mV	slower 1.2x at −100 mV	slower 1.3x	n.d.	(29)
		n.s.*	n.s.* 1.4x at −100 mV	slower* 1.7x	slower*	n.s.*	(30)*
T1620M	DIV S3–S4 loop	n.s.	+10 mV or +4.8 mV	faster	n.d.	n.s.	(26,55,61)
		n.s.*	n.s.* 1.3x at −110 mV or slower	1.3 to 1.6x at −80 mV faster*	n.s.*	n.s.*	(16)*
+β1		n.s.	+10.5 mV	1.2x at −100 mV faster	n.s.	n.s.	(55)*
				3x at −80 mV			(61)
+β1*		n.s.*	n.s.* 1.4x at −100 mV	slower*	n.s.*	n.s.*	(55)*
32–37°C		+10.7 mV* at 32°C	n.s.*	slower 32°C*, −110 mV τfast 2.8x τslow 10x	faster 2x at 37°C	n.d.	(16)*
S1710L +β1	DIV Pore	+18 mV*	−25 mV*	slower*	faster*	n.d.	(32)*
Y1795H +β1*	C-terminal	n.s.*	−10.5 mV*	n.s.*	faster onset*	small increase*	(31)*
1795InsD	C-terminal	+8.1 mV	−7.3 mV	slower	n.s.	n.s.	(53)
(Brugada + LQTS₃) +β1*		n.s.*	−9.7 mV*	1.2x at −100 mV slower* at −120 mV τfast 2.0x τslow 1.3x	faster* τfast 2.3x	1.4%*	(54)*
A1924T	C-terminal	−9 mV	n.s.	n.s.	n.s.	n.d.	(29)

n.s. = no statistically significant change; n.d. = not done. * values found in mammalian cell line expression systems; all other data are from the *Xenopus* oocyte expression system.

195

(T1620M, located in the extracellular linker between S3 and S4 of transmembrane domain IV) *(26)* showed a rightward shift of the steady-state inactivation curve and increased rate of recovery from inactivation; both effects should increase, rather than reduce, Na-channel availability. However, it is now increasingly appreciated that the experimental conditions may play a profound role *(39)*. For instance, temperature-dependence must be considered. Although at 20°C T1620M mutant channels have largely the same electrophysiological properties as wild-type sodium channels (the temperature at which the original studies were performed) *(26)*, they exhibit changes resulting in reduced current when studied at 32°C (a rightward shift of the steady-state activation curve and a reduced rate of recovery from inactivation; Table 1) *(16)*. Another factor to be taken into account is the expression system used. When expressed in *Xenopus* oocytes, *SCN5A* channels with the T1620M mutation have opposite electrophysiological properties compared to those expressed in the mammalian cell line tsA201 *(55)*. Although they have rightward shift of the steady-state inactivation curve and a faster recovery from inactivation (both effects yielding increased sodium channel availability) in *Xenopus* oocytes, the steady-state inactivation curve is unaltered and recovery from inactivation is slower (reducing sodium channel availability) in tsA201 cells. Similarly, for the 1795insD mutation, the steady-state activation is shifted to the right (compared with wild-type) when expressed in *Xenopus* oocytes *(53)*, but is not different from wild-type when expressed in the mammalian cell line HEK-293 *(54)*. And finally, in the case of the R1432G substitution, while expression in *Xenopus* oocytes resulted in a Na$^+$ current with normal gating properties, this substitution was associated with abolishment of membrane expression of the channel in tsA201 cells *(33)*. Taken together, these findings underline that caution must be exercised when attempting to account for the phenotype utilizing experimental studies.

Two other mutations (R1512W and A1924T) have yielded results in patch-clamp studies that are not apparently reconcilable with reduced Na-current. R1512W (located in the cytoplasmic linker between transmembrane domains III and IV) caused a leftward shift of the steady-state activation curve *(29)* and a delayed development of inactivation (both effects should increase Na-current), but, on the other hand, a delayed recovery from inactivation, both in *Xenopus* oocytes and in mammalian cells *(29,30)* (theoretically reduction in Na-current). A1924T (located in the C-terminal tail) caused a leftward shift of the steady-state activation curve. For both mutants, again, some temperature dependence appeared to be present *(29)*. It has been argued that the substantial negative voltage shift of the steady-state activation of mutant channels may lower the action potential threshold thereby increasing excitability, and that the increase in window current of these mutants may increase the depolarizing force early in the course of the action potential *(29,51)*. As a highly speculative hypothesis it has also been suggested that a sufficient increase in window current, as a result of the negative shift of the activation curve of the mutant channels, may lead to depolarizing forces at resting membrane potential. Such depolarizations would lead to a larger fraction of inactivated channels, consequently decreasing the magnitude of the Na$^+$ current during the action potential upstroke *(29,51)*.

MUTATION IN SCN5A AND OTHER PRIMARY ELECTRICAL DISORDERS

Besides the Brugada syndrome, mutations in the cardiac Na-channel have been implicated in other forms of primary electrophysiological disorders, namely the Long QT syndrome and cardiac conduction defects (Fig. 3; *51*). Although Brugada syndrome mutations hasten epicardial repolarization by reducing Na-current, Long QT syndrome-causing *SCN5A* mutations are associated with a "gain-of-function" mechanism either through persistent inward sodium current during the action potential plateau (described for 8 LQTS$_3$ mutations for which expression studies have been carried out) *(51)*, or by an increase in Na$^+$ current during the plateau of the action potential caused by a combination of slowing in rate of inactivation and an increase in the window Na$^+$ current during the final phase of repolarization (caused by a positive shift in voltage dependence of steady-state inactivation), as demonstrated recently for the A1330P mutation associated with a case of Sudden Infant Death Syndrome *(56)*. Both mechanisms delay repolarization thereby prolonging the QT-interval. For the D1790G, the mechanism for QT prolongation is debated. Besides a persistent inward current *(57)* this mutation leads to a negative shift in voltage dependence of inactivation *(58)* and it has been proposed that it may prolong the action potential through a calcium-dependent mechanism *(58)*.

Only 3 mutations causing isolated conduction defects have been reported in *SCN5A* *(59,60)*. One of these mutations, G514C in the DI-DII linker, was associated with diverse gating defects *(59)*. On the other hand, two other mutations (5280delG and IVS22+2T->C; *60*) are expected to produce entirely nonfunctional channels. One would expect that the (clinical) effect of such mutations would mimic that of Brugada syndrome mutations of the same sort, namely IVS7+4insAA and 4196delA, and perhaps also that of R1432G. The fact that they are associated with different clinical manifestations suggests that other factors such as "modifier genes," allele penetrance and developmental factors may also influence the relationship between the phenotype and Na-channel function *(59)*.

Moreover, the three *SCN5A*-related disorders share various clinical features, including conduction defect (conduction defects by definition, Long QT syndrome and Brugada syndrome), nocturnal sudden cardiac death (Brugada syndrome and Long QT syndrome) that in part seems related to bradyarrhythmias, and repolarization disorder (Brugada syndrome and Long QT syndrome). This leads one to view the different clinical presentations of *SCN5A*-related disorders as actually being the outcome of a spectrum of manifestations of cardiac sodium channelopathy resulting from the highly diverse functional behavior of the sodium channel *(51)*.

REFERENCES

1. Alings M, Wilde A. "Brugada" syndrome: clinical data and suggested pathophysiological mechanism. Circulation 1999;99:666–673.
2. Gussak I, Antzelevitch C, Bjerregaard P, Towbin JA, Chaitman BR. The Brugada syndrome: clinical, electrophysiologic and genetic aspects. J Am Coll Cardiol 1999;33:5–15.
3. Brugada P, Brugada J. Right bundle branch block, persistent ST segment elevation and sudden death: A distinct clinical and electrocardiographic syndrome. J Am Coll Cardiol 1992;20:1391–1396.
4. Sumiyoshi M, Nakata Y, Hisaoka T, et al. A case of idiopathic ventricular fibrillation with incomplete right bundle branch block and persistent ST segment elevation. Jpn Heart J 1993;34:661–666.
5. Bjerregaard P, Gussak I, Kotar SL, Gessler JE, Janosik D. Recurrent syncope in a patient with prominent J wave. Am Heart J 1994;127:1426–1430.
6. Miyazaki T, Mitamura H, Miyoshi S, et al. Autonomic and antiarrhythmic drug modulation of ST segment elevation in patients with Brugada syndrome. J Am Coll Cardiol 1996;27:1061–1070.
7. Atarashi H, Ogawa S, Harumi K, et al. for the Idiopathic Ventricular Fibrillation Investigators. Characteristics of patients with right bundle branch block and ST-segment elevation in right precordial leads. Am J Cardiol 1996;78:581–583.

8. Veerakul G, Nademanee K. Dynamic changes in the RBBB and ST-elevation pattern in the right precordial leads observed in patients with idiopathic ventricular fibrillation: evidence of phase 2 repolarization abnormality (abstract). Circulation 1996;94/8 Suppl I:I-626.

9. Brugada J, Brugada P. Further characterization of the syndrome of right bundle branch block, persistent ST-segment elevation, and sudden cardiac death. J Cardiovasc Electrophysiol 1997;8:325–331.

10. Nademanee K. Sudden unexplained death syndrome in Southeast Asia. Am J Cardiol 1997;79:10–11.

11. Matsuo K, Kurita T, Inagaki M, et al. The circadian pattern of the development of ventricular fibrillation in patients with Brugada syndrome. Eur Heart J 1999;20:465–470.

12. Priori SG, Napolitano C, Giordano U, Collisani G, Memmi M. Brugada syndrome and sudden cardiac death in children. Lancet 2000;355:808–809.

13. Wilde A, Düren D. Sudden cardiac death, RBBB, and right precordial ST-segment elevation. Circulation 1999;99:722–723.

14. Yan GX, Antzelevitch C. Cellular basis for the electrocardiographic J wave. Circulation 1996;93:372–379.

15. Yan G-X, Antzelevitch C. Cellular basis for the Brugada Syndrome and other mechanisms of arrhythmogenesis associated with ST-segment elevation. Circulation 1999;100:1660–1666.

16. Dumaine R, Towbin JA, Brugada P, et al. Ionic mechanisms responsible for the electrocardiographic phenotype of the Brugada syndrome are temperature dependent. Circ Res 1999;85(9):803–809.

17. Nabauer M, Beuckelmann DJ, Uberfuhr P, Steinbeck G. Regional differences in current density and rate-dependent properties of the transient outward current in subepicardial and subendocardial myocytes of human left ventricle. Circulation 1996;93:168–177.

18. Wettwer E, Amos GJ, Posival H, Ravens U. Transient outward current in human ventricular myocytes of subepicardial and subendocardial origin. Circ Res 1994;75:473–482.

19. Li GR, Feng J, Yue L, Carrier M. Transmural heterogeneity of action potentials and I_{to1} in myocytes isolated from the human right ventricle. Am J Physiol 1998;275:H369–H377.

20. Krishnan SC, Antzelevitch C. Flecainide-induced arrhythmia in canine ventricular epicardium. Phase 2 reentry? Circulation 1993;87:562–672.

21. Di Diego JM, Sun ZQ, Antzelevitch C. I(to) and action potential notch are smaller in left vs. right canine ventricular epicardium. Am J Physiol 1996;271:H548–H561.

22. Eckhardt L, Kirchhof P, Johna R, Breithardt G, Borggrefe M, Haverkamp W. Transient local changes in right ventricular monophasic action potentials due to ajmaline in a patient with Brugada syndrome. J Cardiovasc Electrophysiol 1999;10:1010–1015.

23. Nomura M, Nada T, Endo J, Kondo Y, Yukinaka M, Saito J, Ito S, Mori H, Nakaya Y, Shinomiya H. Brugada syndrome associated with an autonomic disorder. Heart 1998;80:194–196.

24. Washizuka T, Chinushi M, Niwano S, Aizawa Y. Bifid T waves induced by isoprenaline in a patient with Brugada syndrome. Heart 1998;79:305–307.

25. Krishnan SC. Antzelevitch C. Sodium channel block produces opposite electrophysiological effects in canine ventricular epicardium and endocardium. Circ Res 1991;69:277–291.

26. Chen Q, Kirsch GE, Zhang D, et al. Genetic basis and molecular mechanism for idiopathic ventricular fibrillation. Nature 1998;392:293–296.

27. Priori SG, Napolitano C, Terreni L, et al. Incomplete penetrance and variable response to sodium channel blockade in Brugada's syndrome Eur Heart J 1999;20(Supp):465.

28. Priori SG, Napolitano C, Giordano U, Collisani G, Memmi M. Brugada syndrome and sudden cardiac death in children. Lancet 2000;355:808–809.

29. Rook MB, Bezzina Alshinawi C, Groenewegen WA, et al. Human SCN5A gene mutations alter cardiac sodium channel kinetics and are associated with the Brugada syndrome. Cardiovasc Res 1999;44: 507–517.

30. Deschênes I, Baroudi G, Berthet M, et al. Electrophysiological characterization of SCN5A mutations causing long QT (E1784K) and Brugada (R1512W and R1432G) syndromes. Cardiovasc Res 2000;46:55–65.

31. Rivolta I, Abriel H, Tateyama M, et al. Inherited Brugada and Long QT syndrome mutations of a single residue of the cardiac sodium channel confer distinct channel and clinical phenotypes. J Biol Chem 2001;276:30623–30630.

32. Akai J, Makita N, Sakurada H, et al. A novel SCN5A mutation associated with idiopathic ventricular fibrillation without typical ECG findings of Brugada syndrome. FEBS Letters 2000;479:29–34.

33. Baroudi G, Pouliot V, Denjoy I, Guicheney P, Shrier A, Chahine M. Novel mechanism for Brugada syndrome: Defective surface localization of an SCN5A mutant (R1432G). Circ Res 2001;88:e78–e83.

34. Wilde AAM, Veldkamp MW. What we can learn from individual resuscitated patients. Cardiovasc Res 2000;46:14–16.

35. McNamara DM, Weiss R, Seibel J, et al. Molecular heterogeneity in the Brugada syndrome. Circulation 1998;98:I-456 (Abstract).
36. Priori SG, Napolitano C, Gasparini M, et al. Clinical and genetic heterogeneity of right bundle branch block and ST-segment elevation syndrome: a prospective evaluation of 52 families. Circulation 2000;102:2509–2515.
37. Schulze-Bahr E, Isbrandt D, Eckardt L, Haverkamp W, Breithardt G. How genetic is the 'Brugada-Brugada' syndrome? Eur Heart J 2000;21 Suppl;353 (abstract).
38. Postma AV, Bezzina CR, de Vries JF, Wilde AA, Moorman AF, Mannens MM. Genomic organisation and chromosomal localisation of two members of the KCND ion channel family, KCND2 and KCND3. Human Genetics 2000;106:614–619.
39. Balser JR. Structure and function of the cardiac sodium channels. Cardiovasc Res 1999;42:327–338.
40. Marban E, Yamagishi T, Tomaselli GF. Structure and function of voltage-gated sodium channels. J Physiol 1998;508:647–657.
41. Gellens ME, George AL Jr, Chen LQ, et al. Primary structure and functional expression of the human cardiac tetrodotoxin-insensitive voltage-dependent sodium channel. Proc Natl Acad Sci USA 1992;89:554–558.
42. Wang Q, Li Z, Shen J, Keating MT. Genomic organization of the human SCN5A gene encoding the cardiac sodium channel. Genomics 1996;34:9–16.
43. George AL Jr, Varkony TA, Drabkin HA, et al. Assignment of the human heart tetrodotoxin-resistant voltage-gated Na+ channel alpha-subunit gene (SCN5A) to band 3p21. Cytogenet Cell Genet 1995;68:67–70.
44. Heinemann SH, Terlau H, Stuhmer W, Imoto K, Numa S. Calcium channel characteristics conferred on the sodium channel by single mutations. Nature 1992;356:441–443.
45. Yellen G, Jurman ME, Abramson T, MacKinnon R. Mutations affecting internal TEA blockade identify the pore-forming region of a K+ channel. Science 1991;251:939–942.
46. Stühmer W, Conti F, Suzuki H, et al. Structural parts involved in activation and inactivation of the sodium channel. Nature 1989;339:597–603.
47. Patton DE, West JW, Catterall WA, Goldin AL. Amino acid residues required for fast Na(+)-channel inactivation: charge neutralizations and deletions in then III-IV linker. Proc Natl Acad Sci USA 1992;89:10905–10909.
48. Balser JR, Nuss HB, Chiamvimonvat N, Perez-Garcia MT, Marban E, Tomaselli GF. External pore residue mediates slow inactivation in mu 1 rat skeletal muscle sodium channels. J Physiol 1996;494:431–442.
49. Cummins TR, Sigworth FJ. Impaired slow inactivation in mutant sodium channels. Biophys J 1996;71:227–236.
50. Vilin YY, Makita N, George AL, Ruben PC. Structural determinants of slow inactivation in human cardiac and skeletal muscle sodium channels. Biophys J 1999;77:1384–1393.
51. Bezzina CR, Rook MB, Wilde AAM. Cardiac sodium channel and inherited arrhythmia syndromes. Cardiovasc Res 2001;49:257–271.
52. Zhou Z, Gong Q, Epstein ML, January CT. HERG channel dysfunction in human Long QT Syndrome. J Biol Chem 1998;273:21061–21066.
53. Bezzina C, Veldkamp MW, van den Berg MP, et al. A single sodium channel mutation causing both long QT- and Brugada syndrome. Circ Res 1999;85:1206–1213.
54. Veldkamp MW, Viswanathan PC, Bezzina C, Baartscheer A, Wilde AAM, Balser JR. Two distinct congenital arrhythmias evoked by a multidysfunctional Na+ channel. Circ Res 2000;86:e91–e397.
55. Baroudi G, Carbonneau E, Pouliot V, Chahine M. SCN5A mutation (T1620M) causing Brugada syndrome exhibits different phenotypes when expressed in Xenopus oocytes and mammalian cells. FEBS Lett 2000;467:12–16.
56. Wedekind H, Smits PP, Schulze-Bahr E, et al. De novo mutation in the SCN5A gene associated with early onset of sudden infant death. Circulation 2001;104:1158–1164.
57. Baroudi G, Chahine M. Biophysical phenotypes of SCN5A mutations causing long QT and Brugada syndromes. FEBS Lett 2000;487:224–228.
58. Wehrens XHT, Abriel H, Cabo C, Benhorin J, Kass RS. Arrhythmogenic mechanism of an LQT-3 mutation of the human heart Na+ channel-subunit: A computational analysis. Circulation 2000;102:584–590.

59. Tan HL, Bink-Boelkens MT, Bezzina CR, et al. A sodium-channel mutation causes isolated cardiac conduction disease. Nature 2001;409(6823):1043–1047.
60. Schott JJ, Alshinawi C, Kyndt F, et al. Cardiac conduction defects associate with mutations in SCN5A. Nat Genet 1999;23:20–21.
61. Makita N, Shirai N, Wang DW, et al. Cardiac Na$^+$ channel dysfunction in Brugada syndrome is aggravated by β1–subunit. Circulation 2000;101:54–60.

11

Cellular and Ionic Mechanisms Underlying Arrhythmogenesis

Charles Antzelevitch, PhD,
Alexander Burashnikov, PhD,
and Jose M. Di Diego, MD

INTRODUCTION

The past decade has witnessed remarkable progress in our understanding of the molecular and electrophysiologic mechanisms underlying the development of a variety of cardiac arrhythmias (Table 1). These advances notwithstanding, our appreciation of the basis for many rhythm disturbances is incomplete. This chapter examines the state-of-the-art of our understanding of cellular mechanisms responsible for cardiac arrhythmias, placing them in historical perspective whenever possible.

The mechanisms responsible for active cardiac arrhythmias are generally divided into two major categories:

Enhanced or abnormal impulse formation and Reentry (Fig. 1). Reentry occurs when a propagating impulse fails to die out after normal activation of the heart and persists to reexcite the heart after expiration of the refractory period. Evidence implicating reentry as a mechanism of cardiac arrhythmias stems back to the turn of the previous century *(1–16)*. The mechanisms responsible for abnormal impulse formation include enhanced automaticity and triggered activity. Automaticity can be further subdivided into normal and abnormal and triggered activity, consisting of: Early afterdepolarizations (EADs) and Delayed afterdepolarizations (DADs).

ABNORMAL IMPULSE FORMATION

Normal Automaticity

Automaticity is the property of cardiac cells to generate spontaneous action potentials. Spontaneous activity is the result of diastolic depolarization caused by a net inward

From: *Contemporary Cardiology: Cardiac Repolarization: Bridging Basic and Clinical Science*
Edited by: I. Gussak et al. © Humana Press Inc., Totowa, NJ

Table 1
Mechanisms of Atrial and Ventricular Tachyarrhythmias

Tachyarrhythmia	Mechanism	Rate Range (bpm)
Sinus tachycardia	Automatic (normal)	≥100
Sinus node reentry	Reentry	110–180
Atrial tachycardia	Reentry, Automatic or Triggered (DADs – secondary to digitalis toxicity)	150–240
Atrial flutter	Reentry	240–350 more commonly 300 ± 20
Atrial fibrillation	Reentry Fibrillatory conduction of triggered impulses from pulmonary veins or SVC	260–450
Supraventricular tachycardia— AV nodal reentry	Reentry	120–250 more commonly 150–220
Supraventricular tachycardia— accessory pathway (WPW)	Reentry	140–250 more commonly 150–220
Accelerated idioventricular rhythm	Abnormal automaticity	>60 –
Ventricular tachycardia	Reentry Automatic (rare)	120–300 more commonly 140–240
Right ventricular outflow tract tachycardia	? Triggered (DADs)	120–220
Bundle branch reentry	Reentry	160–250 more commonly 190–240
Torsade de pointes	Precipitated by an EAD-induced triggered beat. Maintained by reentry	>200

bpm=beats per minute; DAD=delayed afterdepolarization; EAD=early afterdepolarization; SVC= superior vena cava; WPW=Wolff-Parkinson-White syndrome.

current flowing during phase 4 of the action potential, which progressively brings the membrane potential to threshold. The sino-atrial (SA) node normally displays the highest intrinsic rate. All other pacemakers are referred to as subsidiary or latent pacemakers, since they take over the function of initiating excitation of the heart only when the SA node is compromised or when impulses of SA nodal-origin fail to propagate.

The ionic mechanism underlying normal SA and atrioventricular (AV) nodes and Purkinje system automaticity include

1. A hyperpolarization-activated inward current (I_f) *(17,18)* and/or
2. decay of outward potassium current (I_K) *(19,20)*.

The contribution of I_f and I_K differs in SA/AV nodes and Purkinje fiber because of the different potential ranges of these two pacemaker types (i.e., –70 to –35 mV and –90 to –65 mV, respectively). The contribution of other voltage-dependent currents may also

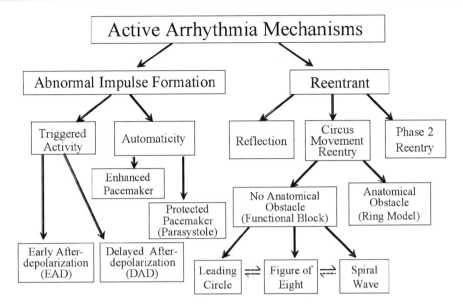

Fig. 1. Classification of active cardiac arrhythmias.

differ among the different cardiac cell types. For example, L-type calcium current (I_{Ca}) participates in the late phase of diastolic depolarization in SA and AV nodes, but not in Purkinje fibers. In atrial pacemaker cells, low voltage-activated T-type I_{Ca}, has been shown to contribute by sarcoplasmic reticulum (SR) calcium release, which, in turn, stimulates the inward sodium calcium exchange current (I_{Na-Ca}) *(21)*. The action potential upstroke is provided largely by the fast sodium current in His-Purkinje system and predominantly by the slow calcium current in SA and AV nodes.

Sympathetic and parasympathetic influences as well as extracellular potassium levels modulate the rate of diastolic depolarization. In general, β adrenergic receptor stimulation increases, whereas muscarinic receptor stimulation reduces, the rate of phase 4 depolarization. In the His-Purkinje system, parasympathetic effects are less apparent than those of the sympathetic system. Although acetylcholine produces little in the way of a direct effect, it can significantly reduce Purkinje automaticity via inhibition of the sympathetic influence, a phenomenon termed accentuated antagonism *(22)*. In all pacemaker cells, an increase of extracellular potassium concentration reduces the rate of diastolic depolarization, while a decrease of extracellular potassium has the opposite effect.

Abnormal Automaticity

Abnormal automaticity or depolarization-induced automaticity is observed under conditions of reduced resting membrane potential, such as ischemia, infarction, or other depolarizing influences (i.e., current injection) (Fig. 2). Abnormal automaticity is experimentally observed in tissues that normally develop diastolic depolarization (i.e., Purkinje fiber), as well as those that normally do not display this feature (e.g., ventricular or atrial working myocardium). Compared to normal automaticity, abnormal automaticity in Purkinje fibers or ventricular and atrial myocardium is more readily suppressed by calcium channel blockers and shows little to no overdrive suppression *(23,24)*. The ionic

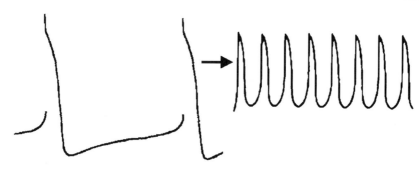

Fig. 2. Transition of normal to abnormal automaticity (depolarization-induced low voltage activity) in a Purkinje fiber.

basis for diastolic depolarization in abnormal automaticity may be similar to that of normal automaticity in SA and AV nodes, consisting of a time-dependent decay of I_K with progressive activation of I_{Ca} *(25,26)*.

The rate of abnormal automaticity is substantially higher than that of normal automaticity and is a sensitive function of resting membrane potential (i.e., the more depolarized resting potential the faster rate). Similar to normal automaticity, abnormal automaticity is enhanced by β-adrenergic agonists and by reduction of external potassium *(23,25)*.

Automaticity as a Mechanism of Cardiac Arrhythmias

Enhanced normal automaticity can be the cause of some, usually benign, cardiac arrhythmias, including sinus tachycardia. Accelerated idioventricular rhythms have been attributed to enhanced normal automaticity in the His-Purkinje system *(27)*. Although automaticity is not responsible for most rapid tachyarrhythmias, it can precipitate or trigger reentrant arrhythmias. The rate of automatic discharge recorded in isolated tissue under artificial experimental conditions may not be representative of the discharge rate to be expected in vivo, where endogenous factors such as catecholamines, histamine, endothelin-1, and other factors, such as stretch, may accelerate automaticity.

Overall, the role of automaticity in experimental and clinical arrhythmias in vivo is not well defined. Although experimental and clinical three-dimensional mapping studies have shown that ventricular arrhythmias arising under conditions of acute ischemia, infarction, heart failure, and other cardiomyopathies can be ascribed to focal mechanisms *(28–32)*, it is often difficult to discern between automatic and focal reentrant (reflection, phase 2 reentry and micro-reentry) mechanisms.

Several recent experimental studies suggest a role for automaticity in cardiac arrhythmias. Haissaguerre and coworkers have shown that atrial fibrillation can be triggered by rapid automaticity arising in the pulmonary veins *(33)*. In addition, myocytes isolated from failing and hypertrophied animal and human hearts have been shown to manifest diastolic depolarization *(34,35)* and to possess enhanced I_f pacemaker current *(36,37)* suggesting that these mechanism contribute to extrasystolic and tachyarrhythmias arising with these pathologies. It is also noteworthy that atrial tissues isolated from patients with atrial fibrillation exhibit increased I_f mRNA levels *(38)*.

Parasystole and Modulated Parasystole

Latent pacemakers throughout the heart are generally reset by the propagating wavefront initiated by the dominant pacemaker and are therefore unable to activate the

Protected Pacemaker

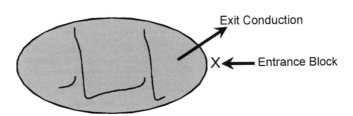

Fig. 3. Classical Parasystole. The ectopic pacemaker is protected from invasion by activity outside the focus (entrance block), but when the pacemaker fires, the impulse generated is able to propagate out of the focus to excite the rest of the myocardium (exit conduction).

heart. An exception to this rule occurs when the pacemaking tissue is somehow protected from the impulse of sinus origin. A region of entrance block arises when cells exhibiting automaticity are surrounded by ischemic, infarcted, or otherwise compromised cardiac tissues that prevent the propagating wave from invading the focus, but which permit the spontaneous beat generated within the automatic focus to exit and activate the rest of the myocardium. A pacemaker region exhibiting entrance block, and exit conduction defines a parasystolic focus (Fig. 3) *(39)*.

The ectopic activity generated by a parasystolic focus is characterized by premature ventricular complexes with variable coupling intervals, fusion beats and inter-ectopic intervals that are multiples of a common denominator. This rhythm is fairly rare. Although it is usually considered benign, any premature ventricular activation can induce malignant ventricular rhythms in the ischemic myocardium or in the presence of a suitable myocardial substrate.

In the late 1970s and early 1980s Moe and coworkers described a variant of classical parasystole, which they termed modulated parasystole *(40–42)*. This variant of the arrhythmia was suggested to result from incomplete entrance block of the parasystolic focus. Electrotonic influences arriving early in the pacemaker cycle delayed, and those arriving late in the cycle, accelerated the firing of the parasystolic pacemaker, so that ventricular activity could entrain the partially protected pacemaker (Fig. 4). As a consequence, at select heart rate, extrasystolic activity generated by the entrained parasystolic pacemaker would mimic reentry, generating extrasystolic activity with fixed coupling (Figs. 5, 6) *(40–52)*.

Afterdepolarizations and Triggered Activity

Oscillations that attend or follow the cardiac action potential and depend on preceding transmembrane activity for their manifestation are referred to as afterdepolarizations *(53)*. They are traditionally divided into two subclasses: Early and delayed. Early afterdepolarizations (EAD) interrupt or retard repolarization during phase 2 and/or phase 3 of the cardiac action potential, whereas delayed afterdepolarizations (DAD) arise after full repolarization. When EAD or DAD amplitude suffices to bring the membrane to its threshold potential, a spontaneous action potential referred to as a triggered response is the result *(54)*. These triggered events may be responsible for extrasystoles and tachyarrhythmias that develop under conditions predisposing to the development of afterdepolarizations.

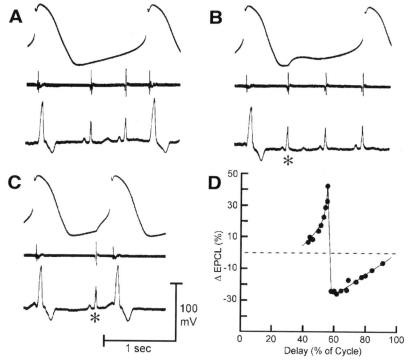

Fig. 4. Electrotonic modulation of a parasystolic pacemaker. Traces were recorded from an experimental model consisting of a sucrose gap preparation in vitro coupled to the heart of an open chest dog. Traces (top to bottom): transmembrane potentials recorded from a distal segment of a Purkinje fiber-sucrose gap preparation, and a right ventricular electrogram and lead II ECG from the in vivo preparation. **(A)** The Purkinje pacemaker was allowed to beat free of any influence from ventricular activation. **(B, C)** Pacemaker activity of the Purkinje is electrotonically influenced by ventricular activation. An electrotonic influence arriving early in the pacemaker cycle delays the next discharge, whereas that arriving late, accelerates the next discharge. **(D)** The electrotonic modulation of pacemaker discharge is described in the form of a phase-response curve. The percentage change in ectopic pacemaker cycle length (EPCL) is plotted as a function of the temporal position of the electrotonic influence in the pacemaker cycle. From *(47)*, with permission.

Early Afterdepolarizations and Triggered Activity

CHARACTERISTICS OF EADS, AND EAD-INDUCED TRIGGERED BEATS

EADs are observed in isolated cardiac tissues exposed to injury *(55)*, altered electrolytes, hypoxia, acidosis *(56,57)*, catecholamines *(58,59)*, pharmacologic agents *(60)*, including antiarrhythmic drugs *(61–65)*. Ventricular hypertrophy and heart failure also predispose to the development of EADs *(35,66,67)*.

EAD characteristics vary as a function of animal species, tissue or cell type and the method by which it is elicited. Although specific mechanisms of EAD induction may differ, a critical prolongation of repolarization accompanies most, but not all, EADs. Figure 7 illustrates the two types of EAD generally encountered in Purkinje fiber. Oscillatory events appearing at potentials positive to −30 mV, are generally referred to as phase 2 EADs. Those occurring at more negative potentials are termed phase 3 EADs. Phase 2 and phase 3 EADs sometimes appear in the same preparation. The right panels show that triggered responses develop when the preparations are paced at slower rates *(64)*. In

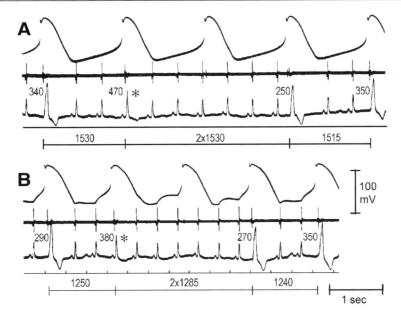

Fig. 5. Patterns of classical Parasystole generated by the experimental model described in Fig. 4 in the absence (**A**) and presence (**B**) of modulating influence from the ventricles. The lowest trace is a stimulus marker. Numbers denote the coupling intervals of the ectopic responses to the preceding normal beats (in ms). Asterisks denote fusion beats. Classical parasystolic features are apparent in both cases. From *(47)*, with permission.

contrast to Purkinje fibers, EAD activity recorded in ventricular preparations are always phase 2 EADs *(68)*.

EAD-induced triggered activity is a sensitive function of stimulation rate. Agents with Class III action generally induce EAD activity at slow stimulation rates and totally suppress EADs at rapid rates *(64,69)*. In contrast, β-adrenergic agonist-induced EADs are fast rate-dependent *(58,59)*. Recent studies have shown that in the presence of I_{Kr} block, β adrenergic agonists and/or acceleration from an initially slow rate transiently facilitate the induction of EAD activity in ventricular M cells, but not in epicardium or endocardium and rarely in Purkinje fibers *(70)*. This biphasic effect is thought to be because of an initial priming of I_{Na-Ca}, which provides electrogenic inward current to sustain the action potential plateau, followed by recruitment of cyclic adenosine monophosphate (cAMP) and Ca^{2+}-activated slowly activating delayed rectifier current (I_{Ks}) which abbreviates action potential duration (APD).

Origin of EADs. Until about a decade ago, our understanding of the EAD was based largely on data obtained from studies involving Purkinje fiber preparations. With few exceptions *(71,72)* EADs were not observed in early experiments involving tissues isolated from the surface of the mammalian ventricle *(73–76)*. More recent studies have demonstrated that although canine epicardial and endocardial tissues generally fail to develop EADs when exposed to APD-prolonging agents, midmyocardial M cells readily develop EAD activity under these conditions *(77)*. Failure of epicardial and endocardial tissues to develop EADs has been ascribed to the presence of a strong I_{Ks} in these cells *(78)*. M cells have a weak I_{Ks} *(78)*, predisposing them to the development of EADs in the presence of I_{Kr} block.

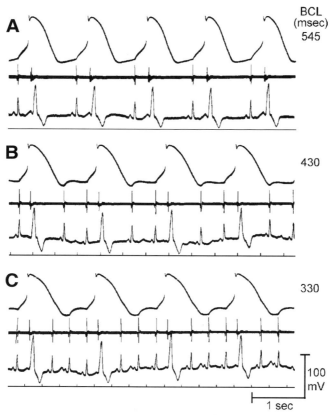

Fig. 6. Records were obtained from the same preparation as in Fig. 5 but at different cycle lengths. At the basic cycle lengths (BCL) shown, the activity generated was characteristic of reentry (fixed coupling of the premature beats to the basic beats). **(A)** Bigeminy; **(B)** Trigeminy; and **(C)** Quadrigeminy. From *(47)*, with permission.

I_{Ks} block with chromanol 293B does not induce EAD in any of the four ventricular cell types *(79)*. However, a combination of I_{Ks} and I_{Kr} block (chromanol 293B + E-4031 or sotalol) induces EAD activity in canine isolated epicardial and endocardial tissues *(80)* as well as in perfused left ventricular wedge preparations *(81)*. The predisposition of cardiac cells to the development of EADs depends principally on the reduced availability of I_{Kr} and I_{Ks} as occurs in many forms of cardiomyopathy. Under these conditions, EADs can appear in any part of the ventricular myocardium.

Three dimensional mapping of torsade de pointes (TdP) arrhythmias in canine experimental models suggest that the extrasystole that initiates TdP can originate from subendocardial, midmyocardium, or subepicardial regions of the left ventricle *(82,83)*. These data point to Purkinje fibers and M cells as the principal sources of EAD-induced triggered activity in vivo. In the presence of combined I_{Kr} and I_{Ks} block, epicardium is often the first to develop an EAD *(80,81)*.

Ionic Mechanisms Responsible for the EAD. EADs are usually associated with a prolongation of the repolarization phase owing to a reduction of net outward current secondary to an increase in inward currents and/or a decrease of outward currents. Most pharmacological interventions associated with EADs can be grouped as acting predominantly through one of four different mechanisms:

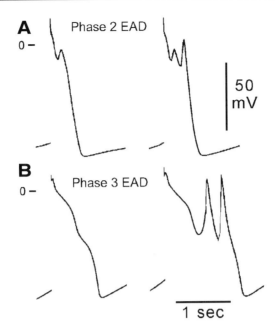

Fig. 7. EAD and triggered activity. Each panel shows intracellular activity simultaneously recorded from a the two ends of a Purkinje preparation pretreated with quinidine. Left panels depict responses displaying only EADs; right panels show responses manifesting triggered activity. (**A**) EAD and triggered activity occurring at the plateau level (phase 2). (**B**) EAD and triggered activity occurring during phase 3. Modified from *(64)*, with permission.

1. A reduction of repolarizing potassium currents (I_{Kr}, class IA and III antiarrhythmic agents; I_{Ks}, chromanol 293B).
2. An increase in the availability of calcium current (I_{Ca}).
3. An increase in the sodium-calcium exchange current because of augmentation of intracellular calcium activity or upregulation of the exchanger (Bay K 8644, catecholamines).
4. An increase in late sodium current (late I_{Na}) (aconitine, anthopleurin-A, and ATX-II).

Combinations of these interventions (i.e., calcium loading and I_{Kr} reduction) may act synergistically to facilitate the development of EADs *(70,76,84,85)*.

The upstroke of the EAD is generally carried by calcium current. There is less agreement on the ionic basis for the critically important conditional phase of the EAD, defined as the period just before the EAD upstroke. Intracellular calcium levels and Na/Ca exchange current play pivotal roles in the conditional phase of isoproterenol-induced EADs *(58,59,86)*. Data from several groups of investigators suggest that intracellular calcium levels do not influence the formation of this phase 2 EADs *(72,87–89)*, whereas other groups have presented strong evidence in support of the influence of intracellular calcium levels in the formation of at least the conditional phase of the EAD *(70,90)*. This discrepancy is in part owing to the type of tissues or cells studied.

There are important differences in the ionic mechanisms of EAD generation in canine Purkinje fibers and ventricular M cells. EADs induced in the canine M cells are exquisitely sensitive to change in intracellular calcium levels, whereas EADs elicited in Purkinje

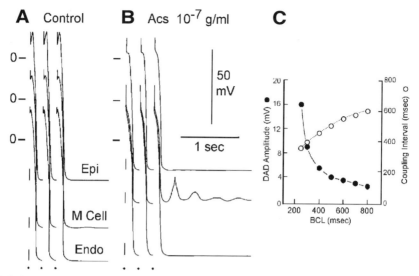

Fig. 8. Digitalis-induced delayed afterdepolarizations in M cells but not epicardium or endocardium. Effects of acetylstrophanthidin (AcS) on transmembrane activity of an epicardial (Epi), endocardial (Endo) and M cell preparation. $[K^+]_o = 4$ mM. **(A)** Control. **(B)** Recorded after 90 min of exposure to 10^{-7} g/ml AcS. Each panel shows the last 3 beats of a train of 10 basic beats elicited at a BCL of 250 ms. Each train is followed by a 3 sec pause. AcS induced prominent DADs in the M cell preparation but not in epicardium or endocardium. **(C)** Rate-dependence of coupling interval and amplitude of the AcS-induced DADs. Measured is the first DAD recorded from the M cell. From *(77)* with permission.

are largely insensitive *(70,91)*. Ryanodine, an agent known to block calcium release from the SR, abolishes EAD activity in canine M cells, but not in Purkinje fibers *(91)*. These distinctions may reflect differences in intracellular calcium handling in M cells, where the SR is well developed, vs Purkinje fibers where the SR is poorly developed.

The Role of EADs in the Development of Cardiac Arrhythmias. As previously discussed, EAD-induced triggered activity is thought to be involved in precipitating TdP under condition of congenital and acquired long QT syndromes (LQTS) *(92,93)*. EAD-like deflections have been observed in ventricular Monophasic Action Potential (MAP) recordings immediately preceding TdP arrhythmias in the clinic as well as in experimental models of LQTS *(74,94–97)*.

EAD activity may also be involved in the genesis of cardiac arrhythmias in cases of hypertrophy and heart failure. These syndromes are commonly associated with prolongation of the ventricular action potential, which predisposes to the development of EADs *(34,35,66,67,98–100)*.

DELAYED AFTERDEPOLARIZATION-INDUCED TRIGGERED ACTIVITY

Delayed afterdepolarizations (DAD) are oscillations of transmembrane activity that occur after full repolarization of the action potential and depend on previous activation of the cell for their manifestation. DADs that reach the threshold potential give rise to spontaneous responses also referred to as triggered activity *(54)*.

Causes and Origin of DAD-Induced Triggered Activity. DADs and DAD-induced triggered activity are observed under conditions that cause large increases in intracellular calcium, $[Ca^{2+}]_i$, such as after exposure to toxic levels of cardiac glycosides (digitalis) *(101–103)* or catecholamines *(58,104–106)*. This activity is also manifest in hypertrophied and failing hearts *(34,66)* as well as in Purkinje fibers surviving myocardial infarction *(107)*. In contrast to EADs, DADs are always induced at relatively rapid rates.

Digitalis-induced DADs and triggered activity have been well characterized in isolated Purkinje fibers *(54)*. In the ventricular myocardium, they are rarely observed in epicardial or endocardial tissues, but readily induced in cells and tissues from the M region. However, DADs are frequently observed in myocytes enzymatically dissociated from ventricular myocardium *(108–110)*. Digitalis, isoproterenol, high $[Ca^{2+}]_0$, or Bay K 8644, a calcium agonist, have been shown to cause DADs and triggered activity in tissues isolated from the M region but not in epicardial or endocardial tissues (Fig. 8) *(77,79,111,112)*. The failure of epicardial and endocardial cells to develop DADs has been ascribed to a high density of I_{Ks} in these tissues *(78)* as compared to M cells where I_{Ks} is small *(78)*. Indeed, reduction of I_{Ks} was recently shown to promote isoproterenol-induced DAD activity in canine and guinea pig endocardium and epicardium *(79,113)*.

Any intervention capable of altering intracellular calcium, either by modifying transsarcolemmal calcium current or by inhibiting SR storage or release of calcium can affect the manifestation of the DAD. DADs can also be modified by interventions capable of directly inhibiting or enhancing I_{ti}. DADs are modified by extracellular K^+, Ca^{2+}, lisophosphoglycerides, and the metabolic factors such as ATP, hypoxia, and pH. Lowering extracellular K^+ (<4 mM) promote DADs, while increasing K^+ attenuates or totally suppresses DADs *(54,114)*. Lisophosphatidylcholine, in concentrations similar to those that accumulate in ischemic myocardium, have been shown to induce DAD activity *(115)*. Elevating extracellular Ca^{2+} promotes DADs *(54)* and an increase of extracellular ATP potentiates isoproterenol-induced DAD *(116)*.

Agents that prolong repolarization such as quinidine and clofilium facilitate the induction of DAD activity by augmenting calcium entry. Recent work indicates that calcium calmodulin (CaM) kinase can facilitate the induction of DADs by augmenting I_{Ca} *(117)*.

Pharmacological agents that affect the release and reuptake of calcium by the SR, including caffeine and ryanodine, can also influence the manifestation of DADs and triggered activity. Low concentrations of caffeine facilitate Ca release from the SR and thus contribute to augmentation of DAD and triggered activity. High concentration of caffeine prevent Ca uptake by the SR and thus abolish I_{ti}, DADs, aftercontractions and triggered activity. Doxorubicin, an anthracycline antibiotic, has been shown to be effective in suppressing digitalis induced DADs, possibly through inhibition of the Na-Ca exchange mechanism *(118)*. Potassium channel activators, like pinacidil, can also suppress DAD and triggered activity by activating ATP-regulated potassium current (I_{K-ATP}) *(109,112)*.

Ionic Mechanisms Responsible for the Development of DADs. DADs and accompanying aftercontractions are caused by oscillatory release of calcium from the SR under calcium overload conditions. The afterdepolarization is believed to be induced by a transient inward current (I_{ti}) generated either by:

1. A nonselective cationic current, I_{ns} *(119,120)*.
2. The activation of an electrogenic Na/Ca exchanger *(119,121–123)*.
3. Calcium-activated Cl^- current *(122,123)*.

All are secondary to the release of Ca from the overloaded SR.

The Role of DAD-Induced Triggered Activity in the Development of Cardiac Arrhythmias. Although a wide variety of studies performed in isolated tissues and cells suggest an important role for DAD-induced triggered activity in the genesis of cardiac arrhythmias, especially bigeminal rhythms and tachyarrhythmias observed in the setting of digitalis toxicity *(54)*, little direct evidence of DAD-induced triggered activity is available in vivo. Consequently, even when triggered activity appears a likely mechanism, it is often impossible to completely rule out other mechanisms (e.g., reentry, enhanced automaticity, and so on).

Clinical arrhythmias suggested to be caused by DAD-induced triggered activity include:

1. *Idiopathic ventricular tachyarrhythmias (124–127)*.
2. *Idioventricular rhythms* - accelerated AV junctional escape rhythms that occur as a result of digitalis toxicity or in a setting of myocardial infarction.

Other possible "DAD-mediated" arrhythmias include exercise-induced adenosine-sensitive ventricular tachycardia (VT) as described by Lerman and Belardinelli *(128)*; repetitive monomorphic VT caused presumably cAMP-mediated triggered activity *(129)*; supraventricular tachycardias, including arrhythmias originating in the coronary sinus *(130)*; some heart failure-related arrhythmias *(32,34,100)*.

REENTRANT ARRHYTHMIAS

Circus Movement Reentry

The circuitous propagation of an impulse around an anatomical or functional obstacle leading to reexcitation of the heart describes a circus movement reentry. Four distinct models of this form of reentry have been described:

1. The ring model.
2. The leading circle model.
3. The figure of 8 model.
4. The spiral wave model.

The ring model of reentry differs from the other three in that an anatomical obstacle is required. The leading circle, figure of 8 and spiral wave models of reentry require only a functional obstacle.

RING MODEL

The ring model, the simplest form of reentry, first emerged as a concept shortly after the turn of the century when A.G. Mayer reported the results of experiments involving the subumbrella tissue of a jellyfish (*Sychomedusa Cassiopea*) *(1,2)*. The muscular disk did not contract until ring-like cuts were made and pressure and a stimulus applied. This caused the disk to "spring into rapid rhythmical pulsation so regular and sustained as to recall the movement of clockwork" *(1)*. Mayer demonstrated similar circus movement excitation in rings cut from the ventricles of turtle hearts, but he did not consider this to be a plausible mechanism for the development of cardiac arrhythmias. His experiments proved valuable in identifying two fundamental conditions necessary for the initiation and maintenance of circus movement excitation:

1. Unidirectional block—the impulse initiating the circulating wave must travel in one direction only.
2. In order for the circus movement to continue, the circuit must be long enough to allow each site in the circuit to recover before the return of the circulating wave.

In 1913, Mines *(3)* developed the concept of circus movement reentry as a mechanism responsible for cardiac arrhythmias *(4)*. Mines confirmed Mayer's observations and suggested that the recirculating wave could be responsible for clinical cases of tachycardia *(3)*. This concept was reinforced *(4)* with Kent's discovery of an extra accessory pathway connecting the atrium and ventricle of a human heart *(131)*. The criteria developed by Mines for identification of circus movement reentry remains in use today:

1. An area of unidirectional block must exist.
2. The excitatory wave progresses along a distinct pathway, returning to its point of origin and then following the same path again.
3. Interruption of the reentrant circuit at any point along its path should terminate the circus movement.

In 1928, Schmitt and Erlanger *(132)* suggested that coupled ventricular extrasystoles in mammalian hearts could arise as a consequence of circus movement reentry within loops composed of terminal Purkinje fibers and ventricular muscle. Using a theoretical model consisting of a Purkinje bundle that divides into two branches which insert distally into ventricular muscle (Fig. 9), they suggested that a region of depression within one of the terminal Purkinje branches could provide for unidirectional block and conduction slow enough to permit successful reexcitation within a loop of limited size (i.e., 10–30 mm). The early investigators recognized that successful reentry could occur only when the impulse was sufficiently delayed in an alternate pathway to allow for expiration of the refractory period in the tissue proximal to the site of unidirectional block. Both conduction velocity and refractoriness determine the success or failure of reentry and the general rule is that the length of the circuit (pathlength) must exceed or equal to that of the wavelength, the wavelength being defined as the product of the conduction velocity and the refractory period or that part of the pathlength occupied by the impulse and refractory to reexcitation. The theoretical minimum pathlength required for development of reentry was initially thought to be quite long. In the early 1970s, micro-reentry within narrowly circumscribed loops was suggested to be within the realm of possibility. Cranefield, Hoffman and coworkers *(133,134)* demonstrated that segments of canine Purkinje fibers which normally display impulse conduction velocities of 2–4 m/sec, can conduct impulses with apparent velocities of 0.01–0.1 m/sec when encased in high K^+ agar. This finding and the demonstration by Sasyniuk and Mendez in 1971 *(135)* of a marked abbreviation of action potential duration and refractoriness in terminal Purkinje fibers just proximal to the site of block, greatly reduced the theoretical limit of the pathlength required for the development of reentry.

Soon after, single and repetitive reentry was reported by Wit and coworkers *(136)* in small loops of canine and bovine conducting tissues bathed in a high K^+ solution containing catecholamines, thus demonstrating reentry over a relatively small path. In some experiments, they used linear unbranched bundles of Purkinje tissue to demonstrate a phenomenon similar to that observed by Schmitt and Erlanger in which slow anterograde conduction of the impulse was at times followed by a retrograde wavefront that produced

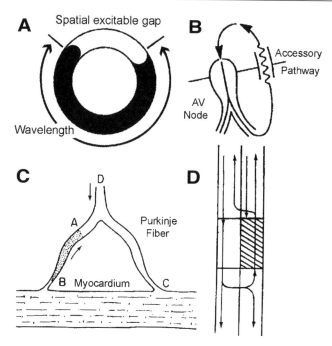

Fig. 9. Ring models of reentry. **(A)** Schematic of a ring model of reentry. **(B)** Mechanism of reentry in the Wolf-Parkinson-White syndrome involving the AV node and an atrioventricular accessory pathway (AP). **(C)** A mechanism for reentry in a Purkinje-muscle loop proposed by Schmitt and Erlanger. The diagram shows a Purkinje bundle **(D)** that divides into two branches, both connected distally to ventricular muscle. Circus movement was considered possible if the stippled segment, A → B, showed unidirectional block. An impulse advancing from D would be blocked at A, but would reach and stimulate the ventricular muscle at C by way of the other terminal branch. The wavefront would then reenter the Purkinje system at B traversing the depressed region slowly so as to arrive at A following expiration of refractoriness. **(D)** Schematic representation of circus movement reentry in a linear bundle of tissue as proposed by Schmitt and Erlanger. The upper pathway contains a depressed zone (shaded) serves as a site of unidirectional block and slow conduction. Anterograde conduction of the impulse is blocked in the upper pathway but succeeds along the lower pathway. Once beyond the zone of depression, the impulse crosses over through lateral connections and reenters through the upper pathway. Panels C and D are from Schmitt and Erlanger *(132)*.

a "return extrasystole" *(137)*. They proposed that the nonstimulated impulse was caused by a circus movement reentry made possible by longitudinal dissociation of the bundle, as in the Schmitt and Erlanger model (Fig. 9). Noting that in many of their experiments "the rapid upstroke within the depressed segment arises after the rapid upstroke of the normal fiber," Wit and coworkers also considered the possibility *(137,138)* that "the reflected impulse that travels slowly backward through the depressed segment is evoked by retrograde depolarization of the cells within the depressed segment by the rapid upstrokes of the cells beyond" *(138)*. Thus arose the suggestion that reexcitation could occur in a single fiber through a mechanism other than circus movement, namely reflection. While both explanations appeared plausible, proof for either was lacking at the time. Direct evidence in support of reflection as a mechanism of reentrant activity did not emerge until the early 1980s, as discussed later.

These pioneering studies led to our understanding of how anatomical obstacles such as the openings of the Venae Cava in the right atrium, an aneurysm in the ventricles, or the presence bypass tract between atria and ventricles (Kent bundle) can form a ring-like path for the development of extrasystoles, tachycardia, and flutter.

LEADING CIRCLE MODEL

The possibility that reentry could be initiated without the involvement of anatomical obstacles and that "natural rings are not essential for the maintenance of circus contractions" was first suggested by Garrey in 1924 *(139)*. Nearly 50 years later, Allessie and coworkers *(140–142)* were the first to provide direct evidence in support of this hypothesis in experiments in which they induced a tachycardia in isolated preparations of rabbit left atria by applying properly timed premature extrastimuli. Using multiple intracellular electrodes, they showed that although the basic beats elicited by stimuli applied near the center of the tissue spread normally throughout the preparation, premature impulses propagate only in the direction of shorter refractory periods. An arc of block thus develops around which the impulse is able to circulate and re-excite the tissue. Recordings near the center of the circus movement showed only subthreshold responses. Thus arose the concept of the leading circle *(142)*, a form of circus movement reentry occurring in structurally uniform myocardium, requiring no anatomic obstacle (Fig. 10). The functionally refractory region that develops at the vortex of the circulating wavefront prevents the centripetal waves from short circuiting the circus movement and thus serves to maintain the reentry. Since the head of the circulating wavefront usually travels on relatively refractory tissue, a fully excitable gap of tissue may not be present; unlike other forms of reentry the leading circle model may not be readily influenced by extraneous impulses initiated in areas outside the reentrant circuit and thus may not be easily entrained.

Kamiyama and coworkers *(143)* later showed that the leading circle mechanism could mediate tachycardia induced in isolated ventricular tissues. Allessie and coworkers *(144)* also described the development of circus movement reentry without the involvement of an anatomic obstacle in a 2 dimensional model of ventricular epicardium created by freezing the endocardial layers of a Langendorf perfused rabbit heart.

Functional arcs or lines of block attending the development of a circus movement reentry were shown to develop in vivo models of canine infarction in which a thin surviving epicardial rim overlies the infarcted ventricle *(9,145–150)*. The lines of block observed during tachycardia are usually oriented parallel to the direction of the myocardial fibers, suggesting that anisotropic conduction properties (faster conduction in the direction parallel to the long axis of the myocardial cells) *(151–153)* also play an important role in defining the functionally refractory zone. Dillon and coworkers *(150)* subsequently showed that the long lines of functional block that sustain reentry in the epicardial rim overlying canine infarction may represent zones of very slow conduction, implying that the dimensions of the area of functional block may in fact be relatively small and may even approach that of the vortex of functional block described by Allessie and coworkers.

FIGURE OF EIGHT MODEL

El-Sherif and coworkers first described the figure of eight model of reentry in the surviving epicardial layer overlying infarction produced by occlusion of the left anterior descending artery in canine hearts in the late 1980s *(14,145–147,154)*. In the figure of eight model, the reentrant beat produces a wavefront that circulates in both directions

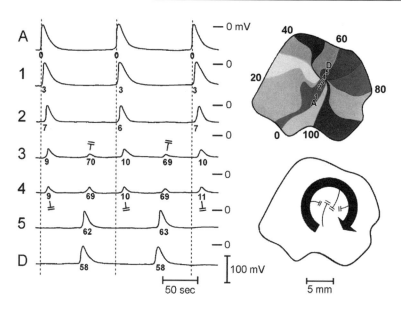

Fig. 10. Leading circle model of reentry. Activation maps during steady-state tachycardia induced by a premature stimulus in an isolated rabbit atrium (upper right). On the left are transmembrane potentials recorded from seven fibers located on a straight line through the center of the circus movement. Note that the central area is activated by centripetal wavelets and that the fibers in the central area show double responses of subnormal amplitude. Both responses are unable to propagate beyond the center, thus preventing the impulse from short-cutting the circuit. The activation pattern is schematically represented, showing the leading circuit and the converging centripetal wavelets. Block is indicated by double bars. From Allessie et al. *(142)*, with permission.

around a long line of functional conduction block (Fig. 11) rejoining on the distal side of the block. The wavefront then breaks through the arc of block to reexcite the tissue proximal to the block. The single arc of block is thus divided into two and the reentrant activation continues as two circulating wavefronts that travel in clockwise and counter-clockwise directions around the two arcs in a pretzel-like configuration. The diameter of the reentrant circuit in the ventricle may be as small as a few millimeters or as large as several centimeters. In 1999, Lin and coworkers *(155)* described a novel quatrefoil-shaped reentry induced by delivering long stimuli during the vulnerable phase in rabbit ventricular myocardium. This pattern, a variant of figure of 8 reentry, consists of two pairs of opposing rotors with all four circuits converging in the center.

SPIRAL WAVES AND ROTORS

The concept of spiral waves, first introduced by Rosenblueth and Weiner in 1946 *(156)*, has attracted a great deal of interest over the past decade. Originally used to describe reentry around an anatomical obstacle *(156)*, the term spiral wave reentry was later adopted to describe circulating waves in the absence of an anatomical obstacle *(157,158)*, similar to the circulating waves of the leading circle mechanism described by Allessie and colleagues *(140,142)*. Spiral wave theory has advanced our understanding of the mechanisms responsible for the functional form of reentry. Although leading circle and spiral wave reentry are considered by some to be similar, a number of distinctions have been suggested *(142,159–161)*. The curvature of the spiral wave is the key to the

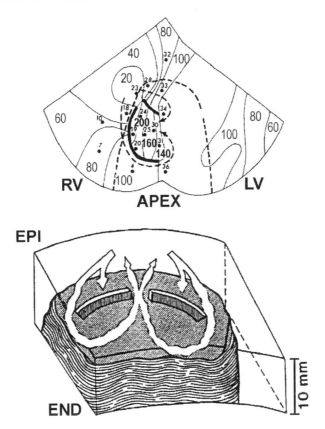

Fig. 11. Figure of eight model of reentry. Isochronal activation map during monomorphic reentrant ventricular tachycardia occurring in the surviving epicardial layer overlying an infarction. Recordings were obtained from the epicardial surface of a canine heart four days after ligation of the left anterior descending coronary artery. Activation isochrones are drawn at 20 ms intervals. The reentrant circuit has a characteristic figure eight activation pattern. Two circulating wavefronts advance in clockwise and counterclockwise directions, respectively, around two zones (arcs) of conduction block (represented by heavy solid lines). The epicardial surface is depicted as if the ventricles were unfolded following a cut from the crux to the apex. A three-dimensional diagrammatic illustration of the ventricular activation pattern during the reentrant tachycardia is shown in the lower panel. RV = right ventricle, LV = left ventricle, EPI = epicardium, END = endocardium. From *(14)*, with permission.

formation of the core *(161)*. The curvature of the wave forms a region of high impedance mismatch (sink-source mismatch), where the current provided by the reentering wavefront (source) is insufficient to charge the capacity and thus excite larger volume of tissue ahead (sink). A prominent curvature of the spiral wave is generally encountered following a wave break, a situation in which a planar wave encounters an obstacle and breaks up into two or more daughter waves. Because it has the greatest curvature, the broken end of the wave moves most slowly. As curvature decreases along the more distal parts of the spiral, propagation speed increases.

    The term spiral wave is usually used to describe reentrant activity in two dimensions. The center of the spiral wave is called the core and the distribution of the core in three dimensions is referred to as the filament (Fig. 12). The three-dimensional form of the spiral wave forms a scroll wave (162). In its simplest form, the scroll wave has a straight filament spanning the ventricular wall (i.e., from epicardium to endocardium). Theoretical studies have described three major scroll wave configurations with curved filaments (L-, U-, and O-shaped) (162), although numerous variations of these three-dimensional filaments in space and time are assumed to exist during cardiac arrhythmias (162).

Anisotropy and anatomical obstacles can substantially modify the characteristics and spatio-temporal behavior of the vortex-like reentries. As anatomical obstacles are introduced approaching a ring model of reentry, the curvature of the wave becomes less of a determinant of the characteristics of the arrhythmia.

Spiral wave activity has been used to explain the electrocardiographic patterns observed during monomorphic and polymorphic cardiac arrhythmias as well as during fibrillation (158,163,164). Monomorphic VT results when the spiral wave is anchored and not able to drift within the ventricular myocardium. In contrast, a polymorphic VT such as that encountered with LQTS-induced TdP is because of a meandering or drifting spiral wave. Ventricular fibrillation (VF) seems to be the most complex representation of rotating spiral waves in the heart. VF is often preceded by VT. VF is thought to develop when a single spiral wave responsible for VT breaks up, leading to the development of multiple spirals that are continuously extinguished and recreated.

There are two basic hypotheses to explain wavebreaks and the formation of multiple wavelets. The classical one is that originally proposed by Moe and colleagues (165) and which has been the dominating concept of atrial fibrillation (AF) and VF for four decades. Moe's multiple-wavelet concept is fundamentally based on spatially inhomogeneous recovery of refractoriness present during fibrillation, which provides the substrate for conduction block and wavefront fragmentation (wave breaks), leading to continuous appearance and disappearance of multiple wandering reentrant wavelets. The other concept of the spiral break-up, called the "Restitution Hypothesis," was formulated less than a decade ago (166). It invokes electrical restitution properties of the myocardium to explain spiral wave instability and breakup during VF. It stipulates that the wavebreak occurs when the slope of the APD restitution curve (determined as the change in APD as a function the preceding diastolic interval) exceed a value of one.

The past two years have witnessed the development of another hypothesis for the maintenance of VF. It suggests that VF can be caused by a single high frequency source, which propagates with variable conduction block to the rest of ventricle (i.e., fibrillatory conduction), leading to VF pattern on the electrocardiogram (ECG) (167–169) (Fig. 13). There may be some variations on these themes. For example, it has been suggested that a single meandering spiral wave could underlie the mechanism of VF (170,171) as in the case of the Brugada syndrome (172). All these concepts of VF maintenance are not mutually exclusive. There are experimental and theoretical data supporting each (166–169,173–177). It is possible that different mechanisms and manifestations of VF may be operative depending on prevailing conditions (species, size of the heart, ischemia, time after the start of VF, and so on).

The ionic basis for the spatio-temporal behavior of reentrant rotor during VF is poorly understood. It was recently shown by Samie et al. (169) that the anterior left ventricular region of the guinea pig heart displays earlier repolarization than right ventricular (RV) free wall during VF and that this region is the usual location of a stable rotor underlying VF in isolated guinea pig heart. Based on measurement of a higher density of background outward current, I_{K1}, in left ventricular (LV) vs RV isolated myocytes, Samie et al. (169)

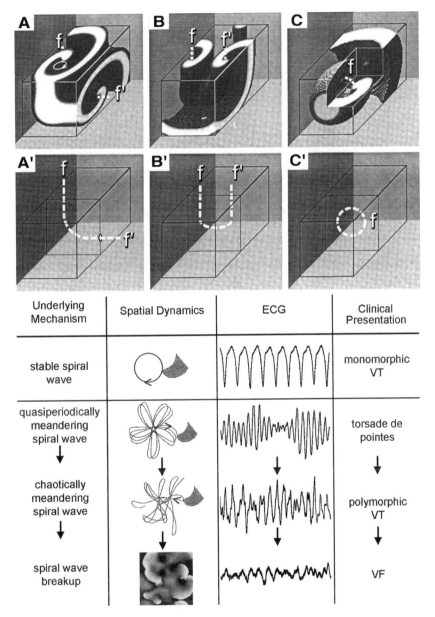

Fig. 12. Schematic representation of basic scroll-type reentry in 3-D and spiral wave phenotypes with their possible clinical manifestations. Upper panel: Basic configurations of vortex-like reentry in three dimensions. A and A', L-shaped scroll wave and filament, respectively. The scroll rotates in a clockwise direction (on the top) about the L-shaped filament (f,f') shown in A'. B and B', U-shaped scroll wave and filament, respectively. C and C', O-shaped wave and filament, respectively. From Pertsov and Jalife, 1995 *(162)* with permission. Bottom panel: Four types of spiral wave phenotypes and associated clinical manifestations. A stable spiral wave mechanism gives rise to monomorphic VT on the ECG. A quasi-periodic meandering spiral wave is responsible for TdP, whereas a chaotically meandering spiral wave is revealed as polymorphic VT. A VF pattern is caused by spiral wave breakup. Second column, spiral wave are shown in gray; the path of their tip are shown as solid lines. From *(164)* with permission.

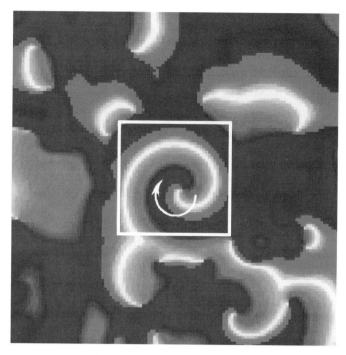

Fig. 13. Schematic representation of a stable high-frequency spiral wave, inducing irregular unstable multiple wavelets (i.e., fibrillatory conduction) in the rest of the ventricle. From Samie et al. 2001 *(169)* with permission.

proposed that the mechanism underlying the primary rotor and wavefront fragmentation may be related to gradients of refractoriness imposed by gradients in I_{K1}. Another recent paper suggests a dominant role of I_{Kr} in wavebreak dynamics during VF *(177)*.

Fibrillatory patterns in the atria have likewise been attributed to multiple wandering reentrant wavelets *(165,178)*, a single stable reentry *(179)*, as well as a focal automatic mechanism firing at a high rate *(33)*.

Reflection

Direct evidence in support of reflection as a mechanism of arrhythmogenesis was first provided by Antzelevitch and coworkers *(43,180)*. The concept of reflection was first suggested by studies of the propagation characteristics of slow action potential responses in K^+-depolarized Purkinje fibers *(133,134,136,138)*. Using strands of Purkinje fiber, Wit and coworkers demonstrated a phenomenon similar to that observed by Schmitt and Erlanger in which slow anterograde conduction of the impulse was at times followed by a retrograde wavefront that produced a "return extrasystole" *(137)*. They proposed that the nonstimulated impulse was caused by circuitous reentry at the level of the syncytial interconnections, made possible by longitudinal dissociation of the bundle, as the most likely explanation for the phenomenon but also suggested the possibility of reflection. Evidence in support of reflection as a mechanism of arrhythmogenesis was provided in the early 1980s *(43,180)*.

Several models of reflection have been developed *(43,47,180,181)*. The first of these involved use of "ion-free" isotonic sucrose solution to create a narrow (1.5–2 mm)

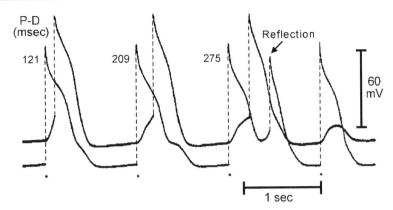

Fig. 14. Delayed transmission and reflection across an inexcitable gap created by superfusion of the central segment of a Purkinje fiber with an "ion-free" isotonic sucrose solution. The two traces were recorded from proximal (P) and distal (D) active segments. P-D conduction time (indicated in the upper portion of the figure, in ms) increased progressively with a 4:3 Wenckebach periodicity. The third stimulated proximal response was followed by a reflection. From Antzelevitch *(45)*, with permission.

central inexcitable zone (gap) in unbranched Purkinje fibers mounted in a three-chamber tissue bath (Fig. 14) *(43)*. In this model, stimulation of the proximal (P) segment elicits an action potential that propagates to the proximal border of the sucrose gap. Active propagation across the sucrose gap is not possible because of the ion-depleted extracellular milieu, but local circuit current continues to flow through the intercellular low resistance pathways (a Ag/AgCl extracellular shunt pathway is provided). This local circuit or electrotonic current, much reduced upon emerging from the gap, slowly discharges the capacity of the distal (D) tissue thus giving rise to a depolarization that manifests as a either subthreshold response (last distal response) or a foot-potential that brings the distal excitable element to its threshold potential (Fig. 15). Active impulse propagation stops and then resumes after a delay that can be as long as several hundred milliseconds. When anterograde (P -> D) transmission time is sufficiently delayed to permit recovery of refractoriness at the proximal end, electrotonic transmission of the impulse in the retrograde direction is able to reexcite the proximal tissue, thus generating a closely coupled reflected reentry. Reflection therefore results from the back and forth electrotonically-mediated transmission of the impulse across the same inexcitable segment; neither longitudinal dissociation nor circus movement need be invoked to explain the phenomenon.

A second model of reflection involves the creation of an inexcitable region permitting delayed conduction by superfusion of a central segment of a Purkinje bundle with a solution designed to mimic the extracellular milieu at a site of ischemia *(180)*. When the K^+ concentration was increased to between 15 and 20 mM, the "ischemic" solution induced major delays in conduction, as long as 500 ms across the 1.5 mm wide "ischemic" central gap. The gap was shown to be largely comprised of an inexcitable cable across which conduction of impulses was electrotonically mediated. The long delays of impulse conduction across the "ischemic" gap permits the development of reflection. When propagation across the gap was mediated by "slow responses," transmission was relatively prompt and reflection did not occur *(180)*.

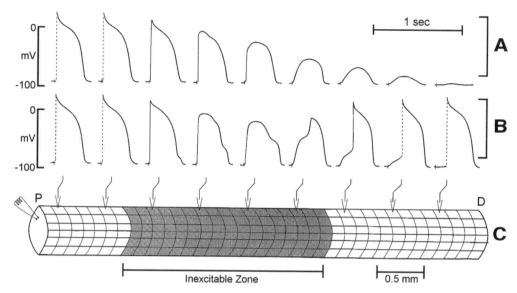

Fig. 15. Discontinuous conduction (**B**) and conduction block (**A**) in a Purkinje strand with a central inexcitable zone (**C**). The schematic illustration is based on transmembrane recordings obtained from canine Purkinje fiber-sucrose gap preparations. An action potential elicited by stimulation of the proximal (P) side of the preparation conducts normally up to the border of the inexcitable zone. Active propagation of the impulse stops at this point, but local circuit current generated by the proximal segment continues to flow through the preparation encountering a cumulative resistance (successive gap junctions). Transmembrane recordings from the first few inexcitable cells show a response not very different from the action potentials recorded in the neighboring excitable cells, in spite of the fact that no ions may be moving across the membrane of these cells. The responses recorded in the inexcitable region are the electrotonic images of activity generated in the proximal excitable segment. The resistive-capacitive properties of the tissue lead to an exponential decline in the amplitude of the transmembrane potential recorded along the length of the inexcitable segment and to a slowing of the rate of change of voltage as a function of time. If, as in panel B, the electrotonic current is sufficient to bring the distal excitable tissue to its threshold potential, an action potential is generated after a step delay imposed by the slow discharge of the capacity of the distal (D) membrane by the electrotonic current (foot-potential). Active conduction of the impulse therefore stops at the proximal border of the inexcitable zone and resumes at the distal border after a step delay that may range from a few to tens or hundreds of milliseconds. Modified from *(297)*, with permission.

Reflected reentry has been demonstrated in isolated atrial and ventricular myocardial tissues as well *(181–183)*. Reflection has also been demonstrated in Purkinje fibers in which a functionally inexcitable zone is created by focal depolarization of the preparation with long duration constant current pulses *(184)*. This phenomenon is also observed in isolated canine Purkinje fibers homogeneously depressed with high K$^+$ solution as well as in branched preparations of "normal" Purkinje fibers *(185)*.

Success or failure of reflection depends critically on the degree to which conduction is delayed in both directions across the functionally inexcitable zone. These transit delays in turn depend on the width of the blocked segment, the intracellular and extracellular resistance to the flow of local circuit current across the inexcitable zone, and the excitability of the distal active site (sink). Because the excitability of cardiac tissues continues to recover for hundreds of milliseconds after an action potential, impulse transmission across the inexcitable zone is a sensitive function of frequency *(43,186–188)*. Consequently, the incidence and patterns of manifest ectopic activity encountered in models of reflection are highly rate-dependent *(45,47,183,187,189)*. Similar rate-dependent changes in extrasystolic activity have been reported in patients with frequent extrasystoles evaluated with Holter recordings *(190)* and in patients evaluated by atrial pacing *(45,191)*. Because reflection can occur within areas of tissue of limited size (as small as 1–2 mm^2), it is likely to appear as focal in origin. Its identification as a mechanism of arrhythmia may be difficult even with very high spatial resolution mapping of the electrical activity of discrete sites. The delineation of delayed impulse conduction mechanisms at discrete sites requires the use of intracellular microelectrode techniques in conjunction with high resolution extracellular mapping techniques. These limitations considered, reflection has been suggested as the mechanism underlying reentrant extrasystolic activity in ventricular tissues excised from a one-day-old infarcted canine heart *(192)* and in a clinical case of incessant ventricular bigeminy in a young patient with no evidence of organic heart disease *(193)*.

Phase 2 Reentry

Phase 2 reentry is another example of a reentrant mechanism that can appear to be of focal origin. Phase 2 reentry occurs when the dome of the epicardial action potential propagates from sites at which it is maintained to sites at which it is abolished, causing local reexcitation of the epicardium and the generation of a closely coupled extrasystole. A more rigorous discussion of phase 2 reentry and its role in the precipitation of VT/VF will follow in the next section.

The Role of Heterogeneity

It is now well established that ventricular myocardium is not homogeneous, as previously thought, but is comprised of at least three electrophysiologically and functionally distinct cell types: Epicardial, M, and endocardial cells. These three ventricular myocardial cell types differ principally with respect to phase 1 and phase 3 repolarization characteristics (Fig. 16). Ventricular epicardial and M, but not endocardial, cells generally display a conspicuous phase 1, due to a prominent 4-aminopyridine (4-AP) sensitive transient outward current (I_{to}), giving the action potential a spike and dome or notched configuration. These regional differences in I_{to}, first suggested on the basis of action potential data *(194)*, have now been directly demonstrated in canine *(195)*, feline *(196)*, rabbit *(197)*, rat *(198)*, and human *(199,200)* ventricular myocytes.

It is not known whether I_{to2}, a calcium-activated component of the transient outward current, differs among the three ventricular myocardial cell types *(201)*. I_{to2}, initially ascribed to a K$^+$ current, is now thought to be primarily due to the calcium-activated chloride current ($I_{Cl(Ca)}$) *(201)*. Myocytes isolated from the epicardial region of the LV wall of the rabbit show a higher density of cAMP-activated chloride current when compared to endocardial myocytes *(202)*.

Dramatic differences in the magnitude of the action potential notch and corresponding differences in I_{to} have also been described between RV and LV epicardium *(203)*. Similar interventricular differences in I_{to} have also been described for canine ventricular M cells *(204)*. As will be discussed later, this distinction is thought to form the basis for why the Brugada syndrome, a channelopathy-mediated form of sudden death, is a RV disease.

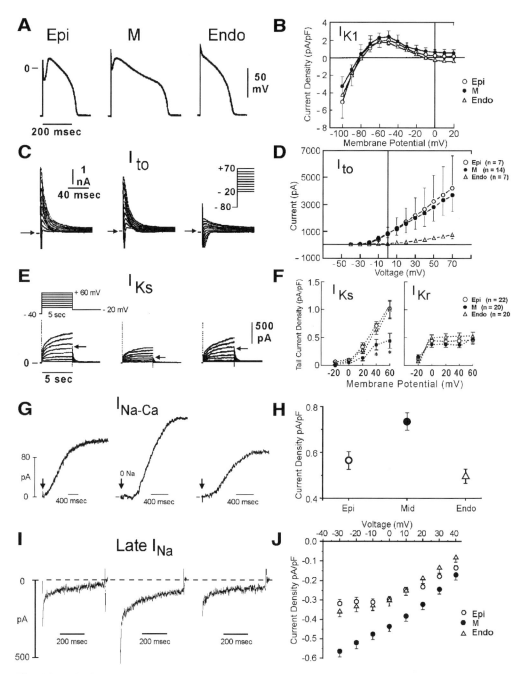

Fig. 16. Ionic distinctions among epicardial, M, and endocardial cells. Action potentials recorded from myocytes isolated from the epicardial, endocardial and M regions of the canine left ventricle. **(B)** I-V relations for I_{K1} in epicardial, endocardial and M region myocytes. Values are mean ± S.D. **(C)** Transient outward current (I_{to}) recorded from the three cell types (current traces recorded during depolarizing steps from a holding potential of –80 mV to test potentials ranging between –20 and +70 mV **(D)** The average peak current-voltage relationship for I_{to} for each of the three cell types. Values are mean ± S.D. **(E)** Voltage-dependent activation of the slowly activating component of the delayed rectifier K^+ current (I_{Ks}) (currents were elicited by the voltage pulse protocol shown in the inset; Na^+-, K^+- and Ca^{2+}- free solution). **(F)** Voltage dependence of I_{Ks} (current remaining after exposure to E-4031) and I_{Kr} (E-4031-sensitive current). Values are mean ± S.E. * $p < 0.05$ compared with Epi or Endo. From references *(78,195,208)* with permission. **(G)** Reverse-mode sodium-calcium exchange currents recorded in potassium- and chloride-free solutions at a

Sandwiched between the surface epicardial and endocardial layers are transitional and M cells. M cells are distinguished by the ability of their action potential to prolong disproportionately relative to the action potential of other ventricular myocardial cells in response to a slowing of rate and/or in response to APD-prolonging agents (Fig. 17) *(111,205,206)*. In the dog, the ionic basis for these features of the M cell include the presence of a smaller slowly activating delayed rectifier current (I_{Ks}) *(78)*, a larger late sodium current (late I_{Na}) *(207)* and a larger Na-Ca exchange current (I_{Na-Ca}) *(208)*. In the canine heart, the rapidly activating delayed rectifier (I_{Kr}) and inward rectifier (I_{K1}) currents are similar in the three transmural cell types. Transmural and apico-basal differences in the density of I_{Kr} channels have been described in the ferret heart *(209)*. I_{Kr} message and channel protein are much larger in the ferret epicardium. I_{Ks} is larger in M cells isolated from the RV vs LV of the dog *(204)*.

M cells are histologically similar to epicardial and endocardial cells. Electrophysiologically and pharmacologically, they appear to be a hybrid between Purkinje and ventricular cells. Like Purkinje fibers, M cells show a prominent APD prolongation and develop EAD in response to I_{Kr} blockers, whereas epicardium and endocardium do not. Like Purkinje fibers, M cells develop DAD in response to agents that calcium load or overload the cardiac cell; epicardium and endocardium do not. Unlike Purkinje fibers, M cells display an APD prolongation in response to I_{Ks} blockers *(79)*; epicardium and endocardium also show an increase in APD in response to I_{Ks} blockers *(79)*. Purkinje and M cells also respond differently to α adrenergic agonists. $α_1$ Adrenoceptor stimulation produces APD prolongation in Purkinje fibers, but abbreviation in M cells, and little or no change in endocardium and epicardium *(210)*.

The distribution of M cells within the ventricular wall has been investigated in greatest detail in the LV of the canine heart. Although transitional cells are found throughout the wall in the canine left ventricle, M cells displaying the longest action potentials (at basic cycle length [BCLs] $\geq$ 2000 ms) are often localized in the deep subendocardium to midmyocardium in the anterior wall, *(211)* deep subepicardium to midmyocardium in the lateral wall *(205)* and throughout the wall in the region of the RV outflow tracts *(212)*. M cells are also present in the deep cell layers of endocardial structures, including papillary muscles, trabeculae, and the interventricular septum *(213)*. Unlike Purkinje fibers, M cells are not found in discrete bundles or islets *(213,214)*, although there is evidence that they may be localized in discrete muscle layers. Cells with the characteristics of M cells have been described in the canine, guinea pig, rabbit, pig, and human ventricles *(68,70,78,82,112,195,205,206,211,213–227)*.

Fig. 16. *(Continued)* voltage of –80 mV. I_{Na-Ca} was maximally activated by switching to sodium-free external solution at the time indicated by the arrow. **(H)** Midmyocardial sodium-calcium exchanger density is 30% greater than endocardial density, calculated as the peak outward I_{Na-Ca} normalized by cell capacitance. Endocardial and epicardial densities were not significantly different. **(I)** TTX-sensitive late sodium current. Cells were held at –80 mV and briefly pulsed to –45 mV to inactivate fast sodium current before stepping to –10 mV. **(J)** Normalized late sodium current measured 300 ms into the test pulse was plotted as a function of test pulse potential. Modified from *(208)* with permission.

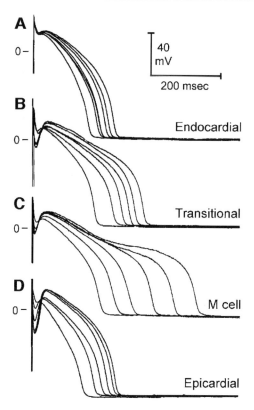

Fig. 17. Transmembrane activity recorded from cells isolated from the epicardial (Epi), M and endocardial (Endo) regions of the canine left ventricle at BCL of 300 to 5000 ms (steady-state conditions). The M and transitional cells were enzymatically dissociated from the midmyocardial region. Deceleration-induced prolongation of APD in M cells is much greater than in epicardial and endocardial cells. The spike and dome morphology is also more accentuated in the epicardial cell.

Amplification of transmural heterogeneities normally present in the early and late phases of the action potential can lead to the development of a variety of arrhythmias, including the Brugada and long QT syndromes and ischemia-induced tachyarrhythmias.

BRUGADA SYNDROME

Sudden cardiac death occurring in individuals with structurally normal hearts accounts for an estimated 3 to 9% of out-of-hospital cases of VF *(228)*. Many of these cases are thought to be due to a primary electrical disease. Prominent among these is the Brugada syndrome, a syndrome characterized by an ST segment elevation in right precordial leads (V_1 to V_3) unrelated to ischemia, electrolyte disturbances or obvious structural heart disease, displaying a RBBB QRS morphology. This electrocardiographic signature was reported as early as 1953, but first described as a distinct clinical entity associated with a high risk of sudden cardiac death by Pedro and Josep Brugada in 1992 *(229–233)*. These characteristics of the Brugada Syndrome are similar, in many cases nearly identical, to those reported by Nademanee and coworkers *(234)* for patients with Sudden Unexpected Death Syndrome (SUDS). Tragically, sudden death from Brugada syndrome is often the first symptom of the disease.

The Brugada syndrome is more commonly diagnosed in males (8:1 ratio of males:females) of Southeast Asian origin. The syndrome is familial, displaying an autosomal dominant mode of transmission with incomplete penetrance. Arrhythmic events are observed at an average age of approx 40, but have been reported in infants over a very wide range of ages, from infants to those in their late 70s (1 to 77 yr). Although structural heart disease must be ruled out by echocardiography and/or magnetic resonance imaging in order to make the diagnosis of Brugada syndrome, postmortem examination has revealed some fatty infiltration into the deep subepicardium in isolated cases. It is noteworthy that a typical ECG pattern and a high risk of sudden arrhythmic death have been reported for a segment of the patient population with structural heart disease in the setting of arrhythmogenic right ventricular cardiomyopathy (ARVC) endemic to the Veneto region of Italy (235). However, the clinical presentation in the vast majority of ARVC patients bears little resemblance to that of the Brugada syndrome. Moreover, ARVC does not appear to be linked to the same chromosomal loci as the Brugada syndrome.

The electrocardiographic signature of the Brugada syndrome is dynamic and often concealed, but can be unmasked by potent sodium channel blockers such as flecainide, ajmaline, procainamide, and psilicainide (236). Although intravenous administration of these agents is most effective in unmasking the syndrome, oral formulations of flecainide have been reported to be effective as well. The specificity of these effects of sodium channel blockers to uncover the syndrome and the prognostic significance of this finding remain to be fully elucidated.

Because of ambiguities concerning the diagnostic criteria for the Brugada syndrome, the incidence remains poorly defined. For these same reasons, it has been difficult to establish what fraction of idiopathic VF cases may be attributable to the Brugada syndrome. Estimates have ranged between 21 and 50% (237–239).

What are the proper diagnostic criteria to be used in identifying the Brugada syndrome? A definitive answer to this question is currently out of reach but will no doubt evolve with time as clinical data become available and as our understanding of the underlying mechanisms advances. The priority that we assign current diagnostics parameters is predicated on our limited clinical knowledge and understanding of the cellular mechanisms responsible for the unique ECG features and arrhythmogenicity of the Brugada syndrome.

The cellular basis for the Brugada syndrome is thought to be because of an outward shift in the ionic current active during phase 1 of the RV epicardial action potential (230,240). A rebalancing of the currents contributing to the early phases of the action potential can accentuate the action potential notch or lead to all-or-none repolarization at the end of phase 1, causing loss of the epicardial action potential dome and marked abbreviation of the action potential at that site. A variety of pathophysiologic conditions (e.g., ischemia, metabolic inhibition, hypothermia, pressure) and some pharmacologic interventions are known to effect these changes in cells in which I_{to} is prominent. Under these pathophysiologic conditions or in response to agents that reduce I_{Na} or I_{Ca} or agents that activate ATP sensitive potassium current (I_{K-ATP}) or augment I_{Kr}, $I_{Cl(Ca)}$, or I_{to}, canine ventricular epicardial cells exhibit an accentuation of the spike and dome morphology of the action potential, resulting in a delay in the development of the dome, secondary to widening of the action potential notch. A further shift in the balance of current leads to loss of the action potential dome and marked abbreviation of the epicardial response. The dome fails to develop because the outward currents flowing at the end of phase 1 overwhelm the inward currents that normally give rise to the secondary upstroke and action potential plateau.

Genetic mutations that affect these same currents are capable of producing the Brugada syndrome. The only gene thus far linked to the syndrome is the α subunit of the cardiac sodium channel gene, SCN5A *(239,241–245)*, the same gene implicated in the LQT3 form of the LQTS. In fact, Bezzina and coworkers *(245)* recently reported a mutation in SCN5A (1795InsD) capable of producing both the Brugada and LQT3 phenotypes. Three types of mutations in SCN5A have been uncovered thus far, and shown to result in:

1. Failure of the sodium channel to express.
2. Reduced current owing to a shift in the voltage- and time-dependence of I_{Na} activation, inactivation or reactivation.
3. Reduced contribution of I_{Na} during the early phases of the action potential due to accelerated inactivation of the sodium channel.

Insertion of two nucleotides (AA) at the 5' end, deletion of a single nucleotide (A) at codon 1397 leading to an in-frame stop codon *(239)* and some missense mutations (R1432G) *(243)* result in disruption of protein formation and failure of channel expression. Other insertion mutations (1795InsD) cause a positive shift of activation and negative shift of inactivation curves resulting in a reduction of I_{Na} *(245)*. In the case of the T1620M missense mutation, inactivation of I_{Na} is accelerated such that I_{to} is left unopposed during phase 1 of the action potential, resulting in a strong predominance of the outward repolarizing current at the end of phase 1, thus providing the substrate for the Brugada syndrome *(242)*. This change in the function of the sodium channel is observed at physiological temperatures, but not at room temperature, typically used in studies of function involving heterologous expression systems. It is interesting that this characteristic of the mutant channel is exaggerated at temperatures above the physiological range, suggesting the possibility that patients with the Brugada syndrome may be at more risk during a febrile state. Several Brugada patients displaying fever-induced polymorphic VT have been identified since the publication of this report. Other mutations such as L567Q, reported by Priori et al. *(244)* to be responsible for the Brugada syndrome in children, also act by importantly accelerating inactivation of I_{Na}. In comparison with T1620M, the dysfunction of the sodium channel with this missense mutation located in the DI-DII linker of SCN5A is less temperature sensitive (Dumaine, Priori, and Antzelevitch, unpublished data). The temperature dependence of most mutations thus far described for the Brugada syndrome is not known because most are expressed in Xenopus Oocytes and studied at room temperature.

In addition to SCN5A, gene mutations that alter the intensity or kinetics of either I_{to}, I_{Kr}, I_{Ks}, I_{K-ATP}, I_{Ca}, or $I_{Cl(Ca)}$ so as to increase the activity of the outward currents and/or diminish that of the inward currents are candidates for the Brugada syndrome. Other candidate genes include those encoding for autonomic receptors that directly modulate ion current density and/or alter the expression of channels in the membrane (e.g., sympathetic control of I_{to}).

The cellular changes believed to underlie the Brugada phenotype are shown in Fig. 18. The presence of an I_{to}-mediated spike and dome morphology or notch in ventricular epicardium, but not endocardium, of larger mammals creates a transmural voltage gradient responsible for the inscription of the electrocardiographic J wave (Osborn wave)

(246). Under normal conditions, the J wave is relatively small, in large part reflecting the LV action potential notch, since that of RV epicardium is usually buried in the QRS. The ST segment is isoelectric because of the absence of transmural voltage gradients at the level of the action potential plateau (Fig. 18A). Accentuation of the RV notch under pathophysiologic conditions is attended by exaggeration of transmural voltage gradients and thus exaggeration of the J wave or J point elevation and/or the appearance of a saddleback configuration of the repolarization waves (Fig. 18B). The development of a prominent J wave can also be construed as an ST segment elevation. Under these conditions, the T wave remains positive because epicardial repolarization precedes repolarization of the cells in the M and endocardial regions. Further accentuation of the notch may be accompanied by a prolongation of the epicardial action potential such that the direction of repolarization across the RV wall and transmural voltage gradients are reversed, thus leading to the development of a coved-type of ST segment elevation and inversion of the T wave (Fig. 18C), typically observed in the ECG of Brugada patients. A delay in epicardial activation may also contribute to inversion of the T wave.

The down-sloping ST segment elevation or accentuated J wave observed in the experimental wedge models often appears as an R', suggesting that the right bundle branch block (RBBB) morphology often encountered in the Brugada ECG may be because of early repolarization of RV epicardium and not to conduction block in the right bundle. Indeed a rigorous application of RBBB criteria reveals that a large majority of RBBB-like morphologies encountered in cases of Brugada syndrome do not fit the criteria *(247)*. Moreover, attempts by Miyazaki and coworkers to record delayed activation of the RV in Brugada patients met with failure *(248)*.

It is interesting to note that although the typical Brugada morphology is present in Fig. 18B,C, the substrate for reentry is not. A further shift in the balance of current leads to loss of the action potential dome at some epicardial sites, which would manifest in the ECG as a further ST segment elevation (Fig. 18D). The loss of the action potential dome in epicardium but not endocardium results in the development of a marked transmural dispersion of repolarization and refractoriness, responsible for the development of a vulnerable window during which a premature impulse or extrasystole can induce a reentrant arrhythmia. Because loss of the action potential dome is epicardium is generally not spatially uniform, we see the development of a striking epicardial dispersion of repolarization (Fig. 18D). Support for these hypotheses derives from experiments involving the arterially perfused RV wedge preparation *(240)*.

Conduction of the action potential dome from sites at which it is maintained to sites at which it is lost causes local reexcitation via a *phase 2 reentry* mechanism, leading to the development of a closely-coupled extrasystole, capable of triggering a circus movement reentry (Figs. 18E, 19) *(240,249)*. The phase 2 reentrant beat fuses with the negative T wave of the basic response. Because the extrasystole originates in epicardium the QRS is largely comprised of a Q wave, which serves to accentuate the negative deflection of the inverted T wave, thus giving the ECG a more symmetrical appearance. This morphology is often observed in the clinic preceding the onset of polymorphic VT.

Phase 2 reentry is observed in canine epicardium exposed to:

1. K^+ channel openers.
2. Sodium channel blockers.
3. Increased $[Ca^{2+}]_o$.

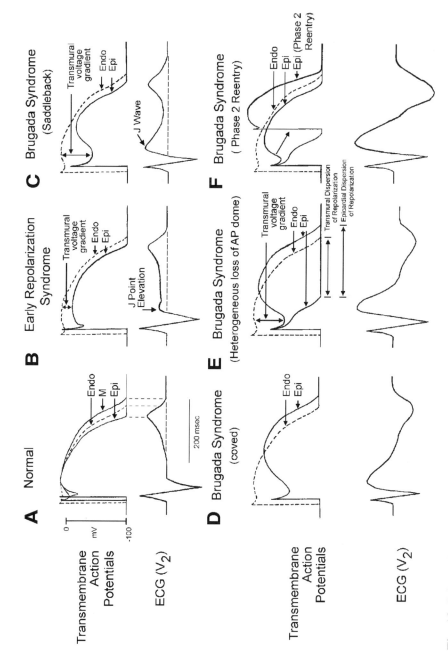

Fig. 18. Schematic representation of right ventricular epicardial action potential changes proposed to underlie the electrocardiographic manifestation of Early Repolarization and Brugada syndromes. From *(232)*, with permission.

230

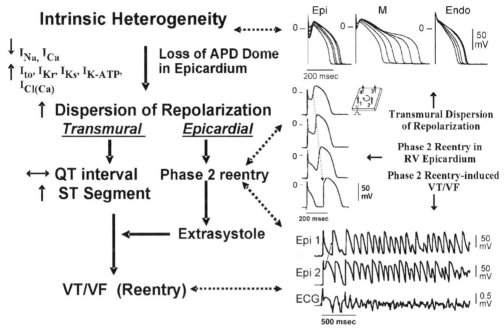

Fig. 19. Cellular mechanisms proposed to underlie arrhythmogenesis in the Brugada syndrome. Modified from *(233)*, with permission.

4. Metabolic inhibition.
5. Simulated ischemia.
6. Local pressure applied to RV epicardium *(250)*.

Phase 2 reentry has been shown to trigger circus movement reentry in isolated sheets of RV epicardium *(249)* as well as in the intact wall of the canine right ventricle *(172,246)*. The arrhythmia commonly takes the form of a polymorphic VT, resembling a rapid TdP, often indistinguishable from VF. In other cases, the experimental model displays monomorphic VT. Both are observed in patients with the Brugada syndrome, although the polymorphic form is much more common.

Local pressure alone applied to a discrete RV site can also produce loss of the action potential, ST segment elevation, phase 2 reentry and VT/VF in the arterially-perfused RV wedge preparation *(240)*. This mechanism may be responsible for the Brugada-like syndrome caused by a mediastinal tumor compressing the RV outflow tract *(251)*.

The mechanism proposed to underlie the Brugada syndrome is one that provides the substrate for the development of circus movement reentry in the form of epicardial and transmural dispersion of repolarization, as well as the trigger for VT/VF in the form of a phase 2 reentrant extrasystole.

The experimental findings suggest a depressed RV epicardial action potential dome as the basis for the accentuated J wave or ST segment elevation and to phase 2 reentry as a trigger for episodes of circus movement reentry responsible for VT and VF in Brugada patients. There are a number of similarities between the conditions that give rise to ST segment elevation and phase 2 reentry in the experimental models and those that attend the appearance of the Brugada syndrome. Accentuation of the action potential notch or loss of the action potential dome in epicardium but not endocardium leads to elevation of the ST segment with either a saddleback or coved appearance, similar to those recorded in patients with the Brugada syndrome (246–248). In Brugada patients, as in the wedge preparation, VT/VF is inducible in the majority of cases. In the wedge preparation, VT/VF is most easily induced by the application of an extrastimulus to the site of briefest refractoriness, always located on the epicardial side. In the clinic, programmed stimulation is most commonly applied to RV endocardium. An epicardial approach is possible via the coronary sinus and it is of interest that in a recent case report VT/VF was shown to be noninducible with endocardial extrastimualtion, but readily inducible using an electrode placed deep within the coronary sinus (252).

In isolated epicardial tissues as well as in wedge preparations, loss of the action potential dome and phase 2 reentry are readily induced in RV preparations, but are more difficult to induce in the left ventricle. These findings are owing to the presence of a much more prominent I_{to} in RV vs LV epicardium and are consistent with the appearance of the ST segment elevation only in right precordial leads in patients with the Brugada syndrome. Normalization of the ST segment in response to an increase in rate is observed in the wedge model as well as in some Brugada patients (248), and is consistent with a decreased availability of I_{to} (because of relatively slow recovery from inactivation) which diminishes the notched configuration of the epicardial action potential. Not all Brugada patients display rate-dependent changes in ST. With some mutations, such as those involving a slowing of reactivation of the sodium channel, or in the presence of sodium channel blockers with strong use-dependence, acceleration may be attended by an ST segment elevation.

Because accentuation of the notch and/or loss of the dome are caused by an outward shift in the balance of currents active at the end of phase 1 (principally I_{to} and I_{Ca}), autonomic neurotransmitters like acetylcholine facilitate these changes in the action potential (253) by suppressing I_{Ca} and/or augmenting potassium current, whereas β adrenergic agonists restore the dome by augmenting I_{Ca}. As a consequence, in the arterially perfused wedge, vagal and sympathetic influences exaggerate and reduce ST segment elevation, respectively (246). Accentuation of the ST segment elevation in patients with the Brugada syndrome following vagal maneuvers and normalization of the ST segment following β adrenergic agents are consistent with these findings (248).

The effect of sodium channel blockers to facilitate loss of the RV epicardial action potential dome in the wedge and in isolated tissues (254) is consistent with their ability to (246) unmask the Brugada syndrome in the clinic (236). Moreover, the linkage of the Brugada syndrome to mutations in SCN5A is consistent with the conduction disturbances that sometimes accompany the Brugada syndrome (255).

Although augmentation of I_{to} may precipitate phase 2 reentry and the Brugada syndrome, it is not a prerequisite. However, the presence of a prominent I_{to} is essential. Because of the pivotal role of I_{to}, agents that inhibit I_{to}, including 4-aminopyridine and quinidine, restore the action potential dome and electrical homogeneity, thus suppressing all arrhythmic activity (172,240). Agents that potently block I_{Na}, but not I_{to} (flecainide, ajmaline, and procainamide), exacerbate or unmask the Brugada syndrome, whereas those with actions to block both I_{Na} and I_{to} (e.g., quinidine and disopyramide) may exert an ameliorative effect (240). The anticholinergic effects of quinidine and disopyramide may also contribute to their effectiveness. An experimental drug that may be useful in the treatment of the Brugada syndrome and other syndromes associated with an ST segment elevation is tedisamil, an agent that blocks a variety of outward potassium currents, including I_{to}.

ISCHEMIA-INDUCED TACHYARRHYTHMIAS

Acute myocardial ischemia is associated with high incidence of malignant ventricular arrhythmias within a few minutes of onset. In large part, heterogeneity in the recovery of excitability within the ischemic myocardium is believed to be the underlying electro-physiologic substrate of the large unstable circus movements that cause reentrant exci-tation. This mechanism has been anticipated to sustain rapid ventricular rhythms during VT and to break into numerous wavelets characteristics of VF. The initial beat of VT or VF is believed to emerge from either small reentrant circuits and/or to be secondary to focal sources (256). The flow of current across the border zone (the boundary between the ischemic and normal myocardium) has been proposed as one of the sites of origin of extrasystolic activity. Injury current is most prominent at the border zone in that this is the site at which voltage gradients between depolarized ischemic cells and adjacent normal myocardial cells is greatest (173,256,257).

Another mechanism suggested to be responsible for the generation of premature beats is phase 2-reentry, discussed above in relation to the Brugada syndrome. Ischemia-induced heterogeneous loss of the epicardial action potential dome in isolated ventricular preparations has been shown to generate extrasystoles that can precipitate monomorphic and polymorphic VT (249,258–260).

At the cellular level, complex ischemia-induced disturbances of ionic homeostasis, depolarization of membrane potential, depression of action potential amplitude, and perturbation of intercellular communication contribute to the changes of impulse propa-gation and dispersion of repolarization, which underlie the increased vulnerability to life-threatening arrhythmias. Increased dispersion of repolarization is owing to differences in repolarization between ischemic and normal zones as well to accentuation of intrinsic transmural heterogeneities of repolarization.

Despite similar changes in resting membrane potential in endocardium and epicar-dium, ischemia decreases action potential amplitude and abbreviates APD more in epi-cardium than in endocardium (258,261,262). Factors believed to contribute to this differential action potential response include differences in membrane responsiveness (261), a greater sensitivity of I_{K-ATP} to ATP depletion in epicardium (263), a greater epicardial depression of the calcium current (264), and the presence of a prominent transient outward current-mediated spike and dome configuration in epicardium but not in endocardium leading to loss of the epicardial action potential dome and marked abbre-viation of epicardial action potential duration (258).

The ECG has long been recognized as an important tool for the diagnosis and local-ization of acute myocardial ischemia and infarction. Under these conditions, changes in the surface ECG are thought to be related to changes in the resting potential, action potential morphology, action potential duration, and/or altered conduction character-istics (265–267). Current thinking regarding the pathophysiological mechanisms of myocardial ischemia-induced changes in the ECG derive principally from theoretical models because attempts to simultaneously record transmembrane action potentials from the ischemic myocardium in vivo are limited to the epicardial surface (268–270). ST-segment elevation is a characteristic ECG manifestation of transmural myocardial ischemia in leads facing the injury (271). Although the mechanisms responsible for such changes have not been experimentally identified, several theoretical models have predicted their correlation with action potential morphology changes *(265,267)*.

The canine ventricular wedge preparation has contributed importantly to our understanding of the cellular basis for ischemia-induced electrocardiographic changes. Transmembrane action potentials recordings in the wedge can be simultaneously recorded from several intramural sites between the endocardium and the epicardium together with a pseudo-ECG, permitting correlation of transmembrane and electrocardiographic activity. Interruption of coronary flow to the wedge leads to electrocardiographic alterations that reproduce the patterns of acute transmural myocardial ischemia observed clinically. The results of these studies indicate that two distinctly different mechanisms involving: 1) a greater depression of the epicardial plateau and/or loss of the epicardial action potential dome (all-or-non repolarization) and 2) a markedly delayed in transmural conduction, underlie, the apparent ST segment elevation encountered during acute ischemia (Di Diego and Antzelevitch, unpublished observations).

The Long QT Syndrome (LQTS)

Exaggeration of intrinsic heterogeneities of ventricular repolarization also contribute to the development of the LQTS. In this case, amplification of differences in final repolarization of the action potential of cells spanning the ventricular wall provide the arrhythmogenic substrate. The congenital and acquired (drug-induced) LQTS are characterized by the development of long QT intervals in the ECG, abnormal T waves and an atypical polymorphic tachycardia known as TdP *(92,272–275)*. Genetic linkage studies have identified several forms of the congenital LQTS caused by mutations in ion channel genes located on chromosomes 3, 7, 11, and 21. Mutations in KvLQT1 and minK (KCNE1) are responsible for defects in the I_{Ks} which underlies the LQT1 and LQT5 forms of LQTS, whereas mutations in HERG and SCN5A are responsible for defects in I_{Kr} and sodium current (I_{Na}) which underlie the LQT2 and LQT3 syndromes. Mutations in a minK-related protein MiRP1 (KCNE2), which associates with HERG to form the I_{Kr} channel, are responsible for the LQT6 form of LQTS *(276)*.

The electrophysiologic, electrocardiographic, and pharmacologic characteristics of the LQT1, LQT2, and LQT3 syndromes were recently studied in the arterially-perfused canine LV wedge preparation. Simultaneous recording of transmembrane activity from epicardial, M, and endocardial or Purkinje sites together with a transmural ECG along the same axis permits correlation of transmembrane and electrocardiographic activity *(211,221,223–225,277)*. The wedge preparation is capable of developing and sustaining a variety of arrhythmias, including TdP. Pharmacologic models that mimic the clinical congenital syndromes with respect to prolongation of the QT interval, T wave morphology, rate dependence of repolarization and response to antiarrhythmic drugs have been developed (Fig. 20) *(211,221,223–225)*.

The I_{Ks} blocker, chromanol 293B, was used to mimic LQT1 and the β adrenergic agonist, isoproterenol, was used to assess β adrenergic influence. I_{Ks} block alone produces a homogeneous prolongation of repolarization and refractoriness across the ventricular wall and does not induce arrhythmias. The addition of isoproterenol causes abbreviation of epicardial and endocardial APD but a prolongation or no change in the APD of the M cell, resulting in a marked augmentation of transmural dispersion of repolarization (TDR) and the development of spontaneous and stimulation-induced TdP *(223)*. These changes give rise to a broad based T wave and the long QT interval char-

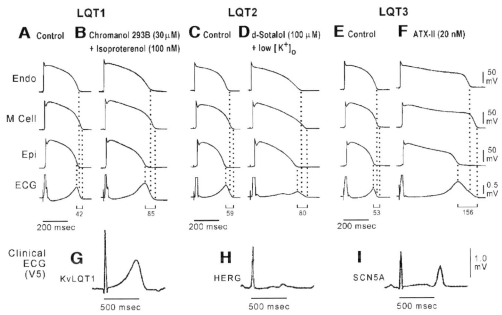

Fig. 20. Transmembrane action potentials and transmural electrocardiograms (ECG) in the LQT1 (**A** and **B**), LQT2 (**C** and **D**), and LQT3 (**E** and **F**) models (arterially-perfused canine left ventricular wedge preparations), and clinical ECG lead V5 of patients with LQT1 (*KvLQT1* defect) (**G**), LQT2 (*HERG* defect) (**H**) and LQT3 (*SCN5A* defect) (**I**) syndromes. Isoproterenol + chromanol 293B—an I_{Ks} blocker, d-sotalol + low $[K^+]_o$, and ATX-II—an agent that slows inactivation of late I_{Na} are used to mimic the LQT1, LQT2 and LQT3 syndromes, respectively. Panels (**A–F**) depict action potentials simultaneously recorded from endocardial (Endo), M and epicardial (Epi) sites together with a transmural ECG. BCL = 2000 ms. In all cases, the peak of the T wave in the ECG is coincident with the repolarization of the epicardial action potential, whereas the end of the T wave is coincident with the repolarization of the M cell action potential. Repolarization of the endocardial cell is intermediate between that of the M cell and epicardial cell. Transmural dispersion of repolarization across the ventricular wall, defined as the difference in the repolarization time between M and epicardial cells, is denoted below the ECG traces. (**B**) Isoproterenol (100 n*M*) in the presence of chromanol 293B (30 μM) produced a preferential prolongation of the APD of the M, resulting in an accentuated transmural dispersion of repolarization and broad-based T waves as commonly seen in LQT1 patients (**G**). (**D**) d-Sotalol (100 μM) in the presence of low potassium (2 m*M*) gives rise to low-amplitude T waves with a notched or bifurcated appearance due to a very significant slowing of repolarization as commonly seen in LQT2 patients (**H**). (**F**) ATX-II (20 n*M*) markedly prolongs the QT interval, widens the T wave, and causes a sharp rise in the dispersion of repolarization. ATX-II also produces a marked delay in onset of the T wave due to relatively large effects of the drug on the APD of epicardium and endocardium, consistent with the late-appearing T wave pattern observed in LQT3 patients (I). Modified from references *(221,223)* with permission.

acteristics of LQT1. The development of TdP in the model requires β adrenergic stimulation, consistent with a high sensitivity of congenital LQTS, LQT1 in particular, to sympathetic stimulation *(274,278–281)*.

The I_{Kr} blocker, d-Sotalol, was used to mimic LQT2 and the most common form of acquired (drug-induced) LQTS. A greater prolongation of the M cell action potential and slowing of phase 3 of the action potential of all three cell types results in a low amplitude T wave, long QT interval, large transmural dispersion of repolarization and the development of spontaneous as well as stimulation-induced TdP. The addition of hypokalemia gives rise to low-amplitude T waves with a deeply notched or bifurcated appearance, similar to those commonly seen in patients with the LQT2 syndrome *(221,225)*. Isoproterenol further exaggerates transmural dispersion of repolarization, thus increasing the incidence of TdP *(86)*.

ATX-II, an agent that increases late I_{Na}, was used to mimic LQT3 *(221)*. ATX-II markedly prolongs the QT interval, delays the onset of the T wave, in some cases also widening it, and produces a sharp rise in transmural dispersion of repolarization as a result of a greater prolongation of the APD of the M cell. The differential effect of ATX-II to prolong the M cell action potential is likely owing to the presence of a larger late sodium current in the M cell *(207)*. ATX-II produces a marked delay in onset of the T wave because of a relatively large effect of the drug on epicardial and endocardial APD. This feature is consistent with the late-appearing T wave (long isoelectric ST segment) observed in patients with the LQT3 syndrome. Also in agreement with the clinical presentation of LQT3, the model displays a steep rate dependence of the QT interval and develops TdP at slow rates. Interestingly, β adrenergic influence in the form of isoproterenol, reduces transmural dispersion of repolarization by abbreviating the APD of the M cell more than that of epicardium or endocardium, and thus reducing the incidence of TdP. Although the β adrenergic blocker propranolol is protective in LQT1 and LQT2 wedge models, it has the opposite effects in LQT3, acting to amplify transmural dispersion and promoting TdP *(86)*.

Torsade de pointes is a life-threatening atypical polymorphic VT commonly associated with LQTS. TdP has been reported in patients receiving potassium channel blockers like d-sotalol and quinidine, usually at slow heart rates or after long pauses. These conditions are similar to those under which these agents induce EADs and triggered activity in isolated Purkinje fibers and M cells, suggesting a role for EAD-induced triggered activity in the genesis of TdP. While EADs may underlie the premature beat that initiates TdP, recent studies provide evidence in support of circus movement reentry as the mechanism responsible for the maintenance of the arrhythmia *(68,82,212,221,223,225, 275,277,282,283)*. In the wedge, TdP develops spontaneously in all three models and can be readily induced by introduction of a single premature beat to the epicardial surface (the site of earliest repolarization) (Fig. 21).

The mechanism responsible for TdP is outlined in Fig. 22. The hypothesis presumes the presence of electrical heterogeneity, principally in the form of transmural dispersion of repolarization, under baseline conditions. The intrinsic heterogeneity is amplified by agents that decrease net repolarizing current by reducing I_{Kr} or I_{Ks} or augmenting late I_{Ca} or late I_{Na} or by ion channel mutations that affect these currents and are responsible for the various forms of LQTS. I_{Kr} blockers and LQT2 mutations or late I_{Na} promoters and LQT3 mutations produce a preferential prolongation of the M cell action potential. As a consequence, the QT interval prolongs and is accompanied by a dramatic increase in transmural dispersion of repolarization. The dispersion of repolarization and refractoriness across the ventricular wall gives rise to a vulnerable window for the development of reentry. The decrease in net repolarizing current can also give rise to EAD-induced triggered activity in M and Purkinje cells, and in some cases in epicardial and endocardial cells, which are responsible for the extrasystole that triggers TdP.

β adrenergic agonists further amplify transmural heterogeneity (transiently) in the case of I_{Kr} and LQT2, but reduce it in the case of late I_{Na} enhancers or LQT3 *(86)*. I_{Ks}

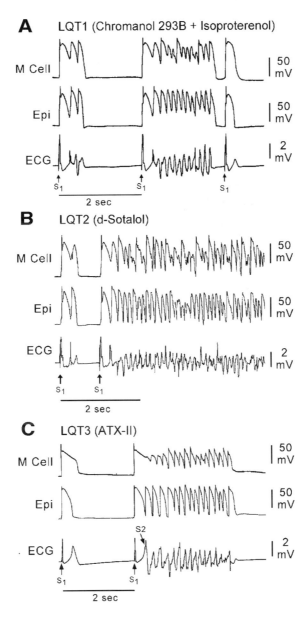

Fig. 21. Polymorphic ventricular tachycardia displaying features of TdP in the LQT1 (**A**), LQT2 (**B**), and LQT3 (**C**) models (arterially-perfused canine left ventricular wedge preparations). Isoproterenol + chromanol 293B, d-sotalol, and ATX-II are used to mimic the 3 LQTS syndromes, respectively. Each trace shows action potentials simultaneously recorded from M and epicardial (Epi) cells together with a transmural ECG. The preparation was paced from the endocardial surface at a BCL of 2000 ms (S1). (**A** and **B**) Spontaneous TdP induced in the LQT1 and LQT2 models, respectively. In both models, the first groupings show spontaneous ventricular premature beat (or couplets) that fail to induce TdP, and a second grouping that show spontaneous premature beats that succeed. The premature response appears to originate in the deep subendocardium (M or Purkinje). (**C**) Programmed electrical stimulation-induces TdP in the LQT3 model. ATX-II produced very significant dispersion of repolarization (first grouping). A single extrastimulus (S2) applied to the epicardial surface at an S1–S2 interval of 320 ms initiates TdP (second grouping). Modified from references *(221,223)* with permission.

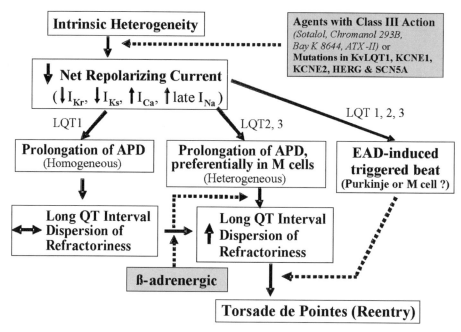

Fig. 22. Proposed cellular and ionic mechanisms for the LQTS.

blockers or LQT1 mutations cause a homogeneous prolongation of APD throughout the ventricular wall, leading to a prolongation of the QT interval but with no increase in transmural dispersion of repolarization. Under these conditions, TdP does not occur spontaneously nor can it be induced by programmed stimulation until a β adrenergic agonist is introduced. The sympathetic agonists dramatically increase transmural dispersion under these conditions by abbreviating the APD of epicardium and endocardium, thus creating a vulnerable window that an EAD-, or DAD-induced triggered response can capture to generate TdP, a circus movement arrhythmia. Recent data suggest that DAD-induced triggered beats may be involved in the initiation of TdP in LQT1 (*79*). I_{Ks} block alone or in combination with β adrenergic stimulation does not induce EADs in epicardium, M cell, endocardium, or Purkinje fibers. However, the combination readily produces DAD and DAD induced triggered activity in ventricular working myocardium (*79*).

Slow Conduction and Reentry

Slow or delayed conduction of the impulse can facilitate the development of reentrant arrhythmias by reducing the wavelength of the reentering wavefront so that it can be accommodated by the available pathlength. Several factors determine the velocity at which an action potential propagates through cardiac tissue. Among these is the intensity of the fast inward sodium current that flows during the upstroke of the action potential and the axial resistance to the flow of local circuit current.

Discontinuities in conduction can give rise to apparently very slow conduction and reentry in cardiac tissues by allowing for the development of prominent step delays in the transmission of impulses at discrete sites. Any agent or agency capable of suppressing the active generator properties of cardiac tissues may diminish excitability to the point of rendering a localized region functionally inexcitable and thus creating a discontinuity in the propagation of the advancing wavefront. Examples include an ion-free, ischemic, or high K⁺ environment *(43,180,181,186,187)* as discussed earlier, as well as electrical blocking current *(184,284,285)*, localized pressure *(186,286)* and localized cooling *(286)*. Inhibition of the inward sodium and calcium currents using blockers of these currents can also create discontinuities in conduction when applied to localized segments *(180)*.

Very slow conduction encountered under these conditions is generally the result of major step delays caused by electrotonically-mediated (saltatory) transmission of impulses across a functionally inexcitable zone (i.e., across a large cumulative axial resistance imposed between two excitable regions) rather than to a uniform or homogeneous slowing of impulse propagation (Fig. 15) *(287)*. The functionally inexcitable zone effectively serves to diminish the electrical coupling between the excitable regions participating in the conduction of the impulse. The decay of the wavefront as it travels across the inexcitable or refractory zone leads to slow activation of the tissue beyond and thus to a step delay in the conduction of the impulse. The resistive barriers created are similar to those encountered with anisotropy *(288)*. With either condition, small changes in the effective impedance to the flow of local circuit current from one excitable element to the next can give rise to major delays in conduction. Conduction delays on the order of tens or hundreds of milliseconds occur when the electrotonic communication between the region already activated (source) and the region awaiting activation (sink) is weak. With progressive electrical uncoupling of source and sink, conduction characteristics become progressively more sensitive to changes in the active and passive membrane properties of both the source and sink *(188)*. Although the importance of the intensity of the source current, as reflected by the action potential amplitude, duration or maximum rate of rise, $(dV/dt)_{max}$, is well appreciated *(107,188,289,290)*, a number of studies suggest that under a variety of conditions the threshold current requirement of the sink (i.e., changes in excitability) *(186,188,290)* may be a more critical determinant of conduction delay (or block).

Discrete step delays of impulse conduction, associated with electrotonic pre-potentials, have been observed in intracellular recordings obtained from human and animal infarcted myocardium *(10,192,291,292)*. Extracellular mapping experiments also have uncovered step delays in the propagation of impulses in canine hearts subjected to acute regional myocardial ischemia *(257)*. These studies lend support to an electrotonic interaction across a high impedance barrier as a mechanism responsible for apparently slow conduction. Nonuniform recovery of refractoriness and geometrical factors also play an important role in determining impulse conduction velocity as well as the success or failure of conduction. Disparity in the recovery of refractoriness has already been discussed as the basis for unidirectional block or the lines of block that develop in response to premature extrasystoles. Disparity of local refractoriness can also contribute to a major slowing of impulse propagation and thus to reentry *(212,230,287,293)*.

Geometry also plays a critically important role. Regions at which the cross-sectional area of interconnected cells increases abruptly are known to be potential sites for the development of unidirectional block or delayed conduction due to an impedance mismatch. Slowing or block of conduction occurs when the impulse propagates in the direction of increasing diameter because the local circuit current provided by the advancing wavefront is insufficient or barely sufficient to charge the capacity of the larger volume of tissue ahead and thus bring the larger mass to its threshold potential. The Purkinje-muscle junction is an example of a site at which unidirectional block and conduction delays are observed *(294–296)*. The pre-excitation (Wolff-Parkinson-White) syndrome is another example, where a thin bundle of tissue (Kent bundle) inserts into a larger ventricular mass.

REFERENCES

1. Mayer AG. Rhythmical pulsations is scyphomedusae. Publication 47 of the Carnegie Institute 1906; 1–62.
2. Mayer AG. Rhythmical pulsations in scyphomedusae. II. Publication 102 of the Carnegie Institute 1908;115–131.
3. Mines GR. On dynamic equilibrium in the heart. J Physiol 1913;46:349–382.
4. Mines GR. On circulating excitations in heart muscles and their possible relation to tachycardia and fibrillation. Trans R Soc Can 1914;8:43–52.
5. Lewis T. The broad features and time-relations of the normal electrocardiogram. Principles of interpretation. In: The Mechanism and Graphic Registration of the Heart Beat. London: Shaw & Sons, Ltd., 1925:44–77.
6. Moe GK. Evidence for reentry as a mechanism for cardiac arrhythmias. Rev Physiol Biochem Pharmacol 1975;72:55–81.
7. Kulbertus HE. In: Kulbertus HE, ed. Reentrant Arrhythmias, Mechanisms and Treatment. Baltimore: University Park Press, 1977.
8. Wit AL, Cranefield PF. Re-entrant excitation as a cause of cardiac arrhythmias. Am J Physiol 1978;235:H1–H17.
9. Wit AL, Allessie MA, Fenoglio JJ, Jr, Bonke FIM, Lammers W, Smeets J. Significance of the endocardial and epicardial border zones in the genesis of myocardial infarction arrhythmias. In: Harrison D, ed. Cardiac Arrhythmias: A Decade of Progress. Boston: GK Hall, 1982:39–68.
10. Spear JF, Moore EN. Mechanisms of cardiac arrhythmias. Annu Rev Physiol 1982;44:485–497.
11. Janse MJ. Reentry rhythms. In: Fozzard HA, Haber E, Jennings RB, Katz AM, Morgan HE, eds. The Heart and Cardiovascular System. New York: Raven Press, 1986:1203–1238.
12. Hoffman BF, Dangman KH. Mechanisms for cardiac arrhythmias. Experientia 1987;43:1049–1056.
13. Antzelevitch C. Reflection as a mechanism of reentrant cardiac arrhythmias. Prog Cardiol 1988; 1:3–16.
14. El-Sherif N. Reentry revisited. PACE 1988;11:1358–1368.
15. Lazzara R, Scherlag BJ. Generation of arrhythmias in myocardial ischemia and infarction. Am J Cardiol 1988;61:20A–26A.
16. Rosen MR. The links between basic and clinical cardiac electrophysiology. Circulation 1988;77: 251–263.
17. DiFrancesco D. The cardiac hyperpolarizing-activated current, I_f. Origins and developments. Prog Biophys Mol Biol 1985;46:163–183.
18. DiFrancesco D. The pacemaker current (I(f)) plays an important role in regulating SA node pacemaker activity. Cardiovasc Res 1995;30:307–308.
19. Vassalle M. Analysis of cardiac pacemaker potential using a "voltage clamp" technique. Am J Physiol 1966;210:1335–1341.
20. Vassalle M. The pacemaker current (I(f)) does not play an important role in regulating SA node pacemaker activity. Cardiovasc Res 1995;30:309–310.
21. Huser J, Blatter LA, Lipsius SL. Intracellular Ca^{2+} release contributes to automaticity in cat atrial pacemaker cells. J Physiol 2000;524 Pt 2:415–422.
22. Levy MN. Sympathetic- Parasympathetic interactions in the heart. Circ Res 1971;29:437–445.
23. Imanishi S, Surawicz B. Automatic activity in depolarized guinea pig ventricular myocardium. Characteristics and mechanisms. Circ Res 1976;39:751–759.
24. Dangman KH, Hoffman BF. Studies on overdrive stimulation of canine cardiac Purkinje fibers: maximal diastolic potential as a determinant of the response. J Am Coll Cardiol 1983;2:1183–1190.
25. Katzung BG, Morgenstern JA. Effects of extracellular potassium on ventricular automaticity and evidence for a pacemaker current in mammalian ventricular myocardium. Circ Res 1977;40:105–111.
26. Pappano AJ, Carmeliet EE. Epinephrine and the pacemaking mechanism at plateau potentials in sheep cardiac Purkinje fibers. Pflugers Arch 1979;382:17–26.

27. Katz LN, Pick A. Clinical Electrocardiography. Part 1. The Arrhythmias. Philadelphia: Lea and Febiger, 1956:224–236.

28. Pogwizd SM, Hoyt RH, Saffitz JE, Corr PB, Cox JL, Cain ME. Reentrant and focal mechanisms underlying ventricular tachycardia in the human heart. Circulation 1992;86:1872–1887.

29. Arnar DO, Bullinga JR, Martins JB. Role of the Purkinje system in spontaneous ventricular tachycardia during acute ischemia in a canine model. Circulation 1997;96:2421–2429.

30. Pogwizd SM. Focal mechanisms underlying ventricular tachycardia during prolonged ischemic cardiomyopathy. Circulation 1994;90:1441–1458.

31. Pogwizd SM. Nonreentrant mechanisms underlying spontaneous ventricular arrhythmias in a model of nonischemic heart failure in rabbits. Circulation 1995;92:1034–1048.

32. Pogwizd SM, McKenzie JP, Cain ME. Mechanisms underlying spontaneous and induced ventricular arrhythmias in patients with idiopathic dilated cardiomyopathy. Circulation 1998;98:2404–2414.

33. Haissaguerre M, Jais P, Shah DC, et al. Spontaneous initiation of atrial fibrillation by ectopic beats originating in the pulmonary veins. N Engl J Med 1998;339:659–666.

34. Vermeulen JT, McGuire MA, Opthof T, et al. Triggered activity and automaticity in ventricular trabeculae of failing human and rabbit hearts. Cardiovasc Res 1994;28:1547–1554.

35. Nuss HB, Kaab S, Kass DA, Tomaselli GF, Marban E. Cellular basis of ventricular arrhythmias and abnormal automaticity in heart failure. Am J Physiol 1999;277:H80–H91.

36. Hoppe UC, Jansen E, Sudkamp M, Beuckelmann DJ. Hyperpolarization-activated inward current in ventricular myocytes from normal and failing human hearts. Circulation 1998;97:55–65.

37. Cerbai E, Barbieri M, Mugelli A. Occurrence and properties of the hyperpolarization-activated current I_f in ventricular myocytes from normotensive and hypertensive rats during aging. Circulation 1996;94:1674–1681.

38. Lai LP, Su MJ, Lin JL, et al. Measurement of funny current (I(f)) channel mRNA in human atrial tissue: correlation with left atrial filling pressure and atrial fibrillation. J Cardiovasc Electrophysiol 1999;10:947–953.

39. Scherf D, Boyd LJ. Three unusual cases of parasystole. Am Heart J 1950;39:650–663.

40. Jalife J, Moe GK. A biological model of parasystole. Am J Cardiol 1979;43:761–772.

41. Jalife J, Antzelevitch C, Moe GK. The case for modulated parasystole. PACE 1982;5:911–926.

42. Moe GK, Jalife J, Mueller WJ, Moe B. A mathematical model of parasystole and its application to clinical arrhythmias. Circulation 1977;56:968–979.

43. Antzelevitch C, Jalife J, Moe GK. Characteristics of reflection as a mechanism of reentrant arrhythmias and its relationship to parasystole. Circulation 1980;61:182–191.

44. Nau GJ, Aldariz AE, Acunzo RS, et al. Modulation of parasystolic activity by nonparasystolic beats. Circulation 1982;66:462–469.

45. Antzelevitch C. Clinical applications of new concepts of parasystole, reflection, and tachycardia. Cardiol Clin 1983;1:39–50.

46. Antzelevitch C, Jalife J, Moe GK. Electrotonic modulation of pacemaker activity. Further biological and mathematical observations on the behavior of modulated parasystole. Circulation 1982;66:1225–1232.

47. Antzelevitch C, Bernstein MJ, Feldman HN, Moe GK. Parasystole, reentry, and tachycardia: A canine preparation of cardiac arrhythmias occurring across inexcitable segments of tissue. Circulation 1983;68:1101–1115.

48. Castellanos A, Melgarejo E, Dubois R, Luceri RM. Modulation of ventricular parasystole by extraneous depolarizations. J Electrocardiol 1984;17:195–198.

49. Jalife J, Moe GK. Effect of electrotonic potentials on pacemaker activity of canine Purkinje fibers in relation to parasystole. Circ Res 1976;39:801–808.

50. Moe GK, Jalife J, Antzelevitch C. Models of parasystole and reentry in isolated Purkinje fibers. Mayo Clin Proc 1982;57 Suppl:14–19.

51. Oreto G, Luzza F, Satullo G, Schamroth L. Modulated ventricular parasystole as a mechanism for concealed bigeminy. Am J Cardiol 1986;58:954–958.

52. Oreto G, Luzza F, Satullo G, Coglitore S, Schamroth L. Sinus modulation of atrial parasystole. Am J Cardiol 1986;58:1097–1099.

53. Cranefield PF. Action potentials, afterpotentials and arrhythmias. Circ Res 1977;41:415–423.

54. Wit AL, Rosen MR. Afterdepolarizations and triggered activity: Distinction from automaticity as an arrhythmogenic mechanism. In: Fozzard HA, et al., eds. The Heart and Cardiovascular System. New York: Raven Press, 1992:2113–2164.

55. Lab MJ. Contraction-excitation feedback in myocardium: Physiologic basis and clinical relevance. Circ Res 1982;50:757–766.

56. Adamantidis MM, Caron JF, Dupuis BA. Triggered activity induced by combined mild hypoxia and acidosis in guinea pig Purkinje fibers. J Mol Cell Cardiol 1986;18:1287–1299.
57. Coraboeuf E, Deroubaix E, Coulombe A. Acidosis-induced abnormal repolarization and repetive activity in isolated dog Purkinje fibers. J Physiol (Paris) 1980;76:97–106.
58. Priori SG, Corr PB. Mechanisms underlying early and delayed afterdepolarizations induced by catecholamines. Am J Physiol 1990;258:H1796–H1805.
59. Volders PGA, Kulcsar A, Vos MA, et al. Similarities between early and delayed afterdepolarizations induced by isoproterenol in canine ventricular myocytes. Cardiovasc Res 1997;34:348–359.
60. Brachmann J, Scherlag BJ, Rosenshtraukh LV, Lazzara R. Bradycardia-dependent triggered activity: Relevance to drug-induced multiform ventricular tachycardia. Circulation 1983;68:846–856.
61. Damiano BP, Rosen MR. Effects of pacing on triggered activity induced by early afterdepolarizations. Circulation 1984;69:1013–1025.
62. El-Sherif N, Zeiler RH, Craelius W, Gough WB, Henkin R. QTU prolongation and polymorphic ventricular tachyarrhythmias due to bradycardia-dependent early afterdepolarizations. Afterdepolarizations and ventricular arrhythmias. Circ Res 1988;63:286–305.
63. January CT, Riddle JM, Salata JJ. A model for early afterdepolarizations: Induction with the Ca^{2+} channel agonist BAY K 8644. Circ Res 1988;62:563–571.
64. Davidenko JM, Cohen L, Goodrow RJ, Antzelevitch C. Quinidine-induced action potential prolongation, early afterdepolarizations, and triggered activity in canine Purkinje fibers. Effects of stimulation rate, potassium, and magnesium. Circulation 1989;79:674–686.
65. Carmeliet E. Electrophysiologic and voltage clamp analysis of the effects of sotalol on isolated cardiac muscle and Purkinje fibers. J Pharmacol Exp Ther 1985;232:817–825.
66. Aronson RS. Afterpotentials and triggered activity in hypertrophied myocardium from rats with renal-hypertension. Circ Res 1981;48:720–727.
67. Volders PG, Sipido KR, Vos MA, Kulcsar A, Verduyn SC, Wellens HJ. Cellular basis of biventricular hypertrophy and arrhythmogenesis in dogs with chronic complete atrioventricular block and acquired torsade de pointes. Circulation 1998;98:1136–1147.
68. Antzelevitch C, Sicouri S. Clinical relevance of cardiac arrhythmias generated by afterdepolarizations: The role of M cells in the generation of U waves, triggered activity and torsade de pointes. J Am Coll Cardiol 1994;23:259–277.
69. Roden DM, Hoffman BF. Action potential prolongation and induction of abnormal automaticity by low quinidine concentrations in canine Purkinje fibers: Relationship to potassium and cycle length. Circ Res 1986;56:857–867.
70. Burashnikov A, Antzelevitch C. Acceleration-induced action potential prolongation and early afterdepolarizations. J Cardiovasc Electrophysiol 1998;9:934–948.
71. Bril A, Faivre JF, Forest MC, et al. Electrophysiological effect of BRL-32872, a novel antiarrhythmic agent with potassium and calcium channel blocking properties, in guinea pig cardiac isolated preparations. J Pharmacol Exp Ther 1995;273:1264–1272.
72. Marban E, Robinson SW, Wier WG. Mechanism of arrhythmogenic delayed and early afterdepolarizations in ferret muscle. J Clin Invest 1986;78:1185–1192.
73. Boutjdir M, El-Sherif N. Pharmacological evaluation of early afterdepolarisations induced by sea anemone toxin (ATXII) in dog heart. Cardiovasc Res 1991;25:815–819.
74. Carlsson L, Abrahamsson C, Drews C, Duker GD. Antiarrhythmic effects of potassium channel openers in rhythm abnormalities related to delayed repolarization in the rabbit. Circulation 1992;85:1491–1500.
75. El-Sherif N, Zeiler RH, Craelius W, Gough WB, Henkin R. QTU prolongation and polymorphic ventricular tachyarrhythmias due to bradycardia-dependent early-afterdepolarizations. Circ Res 1988;63:286–305.
76. Nattel S, Quantz MA. Pharmacological response of quinidine induced early afterdepolarizations in canine cardiac Purkinje fibers: insights into underlying ionic mechanisms. Cardiovasc Res 1988;22:808–817.
77. Sicouri S, Antzelevitch C. Afterdepolarizations and triggered activity develop in a select population of cells (M cells) in canine ventricular myocardium: The effects of acetylstrophanthidin and Bay K 8644. PACE 1991;14:1714–1720.
78. Liu DW, Antzelevitch C. Characteristics of the delayed rectifier current (I_{Kr} and I_{Ks}) in canine ventricular epicardial, midmyocardial and endocardial myocytes: A weaker I_{Ks} contributes to the longer action potential of the M cell. Circ Res 1995;76:351–365.
79. Burashnikov A, Antzelevitch C. Block of I_{Ks} does not induce early afterdepolarization activity but promotes β-adrenergic agonist-induced delayed afterdepolarization activity in canine ventricular myocardium. J Cardiovasc Electrophysiol 2000;11:458–465.

80. Burashnikov A, Antzelevitch C. A prominent I_{Ks} in epicardium and endocardium contributes to the development of transmural dispersion of repolarization but protects against the development of early afterdepolarizations. J Cardiovasc Electrophysiol 2002;13:(in press).

81. Emori T, Antzelevitch C. Cellular basis for complex T waves and arrhythmic activity following combined I(Kr) and I(Ks) block. J Cardiovasc Electrophysiol 2001;12:1369–1378.

82. El-Sherif N, Caref EB, Yin H, Restivo M. The electrophysiological mechanism of ventricular arrhythmias in the long QT syndrome: Tridimensional mapping of activation and recovery patterns. Circ Res 1996;79:474–492.

83. Murakawa Y, Sezaki.K., Yamashita T, Kanese Y, Omata M. Three-dimensional activation sequence of cesium-induced ventricular arrhythmias. Am J Physiol 1997;273:H1377–H1385.

84. Szabo B, Kovacs T, Lazzara R. Role of calcium loading in early afterdepolarizations generated by Cs in canine and guinea pig Purkinge fibers. J Cardiovasc Electrophysiol 1995;6:796–812.

85. Patterson E, Scherlag BJ, Szabo B, Lazzara R. Facilitation of epinephrine-induced afterdepolarizations by class III antiarrhythmic drugs. J Electrocardiol 1997;30:217–224.

86. Shimizu W, Antzelevitch C. Differential effects of beta-adrenergic agonists and antagonists in LQT1, LQT2, and LQT3 models of the long QT syndrome. J Am Coll Cardiol 2000;35:778–786.

87. January CT, Riddle JM. Early afterdepolarizations: mechanism of induction and block: A role for L-type Ca^{2+} current. Circ Res 1989;64:977–990.

88. Zeng J, Rudy Y. Early afterdepolarizations in cardiac myocytes: mechanism and rate dependence. Biophys J 1995;68:949–964.

89. Ming Z, Nordin C, Aronson MD. Role of L-type calcium channel window current in generating current-induced early afterdepolarizations. J Cardiovasc Electrophysiol 1994;5:323–334.

90. Patterson E, Scherlag BJ, Lazzara R. Early afterdepolarizations produced by d,l-sotalol and clofilium. J Cardiovasc Electrophysiol 1997;8:667–678.

91. Burashnikov A, Antzelevitch C. Mechanisms underlying early afterdepolarization activity are different in canine Purkinje and M cell preparations. Role of intracellular calcium. [abstr]. Circulation 1996;94:I-527.

92. Roden DM, Lazzara R, Rosen MR, et al. Multiple mechanisms in the long-QT syndrome: Current knowledge, gaps, and future directions. Circulation 1996;94:1996–2012.

93. Antzelevitch C, Yan GX, Shimizu W, Sicouri S, Eddlestone GT, Zygmunt AC. Electrophysiologic characteristics of M cells and their role in arrhythmias. In: Franz MR, ed. Monophasic Action Potentials: Bridging Cell and Bedside. Armonk, NY: Futura, 2000:583–604.

94. Ben-David J, Zipes DP. Differential response to right and left ansae subclaviae stimulation of early afterdepolarizations and ventricular tachycardia induced by cesium in dogs. Circulation 1988;78:1241–1250.

95. Jackman WM, Friday KJ, Anderson JL, Aliot EM, Clark MA, Lazzara R. The long QT syndromes: A critical review, new clinical observations and a unifying hypothesis. Prog Cardiovasc Dis 1988;31:115–172.

96. Shimizu W, Ohe T, Kurita T, et al. Early afterdepolarizations induced by isoproterenol in patients with congenital long QT syndrome. Circulation 1991;84:1915–1923.

97. Asano Y, Davidenko JM, Baxter WT, Gray RA, Jalife J. Optical mapping of drug-induced polymorphic arrhythmias and torsade de pointes in the isolated rabbit heart. J Am Coll Cardiol 1997;29:831–842.

98. Ben-David J, Zipes DP, Ayers GM, Pride HP. Canine left ventricular hypertrophy predisposes to ventricular tachycardia induction by phase 2 early afterdepolarizations after administration of BAY K 8644. J Am Coll Cardiol 1992;20(7):1576–1584.

99. Beuckelmann DJ, Nabauer M, Erdmann E. Alterations of K^+ currents in isolated human ventricular myocytes from patients with terminal heart failure. Circ Res 1993;73:379–385.

100. Vermeulen JT. Mechanisms of arrhythmias in heart failure. J Cardiovasc Electrophysiol 1998;9:208–221.

101. Ferrier GR, Saunders JH, Mendez C. A cellular mechanism for the generation of ventricular arrhythmias by acetylstrophanthidin. Circ Res 1973;32:600–609.

102. Rosen MR, Gelband H, Merker C, Hoffman BF. Mechanisms of digitalis toxicity—effects of ouabain on phase four of canine Purkinje fiber transmembrane potentials. Circulation 1973;47:681–689.

103. Saunders JH, Ferrier GR, Moe GK. Conduction block associated with transient depolarizations induced by acetylstrophanthidin in isolated canine Purkinje fibers. Circ Res 1973;32:610–617.

104. Rozanski GJ, Lipsius SL. Electrophysiology of functional subsidiary pacemakers in canine right atrium. Am J Physiol 1985;249:H594–H603.

105. Marchi S, Szabo B, Lazzara R. Adrenergic induction of delayed afterdepolarizations in ventricular myocardial cells: Beta-induction and Alpha-Modulation. J Cardiovasc Electrophysiol 1991;2: 476–491.

106. Wit AL, Cranefield PF. Triggered and automatic activity in the canine coronary sinus. Circ Res 1977;41:435–445.

107. Lazzara R, El-Sherif N, Scherlag BJ. Electrophysiological properties of canine Purkinje cells in one-day-old myocardial infarction. Circ Res 1973;33:722–734.

108. Matsuda H, Noma A, Kurachi Y, Irisawa H. Transient depolarizations and spontaneous voltage fluctuations in isolated single cells from guinea pig ventricles. Circ Res 1982;51:142–151.

109. Spinelli W, Sorota S, Siegel MB, Hoffman BF. Antiarrhythmic actions of the ATP-regulated K^+ current activated by pinacidil. Circ Res 1991;68:1127–1137.

110. Belardinelli LL, Isenberg G. Actions of adenosine and isoproterenol on isolated mammalian ventricular myocytes. Circ Res 1983;53(3):287–297.

111. Antzelevitch C, Sicouri S, Litovsky SH, et al. Heterogeneity within the ventricular wall: Electrophysiology and pharmacology of epicardial, endocardial and M cells. Circ Res 1991;69:1427–1449.

112. Sicouri S, Antzelevitch C. Drug-induced afterdepolarizations and triggered activity occur in a discrete subpopulation of ventricular muscle cell (M cells) in the canine heart: Quinidine and Digitalis. J Cardiovasc Electrophysiol 1993;4:48–58.

113. Schreieck J, Wang YG, Gjini V, et al. Differential effect of beta-adrenergic stimulation on the frequency-dependent electrophysiologic actions of the new class III antiarrhythmics dofetilide, ambasilide, and chromanol 293B. J Cardiovasc Electrophysiol 1997;8:1420–1430.

114. Coetzee WA, Opie LH. Effects of components of ischemia and metabolic inhibition on delayed afterdepolarizations in guinea pig papillary muscle. Circ Res 1987;61:157–165.

115. Pogwizd SM, Onufer JR, Kramer JB, Sobel BE, Corr PB. Induction of delayed afterdepolarizations and triggered activity in canine Purkinje fibers by lysophosphoglycerides. Circ Res 1986;59:416–426.

116. Song Y, Belardinelli L. ATP promotes development of afterdepolarizations and triggered activity in cardiac myocytes. Am J Physiol 1994;267:H2005–H2011.

117. Wu Y, Roden DM, Anderson ME. Calmodulin kinase inhibition prevents development of the arrhythmogenic transient inward current. Circ Res 1999;84:906–912.

118. Caroni P, Villani F, Carafoli E. The cardiotoxic antibiotic doxorubicin inhibits the Na^+/Ca^{2+} exchange of dog heart sarcolemmal vesicles. FEBS Lett 1981;130:184–186.

119. Kass RS, Tsien RW, Weingart R. Ionic basis of transient inward current induced by strophanthidin in cardiac Purkinje fibres. J Physiol (Lond) 1978;281:209–226.

120. Cannell MB, Lederer WJ. The arrhythmogenic current I_{TI} in the absence of electrogenic sodium-calcium exchange in sheep cardiac Purkinje fibres. J Physiol (Lond) 1986;374:201–219.

121. Fedida D, Noble D, Rankin AC, Spindler AJ. The arrhythmogenic transient inward current I_{ti} and related contraction in isolated guinea-pig ventricular myocytes. J Physiol (Lond) 1987;392:523–542.

122. Laflamme MA, Becker PL. Ca^{2+}-induced current oscillations in rabbit ventricular myocytes. Circ Res 1996;78:707–716.

123. Zygmunt AC, Goodrow RJ, Weigel CM. I_{NaCa} and $I_{Cl(Ca)}$ contribute to isoproterenol-induced delayed afterdepolarizations in midmyocardial cells. Am J Physiol 1998;275:H1979–H1992.

124. Ritchie AH, Kerr CR, Qi A, Yeung-Lai-Wah JA. Nonsustained ventricular tachycardia arising from the right ventricular outflow tract. Am J Cardiol 1989;64:594–598.

125. Wilber DJ, Blakeman BM, Pifarre R, Scanlon PJ. Catecholamine sensitive right ventricular outflow tract tachycardia: Intraoperative mapping and ablation of a free-wall focus. PACE 1989;12: 1851–1856.

126. Cardinal R, Scherlag BJ, Vermeulen M, Armour JA. Distinct activation patterns of idioventricular rhythms and sympathetically-induced ventricular tachycardias in dogs with atrioventricular block. PACE 1992;15:1300–1316.

127. Cardinal R, Savard P, Armour JA, Nadeau RA, Carson DL, LeBlanc AR. Mapping of ventricular tachycardia induced by thoracic neural stimulation in dogs. Can J Physiol Pharmacol 1986;64: 411–418.

128. Lerman BB, Belardinelli LL, West GA, Berne RM, DiMarco JP. Adenosine-sensitive ventricular tachycardia: Evidence suggesting cyclic AMP-mediated triggered activity. Circulation 1986;74:270–280.

129. Lerman BB, Stein K, Engelstein ED, et al. Mechanism of repetitive monomorphic ventricular tachycardia. Circulation 1995;92:421–429.

130. Ter Keurs HE, Schouten VJA, Bucx JJ, Mulder BM, De Tombe PP. Excitation-contraction coupling in myocardium: implications of calcium release and Na⁺-Ca²⁺ exchange. Can J Physiol Pharmacol 1987;65:619–626.

131. Kent AFS. Observation on the auirculo-ventricular junction of the mammalian heart. Q J Exp Physiol 1913;7:193–197.

132. Schmitt FO, Erlanger J. Directional differences in the conduction of the impulse through heart muscle and their possible relation to extrasystolic and fibrillary contractions. Am J Physiol 1928;87:326–347.

133. Cranefield PF, Hoffman BF. Conduction of the cardiac impulse. II. Summation and inhibition. Circ Res 1971;28:220–233.

134. Cranefield PF, Klein HO, Hoffman BF. Conduction of the cardiac impulse. I. Delay, block and one-way block in depressed Purkinje fibers. Circ Res 1971;28:199–219.

135. Sasyniuk BI, Mendez C. A mechanism for reentry in canine ventricular tissue. Circ Res 1971;28:3–15.

136. Wit AL, Cranefield PF, Hoffman BF. Slow conduction and reentry in the ventricular conducting system. II. Single and sustained circus movement in networks of canine and bovine Purkinje fibers. Circ Res 1972;30:11–22.

137. Wit AL, Hoffman BF, Cranefield PF. Slow conduction and reentry in the ventricular conducting system. I. Return extrasystoles in canine Purkinje fibers. Circ Res 1972;30:1–10.

138. Cranefield PF. The Conduction of the Cardiac Impulse. Mount Kisco, NY: Futura, 1975:153.

139. Garrey WE. Auricular fibrillation. Physiol Rev 1924;4:215–250.

140. Allessie MA, Bonke FIM, Schopman JG. Circus movement in rabbit atrial muscle as a mechanism of tachycardia. Circ Res 1973;33:54–62.

141. Allessie MA, Bonke FIM, Schopman JG. Circus movement in rabbit atrial muscle as a mechanism of tachycardia: II. The role of nonuniform recovery of excitability in the occurrence of unidirectional block as studied with multiple microelectrodes. Circ Res 1976;39:168–177.

142. Allessie MA, Bonke FIM, Schopman JG. Circus movement in rabbit atrial muscle as a mechanism of tachycardia. III. The "leading circle" concept: a new model of circus movement in cardiac tissue without the involvement of an anatomical obstacle. Circ Res 1977;41:9–18.

143. Kamiyama A, Eguchi K, Shibayama R. Circus movement tachycardia induced by a single premature stimulus on the ventricular sheet: Evaluation of the leading circle hypothesis in the canine ventricular muscle. Jpn Circ J 1986;50:65–73.

144. Allessie MA, Schalij MJ, Kirchhof CJ, Boersma L, Huybers M, Hollen J. Experimental electrophysiology and arrhythmogenicity. Anisotropy and ventricular tachycardia. Eur Heart J 1989;10 Suppl E:2–8.

145. El-Sherif N, Smith RA, Evans K. Canine ventricular arrhythmias in the late myocardial infarction period. 8. Epicardial mapping of reentrant circuits. Circ Res 1981;49:255–265.

146. El-Sherif N, Mehra R, Gough WB, Zeiler RH. Ventricular activation pattern of spontaneous and induced ventricular rhythms in canine one-day-old myocardial infarction. Evidence for focal and reentrant mechanisms. Circ Res 1982;51:152–166.

147. Mehra R, Zeiler RH, Gough WB, El-Sherif N. Reentrant ventricular arrhythmias in the late myocardial infarction period. 9. Electrophysiologic-anatomic correlation of reentrant circuits. Circulation 1983;67:11–24.

148. El-Sherif N, Mehra R, Gough WB, Zeiler RH. Reentrant ventricular arrhythmias in the late myocardial infarction period. Interruption of reentrant circuits by cyrothermal techniques. Circulation 1983;68:644–656.

149. Wit AL, Allessie MA, Bonke FIM, Lammers WJEP, Smeets JL, Fenoglio JJ. Electrophysiological mapping to determine the mechanisms of experimental ventricular tachycardia initiated by premature impulses. Experimental approach and initial results demonstrating reentrant excitation. Am J Cardiol 1982;49:166–185.

150. Dillon SM, Allessie MA, Ursell PC, Wit AL. Influences of anisotropic tissue structure on reentrant circuits in the epicardial border zone of subacute canine infarcts. Circ Res 1988;63:182–206.

151. Clerc L. Directional differences of impulse spread in trabecular muscle from mammalian heart. J Physiol (Lond) 1976;255:335–346.

152. Harumi K, Burgess MJ, Abildskov JA. A theoretic model of the T wave. Circulation 1966;34:657–668.

153. Spach MS, Kootsey JM, Sloan JD. Active modulation of electrical coupling between cardiac cells of the dog. A mechanism for transient and steady state variations in conduction velocity. Circ Res 1982;51:347–362.

154. El-Sherif N. The figure 8 model of reentrant excitation in the canine post-infarction heart. In: Zipes DP, Jalife J, eds. Cardiac Electrophysiology and Arrhythmias. New York: Grune and Stratton, 1985:363–378.

155. Lin SF, Roth BJ, Wikswo JP, Jr. Quatrefoil reentry in myocardium: an optical imaging study of the induction mechanism. J Cardiovasc Electrophysiol 1999;10:574–586.
156. Weiner N, Rosenblueth A. The mathematical formulation of the problem of conduction of impulses in a network of connected excitable elements, specifically in cardiac muscle. Arch Inst Cardiol Mex 1946;16:205–265.
157. Davidenko JM, Kent PF, Chialvo DR, Michaels DC, Jalife J. Sustained vortex-like waves in normal isolated ventricular muscle. Proc Natl Acad Sci USA 1990;87:8785–8789.
158. Pertsov AM, Davidenko JM, Salomonsz R, Baxter WT, Jalife J. Spiral waves of excitation underlie reentrant activity in isolated cardiac muscle. Circ Res 1993;72:631–650.
159. Jalife J, Davidenko JM, Michaels DC. A new perspective on the mechanisms of arrhythmias and sudden cardiac death: spiral wave of excitation in heart muscle. J Cardiovasc Electrophysiol 1991;2:S133–S152.
160. Athill CA, Ikeda T, Kim YH, Wu TJ, Fishbein MC, Karagueuzian HS, Chen PS. Transmembrane potential properties at the core of functional reentrant wave fronts in isolated canine right atria. Circulation 1998;98:1556–1567.
161. Jalife J, Delmar M, Davidenko JM, Anumonwo JMB. Basic Cardiac Electrophysiology for the Clinician. Armonk, NY: Futura Publishing, 1999.
162. Pertsov AM, Jalife J. Three-dimensional vortex-like reentry. In: Zipes DP, Jalife J, eds. Cardiac Electrophysiology: From Cell to Bedside. Philadelphia: W.B. Saunders, 1995:403–410.
163. Davidenko JM. Spiral wave activity: a possible common mechanism for polymorphic and monomorphic ventricular tachycardias. J Cardiovasc Electrophysiol 1993;4:730–746.
164. Garfinkel A, Qu Z. Nonlinear dinamics of excitation and propagation in cardiac muscle. In: Zipes DP, Jalife J, eds. Cardiac Electrophysiology: From Cell to Bedside. Philadelphia: W.B. Saunders, 1999: 315–320.
165. Moe GK, Rheinboldt WC, Abildskov JA. A computer model of atrial fibrillation. Am Heart J 1964;67:200–220.
166. Weiss JN, Garfinkel A, Karagueuzian HS, Qu Z, Chen PS. Chaos and the transition to ventricular fibrillation: a new approach to antiarrhythmic drug evaluation. Circulation 1999;99:2819–2826.
167. Chen J, Mandapati R, Berenfeld O, Skanes AC, Jalife J. High-frequency periodic sources underlie ventricular fibrillation in the isolated rabbit heart. Circ Res 2000;86:86–93.
168. Zaitsev AV, Berenfeld O, Mironov SF, Jalife J, Pertsov AM. Distribution of excitation frequencies on the epicardial and endocardial surfaces of fibrillating ventricular wall of the sheep heart. Circ Res 2000;86:408–417.
169. Samie FH, Berenfeld O, Anumonwo J, et al. Rectification of the background potassium current: a determinant of rotor dynamics in ventricular fibrillation. Circ Res 2001;89:1216–1223.
170. Gray RA, Jalife J, Panfilov AV, et al. Mechanisms of cardiac fibrillation. Science 1995;270:1222–1223.
171. Janse MJ, Wilms-Schopman FJG, Coronel R. Ventricular fibrillation is not always due to multiple wavelet reentry. J Cardiovasc Electrophysiol 1995;6:512–521.
172. Antzelevitch C. Ion channels and ventricular arrhythmias. Cellular and ionic mechanisms underlying the Brugada syndrome. Curr Opin Cardiol 1999;14:274–279.
173. Janse MJ, Van Capelle FJL, Morsink H, et al. Flow of "injury" current and patterns of excitation during early ventricular arrhythmias in acute regional myocardial ischemia in isolated porcine and canine hearts. Evidence for two different arrhythmogenic mechanisms. Circ Res 1980;47:151–167.
174. Pogwizd SM, Corr PB. Mechanisms underlying the development of ventricular fibrillation during early myocardial ischemia. Circ Res 1990;66:672–695.
175. Riccio ML, Koller ML, Gilmour RF, Jr. Electrical restitution and spatiotemporal organization during ventricular fibrillation. Circ Res 1999;84:955–963.
176. Rogers JC, Huang JL, Smith WM, Ideker RE. Incidence, evolution, and spatial distribution of functional reentry during ventricular fibrillation in pigs. Circ Res 1999;84:945–954.
177. Choi BR, Liu T, Salama G. The distribution of refractory periods influences the dynamics of ventricular fibrillation. Circ Res 2001;88:E49–E58.
178. Allessie MA, Lammers WJEP, Bonke FIM, Hollen J. Experimental evaluation of Moe's multiple wavelet hypothesis of atrial fibrillation. In: Zipes DP, Jalife J, eds. Cardiac Electrophysiology and Arrhythmias. Grune & Stratton, 1985:265–276.
179. Schuessler RB, Grayson TM, Bromberg BI, Cox JL, Boineau JP. Cholinergically mediated tachyarrhythmias induced by a single extrastimulus in the isolated canine right atrium. Circ Res 1992;71:1254–1267.

180. Antzelevitch C, Moe GK. Electrotonically-mediated delayed conduction and reentry in relation to "slow responses" in mammalian ventricular conducting tissue. Circ Res 1981;49:1129–1139.

181. Rozanski GJ, Jalife J, Moe GK. Reflected reentry in nonhomogeneous ventricular muscle as a mechanism of cardiac arrhythmias. Circulation 1984;69:163–173.

182. Lukas A, Antzelevitch C. Reflected reentry, delayed conduction, and electrotonic inhibition in segmentally depressed atrial tissues. Can J Physiol Pharmacol 1989;67:757–764.

183. Davidenko JM, Antzelevitch C. The effects of milrinone on action potential characteristics, conduction, automaticity, and reflected reentry in isolated myocardial fibers. J Cardiovasc Pharmacol 1985;7:341–349.

184. Rosenthal JE, Ferrier GR. Contribution of variable entrance and exit block in protected foci to arrhythmogenesis in isolated ventricular tissues. Circulation 1983;67:1–8.

185. Antzelevitch C, Lukas A. Reflection and reentry in isolated ventricular tissue. In: Dangman KH, Miura DS, eds. Basic and Clinical Electrophysiology of the Heart. New York: Marcel Dekker, 1991:251–275.

186. Antzelevitch C, Moe GK. Electrotonic inhibition and summation of impulse conduction in mammalian Purkinje fibers. Am J Physiol 1983;245:H42–H53.

187. Jalife J, Moe GK. Excitation, conduction, and reflection of impulses in isolated bovine and canine cardiac Purkinje fibers. Circ Res 1981;49:233–247.

188. Davidenko JM, Antzelevitch C. Electrophysiological mechanisms underlying rate-dependent changes of refractoriness in normal and segmentally depressed canine Purkinje fibers. The characteristics of post-repolarization refractoriness. Circ Res 1986;58:257–268.

189. Davidenko JM, Antzelevitch C. The effects of milrinone on conduction, reflection and automaticity in canine Purkinje fibers. Circulation 1984;69:1026–1035.

190. Winkle RA. The relationship between ventricular ectopic beat frequency and heart rate. Circulation 1982;66:439–446.

191. Nau GJ, Aldariz AE, Acunzo RS, et al. Clinical studies on the mechanism of ventricular arrhythmias. In: Rosenbaum MB, Elizari MV, eds. Frontier of Cardiac Electrophysiology. Amsterdam: Martinus Nijhoff, 1983:239–273.

192. Rosenthal JE. Reflected reentry in depolarized foci with variable conduction impairment in 1 day old infarcted canine cardiac tissue. J Am Coll Cardiol 1988;12:404–411.

193. Van Hemel NM, Swenne CA, De Bakker JMT, Defauw JAM, Guiraudon GM. Epicardial reflection as a cause of incessant ventricular bigeminy. PACE 1988;11:1036–1044.

194. Litovsky SH, Antzelevitch C. Transient outward current prominent in canine ventricular epicardium but not endocardium. Circ Res 1988;62:116–126.

195. Liu DW, Gintant GA, Antzelevitch C. Ionic bases for electrophysiological distinctions among epicardial, midmyocardial, and endocardial myocytes from the free wall of the canine left ventricle. Circ Res 1993;72:671–687.

196. Furukawa T, Myerburg RJ, Furukawa N, Bassett AL, Kimura S. Differences in transient outward currents of feline endocardial and epicardial myocytes. Circ Res 1990;67:1287–1291.

197. Fedida D, Giles WR. Regional variations in action potentials and transient outward current in myocytes isolated from rabbit left ventricle. J Physiol (Lond) 1991;442:191–209.

198. Clark RB, Bouchard RA, Salinas-Stefanon E, Sanchez-Chapula J, Giles WR. Heterogeneity of action potential waveforms and potassium currents in rat ventricle. Cardiovasc Res 1993;27:1795–1709.

199. Wettwer E, Amos GJ, Posival H, Ravens U. Transient outward current in human ventricular myocytes of subepicardial and subendocardial origin. Circ Res 1994;75:473–482.

200. Nabauer M, Beuckelmann DJ, Uberfuhr P, Steinbeck G. Regional differences in current density and rate-dependent properties of the transient outward current in subepicardial and subendocardial myocytes of human left ventricle. Circulation 1996;93:168–177.

201. Zygmunt AC. Intracellular calcium activates chloride current in canine ventricular myocytes. Am J Physiol 1994;267:H1984–H1995.

202. Takano M, Noma A. Distribution of the isoprenaline-induced chloride current in rabbit heart. Pflugers Arch 1992;420:223–226.

203. Di Diego JM, Sun ZQ, Antzelevitch C. I_{to} and action potential notch are smaller in left vs right canine ventricular epicardium. Am J Physiol 1996;271:H548–H561.

204. Volders PG, Sipido KR, Carmeliet E, Spatjens RL, Wellens HJ, Vos MA. Repolarizing K$^+$ currents ITO1 and I_{Ks} are larger in right than left canine ventricular midmyocardium. Circulation 1999;99:206–210.

205. Sicouri S, Antzelevitch C. A subpopulation of cells with unique electrophysiological properties in the deep subepicardium of the canine ventricle: The M cell. Circ Res 1991;68:1729–1741.
206. Anyukhovsky EP, Sosunov EA, Rosen MR. Regional differences in electrophysiologic properties of epicardium, midmyocardium and endocardium: In vitro and in vivo correlations. Circulation 1996;94:1981–1988.
207. Zygmunt AC, Eddlestone GT, Thomas GP, Nesterenko VV, Antzelevitch C. Larger late sodium conductance in M cells contributes to electrical heterogeneity in canine ventricle. Am J Physiol 2001;281:H689–H697.
208. Zygmunt AC, Goodrow RJ, Antzelevitch C. I_{Na-Ca} contributes to electrical heterogeneity within the canine ventricle. Am J Physiol 2000;278:H1671–H1678.
209. Brahmajothi MV, Morales MJ, Reimer KA, Strauss HC. Regional localization of ERG, the channel protein responsible for the rapid component of the delayed rectifier, K^+ current in the ferret heart. Circ Res 1997;81:128–135.
210. Burashnikov A, Antzelevitch C. Differences in the electrophysiologic response of four canine ventricular cell types to a_1-adrenergic agonists. Cardiovasc Res 1999;43:901–908.
211. Yan GX, Shimizu W, Antzelevitch C. Characteristics and distribution of M cells in arterially-perfused canine left ventricular wedge preparations. Circulation 1998;98:1921–1927.
212. Antzelevitch C, Shimizu W, Yan GX, et al. The M cell. Its contribution to the ECG and to normal and abnormal electrical function of the heart. J Cardiovasc Electrophysiol 1999;10:1124–1152.
213. Sicouri S, Antzelevitch C. Electrophysiologic characteristics of M cells in the canine left ventricular free wall. J Cardiovasc Electrophysiol 1995;6:591–603.
214. Sicouri S, Fish J, Antzelevitch C. Distribution of M cells in the canine ventricle. J Cardiovasc Electrophysiol 1994;5:824–837.
215. Stankovicova T, Szilard M, De Scheerder I, Sipido KR. M cells and transmural heterogeneity of action potential configuration in myocytes from the left ventricular wall of the pig heart. Cardiovasc Res 2000;45:952–960.
216. Drouin E, Charpentier F, Gauthier C, Laurent K, Le Marec H. Electrophysiological characteristics of cells spanning the left ventricular wall of human heart: Evidence for the presence of M cells. J Am Coll Cardiol 1995;26:185–192.
217. Weissenburger J, Nesterenko VV, Antzelevitch C. Transmural heterogeneity of ventricular repolarization under baseline and long QT conditions in the canine heart in vivo. Torsades de pointes develops with halothane but not pentobarbital anesthesia. J Cardiovasc Electrophysiol 2000;11:290–304.
218. Sicouri S, Quist M, Antzelevitch C. Evidence for the presence of M cells in the guinea pig ventricle. J Cardiovasc Electrophysiol 1996;7:503–511.
219. Li GR, Feng J, Yue L, Carrier M. Transmural heterogeneity of action potentials and Ito1 in myocytes isolated from the human right ventricle. Am J Physiol 1998;275:H369–H377.
220. Rodriguez-Sinovas A, Cinca J, Tapias A, Armadans L, Tresanchez M, Soler-Soler J. Lack of evidence of M-cells in porcine left ventricular myocardium. Cardiovasc Res 1997;33:307–313.
221. Shimizu W, Antzelevitch C. Sodium channel block with mexiletine is effective in reducing dispersion of repolarization and preventing torsade de pointes in LQT2 and LQT3 models of the long-QT syndrome. Circulation 1997;96:2038–2047.
222. Shimizu W, McMahon B, Antzelevitch C. Sodium pentobarbital reduces transmural dispersion of repolarization and prevents torsade de pointes in models of acquired and congenital long QT syndromes. J Cardiovasc Electrophysiol 1999;10:156–164.
223. Shimizu W, Antzelevitch C. Cellular basis for the electrocardiographic features of the LQT1 form of the long QT syndrome: Effects of b-adrenergic agonists, antagonists and sodium channel blockers on transmural dispersion of repolarization and torsade de pointes. Circulation 1998;98:2314–2322.
224. Shimizu W, Antzelevitch C. Cellular and ionic basis for T-wave alternans under Long QT-conditions. Circulation 1999;99:1499–1507.
225. Yan GX, Antzelevitch C. Cellular basis for the normal T wave and the electrocardiographic manifestations of the long QT syndrome. Circulation 1998;98:1928–1936.
226. Balati B, Varro A, Papp JG. Comparison of the cellular electrophysiological characteristics of canine left ventricular epicardium, M cells, endocardium and Purkinje fibres. Acta Physiol Scand 1998;164:181–190.
227. McIntosh MA, Cobbe SM, Smith GL. Heterogeneous changes in action potential and intracellular Ca^{2+} in left ventricular myocyte sub-types from rabbits with heart failure. Cardiovasc Res 2000;45:397–409.

228. Viskin S, Lesh MD, Eldar M, Fish R, Setbon I, Laniado S, Belhassen B. Mode of onset of malignant ventricular arrhythmias in idiopathic ventricular fibrillation. J Cardiovasc Electrophysiol 1997;8: 1115–1120.

229. Brugada P, Brugada J. Right bundle branch block, persistent ST segment elevation and sudden cardiac death: a distinct clinical and electrocardiographic syndrome: a multicenter report. J Am Coll Cardiol 1992;20:1391–1396.

230. Antzelevitch C, Brugada P, Brugada J, Brugada R, Nademanee K, Towbin JA. The Brugada Syndrome. Armonk, NY: Futura Publishing Company, Inc., 1999:1–99.

231. Alings M, Wilde A. "Brugada" syndrome: clinical data and suggested pathophysiological mechanism. Circulation 1999;99:666–673.

232. Antzelevitch C. The Brugada syndrome: Ionic basis and arrhythmia mechanisms. J Cardiovasc Electrophysiol 2001;12:268–272.

233. Antzelevitch C. The Brugada Syndrome. Diagnostic criteria and cellular mechanisms. Eur Heart J 2001;22:356–363.

234. Nademanee K, Veerakul G, Nimmannit S, et al. Arrhythmogenic marker for the sudden unexplained death syndrome in Thai men. Circulation 1997;96:2595–2600.

235. Corrado D, Buja G, Basso C, Nava A, Thiene G. What is the Brugada syndrome? Cardiol Rev 1999;7:191–195.

236. Brugada R, Brugada J, Antzelevitch C, et al. Sodium channel blockers identify risk for sudden death in patients with ST-segment elevation and right bundle branch block but structurally normal hearts. Circulation 2000;101:510–515.

237. Remme CA, Wever EFD, Wilde AAM, Derksen R, Hauer RNW. Diagnosis and long-term follow-up of Brugada syndrome in patients with idiopathic ventricular fibrillation. Eur Heart J 2001;22:400–409.

238. Viskin S, Fish R, Eldar M, Zeltser D, Lesh MD, Glick A, Belhassen B. Prevalence of the Brugada sign in idiopathic ventricular fibrillation and healthy controls. Heart 2000;84:31–36.

239. Chen Q, Kirsch GE, Zhang D, et al. Genetic basis and molecular mechanisms for idiopathic ventricular fibrillation. Nature 1998;392:293–296.

240. Yan GX, Antzelevitch C. Cellular basis for the Brugada Syndrome and other mechanisms of arrhythmogenesis associated with ST segment elevation. Circulation 1999;100:1660–1666.

241. Rook MB, Alshinawi CB, Groenewegen WA, et al. Human SCN5A gene mutations alter cardiac sodium channel kinetics and are associated with the Brugada syndrome. Cardiovasc Res 1999;44: 507–517.

242. Dumaine R, Towbin JA, Brugada P, et al. Ionic mechanisms responsible for the electrocardiographic phenotype of the Brugada syndrome are temperature dependent. Circ Res 1999;85:803–809.

243. Deschenes I, Baroudi G, Berthet M, et al. Electrophysiological characterization of SCN5A mutations causing long QT (E1784K) and Brugada (R1512W and R1432G) syndromes. Cardiovasc Res 2000;46:55–65.

244. Priori SG, Napolitano C, Glordano U, Collisani G, Memml M. Brugada syndrome and sudden cardiac death in children. Lancet 2000;355:808–809.

245. Bezzina C, Veldkamp MW, van Den Berg MP, et al. A single Na(+) channel mutation causing both long-QT and Brugada syndromes. Circ Res 1999;85:1206–1213.

246. Yan GX, Antzelevitch C. Cellular basis for the electrocardiographic J wave. Circulation 1996;93: 372–379.

247. Gussak I, Antzelevitch C, Bjerregaard P, Towbin JA, Chaitman BR. The Brugada syndrome: clinical, electrophysiological and genetic aspects. J Am Coll Cardiol 1999;33:5–15.

248. Miyazaki T, Mitamura H, Miyoshi S, Soejima K, Aizawa Y, Ogawa S. Autonomic and antiarrhythmic drug modulation of ST segment elevation in patients with Brugada syndrome. J Am Coll Cardiol 1996;27:1061–1070.

249. Lukas A, Antzelevitch C. Phase 2 reentry as a mechanism of initiation of circus movement reentry in canine epicardium exposed to simulated ischemia. The antiarrhythmic effects of 4-aminopyridine. Cardiovasc Res 1996;32:593–603.

250. Antzelevitch C, Dumaine R. Electrical heterogeneity in the heart: Physiological, pharmacological and clinical implications. In: Page E, Fozzard HA, Solaro RJ, eds. Handbook of Physiology. The Heart. New York: Oxford University Press, 2002:654–692.

251. Tarin N, Farre J, Rubio JM, Tunon J, Castro-Dorticos J. Brugada-like electrocardiographic pattern in a patient with a mediastinal tumor. PACE 1999;22:1264–1266.

252. Carlsson J, Erdogan A, Schulte B, Neuzner J, Pitschner HF. Possible role of epicardial left ventricular programmed stimulation in Brugada syndrome. PACE 2001;24:247–249.

253. Litovsky SH, Antzelevitch C. Differences in the electrophysiological response of canine ventricular subendocardium and subepicardium to acetylcholine and isoproterenol. A direct effect of acetylcholine in ventricular myocardium. Circ Res 1990;67:615–627.
254. Krishnan SC, Antzelevitch C. Flecainide-induced arrhythmia in canine ventricular epicardium: Phase 2 Reentry? Circulation 1993;87:562–572.
255. Matsuo K, Shimizu W, Kurita T, et al. Increased dispersion of repolarization time determined by monophasic action potentials in two patients with familial idiopathic ventricular fibrillation. J Cardiovasc Electrophysiol 1998;9:74–83.
256. Janse MJ, Wit AL. Electrophysiological mechanisms of ventricular arrhythmias resulting from myocardial ischemia and infarction. Physiol Rev 1989;69:1049–1169.
257. Janse MJ, Van Capelle FJL. Electrotonic interactions across an inexcitable region as a cause of ectopic activity in acute regional myocardial ischemia. A study in intact porcine and canine hearts and computer models. Circ Res 1982;50:527–537.
258. Lukas A, Antzelevitch C. Differences in the electrophysiological response of canine ventricular epicardium and endocardium to ischemia: Role of the transient outward current. Circulation 1993;88:2903–2915.
259. Di Diego JM, Antzelevitch C. Pinacidil-induced electrical heterogeneity and extrasystolic activity in canine ventricular tissues: Does activation of ATP-regulated potassium current promote phase 2 reentry? Circulation 1993;88:1177–1189.
260. Di Diego JM, Antzelevitch C. High [Ca^{2+}]-induced electrical heterogeneity and extrasystolic activity in isolated canine ventricular epicardium: Phase 2 reentry. Circulation 1994;89:1839–1850.
261. Gilmour RF, Jr, Zipes DP. Different electrophysiological responses of canine endocardium and epicardium to combined hyperkalemia, hypoxia, and acidosis. Circ Res 1980;46:814–825.
262. Kimura S, Bassett AL, Kohya T, Kozlovskis PL, Myerburg RJ. Simultaneous recording of action potentials from endocardium and epicardium during ischemia in the isolated cat ventricle: Relation of temporal electrophysiologic heterogeneities to arrhythmias. Circulation 1986;74:401–409.
263. Furukawa T, Kimura S, Cuevas J, Furukawa N, Bassett AL, Myerburg RJ. Role of cardiac ATP-regulated potassium channels in differential responses of endocardial and epicardial cells to ischemia. Circ Res 1991;68:1693–1702.
264. Kimura S, Bassett AL, Furukawa T, Furukawa N, Myerburg RJ. Differences in the effect of metabolic inhibition on action potentials and calcium currents in endocardial and epicardial cells. Circulation 1991;84:768–777.
265. Miller WT, Geselowitz DB. Simulation studies of the electrogram. 2. Ischemia and infarction. Circ Res 1978; 43:315–323.
266. Miller WT, Geselowitz DB. Simulation studies of the electrocardiogram. 1. The normal heart. Circ Res 1978;43:301–315.
267. Mandel WJ, Burgess MJ, Neville J, Abildskov JA. Analysis of T-wave abnormalities associated with myocardial infarction using a theoretical model. Circulation 1968;38:178–188.
268. Haws CW, Lux RL. Correlation between *in vivo* transmembrane action potential durations and action-recovery intervals from electrograms. Effects of interventions that alter repolarization time. Circulation 1990;81:281–288.
269. Downar E, Janse MJ, Durrer D. The effect of acute coronary artery occlusion on subepicardial transmembrane potentials in the intact porcine heart. Circulation 1977;56:217–224.
270. Ejima J, Martin D, Engle CL, Gettes LS, Kunimoto S, Gettes LS. Ability of activation recovery intervals to assess action potential duration during acute no-flow ischemia in the in situ porcine heart. J Cardiovasc Electrophysiol 1998;9:832–844.
271. Madias JE. The earliest electrocardiographic signs of acute transmural myocardial infarction. J Electrocardiol 1977;10:193–196.
272. Schwartz PJ, Periti M, Malliani A. The long QT syndrome. Am Heart J 1975;89:378–390.
273. Moss AJ, Schwartz PJ, Crampton RS, Locati EH, Carleen E. The long QT syndrome: a prospective international study. Circulation 1985;71:17–21.
274. Zipes DP. The long QT interval syndrome: A Rosetta stone for sympathetic related ventricular tachyarrhythmias. Circulation 1991;84:1414–1419.
275. Shimizu W, Ohe T, Kurita T, et al. Effects of verapamil and propranolol on early afterdepolarizations and ventricular arrhythmias induced by epinephrine in congenital long QT syndrome. J Am Coll Cardiol 1995;26:1299–1309.
276. Abbott GW, Sesti F, Splawski I, et al. MiRP1 forms I_{Kr} potassium channels with HERG and is associated with cardiac arrhythmia. Cell 1999;97:175–187.

277. Antzelevitch C, Sun ZQ, Zhang ZQ, Yan GX. Cellular and ionic mechanisms underlying erythromycin-induced long QT and torsade de pointes. J Am Coll Cardiol 1996;28:1836–1848.

278. Schwartz PJ. The idiopathic long QT syndrome: Progress and questions. Am Heart J 1985;109: 399–411.

279. Moss AJ, Schwartz PJ, Crampton RS, et al. The long QT syndrome: prospective longitudinal study of 328 families. Circulation 1991;84:1136–1144.

280. Crampton RS. Preeminence of the left stellate ganglion in the long QT syndrome. Circulation 1979;59:769–778.

281. Ali RH, Zareba W, Moss A, et al. Clinical and genetic variables associated with acute arousal and nonarousal-related cardiac events among subjects with long QT syndrome. Am J Cardiol 2000;85:457–461.

282. El-Sherif N, Chinushi M, Caref EB, Restivo M. Electrophysiological mechanism of the characteristic electrocardiographic morphology of torsade de pointes tachyarrhythmias in the long-QT syndrome. Detailed analysis of ventricular tridimensional activation patterns. Circulation 1997;96:4392–4399.

283. Akar FG, Yan GX, Antzelevitch C, Rosenbaum DS. Optical maps reveal reentrant mechanism of torsade de pointes based on topography and electrophysiology of mid-myocardial cells [abstr]. Circulation 1997;96(8):I-355.

284. Ferrier GR, Rosenthal JE. Automaticity and entrance block induced by focal depolarization of mammalian ventricular tissues. Circ Res 1980;47:238–248.

285. Wennemark JR, Ruesta VJ, Brody DA. Microelectrode study of delayed conduction in the canine right bundle branch. Circ Res 1968;23:753–769.

286. Downar E, Waxman MB. Depressed conduction and unidirectional block in Purkinje fibers. In: Wellens HJ, Lie KI, Janse MJ, eds. The Conduction System of the Heart. Philadelphia: Lea and Febiger, 1976:393–409.

287. Antzelevitch C, Spach MS. Impulse conduction: continuous and discontinuous. In: Spooner PM, Rosen MR, eds. Foundations of Cardiac Arrhythmias. Basic Concepts: Fundamental Approaches. New York: Marcel Dekker, Inc., 2000:205–241.

288. Spach MS, Miller WT, Geselowitz DB, Barr RC, Kootsey JM, Johnson EA. The discontinuous nature of propagation in normal canine cardiac muscle. Evidence for recurrent discontinuities of intracellular resistance that affect the membrane currents. Circ Res 1981;48:39–54.

289. Antzelevitch C, Jalife J, Moe GK. Frequency-dependent alternations of conduction in Purkinje fibers. A model of phase-4 facilitation and block. In: Rosenbaum MB, Elizari MV, eds. Frontiers of Cardiac Electrophysiology. Amsterdam: Martinus Nijhoff, 1983:397–415.

290. Gilmour RF, Jr., Salata JJ, Zipes DP. Rate-related suppression and facilitation of conduction in isolated canine cardiac Purkinje fibers. Circ Res 1985;57:35–45.

291. Gilmour RF, Jr., Heger JJ, Prystowsky EN, Zipes DP. Cellular electrophysiologic abnormalities of diseased human ventricular myocardium. Am J Cardiol 1983;51:137–144.

292. Gilmour RF, Jr., Zipes DP. Cellular basis for cardiac arrhythmias. Cardiol Clin 1983;1:3–11.

293. Antzelevitch C, Shimizu W, Yan GX. Electrical heterogeneity and the development of arrhythmias. In: Olsson SB, Yuan S, Amlie JP, eds. Dispersion of Ventricular Repolarization: State of the Art. New York: Futura Publishing Company, Inc., 2000:3–21.

294. Gilmour RF, Jr. Phase resetting of circus movement reentry in cardiac tissue. In: Zipes DP, Jalife J, eds. Cardiac Electrophysiology, From Cell to Bedside. New York: WB Saunders, 1989.

295. Matsuda K, Kamiyama A, Hoshi T. Configuration of the transmenbrane action potential at the Purkinje-ventricular fiber junction and its analysis. In: Sano T, Mizuhira V, Matsuda K, eds. Electrophysiology and Ultrastructure of the Heart. New York: Grune & Stratton, 1967:177–187.

296. Overholt ED, Joyner RW, Veenstra RD, Rawling DA, Wiedman R. Unidirectional block between Purkinje and ventricular layers of papillary muscles. Am J Physiol 1984;247:H584–H595.

297. Antzelevitch C. Electrotonus and reflection. In: Rosen MR, Janse MJ, Wit AL, eds. Cardiac Electrophysiology: A Textbook. Mount Kisco, NY: Futura Publishing Company, Inc., 1990:491–516.

Part III

CLINICAL PHYSIOLOGY AND PATHOPHYSIOLOGY OF VENTRICULAR REPOLARIZATION: THEORY AND PRACTICE

Edited by
Stephen C. Hammill, Win-Kuang Shen,
and Ihor Gussak

12 Evaluation of Ventricular Repolarization

The Clinician's Perspective

Jan Němec, MD, Stephen C. Hammill, MD, and Win-Kuang Shen, MD

CONTENTS

INTRODUCTION

The aim of this chapter is to review the methods used to study cardiac repolarization impairment in the clinical setting. The bewildering variety of available techniques testifies to the complexity of ventricular repolarization and to the fact that no fully satisfactory method is currently available. Compared to depolarization, repolarization of cardiac tissue is a more gradual, low-frequency process; even in animal experiments, it has been relatively difficult to study, though the development of optical mapping with voltage dyes and the technique of perfused myocardial wedges have considerably advanced our understanding.

The focus of this chapter will be on the evidence for clinical usefulness of various noninvasive methods to assess repolarization. It is likely that there will be overlaps with other chapters and omissions due to space constraints. For example, although microvoltage T wave alternans (μV-TWA) is reviewed in Chapter 23, it has become such a prominent method of risk stratification that it is difficult to omit in the review on clinical assessment of repolarization. On the other hand, other clinically important topics (such as drug-induced repolarization changes) are discussed very briefly and are treated in more detail elsewhere in the book.

From: *Contemporary Cardiology: Cardiac Repolarization: Bridging Basic and Clinical Science*
Edited by: I. Gussak et al. © Humana Press Inc., Totowa, NJ

NONINVASIVE METHODS TO ASSESS REPOLARIZATION

QT Interval Duration

The measurement of QT interval is undoubtedly the simplest and the most widely used method for repolarization assessment. Although QT interval changes associated with electrolyte derangement and myocarditis have been recognized since the first half of the 20th century, reports on the association between QT prolongation and sudden death date back to the initial description of the autosomal recessive *(1)* and autosomal dominant *(2,3)* forms of congenital long QT syndrome (LQTS). Since then, several papers have been published on the possible significance of QT interval prolongation as a risk marker for sudden death in many other cardiac conditions, ranging from acute coronary syndromes to hypertrophic cardiomyopathy (HCM). However, with the exception of the congenital LQTS and monitoring the effect of class Ia and III antiarrhythmic drugs, there is little consensus regarding its clinical value.

The mechanistic explanation for the link between QT interval prolongation, impaired repolarization of the ventricular myocardium and propensity to ventricular arrhythmias is explained in detail in other chapters of this book. In essence, the QT interval duration approximates the period between the start of depolarization and the end of repolarization of the ventricular myocardium (Fig. 1). Prolonged ventricular repolarization may be associated with increased dispersion of refractoriness and, by implication, increased propensity to reentrant arrhythmias.

EPIDEMIOLOGICAL STUDIES

The relationship between the QT interval duration and mortality has been evaluated in several population-based studies *(4–10)*. While no association between mortality and QT duration was found in the Framingham study *(4)* (5125 patients), most other studies of similar size did report slightly but significantly increased mortality in the groups with the longest QT (QTc) intervals (ranging from QTc>420 to QTc>440 in different studies). At least in some of these studies *(9)*, the increased mortality seemed to result from longer QT duration in subjects with cardiac disease or risk factors for coronary artery disease (CAD) and the association disappeared when subjects with cardiovascular disease were excluded.

CONGENITAL LQTS

Prolongation of the QT interval on surface ECG is the cardinal feature of congenital LQTS. It is accepted that the degree of QT prolongation correlates with the risk of sudden cardiac death (SCD), reflecting a greater degree of repolarization impairment. In a pediatric study performed before the genotyping of LQTS patients became available *(11)*, 38% of patients with QTc $\geq$ 600 ms had cardiac arrest, seizure or syncope during an average follow-up of five years, compared to 7% of those with QTc < 600 ms ($p<0.001$). The data from The International LQTS Registry point in the same direction *(12)*. However, the correlation between the degree of QT prolongation and clinical risk does not appear to be tight. In the same pediatric study, 17 of the 287 patients (6%) had "normal" QT duration (QTc < 440 ms). Six of these 17 subjects presented with serious symptoms. Similar overlap in QT intervals between affected and unaffected subjects was found in a study of three large LQT1 kindreds *(13)*. A particularly high percentage of normal or borderline QT duration may be associated with certain *KCNQ1* or *HERG* mutations—

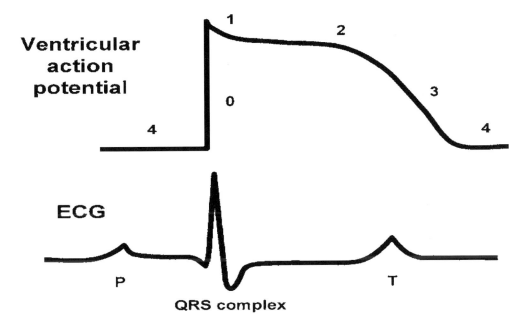

Fig. 1. The relationship between the ventricular action potential and surface ECG is illustrated in this figure. While the QRS complex corresponds to rapid depolarization of ventricular myocytes owing to opening of the cardiac sodium channels (phase 0), isoelectric ST segments roughly reflects the plateau (phase 2) of ventricular action potential. The T wave deflection is generated by different degrees of repolarization among adjacent layers of ventricular myocardium (phase 3). These differences are caused, among else, by variation in densities of certain potassium channels between different layers of the ventricular myocardium. Thus, the QT interval approximates the action potential duration of a ventricular cardiomyocyte.

well over 50% of confirmed gene carriers in certain kindreds *(14)*. The affected members of these families still appear to be at substantial risk of SCD. Although certain therapeutic interventions have been shown to decrease the QT interval duration in LQTS, their clinical feasibility and efficacy remains to be proven *(15–17)*. In summary, prolongation of the QT interval remains the diagnostic gold standard for LQTS, and an excessively prolonged QT interval has been associated with increased risk of SCD. However, its diagnostic and prognostic values are less than optimal.

DRUG-RELATED QT PROLONGATION

The issue of drug-induced repolarization impairment and proarrhythmia has been a focus of considerable interest, especially regarding the "idiosyncratic" reactions to noncardiac drugs like terfenadine. It is now known that a host of widely used noncardiac drugs act as weak blockers of the potassium channel I_{Kr} *(18)*. In a situation of preexisting subclinical repolarization delay, their administration can result in dramatic QT prolongation, but most healthy people are not affected. In contrast, class III antiarrhythmic drugs exhibit a more or less predictable relationship between plasma levels, QT prolongation and risk of proarrhythmia. Both relationships have been best demonstrated for sotalol *(19,20)*, but similar data exist for ibutilide *(21)*. For example, the incidence of serious ventricular arrhythmias was reported to be 0.5% in patients taking sotalol at dose 80–160 mg/d, but 6.8% in patients taking more than 640 mg/d. Maximum QTc was significantly longer in patients on sotalol who eventually developed torsade de pointes (TdP) than in the remaining patients (521 vs 462 ms, $p<0.0001$) *(19)*. On the other hand, certain patients can develop serious ventricular arrhythmias related to sotalol with little QTc prolongation *(22)*. In a study of ibutilide, another antiarrhythmic agent prolonging repolarization, the development of polymorphic ventricular tachycardia (VT) was associated with a significantly more pronounced increase in QT interval compared to the group as a whole (QTc of 529 vs 477 ms; $p<0.02$ for increase from baseline)*(23)*. In clinical practice, increased awareness should be exercised when noncardiac drugs known to prolong the QT interval (Table 1) are used. Concomitant administration of more than one of these drugs should be avoided. When a class Ia or class III antiarrhythmic drug is used for rhythm control, response of the QT interval after initiation of drug therapy should be closely followed. In general, QTc should not exceed 500 ms after the drug has reached a steady-state condition.

CORONARY ARTERY DISEASE

On the cellular level, acute ischemia shortens action potential durations by several mechanisms, with the activation of the potassium current I_{KATP} probably playing the most prominent role; knockout mice lacking this ion channel fail to develop the typical electrocardiogram (ECG) changes during ischemia *(24)*. On the other hand, although QT shortening has been found in the early acute phase (< 12 h) of myocardial infarction (MI) *(25)*, most clinical reports describe QT interval prolongation during acute MI *(26,27)*. This phenomenon has been linked to the increased propensity for arrhythmias in the acute phase of MI. For example, patients who developed VT during the acute phase of MI had significantly longer QTc (434 vs 421 ms) than the other MI patients *(28)*. During acute ischemia due to proximal left anterior descending coronary artery stenosis without MI, QTc prolongation was found in 16 out of 76 patients *(29)*, but no QT prolongation was detected in another study of similar size of patients with unstable angina *(30)*. In a large retrospective study of patients with chronic stable angina, prolonged QTc was associated with sudden death but not with total mortality *(31)*.

Several groups have studied the QT interval and its possible prognostic role in patients after MI; both positive and negative results have been reported. A small (55 post-MI patients) early study found that MI survivors had shorter QTc than patients who died, but longer than normal controls *(32)*. A larger study (865 patients) also found longer QTc in patients who succumbed to cardiac death compared to survivors (471 vs 413 ms, $p<0.001$) *(26)*. In the BHAT trial, 3387 patients within three weeks of MI were randomized to propranolol and placebo. In this study, QTc > 450 ms on baseline ECG conferred approx 55% relative increase in SCD risk compared to the patients with shorter QTc with the relative risk being similar in the propranolol and placebo groups *(33)*.

Although some trials addressing the same issue failed to detect any increased risk of either sudden *(34)* or cardiac *(35)* death associated with QTc prolongation in patients after MI, the meta-analysis of the available data suggests a modest increase in SCD, cardiac mortality, and total mortality related to prolonged QTc *(36)*. However, QTc correlates with other established adverse prognostic factors (left ventricular [LV] dysfunction

Table 1
Examples of Medications Known to Prolong Cardiac Repolarization

Medication Class		Examples
ANTIARRHYTHMICS	Ia	quinidine, procainamide, disopyramide,
	III	sotalol, dofetilide, ibutilide, amiodarone, azimilide, N-acetyl procainamide
	IV	bepridil, terodiline
ANTICANCER DRUGS		amsacrine, doxorubicine, zorubicine
ANTIDEPRESSANTS	tricyclics	amitriptiline, nortriptiline, desipramine, clomipramine, imipramine
	other	citalopram, doxepine, maprotiline, zimelidine
ANTIHISTAMINES	sedating	diphenhydramine, hydroxyzine
	nonsedating	astemizole, loratidine, terfenadine
ANTIMICROBIALS	virostatic	amantadine
	macrolides	erythromycine, clarithromycine, spiramycine, troleandomycine
	quinolones	sparfloxacine, grepafloxacine
	other antibiotics	clindamycine, trimethoprim/ sulfamethoxazole
	antifungals	amphotericine, fluconazole, itraconazole, ketoconazole, miconazole
	antiparasitics	pentamidine, quinine, chloroquine, halofantrine
PSYCHOTROPICS AND RELATED AGENTS	phenothiazines	chlorpromazine, fluphenazine, mesoridazine, prochlorperazine, thioridazine, trifluoperazine
	butyrophenones	haloperidol, droperidol
	other	pimozide, sultopride, sertindole, risperidone, lithium
MISCELLANEOUS		cisapride, probucol, ketanserine, potassium-wasting diuretics (indirectly through hypokalemia)

[a]In most cases, the prolongation is related to I_{Kr} block. A comprehensive list of such medications is available on the Web address www.torsades.org

[37,38], extent of coronary artery disease [39]) and it is unclear whether it provides any additional prognostic information.

MISCELLANEOUS CONDITIONS

Regarding other cardiac disorders associated with SCD, prolonged QT interval has been consistently reported in HCM (40–43). In one study, the QT interval duration was significantly longer in HCM patients than in subjects with LV hypertrophy of a different etiology (44). Although QTc prolongation correlates with LV wall thickness (45), a known SCD risk factor in HCM (46), QTc did not predict SCD in a group of 277 unselected HCM patients (47). Prolonged QT interval has also been noted in patients with aortic stenosis (48).

An interesting prospective study alleges that prolonged QT interval in infants increases the risk of the sudden infant death syndrome (SIDS), raising the possibility that at least some instances of SIDS might actually represent a form of LQTS *(49)*—12 out of 24 SIDS victims had QTc > 440 ms. This possibility has been supported by a case report of a child with LQTS presenting as aborted SIDS *(50)*.

Apart from the situations mentioned above, many other acquired conditions are associated with prolonged QT interval. These include electrolyte derangements, hypothermia, intracranial bleeding, and electrical remodeling related to tachycardia. Most of these are reviewed elsewhere in the book. In contrast, a shortened QT interval is much less common, although several conditions including ischemia shorten action potential duration. The best described situation associated with a shortened QTc interval is hypercalcemia, with opinions differing on the consistency of this association and on the question whether the shortening affects mainly the isoelectric ST segment *(51,52)*. In addition, a possible hereditary syndrome consisting of short QT interval and propensity to cardiac arrhythmias has been described recently *(53)*.

METHODOLOGY

Despite the relative simplicity of QT interval measurement, some aspects of this method have never been standardized. Whereas some of the studies referenced above have used the limb lead II for QT measurement *(54,55)*, the longest QT interval in any of the standard 12 leads has been used by others *(37)*. Yet different papers have measured mean QT interval of all the leads *(35)*, the lead with largest T wave *(34)*, the lead with the sharpest T wave offset *(56)*, QT interval in lead I *(33)* or V2 *(57)*. The study by Cowan et al. *(58)* reported that the QT interval is usually longest when measured in the anteroseptal precordial leads V2 or V3.

There is little doubt that the major source of error in QT interval measurements is the difficulty of the exact determination of T wave offset. This has been recognized for nearly half a century when a complex algorithm for exact separation of the T wave from the U wave was proposed by Lepeshkin and Surawicz *(59)*. While most papers dealing with QT duration still rely on simple manual measurement with real or electronic calipers, several of the more recent articles have used a digitizing board or computer-assisted algorithms. With the proliferation of literature on QT dispersion, the methodology of QT determination seems to have developed into a separate discipline of science *(60)*. It has been shown that the results of QT measurement are affected by the paper speed and ECG gain (longer with 50 mm/s than 25 mm/s, longer with 10 mm/mV than 5 mm/mV) *(61)*. The relative interobserver and intraobserver QT measurement error is close to 5% *(62)*. Surprisingly, the hopes that automatic QT measurement would markedly improve reproducibility have not been realized yet, primarily owing to the availability of different algorithms *(63,64)*. The algorithms most commonly used to determine the T wave offset include the threshold algorithm, where the T wave offset is defined as the instant when the T wave falls under a given threshold which is typically determined based on the T wave peak amplitude. Similarly, the slope (or differential) threshold algorithms define the T wave end as the time when the (negative) T wave slope falls under a threshold level based on the maximal slope *(64)*. The slope intercept algorithms determine the T wave end as the intersection of the baseline with the tangent of the T wave with the maximum negative slope. In addition, different approaches, e.g., one based on T wave curvature *(65)* have been proposed. The variability between QT duration determined by different automatic algorithms is substantial. The correlation between the QT interval determined manually and

Table 2
Examples of Formulas Proposed for Rate Correction of QT Interval.

Reference	Formula	Comment
Bazett (68)	$QTc = \dfrac{QT}{\sqrt{RR}}$	most common; overcorrects for tachycardia
Fridericia (69)	$QTc = \dfrac{QT}{\sqrt[3]{RR}}$	another early formula; uses cubic root instead of square root of HR
Sagie (70)	$QTc = QT + 0.154(1 - RR)$	used in the Framingham Study
Hodges (256)	$QTc = QT + 0.00175(HR - 60)$	another example of linear formula
Sarma (71)	$QTc = QT - 0.0446(1 - e^{2.7(1-RR)})$	an example of exponential formula

[a]QTc is the predicted QT duration at HR 60 bpm. QT, QTc, and RR are given in seconds, HR is given as beats per minute.

automatically is poor (66), which is likely attributable to the error of manual measurements. For both manual and computerized QT interval measurements, low T wave amplitude appears to decrease the precision (61,67).

It has been known for decades that the heart rate (HR) is the major determinant of QT interval duration, which shortens in parallel with cycle length. On the molecular level, this appears to be caused primarily by an incomplete deactivation of the I_{Ks} current during tachycardia, although other factors, such as inhibition of the slow Ca current by an increased cytoplasmic calcium concentration, may also play a role. Because of its HR dependence, some sort of rate correction is needed to label a QT interval "prolonged." The Bazett's formula (68) proposed more than 80 years ago is by far the most common, but many other formulas have been suggested. Among them, the "cubic root" Fridericia's formula (69) and the linear correction used in the Framingham study (70) are the best known, but exponential correction (71) and other more complex techniques have claimed superiority over the Bazett's formula (Table 2). It is appreciated that overall, Bazett's formula overcorrects the QT duration during tachycardia, i.e., the QTc obtained is too long when the RR interval (i.e., the interval between two subsequent R waves) is short (72). The Fridericia formula may provide better correction, but it seems that the optimal form of QT correction differs among normal subjects (73). Moreover, the issue is complicated by the fact that the QT interval response to HR change is not instantaneous but can take several seconds before a new steady-state is reached, so that the optimal rate correction may be different depending on whether the QT interval is recorded when the heart rate is relatively steady or rapidly changing (74). The phenomenon of QT interval hysteresis (75,76) (i.e., QT duration may be different at a given heart rate depending on whether the heart rate is increasing or decreasing) and the case reports of paradoxical QT shortening after a long pause (77,78) indicate that satisfactory QT correction by a formula based on instantaneous HR only may be impossible under certain circumstances.

In addition to HR, several other factors affect the QT duration. Many of them are not associated with disease. This includes genetic variability and changes in autonomic tone. Also, any factor which prolongs ventricular depolarization, such as bundle branch block, prolongs QT duration. It is uncertain how to best handle the latter situation, but measuring JT interval (from the end of QRS complex to the T wave end) instead appears reasonable *(79)*. The fact that QTc is longer in women than in men is well known and is probably caused by the effect of gonadal steroids on ventricular myocardium *(68,80,81)*. There are no differences in QT duration between males and females in childhood, but QT shortens in males during sexual maturation. The exact mechanism of this phenomenon remains to be elucidated; in *Xenopus* oocytes, estradiol suppresses the I_{Ks} current but not other voltage-dependent potassium currents *(82)*. However, the data obtained from castrated males suggest that androgens rather than estrogens are responsible for the gender difference in repolarization duration (and shape) *(83)*. The gender differences in repolarization are likely related to the higher propensity to TdP in females, which has been observed by several authors in congenital *(84,85)* or acquired LQTS *(86,87)*.

For a long time, it was believed that while transmural gradients at the end of the action potential are responsible for the T wave deflection, the U wave is created by a different mechanism, possibly related to the prolonged action potential duration of the Purkinje fibers *(88)*. A more recent theory links U wave to the repolarization of M cells *(89)*. It is generally accepted that the presence of the U wave does not usually signify propensity to arrhythmias and it should not be included in the QT interval measurement, but the differentiation of the U wave from the second component of a morphologically abnormal T wave in the LQTS can be problematic *(90)*. Although hard data are lacking, it seems reasonable to try to separate a "normal," small-amplitude U wave from the end of the T wave, but high-amplitude, abnormal-appearing U waves may be best included in the QT interval measurement *(91)*.

CLINICAL UTILITY

The QT measurement should be routine part of a standard ECG evaluation; many commercial ECGs provide an automatic QT measurement with rate correction. In spite of the reports linking QT interval prolongation to increased risk of arrhythmic, cardiac or total mortality, the correlation appears to be loose and the clinical utility limited in most circumstances. The QT interval determination is most useful in the diagnosis of LQTS, either congenital or acquired, and specifically during initiation of treatment by class III agents. In these settings, the link between the QTc duration is and the arrhythmic risk is well established, although borderline or normal QTc does not indicate negligible risk. In summary, although QT duration without doubt reflects ventricular repolarization, it is a relatively crude measure of this complex process. The major advantage of QT interval determination is its wide availability and ease of measurement.

QT Interval Dispersion, T Wave Morphology, and Related Techniques

INTERLEAD DISPERSION OF QT INTERVALS

The QT dispersion is usually defined as the difference between the longest and the shortest QT interval among the 12 standard ECG leads. It is another conceptually simple technique used frequently for repolarization assessment in a wide range of conditions. Although the observation of different QT interval duration in different leads is nearly as old as the clinical application of ECG *(92)*, the intense interest it has enjoyed recently was sparked by the influential paper by Campbell and associates *(93)* who suggested that QT dispersion measured from the standard ECG might reflect different action potential durations (and, by implication, dispersion of refractoriness) among different regions of ventricular myocardium. It has been appreciated since the 1960s that increased dispersion of refractoriness represents an important mechanism for initiation of reentrant arrhythmias *(94)*. This theoretical concept was supported by animal studies *(95,96)* and, more recently, by the data from perfused myocardial wedges *(97)*. The concept underlying the hope for clinical utility of QT dispersion is the hypothesis that different ECG leads preferentially reflect the electrical activity of the subjacent myocardial tissue. If this was the case, then QT dispersion in surface ECG might approximate refractoriness dispersion measured by more direct methods, e.g., monophasic action potentials (MAPs). This proposition did indeed receive some support from experiments comparing the electrical activity of an animal heart recorded by epicardial electrodes and by electrodes from the surface of a water-filled tank, in which the organ was immersed *(98)*. The MAP data also showed a correlation between MAP dispersion and QT dispersion *(99)*.

The relative simplicity of QT dispersion measurement and its wide availability probably contributed to the copious number of papers analyzing this variable in a wide range of cardiac (and noncardiac) disorders. Although many of the studies showed a value of QT dispersion for risk stratification, several doubts concerning the validity of the underlying concept have appeared *(100)*. The most serious argument against this technique is the contention that QT dispersion does not, in fact, represent regional differences in local repolarization duration, but instead results from a combination of a measurement error and abnormal morphology of the T wave vector loop. This explanation is supported by the reports of poor interobserver and intraobserver reproducibility of QT dispersion determination *(62)* (though acceptable reproducibility was found by others) *(61,101)*. More importantly, simulated ECGs generated by a projection of a single dipole T wave loop into different spatial directions representing ECG leads, were found to have a "QT dispersion" comparable to real ECGs, despite the fact that their underlying "refractoriness dispersion" was by definition zero *(102,103)*. This phenomenon was studied in more detail by Kors et al. *(104)*, who concluded convincingly that QT dispersion is related to different projections of the terminal portion of the T wave vector loop into different ECG leads: A nearly perpendicular lead would appear to have a shorter T wave inscription due to a finite noise level and limited precision of measurement. Thus, increased QT dispersion would reflect, at best, a nonspecific abnormality of T wave loop morphology, and no regional repolarization dispersion needs to be invoked to explain its existence.

Some critics of the method have suggested that the underlying concept was flawed from the beginning, since the 12 ECG leads are not truly independent, but contain redundant information (e.g., lead III can be obtained by subtracting lead I from lead II) and since it is physically impossible for a dipole T wave loop to exhibit any true dispersion in duration. However, there is no *a priori* reason why the electrical field generated by ventricular myocardium should be fully described by the dipole model, and we believe that the initial concept should not have been rejected on the first principles. Nevertheless, the limited data quantifying the deviation from the dipole model indicate that although these deviations do exist and are more pronounced in certain pathological states, they are very small indeed *(105)*. At the current state of knowledge, it appears that the T wave loop can indeed be described by the dipole model with a high degree of precision and that the hypothesis of the relationship between QT dispersion and regional differences in repolarization duration was incorrect. However, that is not the same as stating that QT dispersion contains no useful information at all.

EPIDEMIOLOGICAL STUDIES

The Rotterdam study of more than 5000 subjects showed that in addition to QT duration *(6)*, increased QT dispersion was also a risk marker in the older general population *(106)*. The data derived from the WOSCOPS trial (>6500 middle aged men with elevated cholesterol) also suggest a significant association between increased QT dispersion and risk of death or MI *(107)*, but the reported sensitivity and specificity were quite low. QT dispersion corrected by the Bazett's formula was an independent predictor of cardiovascular mortality in the Strong Heart study of American Indians *(108)*, but since most authors now agree that the rate-dependence of QT interval dispersion is minimal and that it should not be rate-corrected, it is conceivable that prolonged corrected QT dispersion might simply reflect increased HR, a well-established risk for cardiovascular mortality. The mortality increase related to increased QT dispersion in these studies is significant but not dramatic: e.g., in the Rotterdam study, mortality increased by 30% in the patients within the highest tercile of QT dispersion. The most likely explanation is an underlying cardiovascular disease leading to nonspecific T wave abnormalities in these subjects.

CORONARY ARTERY DISEASE

Increased dispersion of QT interval has been reported by several authors both during acute MI and in patients with remote past MI. During acute MI, QT dispersion appears to be highest in the first 1–3 d *(109,110)*. The degree of its prolongation is affected by the location of MI (it is higher in anterior MI) *(111–113)* and the success of thrombolytic treatment (higher with thrombolysis failure) *(113)*. In some *(101,110)* but not all studies *(114,115)*, higher QT dispersion was found in patients who developed serious rhythm disturbances in the acute phase of MI.

Several studies have reported that QT dispersion is higher in patients with remote MI than in healthy subjects, but whether QT dispersion predicts mortality after MI is still controversial. For example, a Finnish study which included 30 subjects with remote MI, history of ventricular fibrillation (VF) and positive electrophysiological (EP) study found that their QT dispersion was significantly higher than in either normal subjects or in CAD patients without documented arrhythmias and negative EP study ($p<0.001$) *(116)*. Several relatively small studies have reached a similar conclusion *(117,118)*, but increased QT dispersion tends to correlate with other established risk markers, including left ventricular ejection fraction (LVEF) *(111,119)* and absence of β-blocker treatment *(33)*, and may not therefore provide independent information.

On the other hand, no relationship between QTc dispersion at the time of hospital discharge and total mortality was detected in the large LIMIT-II study (over 2000 patients) *(109)*. The subsequent decrease in QTc dispersion was less pronounced in the patients who died compared to survivors, though this could again be influenced by differences in HR. Finally, a prospective study enrolling 280 patients with MI *(120)* found that none of the several indices of repolarization dispersion predicted the composite endpoint of death, resuscitated VF or VT, while the traditional risk markers (e.g., decreased LVEF, decreased HR variability) predicted outcome. Methodologically, this is probably the best study available and its negative result casts a serious doubt on the prognostic role of QT dispersion after MI.

Regarding other forms of coronary ischemia, QTc dispersion was found to be prolonged in patients with vasospastic angina compared to subjects with atypical chest pain *(121)* and, among vasospastic angina patients, in those who had experienced cardiac arrest or syncope *(122)*. Most reports on other forms of stable or unstable angina did not find a marked increase in QT dispersion, although successful percutaneous transluminal coronary antioplasty (PTCA) led to a decrease in this quantity in some studies *(123,124)*.

LEFT VENTRICULAR DYSFUNCTION AND HYPERTROPHY

The usefulness of QT dispersion measurement in patients with heart failure or LV dysfunction is also disputed. For example, Barr et al. *(125)* have reported that QT dispersion was higher in the seven heart failure patients who died suddenly (98.6 ms) than in the 21 survivors (53.1 ms) or the 12 patients who died of pump failure (66.7 ms; $p<0.05$). Others have proposed that in a pediatric population, QT dispersion is such a strong mortality predictor that it should be used to prioritize patients on heart transplant waiting list *(126)*. Similar conclusion was reached by other authors *(127,128)*.

In contrast, the bigger UK-HEART study *(129)* (554 patients) found that while *corrected* QT interval dispersion was a univariate predictor of SCD and total mortality in heart failure population, this relationship disappeared when other variables (cardiomegaly, HR and so on) were taken into account. Also, no prognostic information of QT dispersion could be found in the large substudy of the prospective DIAMOND-CHF trial *(130)* which included over 700 patients with advanced chronic heart failure (CHF).

Similarly, increased QT dispersion has been described in HCM *(41,42,105,131)* and higher QT dispersion values have been reported in HCM patients with serious arrhythmic events than in other HCM subjects *(131–133)*. However, the latter finding has not been confirmed in bigger studies *(41,47)*. Increased QT dispersion was also found in patients with LV hypertrophy (LVH) because of hypertension *(134–136)* or aortic stenosis *(137)*, but not in healthy athletes with LVH *(138)*. The QT dispersion in LVH can be decreased by treatment with angiotensin-converting enzyme inhibitors *(139,140)*.

CONGENITAL AND ACQUIRED LQTS

There is little doubt that QT dispersion is prolonged in LQTS *(141)*. The original paper by Day et al. *(93)* measured QT dispersion in patients with congenital or drug-induced LQTS and found that it was longer in patients with ventricular arrhythmias than in the other subjects. Priori et al. reported that QT dispersion was higher in 28 patients with congenital LQTS than in 15 healthy volunteers *(142)*. In addition, QT dispersion was longer in LQTS patients who responded to β-blockade than in those who continued to experience syncope despite the treatment. Finally, the increased QT dispersion in pediatric LQTS patients can be decreased with β-blocker treatment *(143)*. Conversely, epinephrine (but not phenylephrine, a pure α-agonist) was found to increase QT dispersion in LQTS patients *(141)*.

Several authors have attempted to correlate effect of antiarrhythmic drugs with QT dispersion changes. QT dispersion was higher in CAD patients who developed TdP on quinidine treatment than in patients without proarrhythmia *(144)*. Increased QT dispersion was also found to precede serious proarrhythmia in patients treated with sotalol or amiodarone. Correlation between changes in QT dispersion and the efficacy of antiarrhythmic treatment has also been proposed, because shorter QT dispersion was associated with VT noninducibility in patients with prior MI *(145)*.

METHODOLOGY

Some of the methodological issues concerning QT dispersion measurements have been mentioned above. Apart from questions about the ability of this method to actually estimate the dispersion of ventricular refractoriness, several studies have reported poor reproducibility and a wide range of normal values *(91)*. The reproducibility of QT dispersion measurement negatively correlates with T wave amplitude *(61)*. In addition, the measured QT dispersion is affected by posture *(146)* and respiratory phase *(147)*, and by the number of ECG leads analyzed (reasonable correction is possible when some of the 12 leads cannot be analyzed) *(148)*. The fact that the QT dispersion reported in some studies was not obtained from simultaneous 12-lead recordings may have increased the reported values due temporal variability of QT intervals.

Another controversial issue concerns the need for HR correction of QT dispersion. Although many authors have applied Bazett's correction to QT dispersion measurement, nearly all data suggest that this value is relatively heart rate-independent *(149)*. The correction can be confusing since prolonged corrected QT dispersion may result from tachycardia in addition to increased QT dispersion.

CLINICAL UTILITY

Despite the plethora of reports suggesting increased QT dispersion in most cardiac diseases as well as the possible correlation between increased QT dispersion and propensity to SCD, the clinical utility appears very limited for several reasons. First, the available information indicates that QT dispersion is a projection effect reflecting nonspecific changes in the T wave vector loop morphology (e.g., small and rounded vs narrow and elongated) rather than true dispersion in repolarization duration. This does not necessarily mean that QT dispersion does not contain any clinically useful information. However, the initial reports purporting a prognostic value in several conditions have not been confirmed in large prospective studies. The correlation between QT dispersion and prognosis appears to be loose and the prognostic information may not be independent of established risk factors. Finally, the concerns about poor reproducibility and the wide range of normal values reported make routine clinical application of this technique difficult.

These concerns have led several investigators to seek new ways to analyze repolarization abnormalities in a single beat (as opposed to temporal repolarization instability). These range from techniques attempting to assess spatial dispersion of refractoriness to methods that simply claim to quantify what would be labeled "nonspecific repolarization changes" clinically. These include variants of body surface potential mapping *(150)*, measurement of time from T wave peak to T wave end (Tp-Te) *(151,152)*, principal component analysis and its variants *(105,153)*, and certain indices describing T wave morphology, such as "total cosine R-to-T," which reflects the angle between the R wave and T wave vectors *(154)*. The space constraints do not allow detailed discussion of these methods—none has reached a stage of routine clinical application so far, although convincing abnormalities of repolarization using some of these novel methods have been detected in patients with HCM *(155)*, LQTS *(153)* or prior MI *(154)*.

QT Adaptation to HR and Beat-to-Beat QT Variability

General Considerations

Although the techniques described previously concentrated on aspects of repolarization abnormalities which can be detected in a single heartbeat, it has been increasingly recognized that abnormal repolarization can manifest as an abnormal response of QT interval to changing HR in response to pacing, exercise, catecholamine administration or physiological HR changes detectable on ambulatory ECG. The issue of QT interval correction has been briefly discussed before. Most of the reported abnormalities concern increase in QT response to change in HR (slope of QT/RR curve) or increased beat-to-beat variability of the QT interval, which cannot be explained by HR changes.

Changes in QT Interval Adaptation to Heart Rate

Most of the reports dealing with abnormal QT response to HR changes studied patients with congenital or drug-induced repolarization delay. Merri et al. *(156)* analyzed 24-h Holter recordings in congenital LQTS patients and discovered that the RTm interval (measured from R wave peak to T wave peak) depended more steeply on HR than in normal controls (slope of 0.21 vs 0.14, $p<0.003$), so that the repolarization duration changed more for a given HR change (Fig. 2). The difference in RTm duration between LQTS patients and control subjects was more pronounced during bradycardia. They also concluded that β-blockers decreased the slope in normal subjects. Similar result was reached by Emori et al. and by Neyroud et al. *(157,158)*, who also found that the QT/RR slope in normal subjects was higher during daytime than at night, presumably reflecting lower sympathetic tone at night, but that this difference was absent in LQTS patients. During treadmill exercise, Shimizu et al. described a marked increase in *corrected* QT interval in LQTS but not in controls *(159)*. Abnormal repolarization response to exercise was also found in LQTS patients by Krahn et al. *(75)*, who describe exaggerated RT interval hysteresis: In the LQTS group, repolarization was markedly longer during exercise than at the same HR during recovery, again indicating an abnormal response to changes in sympathetic tone. Different repolarization response to HR during recovery and exercise in LQTS patients has been confirmed by Swan et al. *(160)*. In the latter study, which in contrast to the other reports included genetic data, QT interval duration during recovery at HR 100/min provided better discrimination between LQTS and control subjects than QTc at rest.

On the other hand, in a group of six patients with idiopathic ventricular fibrillation, decreased slope of QT/RR dependence in Holter recordings has been found by Tavernier et al. *(161)*; as a group, these patients had slight QTc prolongation on 12-lead ECG, but did not meet classical LQTS criteria.

Gilmour et al. *(162)* studied changes in QT interval prior to TdP in Holter recordings of seven patients with acquired LQTS owing to hypokalemia and/or antiarrhythmic drugs. Decreased slope of QT/RR intervals, indicating diminished QT adaptation, was described prior to TdP onset in four of five patients with multiple TdP episodes.

In HCM, Fei et al. *(163)* have manually measured QT and RR intervals at regular intervals from Holter recordings. They found slightly increased slope of QT/RR dependence in HCM patients, but this parameter did not discriminate the high-risk and low-risk subjects. Treatment with low-dose amiodarone prolonged QT interval but did not affect

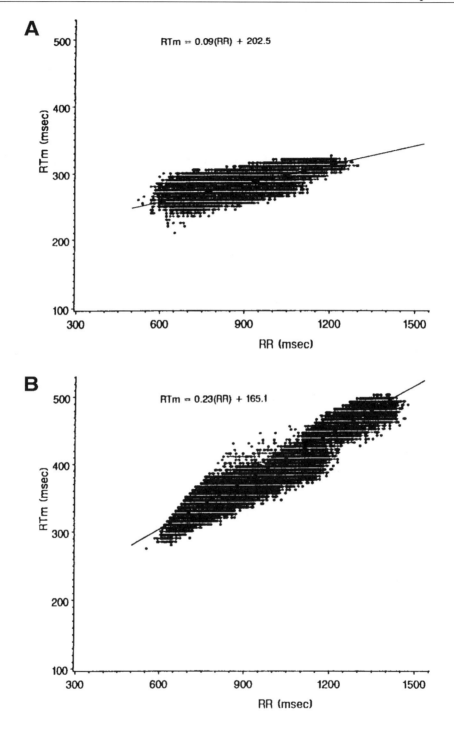

Fig. 2. Scatter plot of RR (X-axis) and RTm (the time interval between the peaks of the R and T waves; *y*-axis) intervals from a normal subject (**A**) and a long QT patient (**B**). Each dot represents a single heartbeat. The RTm intervals in the long QT patients are not only longer, but the slope of the regression line is steeper, indicating higher degree of RTm prolongation for a given degree of RR prolongation. From *(156)* with permission of the American Heart Association (AHA).

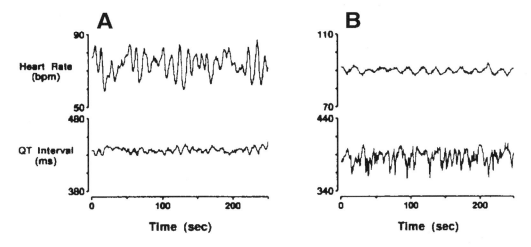

Fig. 3. Increased variability of QT interval in LV dysfunction. Values of HR and QT interval are plotted against time for a normal subject (**A**) and a patient with dilated cardiomyopathy (**B**). In the latter, the beat-to-beat QT variability is increased. This cannot be explained by HR changes, since the HR variability is decreased. From *(167)* with permission of AHA.

the QT/RR slope in these patients. Similarly, exaggerated QT response to HR changes has been reported in patients with LVH because of hypertension, with hypertensive patients without LVH serving as controls *(164)*. In contrast, decreased slope of QT/RR dependence was found prior to episodes of nonsustained VT in HCM patients *(165)*.

Another area of study concerns the beat-to-beat variability of QT interval. Under normal circumstances, this is determined to a large degree by HR variability, since the changes in QT interval in healthy subjects correspond to changes in the preceding RR intervals *(166)*. However, Berger et al. *(167)* have recently reported that in 83 patients with LV dysfunction, QT variability determined from Holter recordings was markedly increased compared to normal subjects, although their HR variability was decreased as expected (Fig. 3). Analogous results have been reported by the same group for patients with HCM *(168)* and patients undergoing EP study because of prior cardiac arrest or sustained VT *(169)*, and by a different group in CAD patients (using 5 min ECG recordings instead of Holter monitoring) *(170)*.

METHODOLOGY

Most of the clinical studies dealing with QT adaptation and variability have used computer-assisted measurements of repolarization. Because of the problems with precise and reproducible detection of T wave end, especially during rapid HR, some authors have decided to use instead the time from Q (or R) wave to the T wave peak, which is easier to detect and seems to contain most of the rate-dependent changes of the QT interval. The issue of different QT duration in steady-state changing HR has been dealt with in several ways, e.g., by selecting and analyzing only steady-state segments. Some form of signal averaging is used in many papers in order to improve signal-to-noise ratio and reliability of T wave detection in ambulatory ECG recordings; this of course precludes true beat-to-beat analysis.

CLINICAL UTILITY

Although both approaches appear promising and high QT variability in HCM may associate with high-risk genotype, there is little data proving they would be useful in prognostic stratification in any cardiac disease. In a retrospective study, QT variability was a better discriminator of high-risk vs low-risk patients referred for EP study *(169)* than many other techniques including microvoltage T wave alternans—confirmation in a prospective study will be necessary before QT variability becomes widely accepted as a risk-stratification tool.

Microvoltage T Wave Alternans

GENERAL CONSIDERATIONS

T wave alternans (TWA) is a form of repolarization segment instability manifested by its alternating morphology between the odd and even beats. In the cases relevant to this discussion, it is caused by an oscillation in action potential duration in a subpopulation of ventricular cardiomyocytes. This phenomenon can be explained on a cellular level by a steep dependence of action potential duration on the preceding diastolic interval (cycle length minus action potential duration) *(171)* and has been occasionally observed on surface ECG in a wide range of conditions *(172–181)*, often related to prolonged repolarization. After the discovery of low-amplitude repolarization oscillations in hypothermia in open chest dogs *(182)* and the relationship of this phenomenon to the ease of VF induction, spectral techniques were applied in humans to detect TWA of an amplitude too low to be appreciated on a regular ECG *(183,184)*. Following the validation of this technique in a prospective study using atrial pacing, attempts to develop a noninvasive technique for microvoltage TWA (μV-TWA) provocation resulted in commercially available treadmill equipment which includes low-noise electrodes and software for TWA analysis *(185)*.

At the same time, further experimental work helped to elucidate the relationship between μV-TWA and VT/VF. When rapid pacing is used to provoke μV-TWA, different myocyte populations initially exhibit "in-phase" oscillations in action potential shape, but with increasing HR, different myocyte populations start to oscillate "out-of-phase" (so called discordant alternans), dramatically enhancing intraventricular dispersion of refractoriness and vulnerability to reentrant arrhythmias *(186)*. The appearance of discordant alternans can be facilitated by the presence of a barrier to conduction (e.g., a scar) *(187)*.

CLINICAL STUDIES

In their classical paper *(183)*, Rosenbaum et al. prospectively studied 83 patients referred for EP study (CAD was the most frequent diagnosis) and found that μV-TWA provoked by atrial pacing was highly predictive of ventricular arrhythmia inducibility and the predictive value of μV-TWA for subsequent event-free survival was similar to EP study. A similar result has been obtained in a study where μV-TWA was induced by means of bicycle exercise *(188)*. The presence of μV-TWA was a better predictor of VT/VF inducibility than signal-averaged ECG in this population, where 10/27 patients had CAD. On the other hand, in a large study of MI patients, none of the 56 patients with exercise-induced μV-TWA died during two year follow-up period *(189)*. Inability to exercise or reach HR>105 bpm was the best predictor of poor outcome in the last study.

In a prospective study of 107 patients with LV dysfunction but no recent MI, arrhythmic events occurred in 11/52 patients with μV-TWA, none of 33 with negative test and in 2/22 with indeterminate result (*p*<0.005) *(190)*. In this population, presence of exercise-induced μV-TWA stratified patients better than any other noninvasive method. In a retrospective study of 60 patients with heart failure owing to nonischemic cardiomyopathy or hypertension, presence of μV-TWA was closely related to history of prior arrhythmic events and to result of EP study *(191)*. Among hypertensive patients, μV-TWA was more common in subjects with LVH *(192)*. A recent paper found that μV-TWA was more common in patients with HCM than in hypertensive patients with similar degree of LVH and that its presence was associated with a high degree of myocardial fiber disarray in biopsy sample *(193)*. An older report found an association between μV-TWA and high-risk clinical features in HCM *(194)*. In dilated cardiomyopathy, μV-TWA predicts occurrence of sustained VT *(195)*. Among the noninvasive markers studied, μV-TWA was the only predictor of appropriate discharge in a group of 95 patients undergoing ICD implantation *(196)*. Finally, in a large prospective study of 313 patients referred for EP study, presence of exercise-induced μV-TWA predicted future arrhythmic event as well as EP study (relative risk 10.9, *p*<0.002) *(197)*.

Interestingly, preliminary data indicate that μV-TWA may be less useful in patients with primary electrical disease: In a large LQT2 kindred, exercise-induced μV-TWA was infrequent and its incidence was not significantly higher in the mutation carriers than in their unaffected relatives *(198)*. Using catecholamine provocation, we have recently found that although μV-TWA was more prevalent in LQTS patients than in controls, its presence failed to identify high-risk subjects *(199)*. Similarly, exercise-induced μV-TWA failed to differentiate patients with Brugada syndrome from healthy controls *(200)*.

METHODOLOGY

It is generally accepted that μV-TWA is usually a rate-dependent phenomenon, which can be detected even in normal hearts during sufficiently short cycle lengths *(201,202)*. The initial technique used clinically for μV-TWA provocation was atrial pacing, but it is rarely used today because of its invasive nature. Measurement of μV-TWA during exercise-induced tachycardia has become the most common technique; split electrodes of special design are used to minimize the noise associated with exercise. Still, some patients are unable to exercise or to comply with the prescribed frequency of pedaling (which may change during the test to avoid interference with the alternans frequency). In others, analysis is precluded by ectopic beats or atrial fibrillation. Some of these issues may be addressed by using dobutamine instead of exercise to induce tachycardia *(203)*, but what is the prognostic impact of "indeterminate" μV-TWA test is unclear. Whether the attempts to induce μV-TWA by ventricular pacing and assessment of other phenomena related to μV-TWA (rate-hysteresis) *(204)* will lead to a test as useful as the other methods remains to be seen.

CLINICAL UTILITY

There is now reasonable evidence that μV-TWA at HR<110 has a similar adverse prognostic significance as inducible VT in patients referred for syncope evaluation and is a good risk stratifier in patients with LV dysfunction or heart failure. More data are needed on patients with recent MI or on subjects with IICM. Although macrovoltage

TWA has been repeatedly detected in LQTS patients, no data support the stratification value of μV-TWA in LQTS or Brugada syndrome at this time.

At this time, the evidence for clinical usefulness of μV-TWA appears to be stronger than for the other methods for repolarization assessment. The fact that the predictive value of μV-TWA may be higher in structural heart disease (where the repolarization abnormality in an isolated cell would likely be relatively mild) than in patients with structurally normal hearts but marked cellular repolarization impairment may mean that μV-TWA elicited by the current methods reflects the presence of obstacles to conduction more than anything else and may thus be a close surrogate of programmed ventricular stimulation.

Related Techniques Detecting Temporal Repolarization Lability

In addition to QT variability, which describes changes in QT duration, and to TWA, which denotes a specific form of T wave shape fluctuation, beat-to-beat changes in T wave morphology not following a TWA pattern have been reported from a LQT3 kindred (205). We have observed a similar phenomenon in LQT patients of different subtypes during catecholamine administration (199).

In this study, 23 LQTS patients (including LQT1, LQT2, and LQT3) and 16 control subjects underwent a protocol involving administration of phenylephrine and increasing rates dobutamine infusion. Ten LQTS patients but none of the controls developed a marked beat-to-beat fluctuation of the ST-T segment (Fig. 4). In one case, this phenomenon preceded an episode of polymorphic VT which required electrical cardioversion. Interestingly, we observed this phenomenon in all three LQTS patients with a history of documented cardiac arrest and in all six patients with history of cardiac arrest or syncope. These data suggest that a periodic T wave lability may be helpful in risk stratification of LQTS patients. The related phenomenon of postextrasystolic U wave augmentation was found to correlate with ventricular arrhythmias in patients without LQTS (206).

Pharmacological Provocation of Repolarization Changes

SODIUM CHANNEL BLOCKADE IN BRUGADA SYNDROME

Diagnostic use of pharmacologic agents to induce repolarization changes is best established in Brugada syndrome. In this condition, the characteristic ECG changes of right bundle branch block (RBBB) morphology and downsloping ST elevation in right precordial leads are often transient; their augmentation by high vagal tone and attenuation during β-adrenergic stimulation has been repeatedly described (207,208). The magnitude of the ECG changes appears to correlate with propensity to VF. Brugada et al. have reported that intravenous administration of sodium channel blockers (procainamide, ajmaline, or flecainide) was highly sensitive and specific for induction of typical ECG changes (209) and can occasionally induce episodes of polymorphic VT. Shimizu et al. (210) confirmed that administration of IV flecainide (but not mexiletine) augments the ECG changes in symptomatic Brugada syndrome patients; 0.15 mV increase in ST displacement measured 20 ms after the end of QRS complex completely separated the 12 patients from normal controls. Interestingly, macrovoltage TWA has also been found in an occasional patient with Brugada syndrome after β-blocker (179) or sodium channel blocker administration (211)—this corresponds to experimental findings during high-grade sodium channel blockade (212). On the other hand, Priori et al. have recently

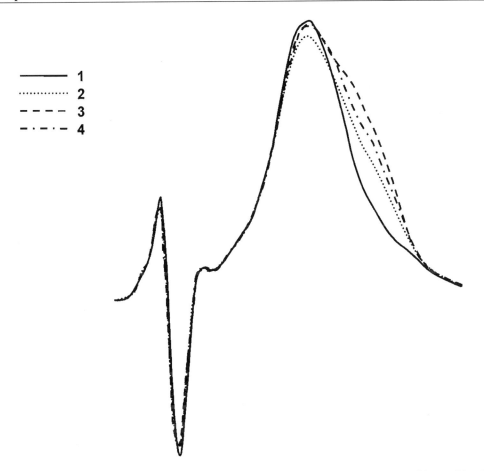

1
2
3
4

Fig. 4. An example of catecholamine-induced T wave lability in a LQTS patient, a 28-yr-old male with LQT2 whose mother died suddenly. During dobutamine infusion (10 μg/kg/min), beat-to-beat fluctuation of the T wave downslope appears. On this figure, 4 consecutive QRST complexes from V4 lead are aligned along the R wave and labeled with different line styles.

reported low sensitivity of flecainide challenge in detection of subclinical mutations carriers in Brugada syndrome kindreds *(213)* as well as positive response in some LQT3 patients *(214)*.

CATECHOLAMINES IN CONGENITAL LQTS

In contrast, although paradoxical QT prolongation and other repolarization changes induced by β-adrenergic stimulation have been frequently reported in LQTS patients, catecholamine challenge has not become standardized and it is not used routinely to establish the diagnosis *(215,216)*. The changes reported include marked QTc prolongation *(216)* (although a degree of QTc prolongation during isoproterenol has also been found in normal subjects) *(159,217)*, changes in T wave morphology *(218)*, temporal lability of T wave shape *(199)*, T wave alternans *(219)*, changes in MAP contour *(218,220,221)* and polymorphic VT *(222)*. It is likely that the response to β-adrenergic stimulation differs between different LQTS subtypes; this is supported by data from animal models of LQTS *(223,224)*.

METHODOLOGY

Both class Ia and Ic agents can be used for ST changes induction in Brugada syndrome. The doses reported are 1 mg/kg for ajmaline, 10 mg/kg for procainamide and 2 mg/kg for disopyramide and flecainide. These drugs can be administered IV over 10 min while ECG is continuously monitored until 30 min after the administration. In the United States, where IV flecainide is not available, procainamide is the usual drug of choice. Defibrillator should be available during the test. Increase in ST segment displacement of 0.15 mV (1.5 mm with the usual ECG gain) has been suggested as the cutoff for positive test.

CLINICAL UTILITY

Flecainide, ajmaline, or procainamide testing seems to be quite useful in uncovering the ECG features of Brugada syndrome and this test may be indicated in most patients in whom idiopathic VT is a diagnostic possibility. The study showing that the test fails to detect some subclinical sodium channel mutation carriers also suggested that the prognosis of these patients is good. Some of the LQT3 patients with ST elevation after flecainide may represent a true overlap between LQTS and Brugada syndrome *(225,226)*. However, it is likely that the specificity of the test is not perfect either, since positive results have been reported in patients with vasospastic angina *(227)* or supraventricular arrhythmias without clinical signs of Brugada syndrome *(228)*. Therefore, the sensitivity and specificity of this useful test should be determined in a larger study.

INVASIVE METHODS OF REPOLARIZATION ASSESSMENT

In essence, two invasive methods are currently available for repolarization assessment: Direct measurement of ventricular refractoriness by serial ventricular stimulation with diastolic interval scanning, and monophasic action potentials (MAPs) recording. Compared to the noninvasive methods, they have the theoretical advantage of higher precision and of measuring local myocardial properties. The former method is technically straightforward but time-consuming. It does not allow detection of rapid changes in refractoriness or simultaneous measurements in different regions of the ventricles.

Programmed Ventricular Stimulation

Programmed ventricular stimulation (PVS) is an important part of an invasive EP study. The technique has become reasonably well standardized *(229)*. The protocol involves direct determination of effective refractory period (ERP) of the ventricular myocardium at the stimulation site (usually the apex and the outflow tract of the right ventricle), typically at the pacing cycle lengths of 600 and 400 ms. However, the clinical endpoint of PVS is usually an induction of sustained monomorphic VT and the information on ERP is rarely used clinically.

ERP correlates well with the APD determined from monophasic action potential recording: As a rule, ERP is a few miliseconds shorter than APD90 (the time from action potential upstroke to the instant in the repolarization phase when the potential differs from baseline by 10% of the maximal action potential amplitude *(230, 231)*. In certain situations, this relationship is altered: Pharmacological sodium channel blockade or decreased sodium channel availability related to ischemia or prior MI can lead to so-called postrepolarization refractoriness (i.e., the refractory period is prolonged beyond full repolarization *(230, 232, 233)*. On the other hand, the ratio between ERP and APD90 appears to decrease in repetitive, short-coupled extrastimuli *(231)*.

Changes in ventricular refractoriness related to drug effects *(230, 234–236)* or auto-nomic changes, such as diurnal variation *(237, 238)* or prolongation related to β-blockade *(239)*, can be readily detected using PVS, but the clinical usefulness of these data is unclear. The same statement applies to repolarization changes attributable to ventricular hypertrophy *(240–242)* or aging *(243)*.

Classically, the induction reentry VT requires the presence of unidirectional conduc-tion block and spatial heterogeneity of refractoriness could facilitate this. Although it is difficult to measure spatial dispersion of refractoriness directly with this technique, the available data do suggest that it increases when multiple extrastimuli (which are typically required for VT induction) are delivered *(244–246)*. Also, it appears that spatial disper-sion of refractoriness is increased in the subjects in whom sustained VT (monomorphic or polymorphic) can be induced *(246–248)*. However, other phenomena (stimulus latency, conduction slowing, anatomic obstacles, and so on) can play a role in VT induc-tion; consequently, this phenomenon is not believed to be useful in repolarization assessment.

Monophasic Action Potentials

MAP recording can be more demanding technically, but suffers from neither of those problems *(249,250)*. The technique has been used in animal experiments for decades. When the low-frequency components of the signal are not removed, its shape (though not its amplitude) closely approximates the local action potential, which has been confirmed in isolated heart studies.

MAP recordings have provided important information on several aspects of ventricu-lar repolarization in humans—for example, they have enabled determination of APD dependence on the preceding diastolic interval *(251)*. Important insight has also been gained using MAPs on several aspects of congenital and acquired LQTS. This includes prolonged MAP duration in LQTS subjects and the observation that MAPs prolong in LQTS patients though not in control subjects during β-adrenergic stimulation *(220)*. Enhancement of dispersion in MAP duration recorded from different ventricular regions *(220,252,253)* and presence of "humps," i.e., upstrokes interrupting the terminal phase of MAP *(254,255)*, which presumably correspond to early afterdepolarizations, has also been consistently found in LQTS patients only.

Despite the fact that MAPs recording is indispensible for research purposes, it has not so far developed into a clinically useful method. Owing in part to the invasive nature of this method, there are insufficient data to conclude that the unique information provided by MAPs recordings is useful for diagnosis or risk-stratification of repolarization disorders.

CLINICAL CONTEXT

As follows from the review provided in the preceding subsections, there are currently three broad clinical settings where systematic evaluation of repolarization abnormalities may have a substantial impact on management.

First, presence of μV-TWA induced by exercise seems to correlate quite well with future arrhythmic risk in several cardiac disorders (prior MI, DCM). In most studies, its value was similar to an invasive EP study. Despite definite technical limitations (e.g., the need for exercise capability and regular heart rate) and knowledge gaps (e.g., role of µV-TWA in HCM), it is conceivable that this noninvasive method may replace the traditional programmed ventricular stimulation in some situations.

The second situation is evaluation of patients with a possible primary electrical disease. This is certainly a complex problem; in some patients, no abnormality is present on standard ECG and no provocation test is available. In the disorders where characteristic ECG changes are typically present, i.e., congenital LQTS and Brugada syndrome, they may be transient or of borderline magnitude. The ECG changes may also not be fully specific—the differentiation between Brugada syndrome and arrhythmogenic right ventricular dysplasia purely by ECG may not be easy (256). In patients without specific resting ECG changes, challenge with iv procainamide may uncover the diagnosis of Brugada syndrome.

The exact role of catecholamine challenge in aiding the diagnosis of congenital LQTS remains uncertain. It is well-known that some mutation carriers are at risk despite normal or near-normal QTc. In some cases, marked paradoxical QT prolongation and/or changes in T wave morphology can be elicited by catecholamine infusion. However, this test has not been standardized and its sensitivity and specificity has not been established. It is likely though unproven that it may be more useful in LQT1 than in LQT3.

Third, the link between drug-induced proarrhythmia and QTc prolongation is undisputed and its monitoring is advisable during initiation of treatment with most class III agents (dofetilide, sotalol). This subject is dealt with in detail in Chapter 14.

The finding that patients differ substantially in their susceptibility to rhythm disturbances in response to an apparently uniform challenge such as a given dose of a class III agent has led to the concept of "repolarization reserve," which could be qualitatively defined as the degree of additional repolarization impairment needed to elicit TdP. Conceptually, perhaps the cleanest examples of decreased repolarization reserve are the subclinical mutations in cardiac potassium channel genes, which do not manifest with syncope or QT prolongation unless the carrier is challenged with a drug which acts as a weak potassium channel blocker. Although such a drug produces mild QT prolongation at most in the majority of normal subjects, it can cause "idiosyncratic" proarrhythmia in the mutation carrier (257). It is likely that a continuous spectrum exists between this situation, overt congenital LQTS (14,258) on one side and common polymorphisms in ion channel genes (259) on the other.

In addition, other components of genetic background affect repolarization (260). The acquired factors which can affect "repolarization reserve" are numerous and include hormonal influences (85,261,262), electrolyte abnormalities, hypothermia, CNS disturbances, drug effects and interactions, along with cardiac conditions such as myocardial ischemia, myocarditis (180), LV dysfunction, and LV hypertrophy.

Most of these situations are discussed in more detail elsewhere in this book. One relatively common condition, which will be mentioned here, is the electrical remodeling of ventricular myocardium caused by longstanding tachycardia.

Clinically, this phenomenon is best described in patients undergoing radiofrequency ablation of the AV node (RFA-AVN) owing to atrial fibrillation with rapid ventricular response. The initial ablations of the AV node were performed in 1980s using a direct current discharge, a method associated with myocardial barotrauma and relatively extensive necrosis. The initial case reports of SCD following AV node ablation were attributed to formation of an arrhythmogenic substrate with this technique. However, since the

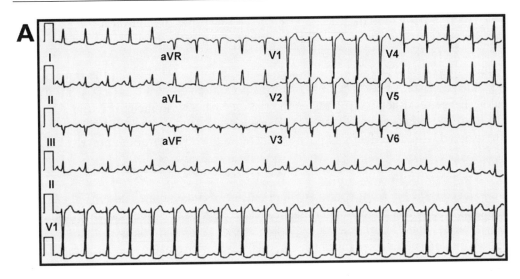

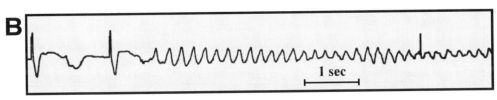

Fig. 5. (A) A 12-lead ECG, prior to AV nodal ablation, showing sinus rhythm of a 52-yr-old woman with a history of asthma, dilated cardiomyopathy, and paroxysmal atrial fibrillation refractory to medical therapy. The heart rate was 118 beats/min. The QT and QTc intervals measured 312 and 437 ms, respectively. **(B)** A single lead rhythm strip showed polymorphic VT (TdP) eight hours after AV nodal ablation and pacemaker implantation. During paced rhythm at 70 beats/min, the QT interval measured 440 ms (not shown). Preceding the episode of polymorphic VT, frequent premature ventricular complexes developed. The tachycardia was initiated during the T wave of a markedly prolonged QT interval (600 ms) of a paced beat following a relative long cycle produced by a postextrasystolic beat. The sensing and pacing functions of the pacemaker were normal *(243)* with permission of Furura Publishing Co.

introduction of RFA-AVN, which allows for creation of small and well delineated lesions, more cases of SCD or resuscitated cardiac arrest have been reported *(263–268)*. TdP or VF was the arrhythmia recorded in documented cases of cardiac arrest (Fig. 5).

It now appears that chronic tachycardia leads to electrical remodeling of ventricular myocardium, which can manifest by QT prolongation or TdP once ventricular rate decreases. The published report of dramatic QT prolongation and TdP after RFA of accessory pathway in paroxysmal junctional reciprocating tachycardia *(269)* strongly suggests that injury of the AV node is not necessary for postablation QT prolongation. The remodeling seems to be reversible and in most instances, rhythm disturbances after RFA-AVN can be prevented by appropriate pacemaker programming *(263,270)*, allowing for gradual decrease in ventricular rate.

Two relatively small studies investigated QT interval duration in patients post RFA-AVN, using patients with primary bradycardia as controls *(271,272)*: Both of them found

QT interval prolongation in patients post RFA-AVN, especially during slow heart rates. This phenomenon resolved within days. These results are corroborated by data from animal experiments *(273)* and human studies *(274)*, which showed that rapid ventricular pacing induces repolarization impairment. On the ion channel level, the limited data available suggest decreased expression of the potassium current I_{to} as a possible explanation. Large retrospective reports on the risk of SCD or cardiac arrest after AV node ablation using direct current discharge *(275)* or RFA *(270)* support the view that the event is associated with other factors known to decrease the repolarization reserve.

CONCLUSION

The last decade has been a period of major advances in our understanding of ventricular repolarization on molecular, cellular, and tissue levels. The plethora of methods used and developed for clinical assessment of ventricular repolarization is a testimony to the lack of simple and universally useful technique. It is certain that the next decade will bring further refinement of these methods. Although steady progress has been made in the clinical assessment of ventricular repolarization, significant effort should be considered in developing clinical tools to assess atrial repolarization as atrial fibrillation has been recognized to be "epidemic" at the turn of the 21st century.

REFERENCES

1. Jervell A, Lange-Nielsen F. Congenital deaf-mutism, functional heart disease with prolongation of the QT interval and sudden death. Am Heart J 1957;54:59–68.
2. Romano C, Gemme G, Pongiglione R. Aritmie cardiache rare dell'eta pediatrica. Clin Pediatr 1963;45:656–683.
3. Ward OC. A new familial cardiac syndrome in children. J Irish Med Assoc 1964;54:103–106.
4. Goldberg RJ, Bengtson J, Chen ZY, Anderson KM, Locati E, Levy D. Duration of the QT interval and total and cardiovascular mortality in healthy persons (The Framingham Heart Study experience). Am J Cardiol 1991;67:55–58.
5. Algra A, Tijssen JG, Roelandt JR, Pool J, Lubsen J. Contribution of the 24 hour electrocardiogram to the prediction of sudden coronary death. Br Heart J 1993;70:421–427.
6. de Bruyne MC, Hoes AW, Kors JA, Hofman A, van Bemmel JH, Grobbee DE. Prolonged QT interval predicts cardiac and all-cause mortality in the elderly. The Rotterdam Study. Eur Heart J 1999;20:278–284.
7. Dekker JM, Schouten EG, Klootwijk P, Pool J, Kromhout D. Association between QT interval and coronary heart disease in middle-aged and elderly men. The Zutphen Study. Circulation 1994;90:779–785.
8. Elming H, Holm E, Jun L, et al. The prognostic value of the QT interval and QT interval dispersion in all-cause and cardiac mortality and morbidity in a population of Danish citizens. Eur Heart J 1998;19:1391–1400.
9. Karjalainen J, Reunanen A, Ristola P, Viitasalo M. QT interval as a cardiac risk factor in a middle aged population. Heart 1997;77:543–548.
10. Schouten EG, Dekker JM, Meppelink P, Kok FJ, Vandenbroucke JP, Pool J. QT interval prolongation predicts cardiovascular mortality in an apparently healthy population. Circulation 1991;84: 1516–1523.
11. Garson AJ, Dick M, Fournier A, Gillette PC, Hamilton R, Kugler JD, Van Hare GF, Vetter V, Vick GW. The long QT syndrome in children. An international study of 287 patients. Circulation 1993;87: 1866–1872.
12. Moss AJ. Measurement of the QT interval and the risk associated with QTc interval prolongation: a review. Am J Cardiol 1993;72:23B–25B.
13. Vincent GM, Timothy KW, Lepert M, Keating M. The spectrum of symptoms and QT intervals in carriers of the gene for the long-QT syndrome. N Engl J Med 1992;327:846–852.

14. Priori SG, Napolitano C, Schwartz PJ. Low penetrance in the long-QT syndrome. Clinical impact. Circulation 1999;99:529–533.

15. Compton SJ, Lux RL, Ramsey MR, Strelich KR, Sanguinetti MC, Green LS, Keating MT, Mason JW. Genetically defined therapy of inherited long-QT syndrome. Correction of abnormal repolarization by potassium. Circulation 1996;94:1018–1022.

16. Priori SG, Napolitano C, Schwartz PJ, Bloise R, Crotti L, Ronchetti E. The elusive link between LQT3 and Brugada syndrome: the role of flecainide challenge. Circulation 2000;102:945–947.

17. Shimizu W, Kurita T, Matsuo K, et al. Improvement of repolarization abnormalities by a K+ channel opener in the LQT1 form of congenital long-QT syndrome. Circulation 1998;97:1581–1588.

18. Mitcheson JS, Chen J, Lin M, Culberson C, Sanguinetti MC. A structural basis for drug-induced long QT syndrome. Proc Natl Acad Sci USA 2000;97:12329–12333.

19. MacNeil DJ, Davies RO, Deitchman D. Clinical safety profile of sotalol in the treatment of arrhythmias. Am J Cardiol 1993;72:44A–50A.

20. Wang T, Bergstrand RH, Thompson KA, Siddoway LA, Duff HJ, Woosley RL, Roden DM. Concentration-dependent pharmacologic properties of sotalol. Am J Cardiol 1986;57:1160–1165.

21. Stambler BS, Wood MA, Ellenbogen KA, Perry KT, Wakefield LK, VanderLugt JT. Efficacy and safety of repeated intravenous doses of ibutilide for rapid conversion of atrial flutter or fibrillation. Ibutilide Repeat Dose Study Investigators. Circulation 1996;94:1613–1621.

22. Chung MK, Schweikert RA, Wilkoff BL, et al. Is hospital admission for initiation of antiarrhythmic therapy with sotalol for atrial arrhythmias required? Yield of in-hospital monitoring and prediction of risk for significant arrhythmia complications. J Am Coll Cardiol 1998;32:169–176.

23. Stambler BS, Wood MA, Ellenbogen KA, Perry KT, Wakefield LK, VanderLugt JT. Efficacy and safety of repeated intravenous doses of ibutilide for rapid conversion of atrial flutter or fibrillation. Ibutilide Repeat Dose Study Investigators. Circulation 1996;94:1613–1621.

24. Li RA, Leppo M, Miki T, Seino S, Marban E. Molecular basis of electrocardiographic ST-segment elevation. Circ Res 2000;87:837–839.

25. Cinca J, Figueras J, Tenorio L, et al. Time course and rate dependence of QT interval changes during noncomplicated acute transmural myocardial infarction in human beings. Am J Cardiol 1981;48:1023–1028.

26. Ahnve S, Gilpin E, Madsen EB, Froelicher V, Henning H, Ross JJ. Prognostic importance of QTc interval at discharge after acute myocardial infarction: a multicenter study of 865 patients. Am Heart J 1984;108:395–400.

27. Doroghazi RM, Childers R. Time-related changes in the QT interval in acute myocardial infarction: possible relation to local hypocalcemia. Am J Cardiol 1978;41:684–688.

28. Ahnve S. QT interval prolongation in acute myocardial infarction. Eur Heart J 1985;6 Suppl D:85–95.

29. Shawl FA, Velasco CE, Goldbaum TS, Forman MB. Effect of coronary angioplasty on electrocardiographic changes in patients with unstable angina secondary to left anterior descending coronary artery disease. J Am Coll Cardiol 1990;16:325–331.

30. Kerr CR, Hacking A, Henning H. Effects of transient myocardial ischemia on the QT interval in man. Can J Cardiol 1987;3:383–386.

31. Puddu PE, Bourassa MG. Prediction of sudden death from QTc interval prolongation in patients with chronic ischemic heart disease. J Electrocardiol 1986;19:203–211.

32. Schwartz PJ, Wolf S. QT interval prolongation as predictor of sudden death in patients with myocardial infarction. Circulation 1978;57:1074–1077.

33. Peters RW, Byington RP, Barker A, Yusuf S. Prognostic value of prolonged ventricular repolarization following myocardial infarction: the BHAT experience. The BHAT Study Group. J Clin Epidemiol 1990;43:167–172.

34. Wheelan K, Mukharji J, Rude RE, et al. Sudden death and its relation to QT-interval prolongation after acute myocardial infarction: two-year follow-up. Am J Cardiol 1986;57:745–750.

35. Ahnve S, Helmers C, Lundman T. QTc intervals at discharge after acute myocardial infarction and long-term prognosis. Acta Med Scand 1980;208:55–60.

36. Davey P. QT interval and mortality from coronary artery disease. Prog Cardiovasc Dis 2000;42:359–384.

37. Juul-Moller S. Corrected QT-interval during one year follow-up after an acute myocardial infarction. Eur Heart J 1986;7:299–304.

38. Davey P. QT interval lengthening in cardiac disease relates more to left ventricular systolic dysfunction than to autonomic function. Eur J Heart Fail 2000;2:265–271.

39. Kramer B, Brill M, Bruhn A, Kubler W. Relationship between the degree of coronary artery disease and of left ventricular function and the duration of the QT-interval in ECG. Eur Heart J 1986;7:14–24.

40. Savelieva I, Yap YG, Yi G, et al. Relation of ventricular repolarization to cardiac cycle length in normal subjects, hypertrophic cardiomyopathy, and patients with myocardial infarction. Clin Cardiol 1999;22:649–654.

41. Yi G, Elliott P, McKenna WJ, et al. QT dispersion and risk factors for sudden cardiac death in patients with hypertrophic cardiomyopathy. Am J Cardiol 1998;82:1514–1519.

42. Dritsas A, Sbarouni E, Gilligan D, Nihoyannopoulos P, Oakley CM. QT-interval abnormalities in hypertrophic cardiomyopathy. Clin Cardiol 1992;15:739–742.

43. Peters S, Rust H, Trummel M, Brattstrom A. Familial hypertrophic cardiomyopathy associated with prolongation of the QT interval. Z Kardiol 2000;89:624–629.

44. Zaidi M, Robert A, Fesler R, Derwael C, Brohet C. Dispersion of ventricular repolarization in hypertrophic cardiomyopathy. J Electrocardiol 1996;29 Suppl:89–94.

45. Dritsas A, Gilligan D, Nihoyannopoulos P, Oakley CM. Amiodarone reduces QT dispersion in patients with hypertrophic cardiomyopathy. Int J Cardiol 1992;36:345–349.

46. Spirito P, Bellone P, Harris KM, Bernabo P, Bruzzi P, Maron BJ. Magnitude of left ventricular hypertrophy and risk of sudden death in hypertrophic cardiomyopathy. N Engl J Med 2000;342:1778–1785.

47. Maron BJ, Leyhe MJ, Casey SA, et al. Assessment of QT dispersion as a prognostic marker for sudden death in a regional nonreferred hypertrophic cardiomyopathy cohort. Am J Cardiol 2001;87:114–115.

48. Ducceschi V, Sarubbi B, D'Andrea A, et al. Increased QT dispersion and other repolarization abnormalities as a possible cause of electrical instability in isolated aortic stenosis. Int J Cardiol 1998;64:57–62.

49. Schwartz PJ, Stramba-Badiale M, Segantini A, et al. Prolongation of the QT interval and the sudden infant death syndrome. N Engl J Med 1998;338:1709–1714.

50. Schwartz PJ, Priori SG, Dumaine R, et al. A molecular link between the sudden infant death syndrome and the long-QT syndrome. N Engl J Med 2000;343:262–267.

51. Ahmed R, Hashiba K. Reliability of QT intervals as indicators of clinical hypercalcemia. Clin Cardiol 1988;11:395–400.

52. Wortsman J, Frank S. The QT interval in clinical hypercalcemia. Clin Cardiol 1981;4:87–90.

53. Gussak I, Brugada P, Brugada J, et al. Idiopathic short QT interval: a new clinical syndrome? Cardiology 2000;94:99–102.

54. Moller M. QT interval in relation to ventricular arrhythmias and sudden cardiac death in postmyocardial infarction patients. Acta Med Scand 1981;210:73–77.

55. Pohjola-Sintonen S, Siltanen P, Haapakoski J. Usefulness of QTc interval on the discharge electrocardiogram for predicting survival after acute myocardial infarction. Am J Cardiol 1986;57:1066–1068.

56. Boudoulas H, Sohn YH, O'Neill W, Brown R, Weissler AM. The QT greater than QS2 syndrome: a new mortality risk indicator in coronary artery disease. Am J Cardiol 1982;50:1229–1235.

57. Tobe TJ, de Langen CD, Crijns HJ, et al. Late potentials, QTc prolongation, and prediction of arrhythmic events after myocardial infarction. Int J Cardiol 1994;46:121–128.

58. Cowan JC, Yusoff K, Moore M, et al. Importance of lead selection in QT interval measurement. Am J Cardiol 1988;61:83–87.

59. Lepeschkin E, Surawicz B. The measurement of the QT interval of the electrocardiogram. Circulation 1952;6:378–388.

60. Batchvarov V, Malik M. Measurement and interpretation of QT dispersion. Prog Cardiovasc Dis 2000;42:325–344.

61. Murray A, McLaughlin NB, Bourke JP, Doig JC, Furniss SS, Campbell RW. Errors in manual measurement of QT intervals. Br Heart J 1994;71:386–390.

62. Kautzner J, Yi G, Camm AJ, Malik M. Short- and long-term reproducibility of QT, QTc, and QT dispersion measurement in healthy subjects. Pacing Clin Electrophysiol 1994;17:928–937.

63. McLaughlin NB, Campbell RW, Murray A. Accuracy of four automatic QT measurement techniques in cardiac patients and healthy subjects. Heart 1996;76:422–426.

64. McLaughlin NB, Campbell RW, Murray A. Comparison of automatic QT measurement techniques in the normal 12 lead electrocardiogram. Br Heart J 1995;74:84–89.

65. Fuller MS, Sandor G, Punske B, et al. Estimates of repolarization dispersion from electrocardiographic measurements. Circulation 2000;102:685–691.

66. Savelieva I, Yi G, Guo X, Hnatkova K, Malik M. Agreement and reproducibility of automatic versus manual measurement of QT interval and QT dispersion. Am J Cardiol 1998;81:471–477.

67. Kors JA, van Herpen G. Measurement error as a source of QT dispersion: a computerised analysis. Heart 1998;80:453–458.

68. Bazett HC. An analysis of the time relations of electrocardiograms. Heart 1920;7:353–370.

69. Fridericia LS. Die Systolendauer im Elektrokardiogramm bei Normalen Menschen und bei Herzkranken. Acta Med Scand 1920;53:469–486.

70. Sagie A, Larson MG, Goldberg RJ, Bengtson JR, Levy D. An improved method for adjusting the QT interval for heart rate (the Framingham Heart Study). Am J Cardiol 1992;70:797–801.

71. Sarma JS, Sarma RJ, Bilitch M, Katz D, Song SL. An exponential formula for heart rate dependence of QT interval during exercise and cardiac pacing in humans: reevaluation of Bazett's formula. Am J Cardiol 1984;54:103–108.

72. Molnar J, Weiss J, Zhang F, Rosenthal JE. Evaluation of five QT correction formulas using a software-assisted method of continuous QT measurement from 24-hour Holter recordings. Am J Cardiol 1996;78:920–926.

73. Malik M. Problems of heart rate correction in assessment of drug-induced QT interval prolongation. J Cardiovasc Electrophysiol 2001;12:411–420.

74. Lande G, Funck-Brentano C, Ghadanfar M, Escande D. Steady-state versus non-steady-state QT-RR relationships in 24-hour Holter recordings. Pacing Clin Electrophysiol 2000;23:293–302.

75. Krahn AD, Klein GJ, Yee R. Hysteresis of the RT interval with exercise: a new marker for the long-QT syndrome? Circulation 1997;96:1551–1556.

76. Sarma JS, Venkataraman SK, Samant DR, Gadgil U. Hysteresis in the human RR-QT relationship during exercise and recovery. Pacing Clin Electrophysiol 1987;10:485–491.

77. Takahashi N, Ito M, Ishida S, et al. Paradoxically shortened QT interval after a prolonged pause. Pacing Clin Electrophysiol 1998;21:1476–1479.

78. Gussak I, Liebl N, Nouri S, Bjerregaard P, Zimmerman F, Chaitman BR. Deceleration-dependent shortening of the QT interval: a new electrocardiographic phenomenon? Clin Cardiol 1999;22:124–126.

79. Zhou SH, Wong S, Rautaharju PM, Karnik N, Calhoun HP. Should the JT rather than the QT interval be used to detect prolongation of ventricular repolarization? An assessment in normal conduction and in ventricular conduction defects. J Electrocardiol 1992;25 Suppl:131–136.

80. Bidoggia H, Maciel JP, Capalozza N, et al. Sex-dependent electrocardiographic pattern of cardiac repolarization. Am Heart J 2000;140:430–436.

81. Rautaharju PM, Zhou SH, Wong S, et al. Sex differences in the evolution of the electrocardiographic QT interval with age. Can J Cardiol 1992;8:690–695.

82. Waldegger S, Lang U, Herzer T, et al. Inhibition of minK protein induced K+ channels in Xenopus oocytes by estrogens. Naunyn Schmiedebergs Arch Pharmacol 1996;354:698–702.

83. Bidoggia H, Maciel JP, Capalozza N, et al. Sex differences on the electrocardiographic pattern of cardiac repolarization: possible role of testosterone. Am Heart J 2000;140:678–683.

84. Locati EH, Zareba W, Moss AJ, et al. Age- and sex-related differences in clinical manifestations in patients with congenital long-QT syndrome. Findings from the international LQTS registry. Circulation 1998;97:2237–2244.

85. Zareba W, Moss AJ, le Cessie S, et al. Risk of cardiac events in family members of patients with long QT syndrome. J Am Coll Cardiol 1995;26:1685–1691.

86. Makkar RR, Fromm BS, Steinman RT, Meissner MD, Lehmann MH. Female gender as a risk factor for torsades de pointes associated with cardiovascular drugs. JAMA 1993;270:2590–2597.

87. Kawasaki R, Machado C, Reinoehl J, et al. Increased propensity of women to develop torsades de pointes during complete heart block. J Cardiovasc Electrophysiol 1995;6:1032–1038.

88. Watanabe Y. Purkinje repolarization as a possible cause of the U wave in the electrocardiogram. Circulation 1975;51:1030–1037.

89. Antzelevitch C, Nesterenko VV, Yan GX. Role of M cells in acquired long QT syndrome, U waves, and torsade de pointes. J Electrocardiol 1995;28 Suppl:131–138.

90. Yan GX, Antzelevitch C. Cellular basis for the normal T wave and the electrocardiographic manifestations of the long-QT syndrome. Circulation 1998;98:1928–1936.

91. Malik M, Batchvarov VN. Measurement, interpretation and clinical potential of QT dispersion. J Am Coll Cardiol 2000;36:1749–1766.

92. Wilson FN, Macleod AG, Barker PS. Determination of the significance of the areas of the ventricular deflections of the electrocardiogram. Am Heart J 1934;10:46–61.

93. Day CP, McComb JM, Campbell RW. QT dispersion: an indication of arrhythmia risk in patients with long QT intervals. Br Heart J 1990;63:342–344.

94. Han J, Millet D, Chizzonitti B, Moe GK. Temporal dispersion of recovery of excitability in atrium and ventricle as a function of heart rate. Am Heart J 1966;71:481–487.

95. Kuo CS, Munakata K, Reddy CP, Surawicz B. Characteristics and possible mechanism of ventricular arrhythmia dependent on the dispersion of action potential durations. Circulation 1983;67:1356–1367.

96. Kuo CS, Atarashi H, Reddy CP, Surawicz B. Dispersion of ventricular repolarization and arrhythmia: study of two consecutive ventricular premature complexes. Circulation 1985;72:370–376.

97. Lukas A, Antzelevich C. Phase 2 reentry as a mechanism of initiation of circus movement reentry in canine epicardium exposed to simulated ischemia. Cardiovasc Res 1996;32:593–603.

98. Zabel M, Portnoy S, Franz MR. Electrocardiographic indexes of dispersion of ventricular repolarization: an isolated heart validation study. J Am Coll Cardiol 1995;25:746–752.

99. Zabel M, Lichtlen PR, Haverich A, Franz MR. Comparison of ECG variables of dispersion of ventricular repolarization with direct myocardial repolarization measurements in the human heart. J Cardiovasc Electrophysiol 1998;9:1279–1284.

100. Malik M. QT dispersion: time for an obituary? Eur Heart J 2000;21:955–957.

101. van de Loo A, Arendts W, Hohnloser SH. Variability of QT dispersion measurements in the surface electrocardiogram in patients with acute myocardial infarction and in normal subjects. Am J Cardiol 1994;74:1113–1118.

102. Lee KW, Kligfield P, Dower GE, Okin PM. QT dispersion, T-wave projection, and heterogeneity of repolarization in patients with coronary artery disease. Am J Cardiol 2001;87:148–151.

103. Macfarlane PW, McLaughlin SC, Rodger JC. Influence of lead selection and population on automated measurement of QT dispersion. Circulation 1998;98:2160–2167.

104. Kors JA, van Herpen G, van Bemmel JH. QT dispersion as an attribute of T-loop morphology. Circulation 1999;99:1458–1463.

105. Malik M, Acar B, Gang Y, Yap YG, Hnatkova K, Camm AJ. QT dispersion does not represent electrocardiographic interlead heterogeneity of ventricular repolarization. J Cardiovasc Electrophysiol 2000;11:835–843.

106. de Bruyne MC, Hoes AW, Kors JA, Hofman A, van Bemmel JH, Grobbee DE. QTc dispersion predicts cardiac mortality in the elderly: the Rotterdam Study. Circulation 1998;97:467–472.

107. Macfarlane PW. QT dispersion—lack of discriminating power. Circulation 1998;98:I–81 (Abstract).

108. Okin PM, Devereux RB, Howard BV, Fabsitz RR, Lee ET, Welty TK. Assessment of QT interval and QT dispersion for prediction of all-cause and cardiovascular mortality in American Indians: The Strong Heart Study. Circulation 2000;101:61–66.

109. Glancy JM, Garratt CJ, Woods KL, de Bono DP. QT dispersion and mortality after myocardial infarction. Lancet 1995;345:945–948.

110. Higham PD, Furniss SS, Campbell RW. QT dispersion and components of the QT interval in ischaemia and infarction. Br Heart J 1995;73:32–36.

111. Ciolli A, Di Lorenzo M, Bevilacqua U, et al. QT dispersion and early arrhythmic risk during acute myocardial infarction. G Ital Cardiol 1999;29:1438–1444.

112. Paventi S, Bevilacqua U, Parafati MA, Di Luzio E, Rossi F, Pelliccioni PR. QT dispersion and early arrhythmic risk during acute myocardial infarction. Angiology 1999;50:209–215.

113. Moreno FL, Villanueva T, Karagounis LA, Anderson JL. Reduction in QT interval dispersion by successful thrombolytic therapy in acute myocardial infarction. TEAM-2 Study Investigators. Circulation 1994;90:94–100.

114. Leitch J, Basta M, Dobson A. QT dispersion does not predict early ventricular fibrillation after acute myocardial infarction. Pacing Clin Electrophysiol 1995;18:45–48.

115. Tomassoni G, Pisano E, Gardner L, Krucoff MW, Natale A. QT prolongation and dispersion in myocardial ischemia and infarction. J Electrocardiol 1998;30 Suppl:187–190.

116. Perkiomaki JS, Koistinen MJ, Yli-Mayry S, Huikuri HV. Dispersion of QT interval in patients with and without susceptibility to ventricular tachyarrhythmias after previous myocardial infarction. J Am Coll Cardiol 1995;26:174–179.

117. Puljevic D, Smalcelj A, Durakovic Z, Goldner V. QT dispersion, daily variations, QT interval adaptation and late potentials as risk markers for ventricular tachycardia. Eur Heart J 1997;18:1343–1349.

118. Trusz-Gluza M, Wozniak-Skowerska I, Giec L, Szydlo K. Dispersion of the QT interval as a predictor of cardiac death in patients with coronary heart disease. Pacing Clin Electrophysiol 1996;19:1900–1904.

119. Endoh Y, Kasanuki H, Ohnishi S, Uno M. Unsuitability of corrected QT dispersion as a marker for ventricular arrhythmias and cardiac sudden death after acute myocardial infarction. Jpn Circ J 1999;63:467–470.

120. Zabel M, Klingenheben T, Franz MR, Hohnloser SH. Assessment of QT dispersion for prediction of mortality or arrhythmic events after myocardial infarction: results of a prospective, long-term follow-up study. Circulation 1998;97:2543–2550.

121. Suzuki M, Nishizaki M, Arita M, et al. Increased QT dispersion in patients with vasospastic angina. Circulation 1998;98:435–440.

122. Parchure N, Batchvarov V, Malik M, Camm AJ, Kaski JC. Increased QT dispersion in patients with Prinzmetal's variant angina and cardiac arrest. Cardiovasc Res 2001;50:379–385.

123. Kelly RF, Parillo JE, Hollenberg SM. Effect of coronary angioplasty on QT dispersion. Am Heart J 1997;134:399–405.

124. Yunus A, Gillis AM, Traboulsi M, et al. Effect of coronary angioplasty on precordial QT dispersion. Am J Cardiol 1997;79:1339–1342.

125. Barr CS, Naas A, Freeman M, Lang CC, Struthers AD. QT dispersion and sudden unexpected death in chronic heart failure. Lancet 1994;343:327–329.

126. Pinsky DJ, Sciacca RR, Steinberg JS. QT dispersion as a marker of risk in patients awaiting heart transplantation. J Am Coll Cardiol 1997;29:1576–1584.

127. Brooksby P, Robinson PJ, Segal R, Klinger G, Pitt B, Cowley AJ. Effects of losartan and captopril on QT dispersion in elderly patients with heart failure. ELITE study group. Lancet 1999;354:395–396.

128. Fu GS, Meissner A, Simon R. Repolarization dispersion and sudden cardiac death in patients with impaired left ventricular function. Eur Heart J 1997;18:281–289.

129. Brooksby P, Batin PD, Nolan J, et al. The relationship between QT intervals and mortality in ambulant patients with chronic heart failure. The United Kingdom heart failure evaluation and assessment of risk trial (UK-HEART). Eur Heart J 1999;20:1335–1341.

130. Brendorp B, Elming H, Jun L, et al. QT dispersion has no prognostic information for patients with advanced congestive heart failure and reduced left ventricular systolic function. Circulation 2001;103:831–835.

131. Miorelli M, Buja G, Melacini P, Fasoli G, Nava A. QT-interval variability in hypertrophic cardiomyopathy patients with cardiac arrest. Int J Cardiol 1994;45:121–127.

132. Buja G, Miorelli M, Turrini P, Melacini P, Nava A. Comparison of QT dispersion in hypertrophic cardiomyopathy between patients with and without ventricular arrhythmias and sudden death. Am J Cardiol 1993;72:973–976.

133. Yetman AT, Hamilton RM, Benson LN, McCrindle BW. Long-term outcome and prognostic determinants in children with hypertrophic cardiomyopathy. J Am Coll Cardiol 1998;32:1943–1950.

134. Perkiomaki JS, Ikaheimo MJ, Pikkujamsa SM, et al. Dispersion of the QT interval and autonomic modulation of heart rate in hypertensive men with and without left ventricular hypertrophy. Hypertension 1996;28:16–21.

135. Dilaveris P, Gialafos E, Poloniecki J, et al. Changes of the T-wave amplitude and angle: an early marker of altered ventricular repolarization in hypertension. Clin Cardiol 2000;23:600–606.

136. Ichkhan K, Molnar J, Somberg J. Relation of left ventricular mass and QT dispersion in patients with systematic hypertension. Am J Cardiol 1997;79:508–511.

137. Darbar D, Cherry CJ, Kerins DM. QT dispersion is reduced after valve replacement in patients with aortic stenosis. Heart 1999;82:15–18.

138. Mayet J, Kanagaratnam P, Shahi M, et al. QT dispersion in athletic left ventricular hypertrophy. Am Heart J 1999;137:678–681.

139. Gonzalez-Juanatey JR, Garcia-Acuna JM, Pose A, et al. Reduction of QT and QTc dispersion during long-term treatment of systemic hypertension with enalapril. Am J Cardiol 1998;81:170–174.

140. Barr CS, Naas AA, Fenwick M, Struthers AD. Enalapril reduces QTc dispersion in mild congestive heart failure secondary to coronary artery disease. Am J Cardiol 1997;79:328–333.

141. Sun ZH, Swan H, Viitasalo M, Toivonen L. Effects of epinephrine and phenylephrine on QT interval dispersion in congenital long QT syndrome. J Am Coll Cardiol 1998;31:1400–1405.

142. Priori SG, Napolitano C, Diehl L, Schwartz PJ. Dispersion of the QT interval. A marker of therapeutic efficacy in the idiopathic long QT syndrome. Circulation 1994;89:1681–1689.

143. Stramba-Badiale M, Goulene K, Schwartz PJ. Effects of beta-adrenergic blockade on dispersion of ventricular repolarization in newborn infants with prolonged QT interval. Am Heart J 1997;134:406–410.

144. Hii JT, Wyse DG, Gillis AM, Duff HJ, Solylo MA, Mitchell LB. Precordial QT interval dispersion as a marker of torsade de pointes. Disparate effects of class Ia antiarrhythmic drugs and amiodarone. Circulation 1992;86:1376–1382.

145. Gillis AM, Traboulsi M, Hii JT, et al. Antiarrhythmic drug effects on QT interval dispersion in patients undergoing electropharmacologic testing for ventricular tachycardia and fibrillation. Am J Cardiol 1998;81:588–593.

146. Yi G, Guo XH, Crook R, Hnatkova K, Camm AJ, Malik M. Computerised measurements of QT dispersion in healthy subjects. Heart 1998;80:459–466.

147. Krupienicz A, Czarnecki R, Adamus J. QT dispersion magnitude is related to the respiratory phase in healthy subjects. Am J Cardiol 1997;80:1232–1234.

148. Hnatkova K, Malik M, Kautzner J, Gang Y, Camm AJ. Adjustment of QT dispersion assessed from 12 lead electrocardiograms for different numbers of analysed electrocardiographic leads: comparison of stability of different methods. Br Heart J 1994;72:390–396.

149. Zabel M, Franz MR, Klingenheben T, Mansion B, Schultheiss HP, Hohnloser SH. Rate-dependence of QT dispersion and the QT interval: comparison of atrial pacing and exercise testing. J Am Coll Cardiol 2000;36:1654–1658.

150. Aiba T, Inagaki M, Shimizu W, et al. Recovery time dispersion measured from 87-lead body surface potential mapping as a predictor of sustained ventricular tachycardia in patients with idiopathic dilated cardiomyopathy. J Cardiovasc Electrophysiol 2000;11:968–974.

151. Lubinski A, Kornacewicz-Jach Z, Wnuk-Wojnar AM, et al. terminal portion of the T wave: a new electrocardiographic marker of risk of ventricular arrhythmias. Pacing Clin Electrophysiol 2000;23:1957–1959.

152. Savelieva I, Yap YG, Yi G, Guo X, Camm AJ, Malik M. Comparative reproducibility of QT, QT peak, and T peak-T end intervals and dispersion in normal subjects, patients with myocardial infarction, and patients with hypertrophic cardiomyopathy. Pacing Clin Electrophysiol 1998;21:2376–2381.

153. Priori SG, Mortara DW, Napolitano C, et al. Evaluation of the spatial aspects of T-wave complexity in the long-QT syndrome. Circulation 1997;96:3006–3012.

154. Zabel M, Acar B, Klingenheben T, Franz MR, Hohnloser SH, Malik M. Analysis of 12-lead T-wave morphology for risk stratification after myocardial infarction. Circulation 2000;102:1252–1257.

155. Yi G, Prasad K, Elliott P, et al. T wave complexity in patients with hypertrophic cardiomyopathy. Pacing Clin Electrophysiol 1998;21:2382–2386.

156. Merri M, Moss AJ, Benhorin J, Locati EH, Alberti M, Badilini F. Relation between ventricular repolarization duration and cardiac cycle length during 24-hour Holter recordings. Findings in normal patients and patients with long QT syndrome. Circulation 1992;85:1816–1821.

157. Emori T, Ohe T, Aihara N, Kurita T, Shimizu W, Kamakura S, Shimomura K. Dynamic relationship between the Q-aT interval and heart rate in patients with long QT syndrome during 24-hour Holter ECG monitoring. Pacing Clin Electrophysiol 1995;18:1909–1918.

158. Neyroud N, Maison-Blanche P, Denjoy I, et al. Diagnostic performance of QT interval variables from 24-h electrocardiography in the long QT syndrome. Eur Heart J 1998;19:158–165.

159. Shimizu W, Ohe T, Kurita T, Shimomura K. Differential response of QTU interval to exercise, isoproterenol, and atrial pacing in patients with congenital long QT syndrome. Pacing Clin Electrophysiol 1991;14:1966–1970.

160. Swan H, Saarinen K, Kontula K, Toivonen L, Viitasalo M. Evaluation of QT interval duration and dispersion and proposed clinical criteria in diagnosis of long QT syndrome in patients with a genetically uniform type of LQT1. J Am Coll Cardiol 1998;32:486–491.

161. Tavernier R, Jordaens L, Haerynck F, Derycke E, Clement DL. Changes in the QT interval and its adaptation to rate, assessed with continuous electrocardiographic recordings in patients with ventricular fibrillation, as compared to normal individuals without arrhythmias. Eur Heart J 1997;18:994–999.

162. Gilmour RFJ, Riccio ML, Locati EH, Maison-Blanche P, Coumel P, Schwartz PJ. Time- and rate-dependent alterations of the QT interval precede the onset of torsade de pointes in patients with acquired QT prolongation. J Am Coll Cardiol 1997;30:209–217.

163. Fei L, Slade AK, Grace AA, Malik M, Camm AJ, McKenna WJ. Ambulatory assessment of the QT interval in patients with hypertrophic cardiomyopathy: risk stratification and effect of low dose amiodarone. Pacing Clin Electrophysiol 1994;17:2222–2227.

164. Singh JP, Johnston J, Sleight P, Bird R, Ryder K, Hart G. Left ventricular hypertrophy in hypertensive patients is associated with abnormal rate adaptation of QT interval. J Am Coll Cardiol 1997;29:778–784.

165. Mezilis NE, Parthenakis FI, Kanakaraki MK, Kanoupakis EM, Vardas PE. QT variability before and after episodes of nonsustained ventricular tachycardia in patients with hypertrophic cardiomyopathy. Pacing Clin Electrophysiol 1998;21:2387–2391.

166. Nollo G, Speranza G, Grasso R, Bonamini R, Mangiardi L, Antolini R. Spontaneous beat-to-beat variability of the ventricular repolarization duration. J Electrocardiol 1992;25:9–17.
167. Berger RD, Kasper EK, Baughman KL, Marban E, Calkins H, Tomaselli GF. Beat-to-beat QT interval variability: novel evidence for repolarization lability in ischemic and nonischemic dilated cardiomyopathy. Circulation 1997;96:1557–1565.
168. Atiga WL, Fananapazir L, McAreavey D, Calkins H, Berger RD. Temporal repolarization lability in hypertrophic cardiomyopathy caused by beta-myosin heavy-chain gene mutations. Circulation 2000;101:1237–1242.
169. Atiga WL, Calkins H, Lawrence JH, Tomaselli GF, Smith JM, Berger RD. Beat-to-beat repolarization lability identifies patients at risk for sudden cardiac death. J Cardiovasc Electrophysiol 1998;9:899–908.
170. Vrtovec B, Starc V, Starc R. Beat-to-beat QT interval variability in coronary patients. J Electrocardiol 2000;33:119–125.
171. Nolasco JB, Dahlen RW. A graphic method for the study of alternation in cardiac action potentials. J Appl Physiol 1968;25:191–196.
172. Bardaji A, Vidal F, Richart C. T wave alternans associated with amiodarone. J Electrocardiol 1993;26:155–157.
173. Chao CL, Chen WJ, Wu CC, Lee YT. Torsade de pointes and T-wave alternans in a patient with brainstem hemorrhage. Int J Cardiol 1995;51:199–201.
174. Ishikawa K, Tateno M. Alternans of the repolarization wave in a case of hypochloremic alkalosis with hypopotassemia. J Electrocardiol 1976;9:75–79.
175. Kleinfeld MJ, Rozanski JJ. Alternans of the ST segment in Prinzmetal's angina. Circulation 1977;55:574–577.
176. Navarro-Lopez F, Cinca J, Sanz G, Periz A, Magrina J, Betriu A. Isolated T wave alternans. Am Heart J 1978;95:369–374.
177. Puletti M, Curione M, Righetti G, Jacobellis G. Alternans of the ST segment and T wave in acute myocardial infarction. J Electrocardiol 1980;13:297–300.
178. Surawicz B. ST-segment, T-wave, and U-wave changes during myocardial ischemia and after myocardial infarction. Can J Cardiol 1986;Suppl A:71A–84A.
179. Tada H, Nogami A, Shimizu W, et al. ST segment and T wave alternans in a patient with Brugada syndrome. Pacing Clin Electrophysiol 2000;23:413–415.
180. Tan KS, Lau YS, Teo WS. T wave alternans and acute rheumatic myocarditis: a case report. Ann Acad Med Singapore 1999;28:455–458.
181. Zareba W, Moss AJ, le Cessie S, Hall WJ. T wave alternans in idiopathic long QT syndrome. J Am Coll Cardiol 1994;23:1541–1546.
182. Adam DR, Smith JM, Akselrod S, Nyberg S, Powell AO, Cohen RJ. Fluctuations in T-wave morphology and susceptibility to ventricular fibrillation. J Electrocardiol 1984;17:209–218.
183. Rosenbaum DS, Jackson LE, Smith JM, Garan H, Ruskin JN, Cohen RJ. Electrical alternans and vulnerability to ventricular arrhythmias. N Engl J Med 1994;330:235–241.
184. Smith JM, Clancy EA, Valeri CR, Ruskin JN, Cohen RJ. Electrical alternans and cardiac electrical instability. Circulation 1988;77:110–121.
185. Hohnloser SH, Klingenheben T, Zabel M, Li YG, Albrecht P, Cohen RJ. T wave alternans during exercise and atrial pacing in humans. J Cardiovasc Electrophysiol 1997;8:987–993.
186. Pastore JM, Girouard SD, Laurita KR, Akar FG, Rosenbaum DS. Mechanism linking T-wave alternans to the genesis of cardiac fibrillation. Circulation 1999;99:1385–1394.
187. Pastore JM, Rosenbaum DS. Role of structural barriers in the mechanism of alternans-induced reentry. Circ Res 2000;87:1157–1163.
188. Estes NA, Michaud G, Zipes DP, et al. Electrical alternans during rest and exercise as predictors of vulnerability to ventricular arrhythmias. Am J Cardiol 1997;80:1314–1318.
189. Tapanainen JM, Still AM, Airaksinen KE, Huikuri HV. Prognostic significance of risk stratifiers of mortality, including T wave alternans, after acute myocardial infarction: results of a prospective follow-up study. J Cardiovasc Electrophysiol 2001;12:645–652.
190. Klingenheben T, Zabel M, D'Agostino RB, Cohen RJ, Hohnloser SH. Predictive value of T-wave alternans for arrhythmic events in patients with congestive heart failure. Lancet 2000;356:651–652.
191. Hennersdorf MG, Perings C, Niebch V, Vester EG, Strauer BE. T wave alternans as a risk predictor in patients with cardiomyopathy and mild-to-moderate heart failure. Pacing Clin Electrophysiol 2000;23:1386–1391.

192. Hennersdorf MG, Niebch V, Perings C, Strauer BE. T wave alternans and ventricular arrhythmias in arterial hypertension. Hypertension 2001;37:199–203.
193. Kon-No Y, Watanabe J, Koseki Y, et al. Microvolt T wave alternans in human cardiac hypertrophy: electrical instability and abnormal myocardial arrangement. J Cardiovasc Electrophysiol 2001;12:759–763.
194. Momiyama Y, Hartikainen J, Nagayoshi H, et al. Exercise-induced T-wave alternans as a marker of high risk in patients with hypertrophic cardiomyopathy. Jpn Circ J 1997;61:650–656.
195. Adachi K, Ohnishi Y, Yokoyama M. Risk stratification for sudden cardiac death in dilated cardiomyopathy using microvolt-level T-wave alternans. Jpn Circ J 2001;65:76–80.
196. Hohnloser SH, Klingenheben T, Li YG, Zabel M, Peetermans J, Cohen RJ. T wave alternans as a predictor of recurrent ventricular tachyarrhythmias in ICD recipients: prospective comparison with conventional risk markers. J Cardiovasc Electrophysiol 1998;9:1258–1268.
197. Gold MR, Bloomfield DM, Anderson KP, et al. A comparison of T-wave alternans, signal averaged electrocardiography and programmed ventricular stimulation for arrhythmia risk stratification. J Am Coll Cardiol 2000;36:2247–2253.
198. Kaufman ES, Priori SG, Napolitano C, et al. Electrocardiographic prediction of abnormal genotype in congenital long QT syndrome: experience in 101 related family members. J Cardiovasc Electrophysiol 2001;12:455–461.
199. Ackerman MJ, Nemec J, Tester DJ, Hejlik J, Shen WK. Catecholamine-provoked T wave lability (TWLI): Identification of a novel index for risk stratification in congenital long QT syndrome. J Am Coll Cardiol 2001;37:505A–505A (Abstract).
200. Ikeda T, Sakurada H, Sakabe K, et al. Assessment of noninvasive markers in identifying patients at risk in the Brugada syndrome: insight into risk stratification. J Am Coll Cardiol 2001;37:1628–1634.
201. Kavesh NG, Shorofsky SR, Sarang SE, Gold MR. Effect of heart rate on T wave alternans. J Cardiovasc Electrophysiol 1998;9:703–708.
202. Rosenbaum DS, Albrecht P, Cohen RJ. Predicting sudden cardiac death from T wave alternans of the surface electrocardiogram: promise and pitfalls. J Cardiovasc Electrophysiol 1996;7:1095–1111.
203. Caffarone A, Martinelli A, Valentini P, Vanoli E. T wave alternans detection during exercise stress test and during dobutamine stress. A comparative study in patients with a recent myocardial infarction. Ital Heart J 2001;2:265–270.
204. Narayan SM, Smith JM. Exploiting rate-related hysteresis in repolarization alternans to improve risk stratification for ventricular tachycardia. J Am Coll Cardiol 2000;35:1485–1492.
205. Couderc JP, Zareba W, Burattini L, Moss AJ. Beat-to-beat repolarization variability in LQTS patients with the SCN5A sodium channel gene mutation. Pacing Clin Electrophysiol 1999;22:1581–1592.
206. Viskin S, Heller K, Barron HV, et al. Postextrasystolic U wave augmentation, a new marker of increased arrhythmic risk in patients without the long QT syndrome. J Am Coll Cardiol 1996;28:1746–1752.
207. Kasanuki H, Ohnishi S, Ohtuka M, et al. Idiopathic ventricular fibrillation induced with vagal activity in patients without obvious heart disease. Circulation 1997;95:2277–2285.
208. Miyazaki T, Mitamura H, Miyoshi S, Soejima K, Aizawa Y, Ogawa S. Autonomic and antiarrhythmic drug modulation of ST segment elevation in patients with Brugada syndrome. J Am Coll Cardiol 1996;27:1061–1070.
209. Brugada R, Brugada J, Antzelevitch C, et al. Sodium channel blockers identify risk for sudden death in patients with ST-segment elevation and right bundle branch block but structurally normal hearts. Circulation 2000;101:510–515.
210. Shimizu W, Antzelevitch C, Suyama K, et al. Effect of sodium channel blockers on ST segment, QRS duration, and corrected QT interval in patients with Brugada syndrome. J Cardiovasc Electrophysiol 2000;11:1320–1329.
211. Chinushi M, Washizuka T, Okumura H, Aizawa Y. Intravenous administration of class I antiarrhythmic drugs induced T wave alternans in a patient with Brugada syndrome. J Cardiovasc Electrophysiol 2001;12:493–495.
212. Tachibana H, Yamaki M, Kubota I, Watanabe T, Yamauchi S, Tomoike H. Intracoronary flecainide induces ST alternans and reentrant arrhythmia on intact canine heart: A role of 4-aminopyridine-sensitive current. Circulation 1999;99:1637–1643.
213. Priori SG, Napolitano C, Gasparini M, et al. Clinical and genetic heterogeneity of right bundle branch block and ST-segment elevation syndrome: A prospective evaluation of 52 families. Circulation 2000;102:2509–2515.

214. Priori SG, Napolitano C, Schwartz PJ, Bloise R, Crotti L, Ronchetti E. The elusive link between LQT3 and Brugada syndrome: the role of flecainide challenge. Circulation 2000;102:945–947.

215. Jackman WM, Friday KJ, Anderson JL, Aliot EM, Clark M, Lazzara R. The long QT syndromes: a critical review, new clinical observations and a unifying hypothesis. Prog Cardiovasc Dis 1988;31: 115–172.

216. Nakagawa M, Iwao T, Ishida S, et al. Dynamics of QT interval in a patient with long QT syndrome and a normal QT interval. Jpn Circ J 1998;62:215–218.

217. Balaji S, Lau YR, Gillette PC. Effect of heart rate on QT interval in children and adolescents. Heart 1997;77:128–129.

218. Shimizu W, Kamakura S, Kurita T, Suyama K, Aihara N, Shimomura K. Influence of epinephrine, propranolol, and atrial pacing on spatial distribution of recovery time measured by body surface mapping in congenital long QT syndrome. J Cardiovasc Electrophysiol 1997;8:1102–1114.

219. Sakurada H, Tejima T, Hiyoshi Y, Motomiya T, Hiraoka M. Association of humps on monophasic action potentials and ST-T alternans in a patient with Romano-Ward syndrome. Pacing Clin Electrophysiol 1991;14:1485–1491.

220. Shimizu W, Ohe T, Kurita T, et al. Early afterdepolarizations induced by isoproterenol in patients with congenital long QT syndrome. Circulation 1991;84:1915–1923.

221. Ohe T, Kurita T, Shimizu W, Emori T, Shimomura K. Induction of TU abnormalities in patients with torsades de pointes. Ann NY Acad Sci 1992;644:178–186.

222. Fujikawa H, Sato Y, Arakawa H, et al. Induction of torsades de pointes by dobutamine infusion in a patient with idiopathic long QT syndrome. Intern Med 1998;37:149–152.

223. Shimizu W, Antzelevitch C. Differential effects of beta-adrenergic agonists and antagonists in LQT1, LQT2 and LQT3 models of the long QT syndrome. J Am Coll Cardiol 2000;35:778–786.

224. Priori SG, Napolitano C, Cantu F, Brown AM, Schwartz PJ. Differential response to Na+ channel blockade, beta-adrenergic stimulation, and rapid pacing in a cellular model mimicking the SCN5A and HERG defects present in the long-QT syndrome. Circ Res 1996;78:1009–1015.

225. Bezzina C, Veldkamp MW, van den Berg MP, et al. A single Na+ channel mutation causing both long-QT and Brugada syndromes. Circ Res 1999;85:1206–1213.

226. Veldkamp MW, Viswanathan PC, Bezzina C, Baartscheer A, Wilde AA, Balser JR. Two distinct congenital arrhythmias evoked by a multidysfunctional Na(+) channel. Circ Res 2000;86:E91–E97.

227. Itoh E, Suzuki K, Tanabe Y. A case of vasospastic angina presenting Brugada-type ECG abnormalities. Jpn Circ J 1999;63:493–495.

228. Fujiki A, Usui M, Nagasawa H, Mizumaki K, Hayashi H, Inoue H. ST segment elevation in the right precordial leads induced with class IC antiarrhythmic drugs: insight into the mechanism of Brugada syndrome. J Cardiovasc Electrophysiol 1999;10:214–218.

229. Buxton AE, Fisher JD, Josephson ME, Lee KL, Pryor DB, Prystowsky EN, Simson MB, DiCarlo L, Echt DS, Packer D: Prevention of sudden death in patients with coronary artery disease: the Multicenter Unsustained Tachycardia Trial (MUSTT). Prog Cardiovasc Dis 1993;36:215–226

230. Haberman RJ, Rials SJ, Stohler JL, Marinchak RA, Kowey PR: Evidence for a reexcitability gap in man after treatment with type I antiarrhythmic drugs. Am Heart J 1993;126:1121–1126

231. Koller BS, Karasik PE, Solomon AJ, Franz MR: Relation between repolarization and refractoriness during programmed electrical stimulation in the human right ventricle. Implications for ventricular tachycardia induction. Circulation 1995;91:2378–2384

232. Pu J, Boyden PA: Alterations of Na+ currents in myocytes from epicardial border zone of the infarcted heart. A possible ionic mechanism for reduced excitability and postrepolarization refractoriness. Circ Res 1997;81:110–119

233. Sutton PM, Taggart P, Opthof T, Coronel R, Trimlett R, Pugsley W, Kallis P: Repolarisation and refractoriness during early ischaemia in humans. Heart 2000;84:365–369

234. Endresen K, Amlie JP, Forfang K: Effects of disopyramide on repolarisation and intraventricular conduction in man. Eur J Clin Pharmacol 1988;3 5:467–474

235. Furukawa T, Rozanski JJ, Moroe K, Gosselin AJ, Lister JW: Efficacy of procainamide on ventricular tachycardia: relation to prolongation of refractoriness and slowing of conduction. Am Heart J 1989; 118:702–708

236. Man KC, Williamson BD, Niebauer M, Daoud E, Bakr O, Strickberger SA, Hummel JD, Kou W, Morady F: Electrophysiologic effects of sotalol and amiodarone in patients with sustained monomorphic ventricular tachycardia. Am J Cardiol 1994;74:1119–1123

237. Huikuri HV, Yli-Mayry S, Linnaluoto MK, Ikaheimo MJ: Diurnal fluctuations in human ventricular and atrial refractoriness. Pacing Clin Electrophysiol 1995; 18:1362–1368

238. Kong TQJ, Goldberger JJ, Parker M, Wang T, Kadish AH: Circadian variation in human ventricular refractoriness. Circulation 1995;92:1507–1516

239. Amlie JP, Refsum H, Landmark KH: Prolonged ventricular refractoriness and action potential duration after beta-adrenoreceptor blockade in the dog heart in situ. J Cardiovasc Pharmacol 1982;4:157–162

240. Jauch W, Hicks MN, Cobbe SM: Effects of contraction-excitation feedback on electrophysiology and arrhythmogenesis in rabbits with experimental left ventricular hypertrophy. Cardiovasc Res 1994;28: 1390–1396

241. Rials SJ, Wu Y, Ford N, Pauletto FJ, Abramson SV, Rubin AM, Marinchak RA, Kowey PR: Effect of left ventricular hypertrophy and its regression on ventricular electrophysiology and vulnerability to inducible arrhythmia in the feline heart. Circulation 1995;91:426–430

242. Wolk R, Sneddon KP, Dempster J, Kane KA, Cobbe SM, Hicks MN: Regional electrophysiological effects of left ventricular hypertrophy in isolated rabbit hearts under normal and ischaemic conditions. Cardiovasc Res 2000;48:120–128

243. Kavanagh KM, Wyse DG, Mitchell LB, Duff HJ: Cardiac refractoriness. Age-dependence in normal subjects. J Electrocardiol 1989;22:221–225

244. Wolk R, Stec S, Kulakowski P: Extrasystolic beats affect transmural electrical dispersion during programmed electrical stimulation. Eur J Clin Invest 2001;31:293–301

245. Shimizu S, Kobayashi Y, Miyauchi Y, Ohmura K, Atarashi H, Takano T: Temporal and spatial dispersion of repolarization during premature impulse propagation in human intact ventricular muscle: comparison between single vs double premature stimulation. Europace 2000;2:201–206

246. Yuan S, Blomstrom-Lundqvist C, Pehrson S, Pripp CM, Wohlfart B, Olsson SB: Dispersion of repolarization following double and triple programmed stimulation. A clinical study using the monophasic action potential recording technique. Eur Heart J 1996; 17:1080–1091

247. Englund A, Andersson M, Bergfeldt L: Dispersion in ventricular repolarization in patients with severe intraventricular conduction disturbances. Pacing Clin Electrophysiol 2001;24:10671075

248. Yuan S, Wohlfart B, Olsson SB, Blomstrom-Lundqvist C: The dispersion of repolarization in patients with ventricular tachycardia. A study using simultaneous monophasic action potential recordings from two sites in the right ventricle. Eur Heart J 1995; 16:68–76

249. Franz MR: Long-term recording of monophasic action potentials from human endocardium. Am J Cardiol 1983;51:1629–1634

250. Franz MR: Monophasic action potential recording, in Zipes DP, Jalife J (eds): Cardiac electrophysiology. From cell to bedside. Philadelphia, W.B.Saunders, 2000, pp 763–770

251. Franz MR, Swerdlow CD, Liem LB, Schaefer J: Cycle length dependence of human action potential duration in vivo. Effects of single extrastimuli, sudden sustained rate acceleration and deceleration, and different steady-state frequencies. J Clin Invest 1988;82:972–979

252. Gavrilescu S, Luca C: Right ventricular monophasic action potentials in patients with long QT syndrome. Br Heart J 1978;40:1014–1018

253. Hirao H, Shimizu W, Kurita T, Suyama K, Aihara N, Kamakura S, Shimomura K: Frequency-dependent electrophysiologic properties of ventricular repolarization in patients with congenital long QT syndrome. J Am Coll Cardiol 1996;28:1269–1277

254. Shimizu W, Ohe T, Kurita T, Tokuda T, Shimomura K: Epinephrine-induced ventricular premature complexes due to early afterdepolarizations and effects of verapamil and propranolol in a patient with congenital long QT syndrome. J Cardiovasc Electrophysiol 1994;5:438–444

255. Shimizu W, Ohe T, Kurita T, Kawade M, Arakaki Y, Aihara N, Kamakura S, Kamiya T, Shimomura K: Effects of verapamil and propranolol on early afterdepolarizations and ventricular arrhythmias induced by epinephrine in congenital long QT syndrome. J Am Coll Cardiol 1995;26:1299–1309

256. Corrado D, Basso C, Buja G, Nava A, Rossi L, Thiene G: Right bundle branch block, right precordial st-segment elevation, and sudden death in young people. Circulation 2001;103:710–717

257. Napolitano C, Schwartz PJ, Brown AM, Ronchetti E, Bianchi L, Pinnavaia A, Acquaro G, Priori SG: Evidence for a cardiac ion channel mutation underlying drug-induced QT prolongation and life-threatening arrhythmias. J Cardiovasc Electrophysiol 2000; 11:691–696

258. Donger C, Denjoy I, Berthet M, Neyroud N, Cruaud C, Bermaceur M, Chivoret G, Schwartz K, Coumel P, Guicheney P: KVLQT1 C-terminal missense mutation causes a forme fruste long-QT syndrome. Circulation 1997;96:2778–2781

259. Sesti F, Abbott GW, Wei J, Murray KT, Saksena S, Schwartz PJ, Priori SG, Roden DM, George ALJ, Goldstein SA: A common polymorphism associated with antibiotic-induced cardiac arrhythmia. Proc Natl Acad Sci U S A 2000;97:10613–10618

260. Friedlander Y, Lapidos T, Simireich R, Kark JD: Genetic and environmental sources of QT interval variability in Israeli families: the kibbutz settlements family study. Clin Genet 1999;56:200–209

261. Rashba EJ, Zareba W, Moss AJ, Hall WJ, Robinson J, Locati EH, Schwartz PJ, Andrews M: Influence of pregnancy on the risk for cardiac events in patients with hereditary long QT syndrome. LQTS Investigators. Circulation 1998;97:451–456

262. Viskin S, Fish R, Roth A, Schwartz PJ, Belhassen B: QT or not QT. N Engl J Med 2000;343:352–356

263. Brandt RR, Shen WK: Bradycardia-induced polymorphic ventricular tachycardia after atrioventricular junction ablation for sinus tachycardia-induced cardiomyopathy. J Cardiovasc Electrophysiol 1995;6:630–633

264. Azar RR, Lippman N, Kluger J: Recurrent polymorphic ventricular tachycardia complicating radiofrequency catheter ablation of the atrioventricular junction. Pacing Clin Electrophysiol 1998; 21:1837–1840

265. Conti JB, Mills RM, Woodard DA, Curtis AB: QT dispersion is a marker for life-threatening ventricular arrhythmias after atrioventricular nodal ablation using radiofrequency energy. Am J Cardiol 1997; 79:1412–1414

266. Morady F, Hasse C, Strickberger SA, Man KC, Daoud E, Bogun F, Goyal R, Harvey M, Knight BP, Weiss R, Bahu M: Long-term follow-up after radiofrequency modification of the atrioventricular node in patients with atrial fibrillation. J Am Coll Cardiol 1997;29:113–121

267. Peters RH, Wever EF, Hauer RN, Wittkampf FH, Robles dME: Bradycardia dependent QT prolongation and ventricular fibrillation following catheter ablation of the atrioventricular junction with radiofrequency energy. Pacing Clin Electrophysiol 1994; 17:108–112

268. Vollmer F, Brembilla-Perrot B, Thiel B: [Polymorphous ventricular tachycardia occurring three months following radiofrequency ablation of the bundle of His]. Ann Cardiol Angeiol (Paris) 1998; 47:109–112

269. Grimm W, Hoffmann J, Menz V, Maisch B: Transient QT prolongation with torsades de pointes tachycardia after ablation of permanent junctional reciprocating tachycardia. J Cardiovasc Electrophysiol 1999;10:1631–1635

270. Ozcan C, Jahangir A, Friedman PA, Patel PJ, Munger TM, Rea RF, Lloyd MA, Packer DL, Hodge DO, Gersh BJ, Hammill SC, Shen WK: Long-term survival after ablation of the atrioventricular node and implantation of a permanent pacemaker in patients with atrial fibrillation. N Engl J Med 2001; 344:1043–1051

271. Cellarier G, Deharo JC, Chalvidan T, Gouvernet J, Peyre JP, Savon N, Djiane P: Prolonged QT interval and altered QT/RR relation early after radiofrequency ablation of the atrioventricular junction. Am J Cardiol 1999;83:1671–4, A7

272. Dizon J, Blitzer M, Rubin D, Coromilas J, Costeas C, Kassotis J, Reiffel J: Time dependent changes in duration of ventricular repolarization after AV node ablation: insights into possible mechanism of postprocedural sudden death. Pacing Clin Electrophysiol 2000;23:1539–1544

273. Satoh T, Zipes DP: Rapid rates during bradycardia prolong ventricular refractoriness and facilitate ventricular tachycardia induction with cesium in dogs. Circulation 1996;94:217–227

274. Krebs ME, Szwed JM, Shinn T, Miles WM, Zipes DP: Short-term rapid ventricular pacing prolongs ventricular refractoriness in patients. J Cardiovasc Electrophysiol 1998;9:1036–1042

275. Evans GT, Scheinman MM, Bardy G, Borggrefe M, Brugada P, Fisher J, Fontaine G, Huang SK, Huang WH, Josephson M: Predictors of in-hospital mortality after DC catheter ablation of atrioventricular junction. Results of a prospective, international, multicenter study. Circulation 1991;84:1924–1937

276. Hodges M, Salerno D, Erlien D: Bazett's QT correction reviewed: evidence that a linear QT correction for heart rate is better. J Am Coll Cardiol 1983; 1:694–694(Abstract)

13   Human Cardiac Repolarization

Philip T. Sager, MD, FACC, FACP

CONTENTS

INTRODUCTION

Modulation of cardiac repolarization is thought to play an important role in the clinical development of many cardiac arrhythmias. In addition, the primary mechanism by which most antiarrhythmic agents exert their beneficial effects appears to be through drug-induced prolongation of repolarization. The evaluation of cardiac repolarization in humans has relied on measurements of the QT interval on the surface EKG or, more recently, tracings of monophasic action potentials (MAP) *(1–3)* recorded from the endocardial surface of the atrium and ventricle during invasive cardiac procedures. These recordings accurately reproduce the temporal sequence of repolarization *(4,5)*. The recording of MAPs has permitted the exploration of physiological perturbations in vivo in humans, the relationship between repolarization and refractoriness, and the effects of antiarrhythmic drugs, and sympathetic stimulation on the human action potential duration. These issues and recording of MAPs will be discussed in this chapter.

MONOPHASIC ACTION POTENTIAL (MAP) RECORDINGS

In order to accurately determine repolarization, it is necessary to obtain high quality MAP recordings that are free of artifacts. This requires a special catheter, expertise in proper positioning of the catheter, an appreciation of the techniques for minimizing artifacts, and adequate recording equipment. The MAP catheter permits recordings of

From: *Contemporary Cardiology: Cardiac Repolarization: Bridging Basic and Clinical Science*
Edited by: I. Gussak et al. © Humana Press Inc., Totowa, NJ

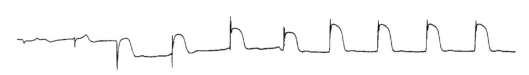

Fig. 1. The left side of the figure shows the MAP catheter recording a local electrogram. Following advancement of the catheter, a partially formed MAP tracing is recorded which quickly matures into a high fidelity action potential recording. Reproduced from *(14)* with permission.

repolarization by exerting pressure at the catheter tip against the endocardium. As the catheter tip is firmly placed against the endocardium, a MAP is displayed (Fig. 1). This results in local depolarization of cells at the catheter tip, thus causing an electrical gradient with the adjacent, nondepolarized cells and a "current of injury." It has been postulated *(5)* that during diastole a sink current is formed from the adjacent normal cells to the depolarized cells at the MAP tip. This gradient presumably reflects the relative changes in the potential of the adjacent cells during periodic cardiac repolarization and repolarization. As the MAP tracings are highly dependent on the interface between mechanically depolarized cells and the catheter tip, recording high-quality tracings requires excellent, stable tissue catheter contact. Most commonly, these recorders are made using the specially designed Franz catheter which has a silver-silver chloride (Ag-AgCl$_2$) electrode pair that permits the hemispherical electrode at the catheter tip to maintain constant pressure against the endocardium during the cardiac cycle, despite movement of the cardiac chambers during systole and diastole *(6–9)*. This is facilitated by the technical innovation of placing a metal spring intraluminal component in the distal aspect of the catheter, helping assure consistent catheter tissue contact.

Monophasic action potential-derived measurements of repolarization have been shown to closely follow the time course of similar determinations made using transmembrane action potential (TAP) recordings *(10)*. In contrast to repolarization, other action potential measurements using MAPs may not be reliable. Specifically, the maximum deflection of phase 0 is not routinely analyzed since the deflection typically overshoots the plateau, a recording artifact. Measurements of dV/dT are slower than those recorded with transmembrane potentials and thus do not accurately reflect this parameter. The slower velocity of the MAP upstroke likely reflects the fact that the MAP recording represents a summation of electrical activity from adjacent cells, and thus depolarization occurs sequentially over time, in contrast to the TAP recording of membrane changes at a single point in a single cell. Several studies, however, have examined the *relative* changes in the upstroke of Phase 0 during ischemia or following the administration of antiarrhythmic drugs and observed that serial changes in this parameter may be of physiologic significance *(8,11,12)*. Thus, whereas the absolute rate of change of phase 0 does not accurately reflect TAP measurements, relative changes owing to physiologic perturbations may be meaningful. Lastly, the amplitude of phase 2 can be easily modified by changing the pressure at the catheter tip and thus is not clinically useful. The ability to record high-quality MAP tracings permits the careful physiologic evaluation of alterations in cardiac physiology, assessment of drug effects, and perturbations in the autonomic nervous system on human repolarization.

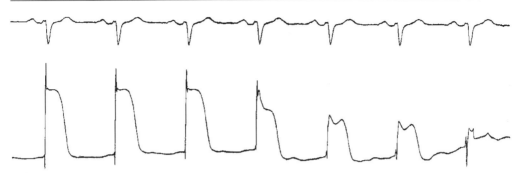

Fig. 2. This figure shows deterioration of the MAP tracing secondary to loss of good MAP-endocardium tissue contact. Reproduced from *(14)* with permission.

It is of paramount importance for the operator to pay special attention to the recording of high-quality MAP tracings, so that cardiac repolarization is accurately represented. Ventricular recordings should be at least 10 mV in amplitude, and those in the atrium should be at least 3 mV in amplitude *(5,13)*. The action potential (AP) should have the typical contour of an AP, with a convex phase 2, a smooth phase 3, and a rapid initial upstroke. In general, extra bumps or apparent depolarizations during phase 3 should not be observed and positive deflections during phase 3 or phase 4 may be separated from artifacts by changing the pressure on the MAP catheter tip. It is easy to misconstrue repolarization artifacts as representing after-depolarizations. Fluctuations in the MAP amplitude beat to beat suggest that catheter contact may be unstable (Fig. 2). The action potential duration (APD) is usually measured at 90% repolarization (APD$_{90}$), since the end of the MAP may be difficult to discern. Further discussion of techniques to record high-quality MAP tracings may be found in ref. *(14)*.

EFFECT OF HEART RATE ON HUMAN REPOLARIZATION

In the normal human myocardium, in the absence of antiarrhythmic agents, there is a close relationship between ventricular repolarization and the effective refractory period. Both of these determinations decrease in a relatively linear fashion over a range of pacing cycle lengths between about 800 ms and 250 ms. At long diastolic intervals there tends to be a plateauing of the APD and effective refractory period (ERP). Measurements of the ERP/APD ratio over this range of cycle lengths are relatively constant with values of approx 0.75 to 0.90. As discussed below, this relationship can be significantly modified by antiarrhythmic drugs or sympathetic stimulation. In fact, being able to determine repolarization and refractoriness at the same cardiac location permits separation of these two parameters during changes in the physiologic milieu.

Measurements of the surface QT interval and the RV monophasic action potential duration have been compared over a range of pacing cycle lengths of 300 ms to 600 ms and found to correlate closely *(15,16)*. In contrast to the situation with the surface QT interval where efforts to create a rate-independent measure of the QT interval have been utilized *(17)*, methodologies to "correct" the APD$_{90}$ for changes in heart rate are not generally utilized and "corrected" values for the human APD$_{90}$ have not been validated. This is a complex issue, as at long diastolic intervals there is a plateauing of the APD$_{90}$ and the QT interval. There are problems with all of the formulas utilized for correcting the QT interval and these fail to take into account many factors. These deficiencies include the fact that the effect of heart rate on repolarization varies significantly from individual to individual *(18)*; That it is difficult to accurately model the effect of heart rate on repolarization during bradycardia; That the formulas do not account for the significant time delay for the QT interval to accommodate to a new value after a significant rate change; That antiarrhythmic drugs can have different effects on repolarization at different heart rates and *(19–21)*; That the cause of the change in heart rate (e.g., sympathetic stimulation) might have direct, rate-independent effects on repolarization. The latter two issues are discussed in detail below and issues regarding surface QT interval correction are discussed in more detail in Chapter 14).

EFFECT OF ISCHEMIA ON REPOLARIZATION

Cardiac ischemia has been closely associated with the development of clinical arrhythmias and the use of MAP recordings has permitted insights into the effects of ischemia on human repolarization. In a cohort of patients undergoing coronary angiography (*n*=26), changes in the MAP duration were evaluated between zones of normal myocardium and zones that became acutely ischemic during rapid atrial pacing *(22)*. Ischemic areas were associated with significant MAP shortening, as compared to the nonischemic areas. These findings confirmed what have been observed on the cellular level during acute ischemia in which the APD shortens. In a second study, Taggart et al. *(22)* examined MAPs during percutaneous coronary angioplasty. Areas of myocardia were subjected to acute ischemia during angioplasty and MAPs recorded from these sites and the APD was compared to nonischemic, nonangioplastied areas. Again, acute shortening of the APD in the ischemic areas was shown, confirming the above findings and demonstrating that acute ischemia increases dispersion of repolarization. Placement of multiple MAP catheters during experiments in which physiologic stimuli are applied can permit determinations of dispersion on repolarization. Lastly, when the effects of dobutamine on repolarization were examined, dispersion of APDs was accentuated during catecholamine administration in humans between normal myocardium and presumably ischemic areas *(23)*.

FREQUENCY-DEPENDENT EFFECTS OF ANTIARRYTHMIC DRUGS ON REPOLARIZATION

Over the last 15 yr, there has been a major shift from the use of Class 1 antiarrhythmic agents to Class 3 drugs that exert their effects primarily by prolonging cardiac repolarization. Such Class 3 drug-induced prolongation of repolarization may terminate a reentrant tachycardia by prolonging the wavelength *(24)* or by altering the dynamics of pivot points *(25)*, preventing tachycardia initiation or the ability of a tachycardia to sustain. However, it has been appreciated that antiarrhythmic drugs may have a decreased ability to prolong repolarization during the rapid heart rates typically associated with many clinical tachycardias and to cause enhanced APD prolongation during relative bradycardia *(26,27)*. This has been termed reverse frequency-dependence. In addition to reverse frequency-dependence possibly limiting a drug's efficacy during tachycardia, this characteristic may also cause excessive QT prolongation and increase the proclivity for torsade de pointes during bradycardia. In addition, the clinical picture is complicated by the fact that autonomic influences, ischemia, acid base alterations, and other factors may alter drug effects on repolarization *(28)*.

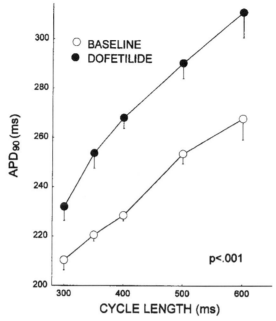

Fig. 3. Graph shows the frequency-dependent effects of dofetilide on the action potential duration (APD$_{90}$). Dofetilide significantly increased the APD$_{90}$ in a reverse-frequency-dependent manner (p<.05). Modified from *(33)* with permission from the American Heart Association and the authors.

The frequency-dependence of antiarrhythmic agents was initially described during single cell recordings of action potentials. Clearly there are major differences between isolated cell preparations and the human in vivo setting (differing ionic currents in different species, loss of cellular coupling *(29)* nonphysiologic temperatures, and so on). Thus, it is important to determine the actions of antiarrhythmic agents in humans and not simply extrapolate the results of single cell or animal studies. As discussed previously, MAP recordings lend themselves to the study of these complex interactions during a variety of pharmacologic and physiologic perturbations. The subheadings below will discuss the frequency-dependent effects on different antiarrhythmic agents.

Dofetilide

Dofetilide is a methanesulfonanilide Class 3 agent *(30–32)* that is a pure blocker of the rapid activating component of the delayed rectifier current (I_{Kr}) and has not been demonstrated to have other significant pharmacologic or adrenergic actions *(24)*. The effects of oral dofetilide on repolarization were examined during serial electrophysiologic studies by Sager et al. *(33)* Right ventricular MAPs were recorded from the RV apex during the patient's baseline drug-free electrophysiologic study during steady-state pacing (cycle lengths of 600 ms, 500 ms, 400 ms, 350 ms, and 300 ms) for at least 150 beats and after steady-state oral dofetilide dosing (0.25 to 0.75 micrograms administered orally every eight hours) for at least five half lives. The APD$_{90}$ was determined along with the right ventricular effective refractory period (RVERP) at the same ventricular site. The QRS duration was determined during steady-state ventricular pacing, as a measure of ventricular conduction *(34)*. The catheter position was determined during the first electrophysiologic study and placed in the same position during the follow-up test.

Dofetilide exerted significant reverse frequency-dependence on the APD_{90}, extending this parameter to a greater degree at longer as compared to shorter paced cycle lengths (Fig. 3). Changes in repolarization were followed by similar changes in the effective refractory period, whereas no effects on ventricular conduction or the $RVERP/APD_{90}$ ratio were observed. These findings are consistent with the demonstration of reverse frequency-dependence observed in experimental isolated cell preparations (35,36). Although the mechanisms of reverse frequency-dependence of dofetilide were not examined in this study, Jurkiewicz and Sanguinetti (32), utilizing voltage clamp studies in isolated guinea pig ventricular myocytes, have examined this issue during rapid pacing. These studies demonstrated that at short diastolic intervals, the slowly activating component of the delayed rectifier potassium current (I_{Ks}) does not have sufficient time to completely deactivate, and that buildup of I_{Ks} offsets the rate-independent block of I_{Kr} by dofetilide, causing enhanced shortening of repolarization during rapid pacing. Other possible mechanisms for dofetilide-induced reverse frequency-dependence include modulation of inward calcium currents (35,37) and extracellular potassium accumulation at short cycle lengths in the intracellular clefts, causing subsequent augmentation of repolarizing potassium current conductance. Interestingly, it may be possible to modify the rate-dependency of pure I_{Kr} blockade. Gjini et al. (28) examined in guinea pig papillary muscle the effects of adding the calcium channel antagonist diltiazem to dofetilide and the frequency-dependency response on repolarization (Fig. 4). Although the addition of diltiazem had little effect during rapid heart rates, it did block excessive prolongation of the APD during relative bradycardia and thus might help prevent torsade de pointes. Thus, the abolition of reverse rate dependent response by adding diltiazem was achieved by decreasing APD prolongation during relative bradycardia, as opposed to prolonging repolarization, during rapid pacing.

The effect of dofetilide on repolarization has also been examined in two other studies. Sedwick et al. (38) examine the effects of intravenous dofetilide over a fairly narrow range of paced cycle lengths (500 to 800 ms) and Yuan et al. (39) examine the effects of intravenous dofetilide at paced cycle lengths of 500 ms and 600 ms. It is not surprising that frequency-dependence was not observed in these studies, since pacing at short cycle lengths was not examined.

Sematilide

The frequency-dependence of sematilide (19), an experimental Class 3 agent that appears to exert its effects by blocking I_{Kr} without other channel or adrenergic effects (19,40,41) was examined in patients undergoing serial electrophysiologic studies utilizing similar methodologies as those described above for dofetilide. As shown in Fig. 5, sematilide significantly prolonged the APD_{90} and these effects were greater during slower pacing (cycle of 600 ms) compared to more rapid pacing (cycle length 300 ms), demonstrating reverse frequency-dependent effects. When the data was analyzed utilizing the diastolic interval, a significant correlation was demonstrated between the diastolic interval for both the percent increase in drug-induced APD_{90} prolongation and the magnitude of the APD_{90} increase, indicating less prolongation of repolarization during shorter as compared to longer diastolic intervals. Changes in refractoriness paralleled changes in repolarization. Effects on conduction and RVERP/APD ratio were not observed, indicating that drug-induced increases in refractoriness were solely secondary to changes in the ventricular repolarization.

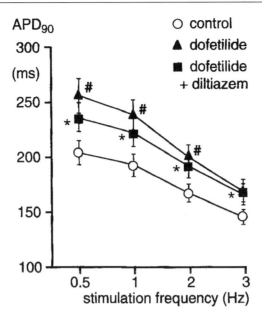

Fig. 4. Shown here is the frequency dependent effect of dofetilide (10 n*M*), a pure Class 3 agent, with or without the presence of a calcium antagonist (diltiazem 10 m*M*) on APD_{90} in isolated guinea pig papillary muscles (*n*=11). Transmembrane APD_{90} was measured using intercellular microelectrode techniques before drug application (control), 30 min after equilibration with dofetilide, and 30 min after exposure to diltiazem, in the continuous presence of dofetilide. Data is expressed as mean ± SEM; # $p <. 01$, dofetilide versus control; *$p < .05$, dofetilide vs dofetilide plus diltiazem. Modified from *(35)* with permission of the *Journal of Cardiovascular Pharmacology.*

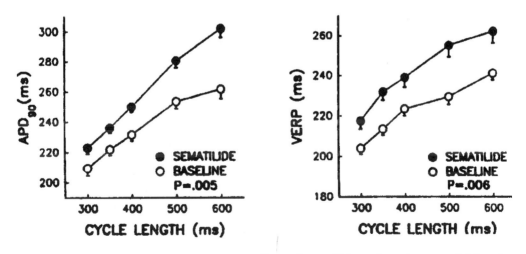

Fig. 5. Graphs show the frequency-dependent effects of sematilide on the action potential duration (APD_{90}) and the right ventricular refractory period (RVERP). Sematilide significantly increased the APD_{90} and the RVERP to a greater extent and longer as compared to shorter paced cycle lengths (*p*<.05, repeated measures ANOVA). Modified from *(19)* with permission from the American Heart Association and the authors.

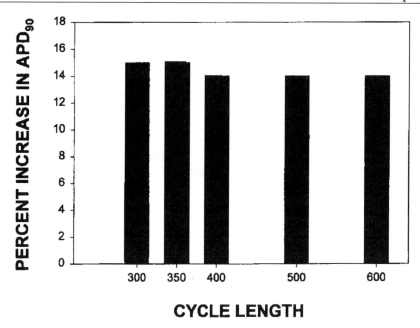

Fig. 6. Plot shows the frequency-dependent effects of d,l-sotalol on the percent increase in repo-larization (APD_{90}). D,l-sotalol prolonged the APD_{90} without frequency-dependent effects. Modi-fied with permission of the *Journal of Cardiovascular Electrophysiology* and the authors from *(42)*.

D,l-Sotalol

Sager et al. *(42)* examined the frequency-dependence of d,l-sotalol in 17 patients during chronic oral therapy (mean dose: 362 ± 21 mg/d). Compared to baseline drug-free values, d,l-sotalol significantly prolonged the APD_{90} by 14–15% at paced cycle lengths of 300 ms to 600 ms ($p < .01$). Thus, in contrast to sematilide and dofetilide, the effects of d,l-sotalol on repolarization were not influenced by the pacing rate (Fig. 6). Interest-ingly, significant, albeit mild, reverse frequency-dependence was observed on the RVERP, though this parameter remained significantly prolonged by 8% at the shortest paced cycle of 300 ms. Effects on conduction or the $RVERP/APD_{90}$ ratio were not observed. The reasons for the lack of frequency-dependence effects on repolarization are unclear. Possible explanations include the fact that d,l-sotalol blocks multiple potassium channels (I_{Kr}, I_{to}, I_{K1}) and/or that the agent's beta-blocking effects may have modulated the frequency-dependent response.

Schmitt et al. *(43)* have reported divergent findings when the effects of intravenous d,l-sotalol on the APD_{90} was examined in humans, demonstrating reverse frequency-depen-dence on repolarization. The apparent discrepancy in the results of these two studies may stem from the fact that the above study examined MAPs after steady-state pacing for 200 beats while Schmitt et al. *(43)* examined MAPs after only 20 beats, a time interval which might not have permitted full APD accommodation to the more rapid pacing rate. In addition, different effects between intravenous and oral drug administration may exist and the type of underlying structural heart disease may also affect the frequency-depen-dent relationship. Schmitt et al. *(28)* have demonstrated in another series of experiments in dogs that d,l-sotalol exerted reverse frequency-dependent effects in normal myocardium, but this phenomenon was not observed in chronically infarcted tissue. Differences in the frequency-dependent effects of quinidine between normal and infarcted dogs on Purkinje fiber APD have also been reported *(44)*.

D-Sotalol

There are limited data examining the frequency-dependent effects of the d-isomer, which is devoid of beta-blocker activity. In six patients, over the paced cycle length of 350–700 ms, the effects of sotalol on the APD appeared to be attenuated during rapid pacing *(45)*.

Amiodarone

Amiodarone is a unique pharmacologic agent that has a relatively high efficacy and a low incidence of torsade de pointes. Experimental studies have demonstrated the relatively unique ability of the agent to prolong repolarization and refractoriness independent of heart rate *(46)*. The effects of an 11 d oral loading regimen of amiodarone on repolarization have been examined *(20)*. In these studies, 19 patients with malignant ventricular arrhythmias underwent an experimental protocol utilizing similar methodologies as those described previously. After amiodarone loading (mean doses 1621 ± 162 mg per day) the APD_{90} increased by 10–13% compared to baseline drug-free values and these increases were independent of the paced cycle length (Fig. 7). While the RVERP did demonstrate mild reverse frequency-dependence ($p=.04$ by ANOVA), the RVERP remained significantly prolonged at the shortest paced cycle length of 300 ms. Importantly, the percent change in the RVERP remained relatively constant. In contrast to the above findings with d,-l sotalol, sematilide, and dofetilide, pacing significantly prolonged the QRS interval in a frequency-dependent manner with greater QRS prolongation during rapid, as compared to slower, pacing. This is consistent with significant sodium channel blockade during rapid pacing. In addition, the RVERP/APD_{90} ratio was significantly increased by amiodarone, indicating that prolongation of the RVERP was secondary to prolongation of repolarization, in addition to other processes (most likely delayed recovery of sodium channels during phase 3 of the action potential). Similar findings have been reported by Hiukuri and Yli-Mayri *(45)*. The finding that amiodarone does not exert frequency-dependent effects on repolarization is most likely multifactorial and may be related to nonselective blockade of potassium repolarizing currents. The absence of reverse frequency-dependence may explain, in part, some of the beneficial effects of amiodarone in preventing reentrant arrhythmias, as well as the low incidence of torsade de pointes, since bradycardia in not associated with exaggerated increases in the APD. The prolongation of the refractoriness, to a greater extent than APD, prolongation may also facilitate the prevention of afterdepolarizations propagating or "triggering," since they may fall within the extended refractory period and thus fail to evoke a response.

Other Class 3 Agents

Ambasilide is an experimental agent that blocks both I_{Ks} and I_{Kr}. As discussed earlier, one explanation for the frequency-dependent effects of Class 3 agents is that at rapid rates I_{Ks} does not have sufficient time to deactivate, and build-up of this current negates the I_{Kr} blocking effects of an antiarrhythmic agent at rapid rates *(32)*. If this hypophysis is true, then it would be expected that ambasilide would not have significant frequency-dependent effects. Indeed, Schmitt et al. *(47)* examined MAP recordings in seven patients

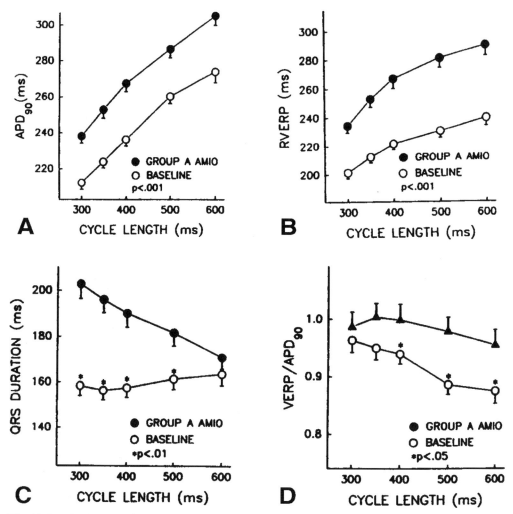

Fig. 7. Graphs show the frequency-dependent effects of amiodarone on electrophysiologic parameters. (**A**) Plot shows the frequency-dependent effect on the APD_{90} demonstrating prolongation of this parameter without frequency-dependent effects. (**B**) Plot shows the frequency-dependent effects of amiodarone on the RVERP demonstrating a mild reverse frequency-dependent effect (there was no significant percent increase in the RVERP as a function of paced cycle length). (**C**) Plot shows the effects of amiodarone on the QRS duration demonstrating significant frequency-dependent prolongation of this parameter during rapid pacing. (**D**) Plot shows the significant increase in the RVERP/APD_{90} ratio during amiodarone therapy ($p<.05$). Reproduced with permission of the American Heart Association and the authors from (20).

receiving ambasilide and demonstrated frequency-independent increases in the APD. Transmembrane recordings from isolated human myocardial tissue have also demonstrated similar findings (48). Thus, blockade of I_{Ks} may result in a more desirable frequency-dependent effect on repolarization as compared to pure I_{Kr} blockade.

Tedisamil is also an experimental Class 3 agent that blocks the transient outward current as well as I_{Kr}. MAP recordings have been assessed in one study and the agents appeared to exert reverse frequency-dependent effects in humans (49).

SYMPATHETIC STIMULATION: EFFECTS ON CLASS 3 DRUG-INDUCED PROLONGATION OF REPOLARIZATION

It is believed that the autonomic nervous system plays an important role in the clinical development of cardiac arrhythmias. Beta-adrenergic blockade following myocardial infarction has been shown to reduce cardiac mortality and arrhythmias *(50,51)*, and increases in sympathetic activity have been associated with clinical arrhythmia development and reduction in the ventricular fibrillation threshold in dogs *(52)*. In addition, sympathetic stimulation, via the administration of epinephrine or isoproterenol, has been shown to significantly attenuate the electrophysiologic actions of Class 1 agents on refractoriness *(38,53–55)*. With the shift from Class 1 to Class 3 agents, determination of the effects of sympathetic stimulation on Class 3 agent-induced changes on repolarization and refractoriness warrant careful attention.

Since it is believed that the clinical benefits of these antiarrhythmic agents are primarily derived from APD prolongation, modulation of this effect by sympathetic stimulation may be of significant clinical importance. Beta-adrenergic catecholamines modulate numerous ionic currents within myocytes and may shorten repolarization by increasing I_{Ks} *(56)*, the chloride current *(57)*, and the sodium-potassium pump current *(58)*. In addition, ventricular conduction may be improved by increasing the fast inward sodium current (I_{Na}). Since many Class 3 agents prolong repolarization by blocking I_{Kr}, catecholamine-induced increases in I_{Ks} and the chloride current might significantly attenuate drug-induced prolongation of repolarization. Pertinent to this issue, in a pivotal study by Sanguinetti et al. *(56)*, E-4031 (a pure I_{Kr} blocker) caused a 50% increase in guinea pig papillary muscle ERP (Fig. 8). However, pretreatment with isoproterenol significantly reduced the refractory period to values significantly below baseline, despite E-4031 administration. The reversal of E-4031's effects on repolarization were shown to be secondary to increases in I_{Ks} and the chloride current, despite the fact that I_{Kr} remained significantly inhibited. In another series of experiments, when left stellate ganglion stimulation was performed in dogs receiving d-sotalol (a blocker of I_{Kr}), drug-induced APD prolongation was markedly attenuated *(59)*.

In a series of experiments, Sager et al. *(42,60)* examined the effects of isoproterenol infusion on drug-induced prolongation of repolarization by sematilide, amiodarone, and d,l-sotalol in humans. In these experiments, patients underwent a drug-free electrophysiologic study with measurements of repolarization as described earlier, a second measurement of repolarization following oral drug administration, and a third measurement during concomitant isoproterenol administration (35 ng/kg per minute after a 12 min equilibration period). All electrophysiologic determinations were made after steady-state pacing (200 beats) at cycle lengths of 300 ms to at least 500 ms. The monophasic action potential recordings were performed at the right ventricular outflow tract and ventricular refractoriness was measured at the same ventricular site. Subjects with recent unstable cardiac syndromes, or those receiving beta-blockers were excluded. All analyses were performed using analysis of variance.

Sematilide

Isoproterenol administration to patients receiving sematilide *(60)* significantly reduced the sinus cycle length from 811±39 ms to 545±36 ms ($p<.001$, n=11) and isoproterenol

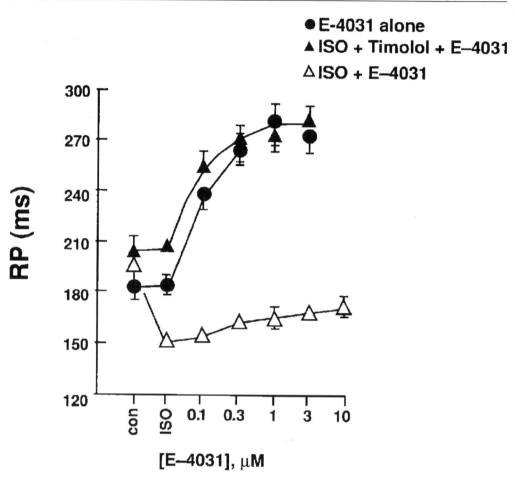

Fig. 8. Graphs show the effects of E-4031 alone, isoproterenol (Iso) plus E-4031, and isoproterenol plus timolol plus E-4031 on the refractory period of isolated guinea pig papillary muscles as a function of E-4031 concentration. E-4031 significantly increased the refractory period and these effects of E-4031 were totally abolished during concomitant isoproterenol administration ($p<.05$). The effects of isoproterenol on E-4031-induced refractory period prolongation were fully reversed after timolol administration ($p<.05$). Published with permission of the American Heart Association from *(56)*.

infusion fully reversed sematilide-induced APD_{90} prolongation to values similar to those obtained at baseline (Fig. 9). More remarkably, isoproterenol fully reversed RVERP to values significantly ($p < .05$) below those obtained at baseline. Thus, isoproterenol-induced effects were greater on refractoriness than on repolarization (confirmed by examining the RVERP/APD_{90} ratio, which was significantly shortened). When the effect of sematilide and sematilide plus isoproterenol on the sustained ventricular tachycardial (VT) cycle was examined in morphologically similar VTs, there was a nonsignificant trend for sematilide to increase the sustained VT cycle length. Isoproterenol significantly shortened the VT cycle length in subjects receiving sematilide and tended to shorten the VT cycle length to values below those obtained at baseline ($p < .06$). In conclusion, isoproterenol fully reversed the effects of sematilide-induced prolongation of APD_{90} and

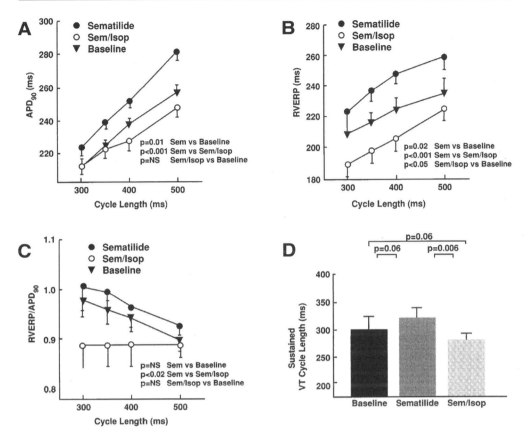

Fig. 9. Graphs show the frequency-dependent effects of sematilide and sematilide plus isoproterenol on electrophysiologic parameters. **(A)** Effects on the APD_{90}. Sematilide-induced APD_{90} prolongation was fully reversed by isoproterenol. **(B)** Effects on the Right Ventricular Refractory Period. Sematilide-Induced RVERP prolongation was reversed by isoproterenol to values significantly below baseline ($p<.05$). **(C)** Plot shows the effects on the ratio of the right ventricular refractory period and action potential duration ($RVERP/APD_{90}$). During isoproterenol administration to patients receiving sematilide the $RVERP/APD_{90}$ ratio was significantly reduced ($p=.02$), secondary to reductions in repolarization as well as to reductions in other factors. **(D)** The effects of sematilide and sematilide plus isoproterenol on the sustained ventricular tachycardia (VT) cycle length. Sematilide mildly increased the sustained VT cycle length ($p=0.06$). Isoproterenol administration to patients receiving sematilide resulted in a significant reduction in the sustained VT cycle length ($p=0.006$) to values that tended to be lower than baseline drug-free values ($p=0.06$). Reproduced with permission from the American Heart Association and the authors from *(60)*.

further reduced the RVERP to values below those obtained in the drug-free state. In addition, isoproterenol reduced the $RVERP/APD_{90}$ ratio, suggesting that the reductions in refractoriness were due, in part, to mechanisms beyond simply shortening the APD_{90}. The reduction in the sustained VT cycle length by isoproterenol might permit transformation of a hemodynamically stable arrhythmia to an unstable tachycardia. Thus, it appears that the electrophysiologic actions of a pure I_{K_1} blocker may be fully reversed during sympathetic stimulation.

Amiodarone

The ability of isoproterenol to modulate amiodarone-induced effects on electrophysiologic parameters was examined in 22 patients *(60)*. Amiodarone significantly increased the sinus cycle length of baseline values (768±26 ms to 871±33 ms) and isoproterenol significantly decreased the sinus cycle by 28% during amiodarone therapy. Thus at the level of the sinus node, the overall reduction in the sinus cycle by isoproterenol was similar to that observed in patients receiving sematilide (266 ms vs 246 ms). However, in contrast to the data with sematilide, amiodarone-induced prolongation of repolarization was attenuated, but not reversed, during isoproterenol administration. In fact, the APD_{90} remained significantly prolonged during isoproterenol administration (Fig. 10) by 4–8 ms at each paced cycle compared to baseline drug-free values (p=.005). In contrast to sematilide, the effects of isoproterenol on refractoriness were similar to those observed on repolarization and changes in the $RVERP/APD_{90}$ ratio were not observed. Interesting, when effects on the paced QRS duration were examined, isoproterenol significantly reduced the QRS duration compared to amiodarone alone by a relatively fixed amount at each cycle length (4–6% reduction, p=005), suggesting that isoproterenol increased the rapid inward sodium current *(61,62)* by a relatively fixed amount. When the effects on morphologically similar VTs were examined, amiodarone significantly prolonged the induced sustained VT cycle length (257±12 ms to 363±19 ms [p < .001] and isoproterenol significantly reduced the sustained VT cycle length to a mean of 329 milliseconds, a value significantly longer than those obtained at baseline [p < .001]). Thus, while some shortening of the VT cycling was observed during isoproterenol administration, the sustained VT cycle length remained significantly prolonged during catecholamine infusion and thus amiodarone might still protect a patient from developing hemodynamically unstable VT during sympathetic stimulation.

Amiodarone's resistance to reversal of the electrophysiologic effects of catecholamine administration are likely multifactorial. Amiodarone nonselectively blocks multiple potassium currents and partial blockade of I_{Ks} (which is increased by catecholamines) may account for some of this resistance. Amiodarone's noncompetitive antiadrenergic effects may also play an important role, though at the level of the sinus node sympathetic stimulation resulted in a significant decrease in heart rate. It has been suggested that adding a beta-blocker to amiodarone may result in a more beneficial patient outcome, and would be expected to further attenuate the effects of catecholamines. The CAMIAT *(63)* and EMIAT *(64)* post-MI trials provided post hoc analyses demonstrating that the greatest benefit on reducing post-MI mortality was observed in patients who received both a beta-blocker and amiodarone.

D,l-Sotalol

In a separate series of experiments, isoproterenol was administered to a cohort of 17 patients receiving d,l-sotalol *(65)*. Isoproterenol only mildly attenuated the drug's effects on repolarization and failed to have an effect on d,l-sotalol induced increases on the RVERP or the $RVERP/APD_{90}$ ratio (Fig. 11). Isoproterenol also had no significant effect on the modest increases in sustained VT cycle length observed during d,l-sotalol administration, compared to the baseline drug-free state. Thus d,l-sotalol was more resistant to amiodarone and sematilide during isoproterenol administration, presumably demonstrating the beneficial effects of more potent beta blockade. Pertinent to the study, Groh

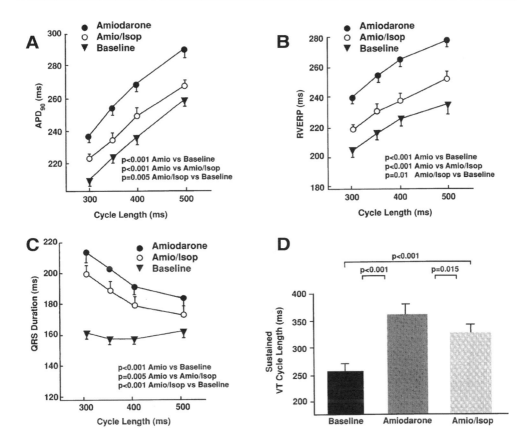

Fig. 10. Graphs show the frequency-dependent effects of amiodarone and amiodarone plus iso-proterenol on electrophysiologic parameters. (**A**) Amiodarone induced prolongation of the APD_{90} was attenuated by isoproterenol but remained significantly prolonged compared to baseline values. (**B**) Amiodarone-induced prolongation of the RVERP was attenuated by isoproterenol but remained significantly prolonged compared to baseline values. (**C**) Plot shows the effects on the conduction as determined by the QRS duration. Isoproterenol administration during amiodarone significantly decreased the QRS duration by a fixed amount of 4–6% independent of the paced cycle length. (**D**) The effects on the sustained ventricular tachycardia (VT) cycle length. The sustained VT cycle length was increased by amiodarone by 107 ms (42%) and decreased by isoproterenol by 34 ms (9%). However, during isoproterenol administration, the sustained VT cycle length still remained markedly prolonged compared with baseline drug-free values (70 ms, 27%). Modified by permission of the American Heart Association and the authors from *(60)*.

et al. *(66)* examined the effects of high dose isoproterenol on myocytes exposed to d,l-sotalol or d-sotalol. D,l-sotalol was significantly more resistant to reversal in this experimental protocol than was d-sotalol. D,l-sotalol demonstrated significantly greater block of repolarizing currents, as compared to d-sotalol, during catecholamine challenge. Studies of whole cell current recordings demonstrated that significant increases in I_{CL} and I_{Ks} overcame blockade of I_{Kr} in the d-sotalol treated myocytes. It appeared that the beta blocking activity associated with the racemic sotalol preparation prevented these increases in repolarizing currents.

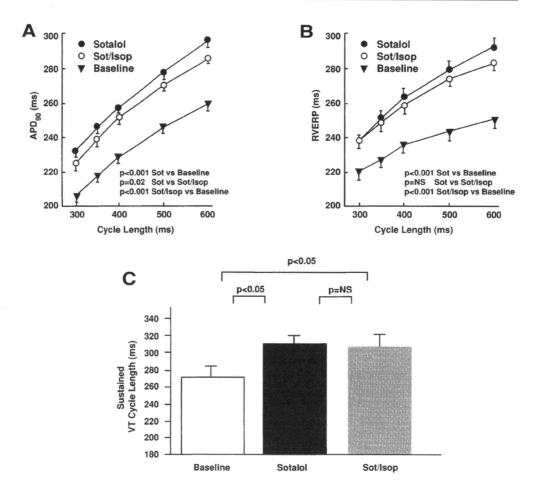

Fig. 11. Graphs show that frequency-dependent effects of d,L-sotalol and d,l-sotalol plus isoproterenol (ISOP) on repolarization (APD$_{90}$, **A**), the right ventricular refractory period (RVERP, **B**), and the sustained VT cycle length (**C**). D,l-sotalol prolonged the APD$_{90}$ without frequency-dependent effects and the drug's effects on repolarization were only mildly attenuated by isoproterenol. D,l-sotalol's effects on the RVERP demonstrated reverse frequency-dependence and overall, isoproterenol's effects on the d,l-sotalol-induced RVERP prolongation were not significant. Sotalol modestly increased the sustained VT cycle length by 32 ms (12%, $p<0.05$). During concomitant administration of isoproterenol the VT cycle length remained unchanged and it remained significantly prolonged compared with baseline drug-free values. Modified with permission of the authors from *(42)*.

CONCLUSIONS

The use of monophasic action potential recordings has permitted the accurate assessment of repolarization in humans and allowed determination of how repolarization is altered by heart rate, ischemia, antiarrhythmic drugs, and sympathetic stimulation. Specifically, ischemia has been shown to shorten repolarization and to increase dispersion within the human ventricle. Different antiarrhythmic agents have varying frequency-dependent effects on repolarization and conduction, which may affect their efficacy and tendency to cause proarrhythmia. Sympathetic stimulation can significantly modify the effects of antiarrhythmic agents on the action potential duration and reverse the beneficial effects of some antiarrhythmic agents. The autonomic nervous system's modulation of Class 3 drug effects is likely to be clinically important.

ACKNOWLEDGMENT

The author wishes to thank Ms. Marcie Aboff for her expert editorial assistance.

REFERENCES

1. Franz MR, Burkhoff D, Spurgeon H, Weisfeldt ML, Lakatta EG. In vitro validation of a new cardiac catheter technique for recording monophasic action potentials. Eur Heart J 1986;7:34–41.
2. Franz MR, Swerdlow CD, Liem LB, Schaefer J. Cycle length dependence of human action potential duration in vivo. Effects of single extrastimuli, sudden sustained rate acceleration and deceleration, and different steady-state frequencies. J Clin Invest 1988;82:972–979.
3. Franz MR, Chin MC, Sharkey HR, Griffin JC, Scheinman MM. A new single catheter technique for simultaneous measurement of action potential duration and refractory period in vivo. J Am Coll Cardiol 1990;16:878–886.
4. Anderson KP, Lux RA, Dustman T. Comparison of QRS morphologies of spontaneous premature ventricular complexes and ventricular tachycardia induced by programmed stimulation. Am Heart J 1990;1:1302–1311.
5. Talajic M, Villemaire C, Nattel S. Electrophysiological effects of alpha-adrenergic stimulation. PACE 1990;13:578–582.
6. Hopson JR, Kienzle MG, Aschoff AM, Shirkey DR. Noninvasive prediction of efficacy of type IA antiarrhythmic drugs by the signal-averaged electrocardiogram in patients with coronary artery disease and sustained ventricular tachycardia. Am J Cardiol 1993;72:288–293.
7. Talajic M, Nattel S, Davies M, McCans J. Attenuation of class 3 and sinus node effects of amiodarone by experimental hypothyroidism. J Cardiovasc Pharmacol 1989;13:447–450.
8. Mason JW, Anderson KP, Freedman RA. Techniques and criteria in electrophysiologic study of ventricular tachycardia. Circulation 1987;75:III125–III133.
9. Nattel S. Relationship between use-dependent effects of antiarrhythmic drugs on conduction and Vmax in canine cardiac Purkinje fibers. J Pharmacol Exp Ther 1987;241:282–288.
10. Shrier A, Dubarsky H, Rosengarten M, Guevara MR, Nattel S, Glass L. Prediction of complex atrioventricular conduction rhythms in humans with use of the atrioventricular nodal recovery curve. Circulation 1987;76:16–205.
11. Duan D, Fermini B, Nattel S. Potassium channel blocking properties of propafenone in rabbit atrial myocytes. J Pharmacol Exp Ther 1993;264:1113–1123.
12. Hopson JR, Kienzle MG. Evaluation of patients with syncope. Separating the 'wheat' from the 'chaff.' Postgrad Med 1992;91:321–328,333,336.
13. Hohnloser SH, Lange HW, Raeder EA, Podrid PJ, Lown B. Short- and long-term therapy with tocainide for malignant ventricular tachyarrhythmias. Circulation 1986;73:143–149.
14. Sager PT. How to record high-quality monophasic avtion potential recordings. Franz MR, ed. Monophasic Action Potentials: Bridging Cell and Bedside. 2002;1[7]:121–135. Armonk, NY: Futura.
15. Subramanian R, Sager P, Shalaby A. Rate-related changes in cardiac repolarization: QT interval versus monophasic action potential duration (Abstract). J Am Coll Cardiol 1999;33:135A.
16. Zabel M, Franz MR, Klingenheben T, Mansion B, Schultheiss HP, Hohnloser SH. Rate-dependence of QT dispersion and the QT interval: comparison of atrial pacing and exercise testing. J Am Coll Cardiol 2000;36[5]:1654–1658.
17. Bazett HC. An analysis of the time-relations of electrocardiograms. Heart 1920;7:353–370.
18. Malik M, Farbom P, Batchvarov V, Hnatkova K, Camm AJ. Relation between QT and RR intervals is highly individual among healthy subjects: implications for heart rate correction of the QT interval. Heart 2002;87[3]:220–228.

19. Sager PT, Nademanee K, Antimisiaris M, et al. Antiarrhythmic effects of selective prolongation of refractoriness. Electrophysiologic actions of sematilide HCl in humans. Circulation 1993;88:1072–1082.

20. Sager PT, Uppal P, Follmer C, Antimisiaris M, Pruitt C, Singh BN. Frequency-dependent electrophysiologic effects of amiodarone in humans. Circulation 1993;88:1063–1071.

21. Malik M. Problems of heart rate correction in assessment of drug-induced QT interval prolongation. J Cardiovasc Electrophysiol 2001;12[4]:411–420.

22. John RM, Taggart PI, Sutton PM, Costa DC, Ell PJ, Swanton H. Endocardial monophasic action potential recordings for the detection of myocardial ischemia in man: a study using atrial pacing stress and myocardial perfusion scintigraphy. Am Heart J 1991;122[6]:1599–1609.

23. John RM, Taggart PI, Sutton PM, Ell PJ, Swanton H. Direct effect of dobutamine on action potential duration in ischemic compared with normal areas in the human ventricle. J Am Coll Cardiol 1992; 20[4]:896–903.

24. Sager PT. New advances in class III antiarrhythmic drug therapy. Curr Opin Cardiol 2000; 15[1]:41–53.

25. Girouard SD, Pastore JM, Laurita KR, Gregory KW, Rosenbaum DS. Optical mapping in a new guinea pig model of ventricular tachycardia reveals mechanisms for multiple wavelengths in a single reentrant circuit. Circulation 1996;93[3]:603–613.

26. Hondeghem LM, Snyders DJ. Class III antiarrhythmic agents have a lot of potential but a long way to go. Reduced effectiveness and dangers of reverse use dependence. Circulation 1990;81:686–690.

27. Nattel S, Zeng FD. Frequency-dependent effects of antiarrhythmic drugs on action potential duration and refractoriness of canine cardiac Purkinje fibers. J Pharmacol Exp Ther 1984;229:283–291.

28. Schmitt C, Beyer T, Karch M, et al. Sotalol exhibits reverse use-dependent action on monophasic action potentials in normal but not in infarcted canine ventricular myocardium. J Cardiovasc Pharmacol 1992;19[4]:487–492.

29. Laurita KR, Girouard SD, Rudy Y, Rosenbaum DS. Role of passive electrical properties during action potential restitution in intact heart. Am J Physiol 1997;273[3 Pt 2]:H1205–H1214.

30. Kiehn J, Wible B, Ficker E, Taglialatela M, Brown AM. Cloned human inward rectifier K+ channel as a target for class III methanesulfonanilides. Circ Res 1995;77[6]:1151–1155.

31. Sager PT. New antiarrhythmic agents. Electrophys Board Rev 1998.

32. Jurkiewicz NK, Sanguinetti MC. Rate-dependent prolongation of cardiac action potentials by a methanesulfonanilide class III antiarrhythmic agent. Specific block of rapidly activating delayed rectifier K+ current by dofetilide. Circ Res 1993;72:75–83.

33. Sager PT. The frequency-dependent effects of dofetilide in humans (Abstract). Circulation 1995; 92:1–774.

34. Ranger S, Talajic M, Lemery R, Roy D, Villemaire C, Nattel S. Kinetics of use-dependent ventricular conduction slowing by antiarrhythmic drugs in humans. Circulation 1991;83:1987–1994.

35. Gjini V, Schreieck J, Korth M, Weyerbrock S, Schomig A, Schmitt C. Frequency dependence in the action of the class III antiarrhythmic drug dofetilide is modulated by altering L-type calcium current and digitalis glucoside. J Cardiovasc Pharmacol 1998;31[1]:95–100.

36. Stroobandt R, Brachmann J, Bourgeois I, Wielders P, Kubler W, Senges J. Simultaneous recording of atrial and ventricular monophasic action potentials: monophasic action potential duration during atrial pacing, ventricular pacing, and ventricular fibrillation. PACE 1985;8:502–511.

37. Li GR, Nattel S. Properties of human atrial ICa at physiological temperatures and relevance to action potential. Am J Physiol 1997;272[1 Pt 2]:H227–H235.

38. Sedgwick ML, Rasmussen HS, Cobb SM. Effects of the class III antiarrhythmic drug dofetilide on ventricular monophasic action potential duration and QT interval dispersion in stable angina pectoris. Am J Cardiol 1992;70;1432–1437.

39. Yuan S, Wohlfart B, Rasmussen HS, Olsson S, Blomstrom-Lundqvist C. Effect of dofetilide on cardiac repolarization in patients with ventricular tachycardia. A study using simultaneous monophasic action potential recordings from two sites in the right ventricle. Eur Heart J 1994;15[4]:514–522.

40. Sager PT, Singh BN. Electrophysiological and pharmacodynamic profile of sematilide HCL. Singh BN, Wellens HJJ, Hiraoka M, eds. Electropharmacological Control of Cardiac Arrhythmias. Mt. Kisco, NY: Futura Publishing Co., Inc., 1994;1:525–534.

41. Lee KS, Tsai TD, Lee EW. Membrane activity of class III antiarrhythmic compounds; a comparison between ibutilide, d-sotalol, E-4031, sematilide and dofetilide. Eur J Pharmacol 1993;234[1]:43–53.

42. Sager PT, Behboodikhah M. Frequency-dependent electrophysiologic effects of d,l-sotalol and quinidine and modulation by beta-adrenergic stimulation. J Cardiovasc Electrophysiol 1996; 7[2]: 102–112.

43. Schmitt C, Brachmann J, Karch M, Waldecker B, Navarette L, Montero M, Beyer T, Kubler W. Reverse use-dependent effects of sotalol demonstrated by recording monophasic action potentials of the right ventricle. Am J Cardiol 1991;68:1183–1187.

44. Montero M, Beyer T, Schmitt C, Kubler W, Brachmann J. Differential effects of quinidine on transmembrane action potentials of normal and infarcted canine Purkinje fibers. J Cardiovasc Pharmacol 1992; 20[2]:304–310.

45. Huikuri HV, Yli-Mayry S. Frequency dependent effects of d-sotalol and amiodarone on the action potential duration of the human right ventricle. Pacing Clin Electrophysiol 1992;15[11 Pt 2]:2103–2107.

46. Anderson KP, Walker R, Dustman T, et al. Rate-related electrophysiologic effects of long-term administration of amiodarone on canine ventricular myocardium in vivo. Circulation 1989;79:948–958.

47. Schmitt C, Karch M, Schreieck J, Weyerbrock S, Plewan A, Schneider MA. Effects of the new class III antiarrhythmic agent ambasilide on monophasic and transmembrane action potential in human ventricular myocardium (Abstract). PACE 1996;19:692.

48. Weyerbrock S, Schreieck J, Karch M, et al. Rate-independent effects of the new class III antiarrhythmic agent ambasilide on transmembrane action potentials in human ventricular endomyocardium. J Cardiovasc Pharmacol 1997;30[5]:571–575.

49. Bargheer K, Bode F, Klein HU, Trappe HJ, Franz MR, Lichtlen PR. Prolongation of monophasic action potential duration and the refractory period in the human heart by tedisamil, a new potassium-blocking agent. Eur Heart J 1994;15[10]:1409–1414.

50. Yusuf S, Wittes J, Friedman L. Overview of results of randomized clinical trials in heart disease. I. Treatments following myocardial infarction. JAMA 1988;260:2088–2093.

51. Olsson G, Rehnqvist N, Sjogren A, Erhardt L, Lundman T. Long-term treatment with metoprolol after myocardial infarction: effect on 3 year mortality and morbidity. J Am Coll Cardiol 1985;5:1428–1437.

52. Parker GW, Michael LH, Hartley CJ, Skinner JE, Entman ML. Central - adrenergic mechanisms may modulate ischemic ventricular fibrillation in pigs. Circ Res 1990;66:259–270.

53. Jazayeri MR, Van Wyhe G, Avitall B, McKinnie J, Tchou P, Akhtar M. Isoproterenol reversal of antiarrhythmic effects in patients with inducible sustained ventricular tachyarrhythmias. J Am Coll Cardiol 1989;14:705–704.

54. Calkins H, Sousa J, el-Atassi R, Schmaltz S, Kadish A, Morady F. Reversal of antiarrhythmic drug effects by epinephrine: quinidine versus amiodarone [see comments]. J Am Coll Cardiol 1992;347–352.

55. Morady F, Kou WH, Kadish AH, Toivonen LK, Kushner JA, Schmaltz S. Effects of epinephrine in patients with an accessory atrioventricular connection treated with quinidine. Am J Cardiol 1988;62: 580–584.

56. Sanguinetti MC, Jurkiewicz NK, Scott A, Siegl PK. Isoproterenol antagonizes prolongation of refractory period by the class III antiarrhythmic agent E-4031 in guinea pig myocytes. Mechanism of action. Circ Res 1991;68:77–84.

57. Harvey RD, Hume JR. Autonomic regulation of a chloride current in heart. Science 1989;244:983–985.

58. Boyett NR, Fedida D. Changes in the electrical activity of dog purkinje fibers at high heart rates. J Physiol (Lond) 1984;350:361–391.

59. Vanoli E, Priori SG, Nakagawa H, et al. Sympathetic activation, ventricular repolarization and Ikr blockade: implications for the antifibrillatory efficacy of potassium channel blocking agents. J Am Coll Cardiol 1995;25[7]:1609–1614.

60. Sager PT, Follmer C, Uppal P, Pruitt C, Godfrey R. The effects of beta-adrenergic stimulation on the frequency-dependent electrophysiologic actions of amiodarone and sematilide. Circulation 1994; 90:1811–1819.

61. Matsuda JJ, Lee H, Shibata EF. Enhancement of rabbit cardiac sodium channels by beta-adrenergic stimulation. Circ Res 1992;70:199–207.

62. Lee HC, Matsuda JJ, Reynertson SI, Martins JB, Shibata EF. Reversal of lidocaine effects on sodium currents by isoproterenol in rabbit hearts and heart cells. J Clin Invest 1993;91:693–701.

63. Cairns JA, Connolly SJ, Roberts R, Gent M. Randomised trial of outcome after myocardial infarction in patients with frequent or repetitive ventricular premature depolarisations: CAMIAT. Canadian Amiodarone Myocardial Infarction Arrhythmia Trial Investigators. Lancet 1997;349[9053]:675–682.

64. Julian DG, Camm AJ, Frangin G, et al. Randomised trial of effect of amiodarone on mortality in patients with left-ventricular dysfunction after recent myocardial infarction: EMIAT. European Myocardial Infarct Amiodarone Trial. Lancet 1997;349[9053]:667–674.

65. Nayebpour M, Talajic M, Villemaire C, Nattel S. Vagal modulation of the rate-dependent properties of the atrioventricular node. Circ Res 1990;67:1152–1166.

66. Groh WJ, Gibson KJ, McAnulty JH, Maylie JG. Beta-adrenergic blocking property of dl-sotalol maintains class III efficacy in guinea pig ventricular muscle after isoproterenol. Circulation 1995; 91:262–264.

14 QT Interval and Its Drug-Induced Prolongation

Wojciech Zareba, MD, PhD,
and Arthur J. Moss, MD

CONTENTS

INTRODUCTION

QT interval prolongation may result from an inherited channelopathy, the long QT syndrome (LQTS), or can be induced by drugs, abnormal electrolyte/metabolic disorders, or other conditions affecting myocardial repolarization *(1–5)*. The LQTS is characterized by prolongation of the QT interval on the electrocardiogram and is associated with an increased propensity to ventricular tachyarrhythmias, that can lead to cardiac events such as syncope, cardiac arrest, or sudden death *(1,2)*. Over the last few decades, clinical observations in LQTS patients as well as clinical and basic science research have led to a better understanding of the role of repolarization in cardiac arrhythmias and cardiac electrophysiology.

Torsades de pointes (TdP) ventricular tachycardia has been recognized as the pathognomonic arrhythmia in congenital forms of LQTS *(1)*. In LQTS patients, the risk of TdP increases significantly with increasing QT interval duration indicating that more advanced repolarization abnormalities lead to more frequent arrhythmias. TdP may also occur with drug-induced delayed repolarization where QT prolongation is considered as a marker or harbinger of proarrhythmic effects of medication *(4)*. Both cardiac and non-cardiac drugs may cause TdP, that may degenerate into ventricular fibrillation and lead to cardiac death *(5)*.

From: *Contemporary Cardiology: Cardiac Repolarization: Bridging Basic and Clinical Science*
Edited by: I. Gussak et al. © Humana Press Inc., Totowa, NJ

In this chapter we aim to provide an overview of current concepts on ventricular repolarization and its pathophysiology especially pertinent to effects of drugs on repolarization, describe clinical and electrocardiographic aspects of QT interval analysis, and clinical and regulatory issues related to drug-induced repolarization abnormalities.

VENTRICULAR REPOLARIZATION

Long QT Syndrome and Identification of Ion Channels that Regulate Ventricular Repolarization

During the last few years, mutations in specific genes encoding cardiac ion channels have been identified in patients with congenital form of LQTS *(3,6)*. These mutations cause alterations in the ion channel proteins leading to abnormalities in ion channel function that prolong ventricular repolarization (Fig. 1). The KVLQT1 (LQT1) gene encodes a potassium channel protein (α-subunit) that when coexpressed with a protein (β-subunit) from the minK (KCNE1; LQT5) gene produces a reduction in the slowly activating, delayed rectifier (repolarizing) potassium current (I_{Ks}). The reduction in I_{Kr} (rapidly activating delayed rectifier) current is caused by mutations in HERG (LQT2) gene regulating the major pore-forming subunit or by mutations in the MiRP1 (LQT6) gene coding putative regulatory subunit of I_{Kr} channel. The SCN5A (LQT3) sodium channel gene mutations cause abnormal inactivation of sodium channel with an inward leakage of sodium ions during repolarization phase contributing to QT prolongation. Only about half of genetically tested patients have mutations found on one of those genes. It is estimated that among patients with known genotype, LQT1 and LQT2 account for the majority (87%) of cases of congenital LQTS, LQT3 accounts for 8%, whereas LQT5 and LQT6 are extremely rare accounting for less than 5% of LQTS cases *(6)*.

Ion Channel Function and Arrhythmogenesis

Identification of specific gene mutations and functional studies of kinetics of ion channels, with their expression in *Xenopus* oocytes or transfected human kidney cells, have provided better understanding of physiology of ion channels and repolarization processes. The physiology of ion channels and associated arrhythmogenic mechanisms are described in other chapters of this book. Here we emphasize the importance of these findings for drug-mediated repolarization abnormalities and arrhythmias.

Although dysfunctions of different ion channels were found to cause inherited forms of LQTS, the HERG channel conducting I_{Kr}, the rapid delayed rectifier current, seems to play a critical role in drug-induced QT prolongation and TdP *(7,8)*. Numerous drugs including some antiarrhythmics, antihistamine, antibiotics, psychotropic, and gastrointestinal prokinetic drugs have been found to block I_{Kr}. The reason for so many different drugs blocking the same channel is found in a different molecular structure and dysfunction of the channel caused by prolonged entrapment of drug molecules in the channel cavity leading to enhanced binding affinity of the drug to the sites in the channel *(7)*. The other potassium channels have protective mechanism (a proline-X-proline sequence in S6 domain) that reduces volume of the channel cavity precluding drug molecules to be trapped there. The HERG channel does not have proline residues in S6 location and therefore this channel is more prone to bind drug molecules inside the channel with subsequent blocking of the channel and reduction in I_{Kr} current. Since not all drugs that block I_{Kr} produce TdP, other mechanisms might be involved in proarrhythmic response

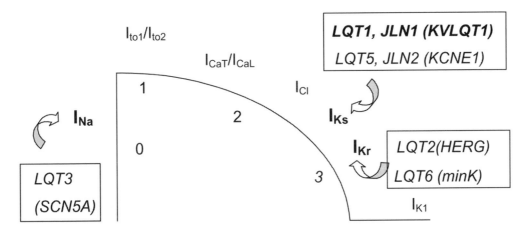

Fig. 1. LQTS genes coding cardiac ion channel genes responsible for conduction of potassium and sodium currents.

including other actions of the drugs. Amiodarone and verapamil are examples of I_{Kr} blockers that are not associated with increased risk of TdP possibly owing to concomitant blocking calcium channels or homogenous prolongation of repolarization in various layers of myocardium.

Transmural dispersion of repolarization seems to play the most important role in arrhythmogenesis in both drug-mediated and congenital forms of LQTS *(9,10)*. There is a physiologic transmural dispersion of repolarization with M cells showing the longest action potential duration, epicardial cells the shortest, and endocardial cells intermediate action potential duration. The magnitude of this physiologic transmural dispersion of repolarization is not sufficient to cause conditions leading to TdP, unless there is selective prolongation of action potential in one of the layers (M cells) owing to action of drugs or to specific genetic mutation. This excessive prolongation increases magnitude of transmural gradient of repolarization, which may cause functional block and reentry in response to a premature beat *(9,10)*.

QT INTERVAL

QT Interval Measurement

The QT interval measured on the ECG is used in clinical medicine to assess global repolarization duration. Although QT interval includes QRS complex (representing ventricular depolarization), the entire QT interval is considered as a measure of repolarization since repolarization process already takes place during QRS complex for early activated regions of myocardium. The QT interval is measured from the onset of QRS complex to the offset of T wave, defined as a deflection point terminating the descending arm of the T wave, usually at the level (or slightly above) isoelectric line. In the presence of separate U wave, QT is measured till the nadir between T and U waves. More difficult situation occurs when T and U waves are merged or when the T wave has a bifid appearance with two components of the T wave. Figure 2 shows different repolarization patterns

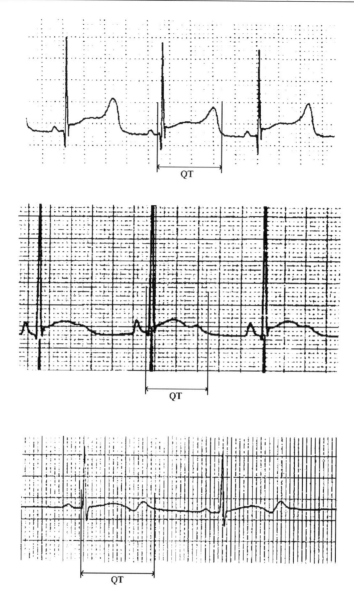

Fig. 2. Examples of complex repolarization patterns with identification of QT intervals.

with respective QT interval identification. In the complex repolarization morphologies some investigators consider the second component of T wave as an enhanced U wave. However, there is no evidence that U waves could reach such proportions. Rather heterogeneous repolarization patterns can contribute to repolarization abnormalities resulting in complex ECG morphologies. The issue of standardization of QT interval measurements has not been solved since a landmark 1952 paper of Lepeschkin and Surawicz *(11)*.

Lead Selection and Interlead Differences in QT Duration

A pertinent question is what lead is the most suitable for QT interval measurement in a 12-lead ECG. The optimal approach should take into account the earliest onset of QRS

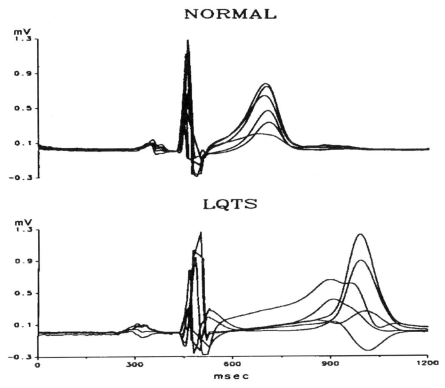

Fig. 3. Superimposition of T waves from precordial leads in normal subject and in a LQTS patient illustrates dispersion of repolarization morphology. Reprinted with permission from *(13)*.

complex in any of 12 leads and the latest offset of T wave in any of the 12 leads, reflecting global duration of repolarization process. This approach is rarely exercised in manual measurements since it is time consuming and in most cases does not provide major benefit on top of routine measurements done in lead II. However, in some cases with borderline QT prolongation careful investigation of repolarization duration and morphology in all leads might help identify QT prolongation and repolarization abnormalities.

Because QT duration varies among recorded leads, the concept of QT dispersion has been applied during the last decade in many research studies with some studies confirming its prognostic value for predicting cardiac events and other studies negating such an association *(12)*. Because of conceptual and methodological limitations of the QT dispersion, this method has not been approved as a standard tool in clinical practice or in drug studies. QT dispersion does provide supportive information about repolarization abnormalities related to nonhomogenous spread of repolarization throughout myocardium. However, manual methods of quantification of QT dispersion show poor reproducibility. Interlead differences in repolarization morphology rather than just QT duration seem to better reflect complexity of repolarization process *(13–15)*. They could be presented in a graphical form showing a superimposition of several leads (Fig. 3) allowing for visualization of heterogeneity of repolarization morphology *(13)*. Interlead differences in repolarization morphology could be quantified utilizing various methods including principal component analysis, area-based analysis of repolarization segment, and other methods. Principal component analysis of the repolarization segment allows quantifying the length (λ1) and width (λ2) of T-wave loop *(14,15)*. The roundness of the T-loop in its preferential plane (λ2/λ1) has been considered as an index of increased T-wave complexity.

Heart Rate Correction of QT Duration

QT duration depends on heart rate and heart rate correction of QT interval is routinely used in clinical practice. In 1920, Bazett described curvilinear association between QT and RR interval and the formula based on his observation (QTc=QT/[RR$^{1/2}$]) is the most frequently used *(16)*. This formula aims to adjust QT interval to the conditions seen for heart rate of 60 bpm. Bazett's QTc formula has limitations of overestimating repolarization duration at fast heart rates and underestimating it at slow heart rates. Subsequently numerous different QTc formulae were proposed and exercised including:

— Fridericia *(17)* *[QT and RR in seconds]:* QTc = QT/RR$^{1/3}$
— Framingham *(18)* *[QT and RR in seconds]:* QTc = QT + 0.154(1 – RR)
— Hodges *(19)* *[QT in seconds]*: QTc = QT + 1.75 (heart rate – 60)
— Rautaharju *(20)* *[QT in milliseconds]:*
    for all females and males <15 and >50 years:
    QTI = QT(HR + 100)/656 ms
    for males 15–50 years:

$$QTI = \frac{100 \times QT}{(656 / (1 + 0.01 HR)) + 0.4\,age - 25}$$

— Karjalainen *(21)* *[QT and RR in milliseconds]*
    for HR<60 $QT_{Nc} = (QT \times 392)/(0.116RR + 277)$
    for HR 60–99 $QT_{Nc} = (QT \times 392)/(0.156RR + 236)$
    for HR ≥100 $QT_{Nc} = (QT \times 392)/(0.384RR + 99)$

All of these formulas tend to adjust well for QT-RR association, however, each has some limitations. Generally speaking, QTc formulae provide good estimation of QT duration at heart rates close to the normal resting range of 55–75 beats per minute (bpm) as observed in the vast majority of ECGs. However, below and above those limits there could be room for misclassification of QTc value. ECGs with heart rates below 55 bpm or above 75–80 bpm are usually recorded using Holter recordings, exercise testing, bedside or event monitors; for those heart rates, QTc correction could be replaced by the analysis of repolarization duration using formulae other than the Bazett correction. Fridericia (cubic) formula is of preference owing to its simplicity of application, although other more complex formulae including Rautaharju's or Karjalajnen's could be used. The problem is that there is insufficient amount of data to determine normal values of QTc utilizing those approaches, including Fridericia.

When comparing ECGs recorded off and on drug, one could utilize other approaches including the analysis of QT for matched RR intervals, QT-RR regression analysis represented by the slope of this relationship, and subject-specific QT-RR relationship plots. When dealing with 24-Holter recordings, identification of matched RR intervals for recordings off and on drugs is frequently possible, and this approach seems to be preferable since it eliminates the need for mathematical correction of QT duration *(22)*. Rarely the drug has major effect on heart rate and makes such a comparison impossible. When performing the analysis of matched RR intervals, ECG data should be analyzed while accounting for circadian rhythm of heart rate and QT duration, (i.e., matched RR intervals off and on drugs should come from separate day or night periods but not mixed together).

The slope of QT-RR relationship has been found to distinguish patients with and without long QT syndrome and therefore this approach could be used to evaluate the effect of the drug on repolarization across various heart rates (23,24). The slope of QT-RR regression line reflects QT dynamicity of repolarization, which could be altered by a disease process or by action of a drug. Therefore the use of this approach is worth considering especially for drugs substantially changing the heart rate.

Since the pattern of RR and QT varies between subjects, French investigators proposed the concept of individual subject-specific QT-RR relationship to study changes in repolarization (25). Recently, Malik et al. (26) promoted the concept of using subject-specific QT-RR relationship to study drug-induced changes in repolarization. Although this approach is interesting it has some practical limitations including labor-intensive and time-consuming analysis.

Automatic Methods for QT Interval Measurements

Increasing use of digital ECG recordings and FDA requirements to submit ECG data from drug studies in digital format make the use of automatic methods of QT analysis more desirable (27,28). There are different methods to automatically identify T wave offset, of which the tangent method is the most popular one. Although fitting tangent to the descending arm of positive T wave (or ascending arm of negative T wave) works well for T waves of normal morphology and normal amplitude, the tangent method is not robust in cases with flat, bifid, or biphasic T waves. The identification of T-wave endpoints using first and second derivatives to ascertain when the repolarization curve crossing the zero line could help in more difficult repolarization patterns. The other approach may consist of an area-based method for quantifying total repolarization duration by measuring the time needed to accumulate a percentage of the T-wave area (29,30). The presence of biphasic T wave, U wave and notched T waves does not affect the accuracy of area-based repolarization measurement, and these time-dependent area parameters may be more robust than the standard QT interval measurements. The time interval from the QRS onset to the time where 90% of the total T-wave area (QT_{A90}) is reached is one of the automatic area-based parameters reflecting QT duration. At present, only limited normative data exist for this parameter.

It is worth emphasizing that automatic QT and QTc measurements provided by ECG manufacturers' algorithms and printed on paper copies of ECG should not be taken for granted. The automatic algorithms operate relatively well in case of normal T-wave morphology, but they are totally unreliable in cases with more complex and abnormal T-wave morphologies. Moreover, automatic algorithms used by different ECG manufacturers utilize different methodology and algorithms for measuring QT interval and therefore they cannot be used uniformly both in clinical practice and in drug studies. There is always a need for validation of automatic QT measurements by an experienced ECG reader.

Normal QTc Values for Age and Gender

QT interval duration varies with age and gender. Table 1 shows proposed normal and abnormal QTc values (using Bazett heart rate correction) by age and gender (31). Women and children have longer duration of repolarization than men.

Table 1
QTc Values by Age and Gender

QTc value (sec)	Children 1–15 yr	Men	Women
Normal	<0.44	<0.43	<0.45
Borderline	0.44–0.46	0.43–0.45	0.45–0.46
Prolonged	>0.46	>0.45	>0.46

Adapted with permission from (31).

Similar observations were reported by Rautaharju et al. (20) indicating that sex-related difference is because of shorter QT duration in men than women at age 15–55 yr, not because of QT prolongation in women (Fig. 4). Suggested factors influencing these differences may include different density of potassium ion channels in male vs females myocardium, effect of female hormones contributing to longer QT duration in women, or possibly effect of male hormones and lower heart rate in men contributing to their shorter QT duration. Sex-related differences in repolarization are also observed for parameters describing T-wave morphology with men having a steeper ascending arm of the T wave than women (32).

Longer QTc duration in women predisposes them to more frequent arrhythmic events in congenital LQTS and acquired forms of QT prolongation. In both circumstances, women account for about 70% of cases of cardiac events, usually from TdP. Several reports describing drug-induced TdP and QTc prolongation demonstrate predominance of women, and female sex is considered as one of risk factors for proarrhythmia.

Relationship Between QT Prolongation and Arrhythmic Risk

Clinical studies of LQTS patients demonstrate (Fig. 5) that risk of arrhythmic events is significantly associated with QT prolongation (1,33). For every 10 ms increase of QTc duration there is 5% exponential increase of the risk of cardiac events (1). Therefore, a patient showing increase in QTc duration from 440 ms to 500 ms has a 34% increase in the risk of cardiac events (60 ms difference indicates $1.05^6 = 1.34$). However, LQTS experience shows that cardiac events can also occur in patients with normal or borderline QTc duration. Genotype-phenotype correlations indicate that about a third of LQTS carriers has normal or borderline QTc values (3). These observations indicate that the magnitude of QTc duration is not the sole factor when evaluating the risk of arrhythmic events, or that lack of QTc prolongation indicates absence of risk of cardiac events. The same logic applies to drug-induced QTc prolongation. Although QTc duration above 500 ms or prolongation by more than 60 ms in response to a drug indicates increased risk of TdP, some drugs may cause smaller QT prolongation which, in suitable conditions (stress, tachycardia, ventricular premature beats with short-long-short series), could lead to TdP (34).

It is noteworthy that not all drugs causing QTc prolongation are arrhythmogenic. Amiodarone is an example of such a drug, for it causes QTc prolongation with minimal evidence for drug-induced TdP. The reason for lack of proarrhythmic effects of certain drugs that prolong the QT interval may be owing to homogenous prolongation of repolarization throughout endocardial, M-cell, and epicardial layers. Whereas drugs that

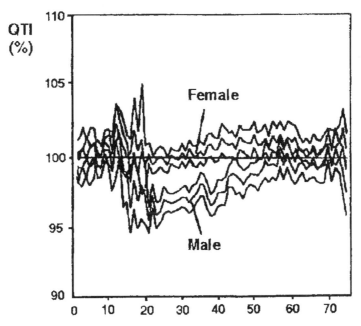

Fig. 4. Age- and sex-related pattern of QTI (QT index by Rautaharju). Reprinted with permission from *(20)*.

prolong QTc duration and cause arrhythmias seem to selectively prolong repolarization in one layer (usually M-cell zone) contributing to transmural heterogeneity of repolarization (and refractoriness). It is this altered cellular electrophysiology and that provides suitable conditions for reentrant arrhythmias *(9,10)*.

Differential effect of drugs on QT interval and risk of cardiac events could also be related to genetic profile of the subjects taking medications. There is a natural biological variation in genes coding specific ion channels, and some of these genetic polymorphism may predispose to drug-induced QT prolongation *(35–37)*. Rarity of drug-induced TdP may indicate that only subjects with specific polymorphism of genes encoding ion channels or encoding enzymes metabolizing these drugs (usually from cytochrome P-450 system) are prone to develop proarrhythmic response to drugs *(38)*.

Changes in T-Wave Morphology

There is a substantial variation in T-wave morphology among LQTS patients. This finding could be related to type of affected ion channel, the magnitude of ion channel dysfunction, as well as other factors including age, heart rate, and the status of autonomic nervous system. The HERG gene mutation encodes the I_{Kr} current (the current most frequently affected by drugs) and is associated with decreased T-wave amplitude with increased presence of notches *(39)*. Similar observations could be done when evaluating drug-induced changes in repolarization. Drugs not only may produce QT prolongation, but also, they may alter repolarization (T wave or TU complex) morphology. However, there are no systematic studies demonstrating the association between quantitative measures of T-wave morphology and risk of arrhythmic events. Drug-induced changes in T-wave morphology reflect changes in transmural gradient of repolarization with propensity to arrhythmogenesis (Fig. 6), as it was elegantly demonstrated by Antzelevitch

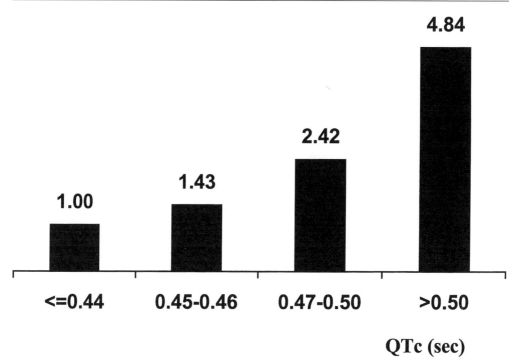

Fig. 5. Odds ratio of cardiac events by QTc duration in LQTS family members off beta-blockers. Adapted with permission from *(33)*.

and coworkers *(40,41)*. Therefore, identification of drug-induced changes in repolarization morphology in clinical studies should always trigger attention since those changes may indicate a propensity to proarrhythmia. Nevertheless, there is no systematic data quantifying repolarization morphology in drug studies.

DRUG-INDUCED QT PROLONGATION

Several cardiac and noncardiac drugs were found to prolong QTc interval duration and cause TdP (Table 2). The majority of them act by blocking I_{Kr} current directly or through their metabolites, other demonstrate such action if administered together with a drug affecting function of the cytochrome P-450 enzymatic system.

Specific Drug-Mediated Repolarization Abnormalities and Arrhythmias

Quinidine is considered as a classical prototype of drug-induced QT prolongation *(42)*. Cases of TdP associated with quinidine administration triggered interest in the entire field of drug-induced arrhythmias and drug-induced QTc prolongation.

Experience with terfenadine highlighted drug interactions (terfenadine + ketoconazole) as a cause for QT prolongation and sudden cardiac death in healthy individuals. Terfenadine, anithistamine agent, blocks the I_{Kr} current (and also it blocks sodium current and L-type calcium channel) causing a mean 6 ms QTc prolongation, which should not have clinical implications *(43)*. Cardiac events were reported in patients taking terfenadine, almost exclusively when used in combination with other medications (ketoconazole, antibiotics) also metabolized by the same enzymatic system of the cyto-

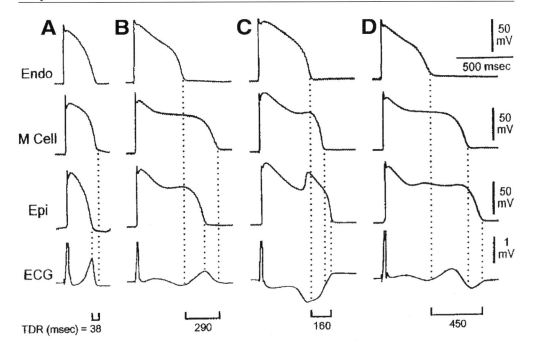

Fig. 6. Transmural dispersion of action potentials and changes in T-wave morphology on ECG. **(A)** Normal T wave with normal transmural gradient of repolarization. **(B)** Biphasic T wave: Increase in transmural gradient with end of endocardial action potential coinciding with negative phase of T wave. **(C)** Inverted T wave: Epicardial layer shows longest repolarization duration contributing to increased and inverted transmural gradient. **(D)** Polyphasic T wave with markedly increased transmural gradient: Negative phases of T wave coincide with end of action potential in endocardial and M cell layers. Reprinted with permission from *(41)*.

chrome P-450 3A4. Such a combination causes increase in plasma concentration of terfenadine owing to inhibition of its metabolism by concomitantly administered drug with subsequent substantial QTc prolongation (>60 ms in majority of reported cases) and torsades de pointes. Broad and uncontrolled use of terfenadine with its potential proarrhythmic potential was the reason for removing this drug from the market.

Cisapride, a gastric prokinetic agent, causes a mild QTc prolongation in healthy subjects. However, when given with drugs inhibiting CYP3A4 function (like clarithromycin, ketoconazole) or in neonates who have limited function of this enzymatic system, there is few-fold increase in plasma concentration of cisapride with consequent 20–30 ms QTc prolongation and propensity to torsades de pointes *(44)*. In neonates, cisapride therapy alone is associated with a 31 ms QTc prolongation. Between 1993 and 1997, 270 cases of adverse events (defined as TdP and/or substantial QTc prolongation) and 70 deaths were reported among 30 million prescriptions written *(45)*. As a result, FDA restricted the use of cisapride by changing its labeling.

Several antipsychotic drugs block I_{Kr} current and cause QTc prolongation (Table 2) and some of them (including thioridazine and phenothiazine) were reported to be associated with sudden death *(46)*. Since psychiatric disorders may predispose to sudden death, it is difficult to determine the causative association between use of these drugs and

Table 2
Drugs That Prolong the QT Interval

Category	Drugs
Antihistamines	astemizole, terfenadine
Anti-infectives	amantadine, clarithromycin, chloroquine, erythromycin, grepafloxacin, moxifloxacin, pentamidine, sparfloxacin, trimethoprim-sulfamethoxazole
Antineoplastics	tamoxifen
Antiarrhythmics	quinidine, sotalol, procainamide, amiodarone, bretylium, disopyramide, flecainide, ibutilide, moricizine, tocainide, dofetilide
Antilipemic agents	probucol
Calcium channel blockers	bepridil
Diuretics	indapamide
Gastrointestinal agents	cisapride
Hormones	fludrocortisone, vasopressin
Antidepressants	amitriptyline, amoxapine, clomipramine, imipramine, nortriptyline, protriptyline
Antipsychotic	chlorpromazine, haloperidol, perphenazine, quetiapine, risperidone, sertindole, thioridazine, ziprasidone, doxepin

arrhythmic events. A systematic study is needed to determine the risk of sudden death and the role of drug-induced arrhythmias in such patients.

Mibefradil, an antihypertensive and antianginal agent blocks primarily T-type calcium channel, but also I_{Kr} and I_{Ks} currents, was removed from the market due to its action on repolarization. Mebefradil is also a potent inhibitor of several enzymatic systems in the liver (CYP3A4, CYP2D6, CYP1A2), and this action contributed to an increased risk of adverse events (47). QT prolongation of mibefradil was mainly due to enhancement of the late phase of the T wave, although some experts claimed that it was a U wave, possibly due to a preferential blocking of specific layers in myocardium (M cell zone) with increased transmural dispersion of repolarization.

Risk Factors Contributing to Drug-Induced QT Prolongation and Susceptibility to Malignant Ventricular Arrhythmias

Table 3 lists clinical factors predisposing to drug-induced QT prolongation and TdP. Female sex is associated with faster resting heart rates and longer QTc intervals than in men, which was already observed by Bazett in 1920s. T-wave morphology is also different by sex with females having longer early phase of repolarization (29) and a less steep ascending arm of T wave (32). Difference in QT and heart rate by sex also contributes to steeper slope of the QT-RR relationship in women than men (48). As shown in Fig. 4, sex-related differences in QTc are age-dependent, with children having similar repolarization duration and pattern regardless of sex; adolescents and adults (15–55 yr) show substantial QTc differences by sex; after age 55 these QTc differences are attenuated. This pattern suggests the role of sex hormones for the appearance of sex-related repolarization changes.

Women account for 70% of cases of drug-induced QT prolongation and TdP indicating that the above sex-related differences in repolarization have clinical implications *(49)*. A similar 70% dominance of women among probands with congenital LQTS further indicates that female gender (in adulthood) is a risk factor for cardiac events *(1)*. There is evidence for variation in drug-induced QT prolongation with the menstrual cycle: Menstruation and the ovulatory phase of the cycle are associated with longer QTc than the luteal phase *(50)*. However, more research is needed to better understand other mechanisms (structural differences in myocardium, protective effect of male hormones) leading to sex-related differences in repolarization.

All individuals regardless of sex have increased risk of proarrhythmia if their baseline QTc is prolonged. This baseline QTc prolongation might be because of specific genetic predisposition (genetic make-up), but more often could be caused by concomitant medical conditions. Patients with heart disorders are most likely to demonstrate QTc prolongation and are also prone to develop drug-induced arrhythmias. Such patients usually are treated with several drugs simultaneously that may be metabolized by the same enzymatic system, thereby increasing the chance of reduced drug metabolism and increased blood levels of a drug. Cardiac patients are frequently receiving diuretics that can cause hypokalemia, a factor further predisposing to QT prolongation and arrhythmias. Presence of bradycardia is another factor that promotes QT prolongation and dispersion of repolarization creating suitable conditions for proarrhythmia. LQT2 patients with mutations in HERG gene are particularly prone to develop arrhythmias at resting heart rates or during bardycardia, a finding that provides evidence for heart rate dependent arrhythmias in I_{Kr} blocking conditions.

Genetic predisposition to drug-induced QT prolongation and proarrhythmia is an attractive but very new and unproven concept. There are some incidental reports suggesting that polymorphisms in genes encoding cardiac ion channels (or in genes encoding enzymatic system in liver) could be more prevalent in patients with drug-induced QT prolongation and TdP *(35–37)*. Polymorphisms of two ion channel genes, minK (LQT5) and MiRP1 (LQT6), were recently found in subjects with proarrhythmic response to a drug. Those two genes encode small proteins regulating function of I_{Ks} and I_{Kr}, respectively. It was shown that polymorphism of MiRP1 may cause a 15% decrease in ion channel function in healthy subject, the magnitude which does not lead to a proarrhythmic response. However, administration of sulfometoxasole (Bactrim), an I_{Kr} blocker, in a subject with this polymorphism was associated with substantial decrease in the ion current density *(37)*. However, systematic analysis of a series of patients with drug-induced QT prolongation showed that they have a similar prevalence of cardiac ion channel gene polymorphisms to control subjects *(51)*.

The combination of several factors (female gender, older age, interaction with another drug, bradycardia, genetic predisposition) is usually needed for TdP to be caused by a drug-prolonging QT interval. This "multiple hit hypothesis" provides at least partial explanation for rarity of drug-induced TdP among millions of patients taking drugs blocking cardiac ion channels.

Magnitude of Drug-Induced QTc Prolongation

There is no universal threshold for QTc prolongation, and each drug has to be analyzed on an individual basis. There is agreement that a QTc prolongation by >30 ms should raise concerns, and with greater concern when the QTc exceeds >60 ms, especially if the QTc prolongs beyond 500 ms.

Table 3
Factors Associated with Increased Risk of QT Prolongation
and Torsades de Pointes

Prolonged QTc
Female sex
Advanced age
Bradycardia
Hypokalemia
Hypomagnesemia
Congestive heart failure (low EF)
Cardiac arrhythmias
Combinations of drugs (cytochrome P450 enzymes inhibitors)
Genetic polymorphisms of gene coding cardiac ion channels or enzymes in
    liver metabolizing drugs

The analysis of the magnitude of QTc prolongation from baseline by a drug should be paralleled by evaluating the absolute value of prolonged QTc. Again, there is no universal threshold but reported cases of drug-induced TdP indicate that almost all of them do occur in subjects with QTc>500 ms. These observations are in agreement (Fig. 5) with data from congenital LQTS studies also showing that QTc > 500 ms is associated with substantial increase in the risk of cardiac events *(33)*.

REGULATORY ASPECTS

Drug regulatory agencies such as the Food and Drug Administration (FDA) in the United States and the Committee for Proprietary Medicinal Products (CPMP) of the European Agency for the Evaluation of Medicinal Products now scrutinize the potential QT prolonging effects of all new drugs undergoing regulatory approval as well as marketed drugs with QT prolongation observed during postmarketing surveillance *(52,53)*. The CPMP has published a document, "Points to Consider: The Assessment of the Potential for QT Interval Prolongation by Non-Cardiovascular Medicinal Products," *(53)* that is already influencing the way electrocardiographic data are collected and analyzed during clinical trials related to regulatory approval.

Each drug has to be evaluated individually after full considerations of risks associated with the drug in relationship to benefit of the drug for the population at risk. Trefenadine was the antihistamine drug broadly used in healthy subjects, and no risk of drug-induced sudden death was acceptable. Some drugs, like ziprasidone, may prolong QT interval and this prolongation is acceptable in patients with schizophrenia, since the drug is extremely effective in the treatment of this serious disorder. The concept of a tolerable risk has to be exercised during evaluation process of each drug under consideration.

Drug testing requires evaluation of the magnitude of mean and range of QT prolongation in studied populations as well as the magnitude and range of QT prolongation in individual subjects. The average QT prolonging effect of a drug may be small in a given population, yet some individuals may experience substantial QT prolongation (if the individual is at higher risk for proarrhythmia or if given simultaneously with another drug affecting its metabolism). The drug needs to be tested vs placebo, the best approach is a crossover design with special emphasis on dose-dependency of QT effects. The analysis of dose-dependency of QT behavior requires serial recordings of 12-lead ECGs or continuous recordings of with 12-lead Holter ECGs. The latter allows for better insight into heart rate dependency of repolarization changes including alterations in T-wave morphology. Postmarketing surveillance is a further important safety tool allowing for identification of drugs that may carry some unexpected risk.

DIGITAL ECG FOR DRUG STUDIES

In the October 2001 issue of the *Annals of Noninvasive Electrocardiology*, the ISHNE Task Force proposed guidelines for evaluating effects of drugs on repolarization. These guidelines rely on combination of manual/visual evaluation of QT duration and increasingly on digital ECG signal processing. There are several benefits of digital ECG data acquisition using both standard resting ECG recordings and 24-h (or even longer) Holter ECG recordings. Especially, continuous access to monitored digital ECG data allows for the analysis of:

1. Dose-dependent effects of a tested drug (and possible arrhythmias).
2. Assessment of adaptation of QT to a wide spectrum of changing heart rates, including night hours.
3. Analysis of dynamic features of repolarization including QT-RR relationship (regression analysis, slope), QT or repolarization morphology variability, or T-wave alternans.
4. Application of novel algorithms for repolarization analyses including automatic area-based approaches or T-wave loop morphology.

Such a comprehensive digital-ECG based approach is likely to improve early identification of drugs that might have proarrhythmic properties.

Digital ECG data acquisition also provides the opportunity to improve quality control of ECG analysis and allows for more comprehensive auditing (review) of ECG interpretation. In particular, FDA is interested in reviewing ECG recordings acquired during drug testing with additional access to interpreter's annotation. This process will permit better document QT measurements and will allow for the inspection of repolarization morphology (TU wave) in single and multiple (superimposed) leads.

Access to digital ECG recordings will provide better opportunity to perform direct comparisons of repolarization duration and morphology when recorded off and on tested drug. The majority of currently used ECG machines record ECG signal in digital format, however, the format of data acquisition and storage is proprietary, and it varies among manufacturers. Similarly, digital acquisition of long-term Holter recordings is replacing analog recordings, but again format of digital ECG data files is diverse among manufacturers of Holter systems. For the above reasons, there is a need to develop uniform standard for ECG/Holter output file allowing universal access to acquired data.

On November 19, 2001, the FDA organized a public meeting focused on "Electronic Interchange Standard for Digital ECG and Similar Data" during which FDA described concrete plans of the agency to request ECG data in a standard digital format whenever ECG information is submitted to FDA by pharmaceutical companies seeking the approval of a drug *(54)*. This requirement calls for development of a standard digital format which will have to be used instead of proprietary manufacturer's digital formats. FDA task force proposed an XML file format, which is receiving wide approval for short-term (standard)

ECG recordings and can be used for long-term recordings. These requirements aiming to implement a standardized system for submitting ECG data to FDA will have several implications. Most importantly, digital electrocardiology will enter a new era with benefits not only for regulatory approval, but also for clinical and research activities.

SUMMARY

Drug-induced QT interval prolongation is associated with an increased probability of TdP and arrhythmic sudden death. The mechanisms of drug-mediated repolarization abnormalities have received new insight from research focused on pharmacological models and clinical observations in patients with the long QT syndrome. Functional and structural abnormalities in HERG channel for I_{Kr} current together with transmural heterogeneity of repolarization create conditions for QT prolongation and proarrhythmic responses to a drug. Careful evaluation of ECGs for QT prolonging effects of tested drugs allows for early identification of compounds that may be associated with adverse events. Similarly clinical analysis of repolarization patterns during drug therapy may help identify an elevated risk for proarrhythmia. Drug-induced QTc prolongation by over 60 ms or above 500 ms in an individual subject should raise major concerns about safety of the drug. Major regulatory and research efforts aim to identify drugs that can cause adverse effects in form of QTc prolongation, episodes of TdP, or sudden death.

REFERENCES

1. Moss AJ, Schwartz PJ, Crampton RS, et al. The long QT syndrome: Prospective longitudinal study of 328 families. Circulation 1991;84:1136–1144.
2. Schwartz PJ, Moss AJ, Vincent GM, Crampton RS. Diagnostic criteria for the long QT syndrome. An update. Circulation 1993;88:782–784.
3. Zareba W, Moss AJ, Schwartz PJ, et al. Influence of the genotype on the clinical course of the long QT syndrome. N Engl J Med 1998;339:960–965.
4. Locati EH, Maison-Blanche P, Dejode P, Cauchemez B, Coumel P. Spontaneous sequences of onset of torsade de pointes in patients with acquired prolonged repolarization: quantitative analysis of Holter recording. J Am Coll Cardiol 1995;25:1564–1575.
5. Roden DM. Acquired long QT syndromes and the risk of proarrhythmia. J Cardiovasc Electrophysiol 2000;11:938–940.
6. Splawski I, Shen J, Timothy KW, et al. Spectrum of mutations in long-QT syndrome genes. KCNQ1, HERG, SCN5A, KCNE1, and KCNE2. Circulation 2000;102:1178–1185.
7. Mitcheson JS, Chen JL, Culberson C, Sanguinetti MC. A structural basis for drug-induced long QT syndrome. Proc Natl Acad Sci USA 2000;24:97.
8. Yang T, Snyders D, Roden DM. Drug block of I(kr): model systems and relevance to human arrhythmias. Cardiovasc Pharmacol 2001;38:737–744.
9. Fadi AG, Yan GX, Antzelevitch C, Rosenbaum DS. Unique topographical distribution of M cells underlies reentrant mechanism of torsade de pointes in the long-QT syndrome. Circulation 2002;105:1247–1253.
10. Antzelevitch C, Fish J. Electrical heterogeneity within the ventricular wall. Basic Res Cardiol 2001;96:517–527.
11. Lepeschkin E, Surawicz B. The measurement of the QT interval of the electrocardiogram. Circulation 1952;6:378–388.
12. Zareba W. Dispersion of repolarization: time to move beyond QT dispersion. Ann Noninvasive Electrocardiol 2000;5:373–381.
13. Benhorin J, Merri M, Alberti M, et al. The long QT syndrome: New electrocardiographic characteristics. Circulation 1990;82:521–527.
14. Badilini F, Fayn J, Maison-Blanche P, et al. Quantitative aspects of ventricular repolarization: relationship between three-dimentional T wave loop morphology and scalar QT dispersion. ANE 1997;2:146–157.

15. Priori SG, Mortara DW, Napolitano C, et al. Evaluation of the spatial aspects of T-wave complexity in the long-QT syndrome. Circulation 1997;96:3006–3012.
16. Bazett HC. An analysis of time relations of electrocardiograms. Heart 1920;7:353–367.
17. Fridericia LS. Duration of systole in electrocardiogram. Acta Med Scandinav 1920;53:469.
18. Sagie A, Larson MG, Goldberg RJ, Bengtson JR, Levy D. An improved method for adjusting the QT interval for heart rate (the Framingham Heart Study). Am J Cardiol 1992;70:797–801.
19. Hodges M, Salerno D, Erlien D. Bazett's QT correction reviewed: Evidence that alinear QT correction for heart rate is better. J Am Coll Cardiol 1983;1:694.
20. Rautaharju PM, Zhou SH, Wong S, et al. Sex differences in the evolution of electrocardiographic QT interval with age. Can J Cardiol 1992;8:690–695.
21. Karjalainen J, Viitasalo M, Manttari M. Relation between QT intervals and heart rates from 40– to 120 beats/min in rest electrocardiogram of men and a simple method to adjust QT interval values. J Am Coll Cardiol 1994;23:1547–1553.
22. Badilini F, Maison-Blanche P, Childers R, Coumel P. QT interval analysis on ambulatory electrocardiogram recordings: a selective beat averaging approach. Med Biol Eng Comput 1999;37(1):71–79.
23. Neyroud N, Maison-Blanche P, Denjoy I, et al. Diagnostic performance of QT interval variables from 24-h electrocardiography in the long QT syndrome. Eur Heart J 1998;19:158–165.
24. Zareba W, Moss AJ, Rosero SZ, Hajj-Ali R, Konecki JA, Andrews M. Electrocardiographic findings in patients with Diphenhydramine overdose. Am J Cardiol 1997;80:1168–1173.
25. Demolis JL, Funck-Brentano C, Ropers J, Ghadanfar M, Nichols DJ, Jaillon P. Influence of dofetilide on QT-interval duration and dispersion at various heart rates during exercise in humans. Circulation 1996;94:1592–1599.
26. Malik M. Problems of heart rate correction in assessment of drug-induced QT interval prolongation. J Cardiovasc Electrophysiol 2001;12:411–420.
27. Moss ANE, Moss AJ, Zareba W, Benhorin J, et al. ISHNE Guidelines for Electrocardiographic Evaluation of Drug-related QT Prolongation and Other Alterations in Ventricular Repolarization: Task Force Summary Annals of Noninvasive Electrocardiol 2001;6:333–341.
28. Zareba W. New era for digital ECG: FDA requires digital ECG submission for tested drugs. ANE 2002;7:1–3.
29. Merri M, Benhorin J, Alberti M, Locati E. Moss AJ. Electrocardiographic quantitation of ventricular repolarization. Circulation 1989;80:1301–1308.
30. Zareba W, Moss AJ, Konecki J. TU wave area-derived measures of repolarization dispersion in the long QT syndrome. J Electrocardiol 1998;30(suppl):191–195.
31. Moss AJ, Robinson J. Clinical features of the idiopathic long QT syndrome. Circulation 1992;85(1 Suppl):I140–I144.
32. Lehmann, MH, Yang, H. Sexual dimorphism in the electrocardiographic dynamics of human ventricular repolarization: characterization in true time domain. Circulation 2001;104:32–38.
33. Zareba W, Moss AJ, le Cessie S. Risk of cardiac events in family members of patients with long QT syndrome. J Am Coll Cardiol 1995;26:1685–1691.
34. Monahan BP, Ferguson CL, Killeavy ES, et al. Torsades de pointes occurring in association with terfenadine use. JAMA 1990;264:2788–2790.
35. Napolitano C, Priori SG, Schwartz PJ, et al. Identification of a long QT syndrome molecular defect in drug-induced torsades de pointes. Circulation 1997;96:I–211.
36. Schultz-Bahr E, Haverkamp W, Hordt M, et al. Do mutations in cardiac ion channel genes predispose to drug-induced (acquired) long QT syndrome? Circulation 1997;96:I–211.
37. Sesti F, Abbott GW, Wei J, et al. A common polymorphism associated with antibiotic-induced cardiac arrhythmia. Proc Natl Acad Sci USA 2000;97:10613–10618.
38. Flockhart DA, Tanus-Santos JE. Implications of Cytochrome P450 interactions when prescribing medication for hypertension. Arch of Intern Med 2002;162:405–412.
39. Moss AJ, Zareba W, Benhorin J, et al. Electrocardiographic T-wave patterns in genetically distinct forms of the hereditary long QT syndrome. Circulation 1995;92:2929–2934.
40. Yan GX, Antzelevitch C. Cellular basis for the normal T wave and the electrocardiographic manifestations of the long-QT syndrome. Circulation 1998;98:1928–1936.
41. Emori T, Antzelevitch C. Cellular basis for complex T waves and arrhythmic activity following combined I_{Kr} and I_{Ks} block. J Cardiovasc Electrophysiol 2001;12:1369–1378.
42. Grace AA, Camm AJ. Quinidine. New Engl J Med 1998;338:35–44.

43. Pratt CM, Euberg S, Morganroth J, et al. Dose-response relation between terfenadine (Seldane) and the QTc interval on the scalar electrocardiogram: distinguishing a drug effect from spontaneous variability. Am Heart J 1996;131:472–480.

44. van Haarst AD, van't Klooster GAE, van Gerven JME, et al. The influence of cisparide and clarithromycin on QT intervals in healthy volunteers. Clin Pharmacol Ther 1998;64:542–546.

45. Walker AM, Szneke P, Weatherby LB, et al. The risk of serious cardiac arrhythmias among cisapride users in the United Kingdom and Canada. Am J Med 1999;107:356–362.

46. Glassman AH, Bigger JT Jr. Antipsychotic drugs: prolonged QTc interval, torsade de point sudden death. Am J Psychiatry 2001;158:1774–1782.

47. Krayenbuhl JC, Vozeh S, Kondo-Oestreicher M, et al. Drug-drug interaction of new active substances: mibefradil example. Eur J Clin Pharmacol 1999;55:559–565.

48. Stramba-Badiale M, Locati EH, Martinelli A, Courville J, Schwartz PJ. Effects of gender on the relation between ventricular repolarization and cardiac cycle length during 24-hour Holter recordings. Eur Heart J 1997;18:1000–1006.

49. Makkar RR, Fromm BS, Steinman RT, Meissner MD, Lehmann MH. Female gender as a risk factor for torsade de pointe associated with cardiovascular drugs. JAMA 1993;270:2590–2597.

50. Rodriguez I, Kilborn MJ, Liu XK, Pezzullo JC, Woolsey RL. Drug-induced QT prolongation in women during the menstrual cycle. JAMA 2001;285:1322–1326.

51. Yang P, Kanki H, Drolet B, et al. Allelic variants in long QT disease genes in patients with drug-associated torsades de pointes. Circulation 2002;105:1943–1948.

52. Haverkamp W, Breithardt G, Camm AJ, et al. The potential for QT prolongation and proarrhythmia by non-antiarrhythmic drugs. Clinical and regulatory implications. Cardiovasc Res 2000;47:219–233.

53. Committee for Proprietary Medicinal Products. Points to Consider: The Assessment of the Potential for QT Interval Prolongation by Non-Cardiovascular Medicinal Products. The European Agency for the Evaluation of Medicinal Products. December, 1997.

54. FDA website containing information about November 19 meeting and "Proposed Standard for Exchange of Electrocardiographic and Other Time-Series Data": http://www.fda.gov/cder/regulatory/ersr/default.htm

15

Neuro-Mediated Repolarization Abnormalities

Philippe Coumel, MD, FESC,
and Pierre Maison-Blanche, MD

CONTENTS

INTRODUCTION

Physiology implies adaptative variations to environmental conditions so that it is characterized by flexibility. Variations of state are more important than the baseline state itself because they reflect the impact of the modulating factors, essentially formed in the field of ventricular repolarization by cardiac rate and the autonomic nervous system. Studies were mainly devoted to QT duration, an already difficult but very promising field. Studying the QT interval should not be restricted to the static aspect of its duration. QT length forms on its own a limited information if not considered in the context of its environment that conditions its dynamicity. The basic difficulty of studying the physiology of the QT interval is that ventricular repolarization mainly depends on cardiac cycle length (RR Interval), but both QT and RR variables are in fact modulated by rate-independent factors, particularly the autonomic nervous system. Finally, because the repolarization phase on the surface ECG results from the algebraic sum of the action potentials of the multiple layers of myocardial fibers, the morphology of the slow phase of the ECG probably is more important than the QT interval because it really reflects the electrical activity of myriads of cells. Presently however, the morphology of ventricular repolarization cannot be adequately quantified.

SIGNIFICANCE OF QT DYNAMICITY VS QT CORRECTION

Using a formula to evaluate QT modulation looks meaningless when one considers Fig. 1, because no rate formula will ever help to compensate for circadian QT changes

From: *Contemporary Cardiology: Cardiac Repolarization: Bridging Basic and Clinical Science*
Edited by: I. Gussak et al. © Humana Press Inc., Totowa, NJ

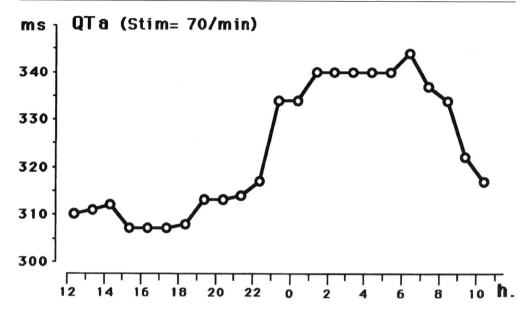

Fig. 1. Evidence of rate-independent circadian modulation of QT duration. In a regularly paced patient with fixed-rate implanted pacemaker at 70 beats/min-1 QT durations longer at night than at daytime by some 30 ms. No formula will ever offer any satisfactory rate correction for a phenomenon that is not rate-dependent. It is no more meaningful to study the variations of any corrected QT over 24 h.

evaluated at identical RR intervals. Circadian changes owing to autonomic influences are normally present notwithstanding a fixed paced cardiac rate in an implanted patient. There is a fundamental difference between what is familiar to the cardiologist, i.e., *QT correction*, and what is in essence a quite different concept, that is, *QT dynamicity*. Many studies repeatedly called for attention on the limitations and pitfalls of the supposedly universal Bazett formula *(1)* often proposing nothing more than other population specific formulas *(2–4)*. In fact, the best evidence that no formula can make a population of individuals homogeneous is suggested by the persistance of circadian variations of the corrected QT interval *(5)*. This is nonsense for a formula that is supposed to correct for rate: Malik showed that the correction, if any, should be different for each individual *(6)*. Each individual is actually characterized by his own heart rate dependence, and this is precisely where the concept of QT dynamicity starts. QT correction aims at comparing static values of QT in a population, whereas QT dynamicity aims at studying QT changes in individuals. On the other hand, a complete autonomic blockade would not abolish the rate-dependent changes of the QT interval but it may modify them. In short, QT correction is a concept which is exactly opposite to QT dynamicity.

THEORETICAL CONSIDERATIONS

Restitution Curve

For the physiologists, the time course of action potential recovery as a function of the interval between a steady-state response and a subsequent test response is known as the electrical restitution curve. Franz *(7)* used the monophasic action potential technique

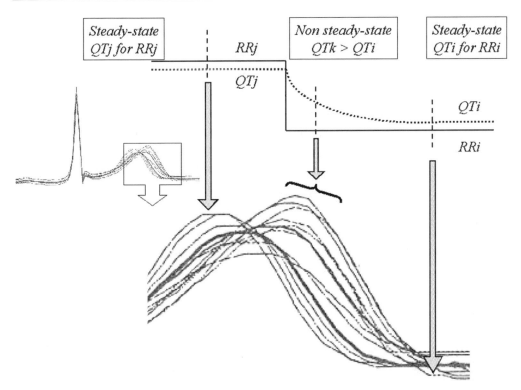

Fig. 2. QT adaptation of a stepwise increase of cycle length. The QT duration is precisely studied during the 60 s following a sudden increase of the paced RR cycle: the steady-state ***RRj*** cycle length is followed by another steady-state with a longer ***RRi***. It takes about 1 minute for the short ***QTj*** duration to reach the new stable ***QTi*** value. Measuring QT interval on a beat-by-beat basis does not take into account such a physiological phenomenon.

called attention on the latency time that exists in the QT adaptation after a sudden heart rate change, a phenomenon frequently studied *(8–10)*. The QT interval adapts to a stepwise change in pacing rate in two phases: A fast adaptation with more than 50% of the QT changes completed in less than one minute, and a slow adaptation which takes up to several minutes (Fig. 2). In addition, a "hysteresis" effect was demonstrated as the QT interval adapted faster when the pacing rate was increased than when it was decreased *(10)*. The time course of QT changes that starts with the first different RR interval, and the hysteresis were reported to be independent from the magnitude of heart rate change and of the baseline heart rate from which the change took place. The mechanism of the apparent delay in QT adaptation, which also applies to its equivalent of monophasic action potential and effective refractory period *(11)* is obscure. However an important practical consequence is that it is not meaningful to study the QT interval solely as a function of the preceding RR interval if one has no information on the heart rate during at least the preceding minute (Fig. 3). Respecting the condition of a stable RR interval before measuring QT results in a very high correlation coefficient between the two variables *(12)*, and comparing the QT/RR slopes obtained after the last RR interval or after a one-minute stability of the heart rate constantly shows that the slope of the regression line is constantly steeper in the latter situation *(13)*.

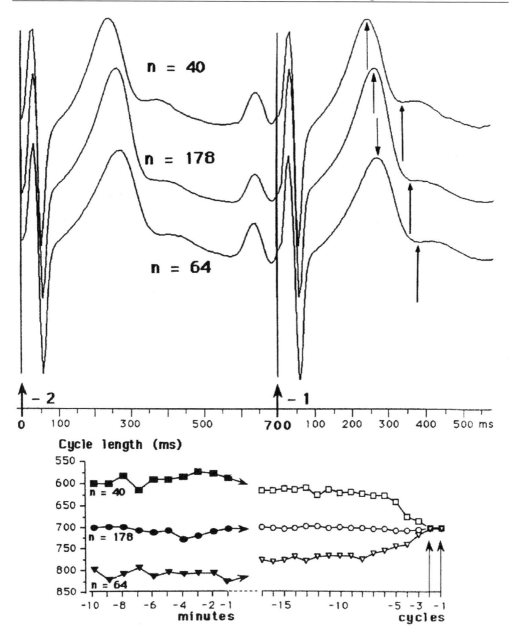

Fig. 3. Influence of the preceding heart rate on the QT interval. Three populations of QRS-T complexes have been selected from a two-hour Holter recording in such a way that the last RR cycle is identical (700 ms) in the three averaged templates. The difference between the populations resides in the preceding mean RR values during the 15 cycles and up to the 10 min preceding the measured QT interval. The shorter (600 ms, *n*=40) or longer (800 ms, *n*=64) populations of RR cycles compared to the "stable" 700 ms (*n*=170) template clearly explains why the last QT interval differs by as much as 20 ms from the reference, with even greater differences for the corrected QT (Bazett).

Rate-Independent Modulation of the QT Interval

Analyzing the mechanisms of the modulation of the ventricular repolarization from the point of view of fundamental electrophysiology forms a fascinating and very complex field *(14)*. Indeed the heart rate and the autonomic nervous system are the main operative factors, but they are not alone. Age and sex have been largely investigated in the literature *(11,15–18)* and the results are quite consistent. The QT duration is longer by an average of about 20 ms in women than in men, and in fact it is correct to say that it becomes shorter in men after puberty *(16)* as a result of hormonal differenciation and perhaps other indirect ionic mechanisms *(19)*. Rate-dependence is more marked in women than in men, but aging decreases it in both, as well as the physiological difference between steeper slopes at daytime and smaller values at night. These rate-independent factors probably explain the individual profile of the rate-dependence.

PRACTICAL CONSIDERATIONS

Quantification of Ventricular Repolarization

The concept of QT dynamicity as a tool to evaluate ventricular repolarization changes is now widely accepted. However, the impact of the concept in the medical community remains limited, probably for practical considerations. Every cardiologist knows how difficult the determination of the QT interval is on the surface ECG, and the phenomenon of QT dispersion in conventional electrocardiography illustrates how the duration of a single vectorcardiographic T-wave loop may look different when measured in several projections in the frontal or horizontal planes *(20)*. The common standards for quantitative electrocardiography (CSE) working project conducted in the late 80s by Joss Willems perfectly illustrates the challenge to determine where the QRS complex starts and where the T wave ends. Among experts, regardless of the data quality, regardless of the method used (paper ECG or on screen evaluation), the localization of the ECG points may vary up to 10 ms. The more recent studies on QT dispersion confirmed the poor reproducibility of manual measurements *(21,22)*.

To make the challenge even more complex, beat-to-beat variations of the T-wave morphology exist and may trouble the evaluation. They were commonly described as a consequence of short-long-short cycle length sequences particularly in the long QT syndrome but in fact they are not limited to this particular situation. The T-wave alternans is the subject of particular attention *(23, 24)* and sensitive techniques like spectral analysis also suggest that beat-to-beat varitions of QT duration exist *(25, 26)*. They can detect the respiratory-related oscillations well-identified in the domain of heart rate variability. A trivial example like Fig. 4 clearly shows that in the context of an atrial fibrillation with an irregular ventricular response, the preceding RR interval conditions the morphology of the T wave of the following ventricular complex. Not only the last RR interval, but the preceding cycles as well condition the amplitude of the T wave. In fact, the real question may be to decide whether the change in QT duration is real or only apparent, and to which extent the QT measurement is dependent on the T-wave morphology. It is difficult to reconcile the apparent cycle-to-cycle changes in QT duration with the above-mentioned lagtime of about one minute necessary for the QT duration to adapt to sudden heart rate changes.

Characterization of QT dynamicity is based on the assumption that multiple ECG taken by the same individual can be reliably measured. Because they are by definition

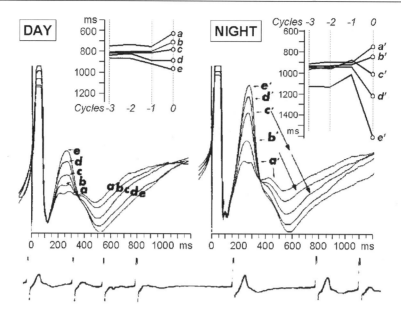

Fig. 4. Beat-to-beat variations of the morphology of ventricular repolarization. In a patient with atrial fibrillation, the bottom tracing shows that the T-wave morphology is very unstable from beat-to-beat, with an increase amplitude of the T wave following longer RR intervals. To further study this phenomenon, a selection algorithm allows for comparing populations of QRS-T complexes that essentially differ by the last RR cycle length. The longer the cycle from *a* to *e* at daytime, or from *a'* to *e'* at night, the taller the T wave. Conceivably, these morphological changes may be responsible for changes in the apparent QT duration.

taken in a variable environment such as different physical activities, not only in resting position, the amount of technical difficulty is obvious. However, modern digitized quantitative ECG technique can overcome that hurdle. The key tools are, on one hand, averaging technique to reduce the muscle noise and, on the other, serial approach. The background for serial ECG analysis is that an ECG waveform variation is much easier to calculate than the absolute value of each individual waveform.

Long-term ECG data streams and, in particular, ambulatory 24-h recording form the best tools to explore the dynamicity of ventricular repolarization. Merri et al. *(25)* measuring the RTm interval (the time interval between the peak of the R wave and the peak of the T wave) or Laguna et al. *(28)* measuring the end of the T wave on a beat-to-beat basis required the removal of low quality data, so that up to 20% of cardiac complexes had to be rejected. However, a common situation is that the ECG segments that are most likely to contain valuable information on QT during daily activity or exercise are precisely those containing artifacts. Thus, a possible consequence of using too strict rejecting procedures is to eliminate the data that are most relevant clinically. When an averaging procedure is implemented, low-noise templates can be obtained even from artifacted ambulatory ECG data. In our experience *(29)*, a lower limit of 50 beats is sufficient to obtain quite analyzable signals. Many softwares concentrate on measuring the QTm (or QTa) interval because the wave apex looks easier to detect, which does not necessarily mean that it is. QTa and QTo (or QT end) intervals are considered equivalent. Still, a usual (though rarely quoted) observation is that the relationships between QTa and QTo vary

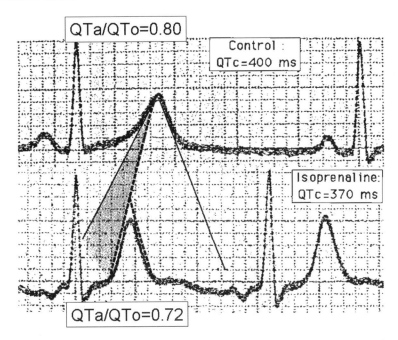

Fig. 5. Effect of isoprenaline infusion on the T-wave morphology. Humoral adrenergic stimulation modifies the time relationships between the apex and the end of the T wave. They can be evaluated from the QTa/QTo ratio that tends to diminish. The physiological assymmetry of the T wave disappears because of a steeper ascending limb whereas the descending limb is unchanged.

with the amount of adrenergic stimulation so that the physiological asymmetry of the ascending and descending limbs of the T wave and the QTa/QTo ratio tend to diminish (Fig. 5). This is consistent with steeper regression lines for QTm/RR than for QTo/RR a different behavior that is more marked at daytime than at night.

Modulation of QT/RR: Heart Rate and Autonomic Nervous System

NONSELECTIVE APPROACHES

The basic difficulty of studying the physiology of QT and RR relationship is that both variables are modulated by the autonomic nervous system. As a result, QT modification of autonomic origin are by definition nonselective because the effect of heart rate acceleration cannot be distinguished from proper autonomic influences on repolarization. Taken together, nonselective approaches of QT dynamicity propose nonlinear relationships between QT and RR. The reason they share this is that they are mixing at least two (probably several) factors of modulation and behavior. In fact every time a selective evaluation of the two main modulating factors (the rate and the autonomics) is performed, the QT/RR relationships appear linear. However, the slopes of the regression lines differ according to the factor studied. Mathematically, the combination of linear regressions with different slopes produces an exponential pattern of the regression.

The lack of selectivity forms the basic pitfall of studies using exercise or pharmacologic agents to propose new formulas for QT correction *(30–35)*. In fact they reflect QT dynamicity in conditions strictly limited to the protocol used, thus illustrating Levy's

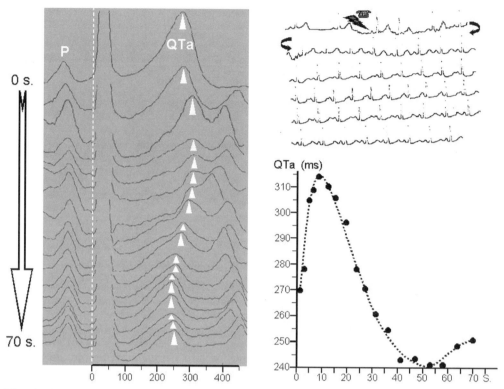

Fig. 6. Short-term effect of stress on ventricular repolarization. In a normal subject a stressful arousal from sleep by a telephone call provokes a sudden heart rate acceleration, and the QT interval (QTapex) can be adequately followed over 70 s. The QT duration actually increases during the first 20 s before adapting after a timelag of 50 s. This paradoxical QT change suggests that the electrophysiological status of the myocardium may be very unstable and most probably inhomogeneous thus setting the stage for potential arrhythmias (*see* Figs. 10 and 11).

reflections on these matters *(36)*. Protocols should be strictly defined, and in particular they should respect at least the minimal condition of sufficiently long plateaus (more than one minute) in order not to be in a permanent unstable situation of QT adaptation *(37)*. For instance, one should also recall that any adrenergic stimulation first induces a paradoxical QT lengthening *(31,32)* well exemplified in Fig. 6. Another supposedly selective approach is the Valsalva maneuver *(38)*. Not only is it much more complex than realized when it is not familiar *(39)* but it is clearly difficult to obtain any steady-state in the various steps of the investigation that are supposed to alternate vagal and sympathetic influences. Compared to exercise, the tilt test offers the advantage of avoiding too large heart rate variations thus permitting comparison of two well-defined situations opposing rest and adrenergic stimulation *(40)*. Using this method at identical rates, we can confirm that QT shortened in the standing compared to supine position (363 ± 15 vs 387 ± 14 ms, $p<0.01$). Whereas the Fridericia formula decreased it using the Bazett formula to correct the QT interval at different rates increased the corrected value.

SELECTIVE APPROACHES

Selective approaches aim at dissociating as much as possible the proper effect of cardiac frequency from the autonomic influences. Controlling the heart rate can be done using clinical electrophysiology with the inherent limitations of invasive and short-term investigations, or in chronically-implanted patients which form clearly restricted cohorts of patients rather than subjects. The Holter technique does not have such limitations but it supposes an adequate selection of the data.

Pacing. Pacing at fixed rates is the most convenient way to investigate specifically the rate dependence *(41–47)*. By so doing, one is able to draw the QT/RR regression line and to determine its slope, which is a characteristic of the underlying cell. When studied in its purest aspect, i.e., by atrial pacing, the QT/RR relationships were found linear by Ahnve *(41)* but in fact the initial study included only two pacing rates (90 and 130/min) compared with the basic rate of 65/min. The result concerning 13 healthy subjects, expressed in terms of difference of QT duration between the rates of 90 and 130/min, was 35 ms ± 26 (mean ± SD) which approximately corresponds to a regression line slope value of 0.165. Milne's results *(42)* very well match at the time these values as well as the data of 10 subjects studied by Dickuth *(43)* with a QT/RR slope of about 0.160. Based on paced RR intervals ranging from 400 to 600 ms, the 10 subjects studied by Cappato *(44)* had an average slope of 0.220, but it should be noted that they were significantly younger than the Ahnve's subjects (mean age 42 yr vs 67.5 yr), and the short-term (a few seconds) stepwise protocol may not have included sufficient steady-state periods. The same probably applies to Fananapazir's results *(45)* with the additional remark that atrial pacing provokes greater QT changes than ventricular pacing. Interestingly, the reality and practical consequence of the "memory phenomenon," which explains the timelag of about one minute was verified in the rate-responsive pacemakers based on QT monitoring *(46,47)*. Another interest of investigating chronically-implanted patients is that variations can be investigated over the 24-h period *(47)*.

Selecting the Data from 24-H Recordings. Holter monitoring is particularly adapted to studying noninvasive QT physiology because it allows consideration of QRS-T complexes or templates selected according to either the rate or the time so that the influence of these factors can be studied independently. Figure 7 displays the two dimensions of the investigations, with a particular emphasis on the fact that a fixed RR interval is responsible for different QT durations according to the distribution overtime. The active and the sleeping periods should be considered separately *(48,49)* with a particular reference to the awakening period, and the disappearance of the differences in transplanted hearts is the best evidence of the autonomic modulation *(50,51)*. Direct comparison of QT intervals at similar heart rates was proposed to avoid the use of correction formulas *(49–53)* but one realizes how important it is to consider these rate-dependent values as a function of time. Finally, the concept of selection of stable heart rate segments for QT analysis has been introduced and, if they can be identified by visual inspection of the RR tachograms, using selection algorithms certainly is more accurate *(54)*. There is a significant difference between the day and the night slopes, the latter being less steep than the former (Fig. 8) *(12)*. Respecting the condition of a stable heart rate during the preceding minute is the condition for obtaining high correlation coefficients (>0.90) so that apparently small differences are significant. Not only this steady-state use of templates transforms the cloud of multiple points in well-aligned values, but both day and night regression lines are steeper than the nonsteady-state data *(13)*. Finally, mixing diurnal and nocturnal QT values at identical rates has the same blurring effect as nonsteady-state approaches that not only masks the circadian influences but makes less steep the slope of the 24-hour QT-RR regression line *(54)*.

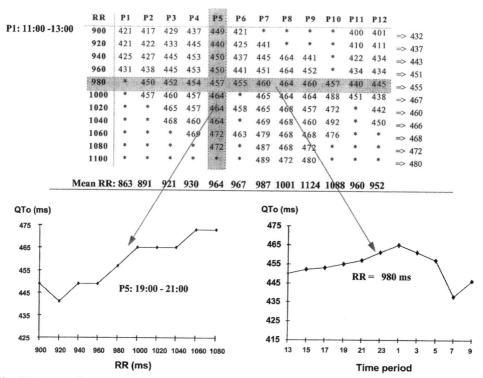

P1: 11:00 -13:00	RR	P1	P2	P3	P4	P5	P6	P7	P8	P9	P10	P11	P12	
	900	421	417	429	437	449	421	*	*	*	*	400	401	=> 432
	920	421	422	433	445	440	425	441	*	*	*	410	411	=> 437
	940	425	427	445	453	450	437	445	464	441	*	422	434	=> 443
	960	431	438	445	453	450	441	451	464	452	*	434	434	=> 451
	980	*	450	452	454	457	455	460	464	460	457	440	445	=> 455
	1000	*	457	460	457	464	*	465	464	464	488	451	438	=> 467
	1020	*	*	465	457	464	458	465	468	457	472	*	442	=> 460
	1040	*	*	468	460	464	*	469	468	460	492	*	450	=> 466
	1060	*	*	*	469	472	463	479	468	468	476	*	*	=> 468
	1080	*	*	*	*	472	*	487	468	472	*	*	*	=> 472
	1100	*	*	*	*	*	*	489	472	480	*	*	*	=> 480

Mean RR: 863 891 921 930 964 967 987 1001 1124 1088 960 952

QTo (ms)

475
465
455
445
435
425

P5: 19:00 - 21:00

900 920 940 960 980 1000 1020 1040 1060 1080

RR (ms)

QTo (ms)

475
465
455
445
435
425
415

RR = 980 ms

13 15 17 19 21 23 1 3 5 7 9

Time period

Fig. 7. The two dimensions of ventricular repolarization duration. The table is extracted from QT trend analysis of a 24-h period in a normal subject. The 24 h are divided in 12 two-hour periods, within which the QT intervals at increasing stable heart rates are given. A column of the table for a fixed period is displayed in the left lower diagram (thus providing QT/RR relation within the selected period). A row of QT values at a fixed RR interval over the time periods is displayed in the right lower diagram, with shorter values at daytime compared to night.

Circadian variations of the QT interval are agreed upon by the various authors although with variable expressions of the results. Speaking of QT/RR slopes is more meaningful although less practical for the clinician than values of QT duration at different rates but the latter can be easily drawn from the regression lines. To avoid using the questionable concept of corrected QT values, the authors often prefer to speak of QT duration effectively measured from Holter recordings at the actual (or sometimes extrapolated) heart rate of 60/min. The "ΔQT" values expressing the difference between day and night are quite consistent in normals: 19 ms for Browne *(48)*, 18 ms for Viitasolo *(52)*, 16 ms for Murakawa *(53)*, and 19 ms in our own initial experience *(54)*. Aging tends to alter this circadian flexibility: A comparison of 11 young (31 ± 6 yr) and older (58 ± 10) normal subjects showed a significantly greater nocturnal lengthening in young people (33 vs 19 ms). Bexton's *(51)* findings are consistent with the preceding values, the difference being that the changes of the QT interval were assessed from Holter recordings of patients who were pacemaker-dependent.

The Autonomic Modulation of the QT Interval

The long-term circadian modulation we have just studied is one facet of the influence of the autonomic nervous system on ventricular repolarization. There is numerous, and

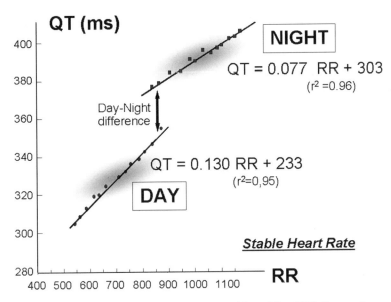

Fig. 8. QT analysis over the 24-h period in a normal subject. The QRS-T complexes are selected for analysis on the basis of a stable heart rate during the preceding minute (the mean RR cycle does not differ by more than 15 ms from the last cycle preceding the measured QT interval). This explains the very high correlation coefficient of the linear regression line of the rate-selected templates during the day (defined as the 8 consecutive faster hours) and the night (4 consecutive slower hours) periods. The ovals represent the usual cloudy pattern of beat-by-beat analysis, another mode of analysis without "stable heart rate" approach. The great axis of the ovals is less steep and the day to night difference of the slopes is less marked. The day-to-night difference of about 20 ms at a common cycle of 800–900 ms can be calculated from the actually available data.

often conflicting, data in the literature concerning the autonomic influences, which are probably largely explained by the variety of the conditions and study protocols. Another factor of confusion is that authors are using either actual or corrected QT values. This formula over- or underestimates the QT value according to slow or fast heart rates and combines with the proper action of pharmacological agents on the heart rate, thus making the situation extremely confusing.

Some studies tried to eliminate the role of heart rate by comparing different situations of autonomic blockade but including the same heart rate through various individuals *(56)*. By so doing however, the authors eliminate any possibility of interindividual comparison *(6)*, very risky in this type of study in which individuals react to pharmacodynamic agents as a function of their own vago-sympathetic balance *(57)*. With these reservations, it was found that sympathetic stimulation prolongs the QTc interval whereas beta-blockade shortens it. The same applies to alpha-adrenergic stimulation, but parasympathetic blockade also prolonged the QTc. Browne *(48)* found opposite results, discovering that propranolol prolongs the QTc whereas autonomic blockade lengthens it. For Bellavere et al. *(58)*, using the Valsalva maneuver in diabetics, the QT interval is prolonged in case of neuropathy supposedly affecting predominantly the vagus.

One is tempted to trust more the experiments in which the rate is controlled by pacing *(41,43–47,59,60)*. This is a favorable situation for studying the slope QT/RR relationship, with the limitation that the exploration is only valid for daytime. For Ahnve *(41)*, propranolol causes no significant change in the QT interval when heart rate is held constant. In contrast, atropine produces rate independent reductions of QT interval (5%) in subjects with beta-adrenergic blockade ($p<0.05$). He concluded that cholinergic activity has a direct influence on the ventricular repolarization. For Cappato *(60)* the QT/RR slope (0.22±0.12) is not changed by beta-blockade but is significantly lower after autonomic blockade (0.10±0.4) and he concludes that the vagal influences are likely to be directly exerted on the ventricular substrate. QTc was significantly shorter in this experiment after beta-blockade than at baseline, whereas there was no significant differences after autonomic blockade. But for the same cycle length beta-blockade did prolong the QT and autonomic blockade did shorten it. Most studies dealing with propranolol confirm that it is substantially unable to modify QT duration in short-term experiments *(45,48,52)*. However, 20 yr ago it was established that if the acute intravenous administration of metoprolol had no detectable effect, chronic treatment caused a significant increase of the QT interval during atrial stimulation *(61)*. Furthermore, we recently showed that the effect of beta-blockers on the QT interval is circadian dependent *(57)*. QT rate-dependency (0,216 [0.195–0.236]) was significantly reduced by atenolol (0.180 [0,162–0.198] $p<0.01$) at daytime but not at night. Thus, the effects of beta-blockers depend on the circadian variations of the sympathetic drive and the circulating catecholamines, and it is not indifferent whether they are tested in basic conditions or at exercise, or using other approaches for testing the autonomic nervous system. Arrowood tried to distinguish the influence of increased circulating catecholamines from myocardial efferent stimulation, by comparing the effect of exercise and reflex stimulation in cardiac transplant patients and normal control subjects *(62)*. The QT/RR relationship did not differ between the groups at exercise, and cold pressor test and Valsalva maneuvers did not modify the QT interval whereas the heart rate was accelerated only in normals.

It is not easy to reconcile the data obtained in so many different conditions of experiments that essentially refer to adrenergic stimulation. One should recall however the concept of accentuated vagal antagonism *(63)* and its applications *(64)*. The steeper QT/RR slope on Holter recordings during daytime compared to night is in apparent discordance with the effect of atropine or beta-blockers on regression lines, that are not consistent in the literature. That Cappato et al. *(60)* find no effect of beta-blockade on QT/RR slopes whereas complete autonomic blockade tend to make steeper the slopes when the relationship is explored by pacing at daytime may look nonconsistent with the Holter findings we just mentioned. However, if the proper action of the vagus is looked as permanently counteracting the sympathetics, the concept of accentuated vagal antagonism implies that, as the adrenergic drive is higher at daytime, logically the vagal tone also should be higher than at night, which does not preclude its relative predominance at night. Cycle length, QT duration, and QT/RR modulation through humoral and neurogenic influences are complex and it is quite difficult to dissociate the various factors even in complex experiments *(65)*, and even more so in the clinical situation. If QT duration seems to depend on the amount of circulating catecholamines, QT dynamicity may not be modulated in the same way and may well depend on the vagal drive.

QT Dynamicity and the Arrhythmia Risk

A common behavior of practically all heart diseases is that they are marked by an increased QT duration and a steeper QT/RR relationship. It is not clear however whether the rate-dependence of ventricular repolarization, an intrinsic characteristic of myocardial fiber, or its modulation by the autonomic nervous system, or a combination of the two, are responsible for this situation. The question of a relationship between the arrhythmia risk including sudden death, and QT changes was for the first time evoked by Schwartz *(66)*, and the alteration of the autonomic nervous system after myocardial infarction also is a well-established fact *(67)*. However, the relationship between these two parameters does not seem to be direct if one refers to Algra's study that more or less closed a long controversy when he showed that QT prolongation was indeed a prognostic marker only in the context of the absence of heart failure *(68)*. This is not in contradiction with the vast literature that established the role of the adrenergic stimulation and the decrease of heart rate variability as reliable markers of poor prognosis in heart disease. Only a very few studies compared the performances of the two markers, QT dynamicity and heart rate variability, when we had the opportunity to do so on two occasions *(69,70)*. We compared two cohorts of patients with an old myocardial infarction, using a collective of patients already studied by Huikuri *(71)* in terms of heart rate variability. Patients with ventricular tachyarrhythmias during the follow-up were matched with patients without complications but not different in age, sex, NYHA functional class, left ventricular ejection fraction, and beta-blocking treatment. There was no difference in the QTc value whatever the circadian period. Patients with ventricular tachyarrhythmias and/or cardiac arrest at the outcome differed from controls by a steeper QT/RR slope, and a reduced difference between daytime and nighttime slopes. The difference was even more pronounced after awakening and the significance was more marked for QT dynamicity than for heart rate variability *(69)*. More recently we had the same experience using the collective of patients of the EMIAT study, and again, as markers of sudden death, the performance of QT dynamicity exceeded that of heart rate variability *(70)*.

Although they are fundamentally different in terms of intrinsic myocardial impairment and autonomic abnormalities, it is striking to observe that coronary artery disease *(72)*, diabetes mellitus with its predominant vagal impairment *(58,73)*, heart failure with its predominant adrenergic stimulation *(74)*, and even the long QT syndrome with its pure channelopathy *(75)* have a common increase in the rate-dependence of the QT interval, a decrease (sometimes an inversion) of the slope differences between day and night, and an increased risk of sudden death. Figures 9 to 11 may offer a common hypothesis to link this situation with the risk of arrhythmias according to the electrophysiological concepts of inhomogeneity as a powerful arrhythmogenic factor. The diagram of Fig. 9 shows the consequence of a steeper QT/RR relationship, with a biphasic QT behavior according to heart rate changes. What is of importance is not that much the absolute value of the QT interval at this or that rate, or of any more or less corrected QT interval. It is clearly apparent in Fig. 9 where the QT intervals between groups of normal and diseased patients become different only at either slow or fast heart rates. The more different the slopes, the larger the zones of significant differences in the QT intervals. Occasionally, this figure shows how meaningless the notion of corrected QT interval is, because it tends to blunt differences which precisely form the main interest of measuring the QT interval dynamicity. QT duration in itself is no more informative than QTc, because it can be either longer or shorter in at-risk patients compared to controls, just depending on the rate at which it is measured. Rather, what probably is of crucial importance are changes of QT according to heart rate variations, and their potential absence of homogeneity in a diseased myocardium. When the RR interval is long, that is, at slower rates, the QT interval is longer in groups at risk compared to normals, but it becomes shorter when the heart rate

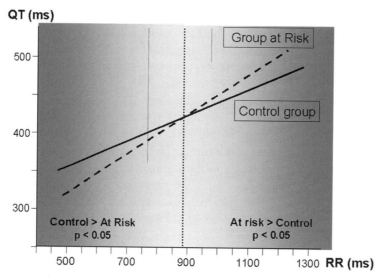

Fig. 9. Consequences of the behavior of QT dynamicity. The steeper slope QT/RR relationship in patients at risk compared to controls explains why QT values may look shorter, longer, or not different, depending on the heart rate at which they were measured. In the example of the figure, QT intervals are equal at a 900 ms cycle length. What really matters in fact is that any sudden heart rate acceleration or slowing may make significantly different the QT values in the diseased group.

accelerates, so that discrepancies may appear in the conduction properties and refractory periods of neighboring myocardial cells, thus setting the stage for arrhythmias. The more sudden the heart rate changes, the more marked the discordance in the adaptation, and one notes the striking similarity between the QT changes observed in Fig. 6 and the occurrence of torsade de pointes and ventricular fibrillation in Fig. 10. In both cases the stress is provoked by a telephone call delivered at night, and the same time interval of about 10 to 15 s intervenes between the starting point of the sinus acceleration and the maximal QT changes (Fig. 6) or the onset of arrhythmias (Fig. 10). Finally, the curious relationships we observe between QT adaptation, QT dynamicity, and the onset of arrhythmias seems also to extend to the acquired forms of the long QT syndrome the torsades de pointes of which are apparently triggered by a short-term sympathetic stimulation (Fig. 11) *(76)*.

The congenital Long QT Syndrome (LQTS) is the prototype of a clinical entity associated with an abnormal repolarization but with a preserved myocardial function. The controversy regarding the "sympathetic imbalance" hypothesis as the basic abnormality was ended by the identification of the genes encoding ion channels involved in the genesis of ventricular repolarization. Mutations on those genes produce either gain or loss of the cellular function and explain the prolongation or the abnormalities of the QT interval in LQTS *(77)*. Still, the well-known deleterious effects of sympathetic influences reported for more than 40 yr have been highlighted by a recent report on 670 symptomatic genotyped LQTS patients. Lethal arrhythmias occur under specific circumstances in a gene-specific manner and sympathetic stimulation (Fig. 11) is the trigger for the vast majority of LQT1 patients with an impaired slow component of the delayed rectifier potassium current Iks, in contrast with LQT2 or LQT3. The facilitation of arrhythmias

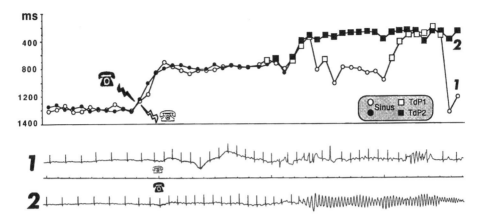

Fig. 10. Arrhythmogenic effect of stress in a patient with the long QT syndrome. Two telephone calls are delivered at night to a patient with the long QT syndrome and a history of syncope. In both cases the strong neurogenic sympathetic stimulation is immediately heralded by the sinus acceleration, and a lagtime of 10–15 s is necessary for the venticular arrhythmia to fire in the form of a run of premature beats ("TdP1") or a ventricular fibrillation necessitating a resuscitation (TdP2). This delay of 10–15 s between the sympathetic stimulation and the tachyarrhythmia recalls the time course of the paradoxical QT lengthening in Fig. 5.

by adrenergic influences have obvious implications for therapy but also for phenotypic characterization. The spectrum of QT interval duration is large even in a genetically homogenous population with a mutation on Iks.

QT dynamicity as a potential diagnostic index has been used in many studies. Swan et al. showed that the difference in QT intervals between LQT1 patients and healthy subjects was more pronounced after physical effort, which is a way to express an increased dynamicity, based on a nonselective approach *(78)*. This is also our experience with Holter. For instance, in a homogeneous database of 68 LQT1 carriers and 54 nonaffected family members (unpublished data) we found that the QT/RR slopes were significantly increased at night but only moderately impaired during the day (Fig. 12). There is a reverse circadian pattern of QT dynamicity. The increased nocturnal QT/RR ratio reflects the basically altered rate-dependence of the myocardial cells that probably is the marker of the channelopathy. But there is also a reversed pattern of diurnal slopes in affected patients, this characteristic being more marked in symptomatic than in asymptomatic carriers (though not reaching a statistical significance). The role of the autonomic nervous system in the long QT probably is the modulation of the cardiac ion channel impairment *(79)*. The phenotypic expression among carriers of the same mutation is quite variable so the question about the role of a modifier gene is raised. Preliminary data showed that heart rate variability, a marker of autonomic nervous system activity is under genetic control *(80)*. It suggests than an interaction between electrical abnormalties owing to mutations on genes coding repolarization channels and genetic variability in the autonomic nervous system may be important. For the clinician, a clear difference should be made in the modalities of adrenergic stimulation. Adrenergic stimulation because of stress or emotion is much more deleterious than exercise or catecholamine infusion, with the noticeable exception of the catecholaminergic ventricular tachyarrhythmias *(81)*. The

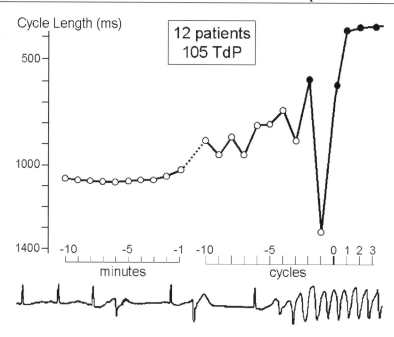

Fig. 11. Acquired long QT syndrome and the role of sympathetic stimulation. A total of 105 attacks of torsades de pointes were collected in the Holter recordings of 12 patients with an acquired long QT syndrome. They were studied in terms of cycle length over the 10 cycles preceding the arrhythmia onset, and mean cycle length over the preceding 10 min. The role of pauses and long-short phenomena as triggers of torsades de pointes is expressed by the more and more marked alternating pattern of the cardiac cycles. In particular, the short cycle "minus 2" always corresponds to a ventricular premature beat (solid circle), whereas cycle "minus 1" represents the post-extrasystolic pause (open cycle) that precedes the torsade de pointes (solid circles). A trend of increasing heart rate already detectable during the last minute preceding the arrhythmia onset is clearly visible during the 10 last cycles, thus suggesting the favoring role of a sympathetic stimulation, with a 10–20 s time course recalling that observed in Figs. 5 and 10.

reason probably is that stimulation via sympathetic nerves is much more sudden and unequally distributed within the myocardial fibers thus favoring the inhomogeneity of electrophysiological effects, an essential arrhythmogenic factor. This applies to the long QT syndrome, and the example of Fig. 13 is in this regard quite rare because this patient with a Jervell and Lange-Nielsen form of the syndrome reacted immediately to isoprenaline infusion by developing electrical alternans and torsades de pointes.

QT Dynamicity and Drugs

Many studies have shown that the action potential prolongation observed with class III antiarrhythmic agents is more pronounced at slow heart rates. This effect is referred to as reverse frequency-dependence. It is an important issue for the clinical use of class III drugs, for both efficacy and safety view points (82–83). Amiodarone forms an exception in terms of efficacy as well as rarity of torsades de pointes. Hondeghem (84) recently suggested that triangulation of the action potential was essential to discern arrhythmogenic drugs. This tends to confirm that simply looking at QT duration is a rustic

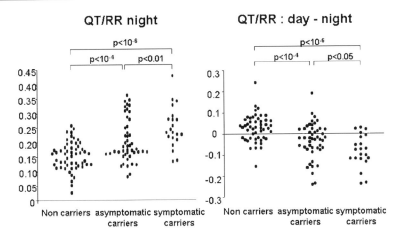

Fig. 12. Particular behavior of QT dynamicity in the congenital LQT1 syndrome. The circadian behavior of QT dynamicity was evaluated from Holter recordings in genotyped families with LQT1 syndrome, and the comparison was made between noncarriers on the one hand, and asymptomatic and symptomatic carriers on the other hand. The normal contrast between a steeper QT/RR ratio at daytime is present in noncarrier individuals, it tends to reverse in asymptomatic carriers, and the reversion is even more apparent in symptomatic patients. The overlap between the various populations suggests that this marker is not the only cause in the determinism of arrhythmias.

approach compared to what should be done, i.e., looking at morphological changes of ventricular repolarization.

Kadish et al. *(85)* examined the QT variability and specifically the rate-dependence of the QT interval in patients with torsade de pointes while taking class IA antiarrhythmic agents. These patients were compared to control sex-matched patients receiving type IA antiarrhythmic agents. The QT shortening at exercise tended to be greater in the control patients when compared to the torsade group although a similar decrease in cycle length was observed in both groups. Thus, the QTc interval is paradoxically prolonged at high rates in patients with a proarrhythmic effect. The authors concluded that exercise testing may be a useful noninvasive screening test to predict which patients are at risk of developing torsade de pointes under type IA drug therapy. A few years later, Buckingham et al. *(86)* confirmed these results using 24-h ambulatory ECG. In this study, it was specifically hypothesized that extremes of heart rates observed during Holter recordings could reflect various autonomic tone activities. Mean QTc at lower heart rates were comparable between patients and controls (413 ± 100 ms vs 420 ± 72 ms, NS). At maximal heart rates, the QTc rose up to 555 ± 22 ms in patients and up to 439 ± 11 ms in controls ($p = 0.001$). Then, the rise in the QTc length from minimal to maximal heart rate during ambulatory ECG could identify patients with drug-induced torsade de pointes (sensitivity of 70% and specificity of 89%), an observation that strikingly recalls that of Swan et al. *(78)* although with a different approach in different patients.

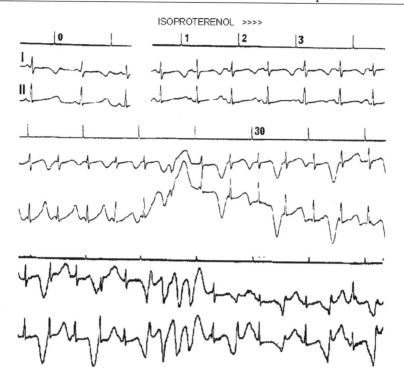

Fig. 13. Isoproterenol-induced electrical alternans and ventricular arrhythmias in a 11-yr-old patient with a JLN syndrome. It takes only 30 s to induce electrical alternans and the first attack of torsade de pointes a rare behavior in the congenital long QT syndrome. Note that electrical alternans is triggered by the pause following a ventricular premature beat.

CONCLUSION: FUTURE AND LIMITATIONS OF QT DYNAMICITY

Improvement of the techniques of analysis of the ECG signal not only refined the investigation of the QT interval but in fact completely renewed the way we can investigate ventricular repolarization. The morphology of QT still remains difficult to evaluate and interpret. We are well equipped to study QT dynamicity and we have to learn how to use this tool correctly which in fact covers two important phenomena: The rate-dependence of ventricular repolarization, and the modulation of this rate-dependence by the autonomic nervous system.

We should be conscious of how much our tools are still imperfect. Measuring the QT interval means looking at the repolarization duration of this particular group of cells that repolarizes last, either because their action potential lasted longer or because it started later than in any other region of the ventricular myocardium, or both. In fact, ideally we should consider repolarization in a global way, and for the moment we can just use the apex and the end of the T wave as fiducial points. This is already sufficient, however, to realize that they do not follow the same rules. Clearly, important progress will come from taking into account the ST-T wave morphology and its variations. When looking at the phenomenon of T wave alternans, we are just at the beginning of this process.

REFERENCES

1. Bazett HC. An analysis of the time-relations of electrocardiograms. Heart 1920;7:353–370.
2. Kovaks SJ Jr. The duration of the QT interval as a function of heart rate: a derivation based on physical principles and a comparison to measured values. Am Heart J 1985;110:972–978.
3. Puddu PE, Jouve R, Mariotti S, et al. Evaluation of 10 QT prediction formulas in 881 middle-aged men from the Seven Countries Study: emphasis on the cubic root Fridericia's equation. J Electrocardiol 1988;21:219–229.
4. Sagie A, Larson MG, Goldberg RJ, Bengston JR, Levy D. An improved method for adjusting the QT interval for heart rate. (The Framingham Heart Study). Am J Cardiol 1992;70:797–801.
5. Ong JJC, Sarma JSM, Levin SR, Singh BM. Circadian rhythmicity of heart rate and QTc interval in diabetic autonomic neuropathy: implications for the mechanism of sudden death. Am Heart J 1993;125:744–752.
6. Malik M, Färbom P, Batchvarov V, Hnatkova K, Camm AJ. The relationship between QT and RR intervals is highly individual among healthy subjects. Implications for heart rate correction of the QT interval. Heart 2002;87:220–228.
7. Franz MR, Swerdlow CD, Liem LB, Schaefer J. Cycle length dependence of human action potential duration in vivo: effects of single extrastimuli, sudden sustained rate acceleration and deceleration, and different steady state frequency. J Clin Invest 1988;82:972–979.
8. Attwell D, Cohen I, Eisen DA. The effect of heart rate on the action potential duration of guinea-pig and human ventricular muscle. J Physiol (Lond) 1981;313:439–461.
9. Elharrar V, Surawicz B. Cycle length effect on restitution of action potential duration in dog cardiac fibers. Am J Physiol 1983;244:H782–H792.
10. Lau CP, Freedman AR, Fleming S, Malik MM, Camm AJ, Ward DE. Hysteresis of the ventricular paced QT interval in response to abrupt changes in pacing rate. Cardiovasc Res 1988;22:67–72.
11. Morgan JM, Cunningham AJ, Rowland E. Relationship of the effective refractory period and monophasic action potential duration after a step increased in pacing frequency. PACE 1990;13:1002–1008.
12. Extramiana F, Maison-Blanche P, Badilini F, Pinoteau J, Deseo T, Coumel P. Circadian modulation of QT rate dependence in healthy volunteers: gender and age differences. J Electrocardiol 1999;32:33–43.
13. Lande G, Funck-Brentano C, Ghadanfar M, Escande D. Steady-state versus non-steady-state QT-RR relationship in 24-hour Holter recordings. Pacing Clin Electrophys 2000;23:293–302.
14. Rosen MR, Heck CD, Steinberg SF. Autonomic modulation of cellular repolarization and of the electrocardiographic QT interval. J Cardiovasc Electrophysiol 1992;3:487–499.
15. Merri M, Benhorin J, Alberti M, Locati E, Moss AJ. Electrocardiographic quantitation of ventricular repolarization. Circulation 1989;80:1301–1308.
16. Rautaharju PM, Zhou SH, Wong S, et al. Sex differences in the evolution of the electrocardiographic QT interval with age. Can J Cardiol 1992;8:690–695.
17. Mayuga KA, Parker M, Sukthander ND, Perlowski A, Schwartz JB, Kadish AH. Effects of age and gender on the QT response to exercise. Am J Cardiol 2001;87:163–167.
18. Taneja T, Larsen J, Goldberger J, Kadish A. Age, gender, and autonomic tone effects on surface electrocardiographic indices of ventricular repolarization. ANE 2001;6:290–297.
19. Drici MD, Burklow TR, Haridasse V, Glazer RI, Woosley RL. Sex hormones prolong the QT interval and downregulate potassium channel expression in the rabbit heart. Circulation 1996;94:1471–1474.
20. Coumel P, Maison-Blanche P, Badilini F. Dispersion of ventricular repolarization. Reality? Illusion? Significance? Circulation 1998;97:2491–2493.
21. Alberti M, Merri M, Ward DEE, Camm AJ. QT dispersion. Problems of methodology and clinical significance. J Cardiovasc Electrophysiol 1994;5:672–685.
22. Kautzner J, Gang Y, Kishore AGR, et al. Interobserver reproducibility of QT interval and QT dispersion in patients after acute myocardial infarction. ANE 1996;1:363–374.
23. Rosenbaum DS, Jackson LE, Smith JM, Garan H, Ruskin JN, Cohen RJ. Electrical alternans and vulnerability to ventricular arrhythmias. N Engl J Med 1994;330:235–241.
24. Rosenbaum DS, Kaplan DT, Kanai A, et al. Repolarization inhomogeneities in ventricular myocardium change dynamically with abrupt cycle length shortening. Circulation 1991;84:1333–1345.
25. Merri M, Moss A, Benhorin J, Locati E, Alberti M, Badilini F. Relation between ventricular repolarization duration and cardiac cycle length during 24-hour Holter recordings. Circulation 1992;85:1816–1821.
26. Nollo G, Speranza G, Grasso R, Bonamini R, Mangiardi L, Antolini R. Spontaneous beat-to-beat variability of the ventricular repolarization duration. J Electrocardiol 1992;25.9–17.

27. Willems JL, Abreu-Lima C, Arnaud P, et al. The diagnostic performance of computer programs for the interpretation of electrocardiograms. N Engl J Med 1991;325:1767–1773.

28. Laguna P, Thakor NV, Caminal P, et al. New algorithm for QT interval analysis in 24-hour Holter ECG: performance and application. Med Biol Eng Comput 1990;28:67–73.

29. Badilini F, Maison-Blanche P, Childers R, Coumel P. QT interval analysis on ambulatory ECG recordings: a selective beat averaging approach. Med Biol Eng Computer 1999;37:71–79.

30. O'Donnell J, Knoebel S, Lovelace D, McHenry P. Computer quantification of QT and terminal T wave (aT-eT) intervals during exercise: methodology and results in normal men. Am J Cardiol 1981;47:1168–1172.

31. Abildskov JA. Adrenergic effects on the QT interval of the electrocardiogram. Am Heart J 1976;92:206–212.

32. Coghlan JG, Madden B, Norrell MN, et al. Paradoxical early lengthening and subsequent linear shortening of the QT interval in response to exercise. Eur Heart J 1992;13:1325–1328.

33. Akhras F, Rickards AF. The relationship between QT interval and heart rate during physiological exercise and pacing. Jpn Heart J 1980;22:345–351.

34. Sarma JSM, Sarma RJ, Bilitch M, Katz D, Song SL. An exponential formula for heart rate dependence of QT interval during exercise and cardiac pacing in humans: reevaluation of Bazett's formula. Am J Cardiol 1984;54:103–108.

35. Lecocq B, Lecocq V, Jaillon P. Physiologic relation between cardiac cycle and QT duration in healthy volunteers. Am J Cardiol 1989;63:481–486.

36. Levy MN. Neural control of the heart: the importance of being ignorant. J Cardiovasc Electrophysiol 1995;6:283–293.

37. Lax KG, Okin PM, Kligfield P. Electrocardiographic repolarization measurements at rest and during exercise in normal subjects and in patients with coronary artery disease. Am Heart J 1994;128:271–280.

38. Butrous GS, Butrous MS, Camm AJ. Dynamic interactions between heart rate and autonomic neural activities on the QT interval. In "Clinical aspects of ventricular repolarization," GS Butrous and PJ Schwartz, eds, Farrand Press, London 1989;139–150.

39. Eckberg DL, Sleight P. Valsalva's manoeuvre. In "Human baroreflexes in health and diseases. Eckberg DL, Sleight P, eds, Clarendon Press, Oxford 1992;61–77.

40. Badilini F, Maison-Blanche P, Spaulding R, Palma M, Coumel P. Analysis of QT interval during passive tilt test: comparison of different correction formula. Computers in Cardiology 1998;25:713–716.

41. Ahnve S, Vallin M. Influence of heart rate and inhibition of autonomic tone on the QT interval in man. Circulation 1982;65:435–439.

42. Milne JR, Ward DE, Spurrell RAJ, Camm AJ. The ventricular paced QT interval. The effects of rate and exercise. Pace 1982;5:352–358.

43. Dickhuth HH, Bluemner E, Auchschwelk W, Zehnder M, Irmer M, Meinertz T. The relationship between heart rate and QT interval during atrial stimulation. PACE 1991;14:793–799.

44. Cappato R, Alboni P, Pedroni P, Gilli G, Antonioli G. Sympathetic and vagal influences on rate-dependent changes of QT interval in healthy subjects. Am J Cardiol 1991;68:1188–1193.

45. Fananapazir L, Bennett DH, Faragher EB. Contribution of heart rate to QT interval shortening during exercise. Eur Heart J 1983;4:265–271.

46. Rickards AF, Norman J. Relation between QT interval and heart rate: new design of physiologically adaptative cardiac pacemakers. Br Heart J 1981;45:56–61.

47. Horstmann E, Koenn B. Temporal relationship between exercise and QT shortening in patients with QT pacemakers. PACE 1989;12:1080–1084.

48. Browne KF, Prystowsky EN, Heger JJ, Zipes DP. Modulation of the QT interval by the autonomic nervous system. PACE 1983;6:1050–1055.

49. Browne KF, Zipes DP, Heger JJ, Prystowsky EN. Prolongation of the QT interval in man during sleep. Am J Cardiol 1983;52:55–59.

50. Alexopoulos D, Rynkiewiez A, Yusuf S, Johnston JA, Sleight P, Yacoub MH. Diurnal variation of QT interval after cardiac transplantation. Am J Cardiol 1988;61:482–485.

51. Bexton RS, Vallin HO, Camm AL. Diurnal variation of the QT interval in influence of the autonomic nervous system. Br Heart J 1986;55:253–258.

52. Viitasalo M, Karjalainen J. QT intervals at heart rates from 50 to 120 beats per minute during 24-hour electrocardiographic recordings in 100 healthy men. Effects of atenolol. Circulation 1992;86:1439–1442.

53. Murakawa Y, Inoue H, Nozaki A, Sugimoto T. Role of sympatho-vagal interaction in diurnal variation of QT interval. Am J Cardiol 1992;69:339–343.

54. Coumel P, Fayn J, Maison-Blanche P, Rubel P. Clinical relevance of assessing QT dynamicity in Holter recordings. J Electrocardiology 1994;27:62–66.

55. Maison-Blanche P, Catuli D, Fayn J, Coumel P. QT interval, heart rate and ventricular arrhythmias. In "Non-invasive Electrocardiology. Clinical Aspects of Holter Monitoring," Moss AJ, Stern S, eds, WB Saunders Company Ltd, London, Philadelphia 1995;383–404.

56. Ahmed MW, Kadish AH, Goldberger JJ. Autonomic effects on the QT intereval. ANE 1996;1:44–153.

57. Extramiana F, Tavernier R, Maison-Blanche P, et al. Repolarisation ventriculaire et enregistrement Holter. Role du blocage sympathique sur le physiologie de la relation QT/RR. Arch Mal Cœur 2000;93:1277–1283.

58. Bellavere F, Ferri M, Guarini L, et al. Prolonged QT period in diabeticc autonomic neuropathy: a possible role in sudden cardiac death? Br Heart J 1988;59:379–383.

59. Ahnve S. Correction of the QT interval for heart rate: review of different formulas and the use of Bazett's formula in myocardial infarction. Am Heart J 1985;109:568–573

60. Cappato R, Alboni P, Codecà L, Guardigli G, Toselli T, Antonioli GE. Direct and autonomically mediated effects of oral quinidine on RR/QT relation after an abrupt increase in heart rate. J Am Coll Cardiol 1993;22:99–105.

61. Edvarsson N, Olsson SB. Effects of acute and chronic beta-receptor blockade on ventricular repolarisation in man. Br Heart J 1981;45:628–636.

62. Arrowood JA, Kline J, Simpson PM, et al. Modulation on the QT interval: effect of graded exercise and reflex cardiovascular stimulation. J Appl Physiol 1993;75:2217–2223.

63. Levy MN. Sympathetic-parasympathetic actions in the heart. Circ Res 1971;29:437–445.

64. Morady F, Kou WH, Nelson SD, et al. Accentuated antagonism between beta-adrenergic and vagal effects on ventricular refractoriness in humans. Circulation 1988;77:289–297.

65. Zaza A, Malfatto G, Schwartz PJ. Sympathetic modulation of the relation between ventricular repolarization and cycle length. Circ Res 1991;68:1191–1203.

66. Schwartz PJ, Wolf S. QT interval prolongation as predictor of sudden death in patients with myocardial infaction. Circulation 1978;57(6):1074–1077.

67. Schwartz PJ, Zaza A, Pala M, Locati E, Beria G, Zanchetti A. Baroreflex sensitivity and its evolution during the first year after myocardial infarction. J Am Coll Cardiol 1988;12:629–636.

68. Algra A, Tijssen JGP, Roelandt JRTC, et al. QT interval variables from 24-hour electrocardiography and the two year risk of sudden death. Br Heart J 1993;70:43–48.

69. Extramiana F, Neyroud N, Huikuri H, et al. QT interval and arrhythmic risk assessment after myocardial infarction. Am J Cardiol 1999;83:266–269.

70. Milliez P, Leenhardt A, Maison Blanche P, et al. Arrhythmic death in the EMIAT trial: role of ventricular repolarization dynamicity as a new discriminant risk marker (Abstract). Eur Heart J 1999;20–I:160.

71. Huikuri HV, Koistinen MJ, Yü-Mayry S, et al. Impaired low frequency oscillations of heart rate in patients with prior acute myocardial infarction and life-threatening arrhythmias. Am J Cardiol 1995;76:56–60.

72. Murakawa Y, Ajiki K, Usui M, Yamashita T, Oikawa N, Inoue H. Parasympathetic activity is a major modulator of the circadian variability of heart rate in healthy subjects and in patients with coronary artery disease or diabetes mellitus. Am Heart J 1993;126:108–114.

73. Coumel P, Johnson N, Extramiana F, Maison-Blanche P, Valensi P. Modulation de l'électrocardiogramme et troubles du rythme chez le diabètique. Arch Mal Coeur 2000;93(IV):59–66.

74. Pellerin D, Maison-Blanche P, Extramiana F, et al. Autonomic influences on ventricular repolarization in congestive heart failure. J Electrocardiol 2001;34:35–40.

75. Neyroud N, Maison-Blanche P, Denjoy I, et al. Diagnostic performance of QT interval variables from 24-h electrocardiography in the long QT syndrome. Eur Heart J 1998;19:158–165.

76. Locati EH, Maison-Blanche P, Dejode P, Cauchemez B, Coumel P. Spontaneous sequences of onset of torsades de pointes in patients with acquired prolonged repolarization: quantitative analysis of Holter recordings. J Am Coll Cardiol 1995;25:1564–1575.

77. Schwartz PJ, Priori S, Spazzolini C, et al. Genotype-Phenotype correlation in the Long QT syndrome. Gene specific triggers for life-threatening arrhythmias. Circulation 2001;103:89–95.

78. Swan H, Viitasalo M, Piippo K, et al. Sinus node function and ventricular repolarization during exercise stress test in Long QT syndrome patients with KvLQT1 and HERG potassium channel defects. J Am Coll Cardiol 1999;34:823–829.

79. Schwartz PJ. Another role for the sympathetic nervous sytem in the Long QT syndrome? J Cardiovasc Electrophysiol 2001;12:500–502.

80. Singh JP, Larson MG, O'Donnell CJ, et al. Heritability of heart rate variability. The Framingham Heart Study. Circulation 1999;99:2251–2254.
81. Leenhardt A, Lucet V, Denjoy I, Grau F, DoNgoc D, Coumel P. Catecholaminergic polymorphic ventricular tachycardia in children: a 7-year follow-up of 21 patients. Circulation 1995;91:1512–1519.
82. Funck-Brentano C, Kibleur Y, Le Coz F, et al. Rate dependence of sotalol-induced prolongation of ventricular repolarization during exercise in humans. Circulation 1991;83:536–545.
83. Lande G, Maison-Blanche P, Fayn J, et al. Dynamic analysis of dofetilide-induced changes in ventricular repolarization. Clin Pharmacol Ther 1998;64:312–321.
84. Hondeghem, et al. Instability and triangulation of the action potential predict serious proarrhythmia, but action potential duration prolongation is antiarrhythmic. Circulation 2001;103:2004–2010.
85. Kadish AH, Weisman HF, Veltri EP, et al. Paradoxical effects of exercise on the QT interval in patients with polymorphic ventricular tachycardia receiving type Ia antiarrhythmic agents. Circulation 1990;81:14–19.
86. Buckingham TA, Bhutto ZR, Telfer EA, et al. Differences in corrected QT intervals at minimal and maximal heart rates may identify patients at risk for torsades de pointes during treatment with antiarrhythmic drugs. J Cardiovasc Electrophysiol 1994;5:408–411.

16 The Electrophysiologic Matrix
Equilibrium and Arnsdorf's Paradox

Morton F. Arnsdorf, MD, MACC

CONTENTS

INTRODUCTION
ELECTROPHYSIOLOGIC EQUILIBRIA AND THE MATRICAL CONCEPT
    OF CARDIAC EXCITABILITY
CURRENT PERSPECTIVES ON THE ELECTROPHYSIOLOGIC MATRIX
CLINICAL IMPLICATIONS
THE ELECTROPHYSIOLOGIC UNIVERSE AND THE ELECTROCARDIOGRAM:
    THE EXTRACELLULARLY RECORDED POTENTIAL WITH EMPHASIS
    ON THE DIASTOLIC ELECTROCARDIOGRAM
RECOMMENDATIONS FOR FUTURE RESEARCH
REFERENCES

INTRODUCTION

The heart beat results from a tightly controlled flow of ions of several species through specialized channels in the cell membrane, within the myoplasm, through the gap junctions that connect the cells, and through the extracellular space. Impulse propagation is importantly affected by the structure of the cell membrane, the distribution of gap junctions, and the characteristics of the extracellular space as well as by neurohumoral influences and other feedback mechanisms. The objectives of this chapter are several.

At the urging of the editors, we will revisit the Paradox which for complicated reasons I claimed as my own in 1990. The seeming Paradox is that the multiplicities, discontinuities, dynamic interactions, and other complexities that exist in and among the determinants of cardiac excitability should result in unpredictably complex behavior, yet, electrophysiologic events usually are coordinated sufficiently to produce predictable outcomes. In other words, there is order in this seeming chaos. Resolution of the paradox resides in the self-organization of the electrophysiologic universe which moves as a system in response to normal, pathophysiologic and pharmacologic influences. The reproducibility of the change or changes in the system and the movement of the electrophysiologic universe as a system results, therefore, in predictability of the type of change expected. The change in electrophysiologic matrices as a system has a number of important clinical implications concerning arrhythmogenesis, antiarrhythmic drug effects, and proarrhythmia. The movement as a system also provides a fresh look at

From: *Contemporary Cardiology: Cardiac Repolarization: Bridging Basic and Clinical Science*
Edited by: I. Gussak et al. © Humana Press Inc., Totowa, NJ

351

predominant drug actions and the resulting empirical usefulness of scientifically shaky clinical classifications of antiarrhythmic agents. Finally, the change as a system also explains in large part the seeming empirical usefulness of very simplified electrocardiographic measurements during electrical diastole that are being used to assess ischemia and stratify patient risk.

In this chapter, we will consider first the concept of cardiac excitability as a dynamic system that depends on the individual and sequential regenerative depolarization of cells and communication between cells to cause the normal, orderly propagation of electrical impulses throughout the heart which, in turn, elicits the coordinated mechanical contraction required for an efficient cardiac output. This concept has been considered recently in great detail *(1)*. Second, given the theme of this book, more emphasis will be placed on repolarization as an important determinant of normal and abnormal cardiac excitability. Finally, we will revisit the electrocardiographic manifestations of repolarization, focussing on the genesis of changes in the TQ-ST segment, the QT interval, and other measurements made during electrical diastole in the context of our proposed electrophysiologic universe.

ELECTROPHYSIOLOGIC EQUILIBRIA AND THE MATRICAL CONCEPT OF CARDIAC EXCITABILITY

Passive and Active Cellular Properties

The electrophysiologic universe is very complex and consists of sources that provide current flow of various types, several ionic channels with differing properties and selectivities that allow the appropriate currents to flow that are necessary for depolarization and repolarization, sinks into which the current flow, linkages between cells that include another type of specialized channels called gap junctions, nonconductive tissues between cells that facilitate impulse propagation in one direction over another, and energy-requiring pumps that maintain the electrochemical gradients necessary for the electrical events. It is useful, although not strictly accurate, to consider cellular properties as being either passive or active. Conceptually, passive properties can be considered the *sink* into which currents flow, whereas active properties can be considered the *source* for the current.

Passive properties are more or less constant and are characterized by a response proportional to the stimulus. Few properties, however, are truly passive. Ionic activities within and outside the cell as well as membrane capacitance are usually considered passive properties, but the ionic activities are dynamic and depend on energy-requiring pumps whereas the membrane capacitance can be influenced by insertions into the cell membrane including metabolites of ischemia and drugs. The flow of ionic currents and molecules from cell to cell is regulated by a longitudinal resistances that are also generally considered passive. The gap junctions control most of the conductance between cells and, like other channels, open and close in response to stimuli, but sufficiently slowly to render their effects constant. The effects of passive properties are often approximately *linear* for small stimuli, and, therefore, can be described by Ohm's Law ($V = IR = I/G$ where V is voltage, I is current, R is resistance and G is conductance, the reciprocal of resistance). The relationship between current and resistance becomes *nonlinear* for larger stimuli in the range of transmembrane potentials between the resting or maximal diastolic potential and threshold.

Active properties are nonlinear and, further, have a response out of proportion to the stimulus. The changes in ionic conductances which are dependent on the transmembrane voltage, V_m, and on time and are responsible for the depolarization and repolarization of the action potential are considered active properties. Subthreshold responses in V_m to steps in intracellular current injection, as mentioned, are nonlinear, but are *continuous* until the threshold is attained when there is a sudden explosive, *discontinuous* response to a stimulus of the same magnitude.

It is beyond the scope of this chapter to consider in detail, the currents responsible for regenerative depolarization and repolarization. A brief summary, however, is in order to prepare a background for the discussion of this chapter. The phase or regenerative depolarization (phase 0) is determined mainly by the properties of the inward sodium current, i_{Na}, and to a lesser extent by Ca^{2+} currents in the so-called *fast response* tissues which include the atria, the cells of Purkinje fibers, ventricles and accessory bypass tracts. In the so-called *slow response* tissues of the sinoatrial (SA) and atrioventricular (AV) nodes, the kinetically fast i_{Na} is not evident. This is so either because V_m rests at around −60 mV, at which potential i_{Na} is completely inactivated and therefore eliminated functionally, or because fast Na^+ channels are simply not expressed. Instead, phase 0 depolarization is dominantly owing a current called i_{Ca}, carried by a Ca^{2+} channel (L-type) which can be blocked by phenylalkylamines (e.g., verapamil) and by dihydropyridines (e.g., nifedipine). This current is sometimes called the "slow inward" current, i_{si}. Fast response tissues can behave like slow response tissues, if they are depolarized by injury, or treated with drugs modifying the kinetics and states of the fast Na^+ channel. In these cases, standing Na^+ channel inactivation without recovery occurs. Action potentials developed by fast tissues in these states depend on i_{Ca}.

The plateau phase and repolarization of the action potential is a complex process, and this process is considered in detail in other chapters. An initial rapid repolarization is seen in fast response tissues, which may inscribe a notch (phase 1), and results from the rapid early decay of the Na^+ current combined with activation of transient outward currents carried by a voltage activated transient outward K^+ current, a calcium activated transient outward Cl^- current, and electrogenic Na-Ca exchange. Membrane resistance is relatively high during the plateau phase (phase 2) during which slowly decaying late residual depolarizing inward currents through Na^+ and Ca^{2+} channels are balanced against voltage- and time-dependent activating repolarizing outward K^+ currents carried by the slow and rapidly activating delayed rectifier K^+ channels. Rapid repolarization occurs during phase 3 when the balance of the repolarizing currents gain the upper hand and the inward rectifier K^+ channels provide a final assist to repolarize the membrane. Repolarization in the slow response tissues also reflects a balance between inward depolarizing and outward repolarizing currents. Some characteristics of the so-called fast and slow response tissues are listed in Table 1. Currents important to depolarization and repolarization in fast response tissues are diagrammatically shown in Panel A of Fig. 1.

The Electrophysiologic Matrix During Repolarization

A premise that we will return to later in this chapter is that electrophysiologic events can be discussed in terms of there being a matrix of interacting cellular electrophysiologic properties that determines normal cardiac excitability. This normal matrix represents a stable dynamic electrophysiologic equilibrium that is maintained by homeostatic feed-

Table 1
Selected Electrophysiologic Characteristics of So-Called Fast and Slow Response Tissues

Properties	Fast Response Tissues	Slow Response Tissues
Geographic Location	Atrial tissues; Purkinje fibers of the infranodal specialized conduction system; ventriclular myocardium; AV bypass tracts (accessory pathways)	SA and AV nodes; perhaps valves and coronary sinus. Depolarized "fast" response tissues in which sodium channels are inactivated and phase 0 depends on calcium current.
Normal resting potential (V_r)	–80 to –95 mV	–40 to –65 mV
Subthreshold conductance	Primarily components of potassium conductance, particularly g_{K1}	Probably a component of gK
Current responsible for phase 0 (rapid depolarization)	Kinetically rapid transient inward sodium current (i_{Na})	Predominantly i_{Ca} through L-type channel (can be a mixed current with Na^+) often called "slow inward current" (i_{si})
Phase 0 channel kinetics activation and if inactivation	Rapid and transient.	Slow, and the activation is multistep
Maximal rate of rise of phase 0 (dV/dt_{max}) or ($\dot{V}_{max}$)	300–1000 V/sec	1–50 V/sec
Peak overshoot (V_{os})	+20 to +40 mV	–5 to +20 mV
Action potential amplitude	90 to 135 mV	30 to 70 mV
Properties importantly dependent on the interaction between active and passive properties		
"Threshold" voltage (V_{th})	–60 to –75 mV	–40 to –60 mV
Conduction	Rapid. 0.5 to 5 m/sec	Slow. 0.01 to 0.1 m/sec
Safety factor	High source over sink	Low source over sink
Refractoriness and reactivation	Partial reactivation during phase 3 with complete reactivation in normal tissue 10 to 50 ms after return to normal V_r	Partial and complete reactivation returns after attainment of V_r (> 100 ms)
Relationship of rate to:		
Action potential duration	Marked change	Slight change
Refractory period duration	Steep curve	"Flat" curve
Threshold	Independent	Varies directly with frequency
Conduction velocity	Independent	Decays with frequency
Characteristics conducive to reentry	Only with inactivation of sodium system with marked slowing of conduction velocity	Present even in normally i_{Ca} tissues (SA and AV nodes)
Automaticity	Yes. Depends on changing balance between inward currents and an increasing outward i_K	Yes
Automaticity depressed by physiologic increases in $[K^+]_o$	Yes	No to slightly

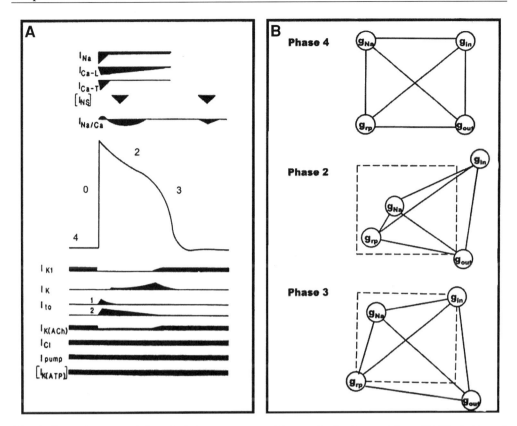

Fig. 1. The action potential, underlying currents and the repolarization matrices. (**A**) The left panel schematically illustrates the action potential and the contributing currents in cardiac myocytes. The approximate time courses of the currents associated with channels and pumps are quantitatively indicated, but no effort is made to compare the magnitude of one current with another. The inward depolarizing currents are shown in the upper portion of the panel and include the kinetically rapid inward sodium current (I_{Na}) that is responsible for phase 0, the L- and T- type calcium currents (I_{Ca-L}, I_{Ca-T}, respectively), a nonspecific inward current (I_{NS} and a current resulting from sodium-calcium exchange ($I_{Na/Ca}$). The outward repolarizing currents are shown in the lower portion of the panel and include the inwardly rectifying K$^+$ current (I_{K1}), the delayed rectifier current (I_K), and the voltage-dependent transient outward current (I_{to}). The heavy bars associated with the chloride, pump, and I$_{K(ATP)}$ vary with pathophysiologic conditions and so are represented by a constant magnitude. This panel was adapted from The Sicilian Gambit I *(23)*. (**B**) The right panel is a simplified matrix of conductances important in repolarization during phase 4 (the resting potential), phase 2 (slow repolarization) and phase 3 (rapid repolarization). The conductances important to maintaining the resting potential, mainly g_{K1}, are contained in the term g_{rp}; g_{Na} is the conductance responsible for the flow of I_{Na}; g_{in} is the lumped conductance of the several inward depolarizing currents important in maintaining the plateau that are shown in the upper portion of the left panel; and g_{out} is the lumped conductances of the several outward repolarizing currents that return the membrane potential back to phase 4. Bonds connecting the elements indicate interactions and mutual dependencies. The square indicates the normal situation during phase 4. A shift of the element towards the center of the rectangle represents a decrease and a shift outwards an increase in the quantity.

back mechanisms. The matrix is impossibly complex since it represents a multidimensional model of all the active and passive properties that determine cardiac excitability and impulse propagation. But, the matrices can be simplified to illustrate specific points. In this section of the chapter, we will develop a simple matrix that represents the electrophysiologic universe during repolarization.

Panel B in Fig. 1 is a simplified matrix of conductances important in repolarization during phase 4 (the resting potential), phase 2 (slow repolarization) and phase 3 (rapid repolarization). During phase 4, four lumped conductances, each represented by a circle, are positioned at each corner of a square. The square represents the normal lumped conductance at the resting potential, V_r, during phase 4. Bonds connecting the elements indicate interactions and mutual interdependencies.

The conductances important to maintaining the resting potential, mainly g_{K1}, are contained in the term g_{rp}. The channel conductance responsible for the flow of I_{Na} is g_{Na}. As has been discussed, several conductances are responsible for the inward depolarizing currents that contribute to the maintenance of the plateau and are depicted in the upper portion of Panel A, and in this illustration we have lumped these several conductances into the term g_{in}. Similarly, g_{out} represents the lumped conductances of the several outward repolarizing currents shown in the lower portion of Panel A that strive to bring the membrane potential back to phase 4. A shift of the element toward the center of the rectangle represents a decrease and a shift outward an increase in the quantity.

In phase 4, the lumped conductances are in balance and are maintained by normal homeostatic mechanisms. During phase 0 (not shown), g_{Na} becomes maximal and sodium current rushes into the cell. V_m rapidly becomes less negative and finally positive as the equilibrium potential for sodium is approached. The sodium channel rapidly closes and refractory, which is the basis for the absolute refractory period.

During phase 2 repolarization that constitutes the plateau of the action potential, the sodium channel is inactivated and g_{Na} is virtually zero, thereby preventing any flow of sodium current into the cell. As shown in the diagram, this can be depicted by moving g_{Na} to nearly the center of the square. The conductances that determine the resting potential decrease, but not relatively as much as the sodium conductance, so g_{rp} is moved only a small distance inside the rectangle. The inward depolarizing currents responsible for maintaining the plateau increase as compared to the situation in phase 4, and this is depicted by moving g_{in} outside the square. The repolarizing outward currents also begin to increase, but since the depolarizing inward currents outbalance the outward repolarizing currents, g_{out} is moved outside the rectangle, but less than g_{in}.

During phase 3, g_{Na} is beginning to move back to its normal diastolic position. At some time during phase 3, the sodium channels are sufficiently reactivated that a stimulus can elicit an action potential, but usually it is a somewhat attenuated action potential. This is the basis for the relative refractory period. Full recovery of the sodium channel usually does occur shortly before the return to phase 4. During phase 3, the inward repolarizing currents that have maintained the plateau and the currents responsible for the normal resting potential have returned to their normal values, and this is depicted by g_{in} and g_{rp} returning to their positions at the corner of the square. Some components of g_{in}, such as the conductance of the inward calcium current may not fully reactivate until well into phase 4 since there may be a time- as well as a voltage-dependent component to reactivation. On full repolarization, the situation once again becomes that of phase 4.

Matrices of greater or lesser complexity can be created. The "normal" phase 4 matrix shown in panel B of Fig. 2 has six components, but it could have many more since each

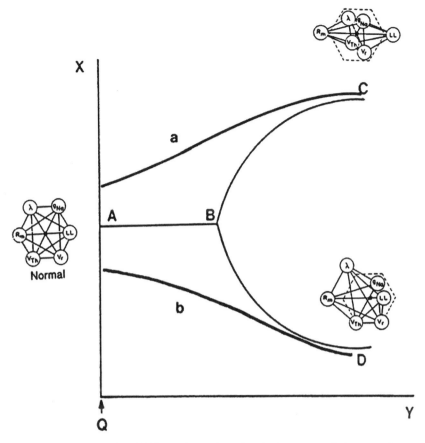

Fig. 2. Bifurcations and assisted bifurcations. At point A, the system is in a steady-state with the equilibrium maintained by feedback mechanisms. The "normal" matrix at point A contains more elements than the four-component "normal" phase 4 matrix in Fig. 1 and contains active and passive cellular electrophysiologic properties which determine cardiac excitability. The elements include resting potential (V_r), threshold voltage (V_{th}), sodium conductance (g_{Na}), membrane resistance (R_m), length constant (λ), and liminal length (LL). Each element in turn depends on a set of more basic processes. The bonds connecting the elements indicate interactions and mutual dependencies. A normal state is indicated by the regular hexagonal shape. When quantities represented in the matrix change, the matrix changes shape; when a quantity decreases, the corresponding element shifts toward the center of the hexagon; when the quantity increases, the corresponding element shifts away from the center. One or more controlling parameters drives the system from left to right. At point B, the system becomes unstable and moves to a new equilibrium at either points C or D. The value of one or more parameters along the x-axis will assist the bifurcation to either point C or D (pathways a and b, respectively). Quinidine (Q) is applied at time = 0. See text for discussion. From Arnsdorf *(17)*.

lumped conductance contains several individual conductances which, in turn, contain a number of other determinants. The "normal" matrix at point A in Fig. 2 represents the same situation as shown in Fig. 1B during phase 4, but additional elements are included in this depiction. The elements include resting potential, V_r, which is the end result of the lump conductances g_{rp}. It also includes some passive cellular properties and some properties that depend both on passive and active properties. The plasma membrane is a thin, phospholipid bilayer that separates aqueous phases inside and outside the cells. They can store charge as an electrical capacitor and can act as an insulator to limit the leakage of ions into and out of the cell. The resistance of the insulation, a passive property, is called the membrane resistance, R_m, and is expressed as ohms. Current flow within the cell affects neighboring cells, and the distance over which current influences the neighboring cells is called the length constant, λ, and is described in millimeters. As will be described later, λ is a function of the leakiness of the membrane, the resistance within the cell and between cells across gap junctions, and the extracellular resistance.

The excitable cell must be depolarized beyond a certain voltage to permit regenerative production of an action potential, and this has been called the threshold voltage, V_{th}. Fozzard and Schoenberg *(2)* applied the concept of liminal length to excitability in cardiac tissues. The liminal length *(LL)* is that amount of tissue that must be raised above threshold to overcome the effects of the outward repolarizing current from neighboring tissues in order for a regenerative action potential to occur. The liminal length depends on a number of factors and is directly proportional to the charge threshold and inversely proportional to radius, capacitance, length constant, and the threshold potential (for greater detail, see our recent discussion, *1*).

Each element in turn depends on a set of more basic processes that can be included in or omitted depending on the focus of the discussion or of an experiment. As was true in Fig. 1, the bonds connecting the elements indicate interactions and mutual dependencies. In this more complex model, a normal state is indicated by the regular hexagonal shape. When quantities represented in the matrix change, the matrix changes shape; when a quantity decreases, the corresponding element shifts toward the center of the hexagon; when the quantity increases, the corresponding element shifts away from the center.

Matrices and Systems: Depiction of Nonlinear and Discontinuous Events

As already discussed, sometimes electrophysiologic events can be approximately linear, but are more commonly nonlinear. They can be continuous or discontinuous. The nonlinear nature of a system is frequently evident, as, for example, in the regenerative depolarization of the action potential during phase 0. Nonlinear and discontinuous events are quite common in response to stimuli and may demonstrate, for example, bifurcations, bistability, and hysteresis.

BIFURCATIONS AND ASSISTED BIFURCATIONS

In bifurcations, the character of the response evolves in time, or as a parameter is changed, in a specific sequence. In our experimental work, we frequently have seen an electrophysiologic matrix that is maintained in a dynamic equilibrium by complex feedback systems give way, often explosively, to disequilibrium, and then to self-organize into a new equilibrium. Bifurcation diagrams are frequently used to depict such events (see, for example, *3*). Consider the bifurcation diagram in Fig. 2. At point A, the system is in a dynamic equilibrium. Beginning at point A, some condition changes and carries the system along the *y*-axis until point B is reached. Between points A and B, homeostatic feedback mechanisms have maintained the steady-state. At point B, however, these mechanisms fail, the system becomes unstable, and there is a transition to a new equilibrium at C or perhaps at D. Given the choice of moving from point B to points C or D, the parameter along the *x*-axis assists in determining the path taken (lower case a or b); and this is termed an *assisted bifurcation*.

Figure 2 is based on some of our experiments on quinidine *(4)*. Quinidine superfusion of the Purkinje fiber is indicated by the arrow at Q. The system is being driven from left to right along the *y*-axis. At a $[K]_o$ of 5.4 mM, quinidine produced a matrical configuration that increased excitability in all experiments (pathway b to steady-state D in Fig. 2B). This change resulted from a substantial increase in membrane resistance, R_m, and λ despite a slight decrease in the marker for g_{Na}. At a $[K]_o$ of 8 mM, quinidine could either increase or decrease excitability depending whether the net excitability was determined primarily by the altered passive or active properties. At a $[K]_o$ of 12 mM, quinidine produced a matrical configuration that decreased excitability in all experiments (pathway a to steady-state C in Fig. 2B). Given the choice of moving from point B to points C or D, the decision is *assisted* by the level of $[K]_o$.

Bifurcations, particularly those assisted by conditions, occur commonly in clinical electrophysiology, and that this is an important principle in arrhythmogenesis and in the actions of antiarrhythmic drugs (*see 1,5–7*, and original articles cited in these reviews). We will return to this theme in several sections that follow.

BISTABILITIES

Bistable systems are characterized by a stimulus causing two or more kinds of response; for example, a propagated response and the initiation of triggered activity. It should be recalled that membrane resistance increases nonlinearly as a function of voltage. To demonstrate this point and for historical interest, I have included an illustration from Sylvio Weidmann's classic publication in 1951 *(8)*. Figure 3 is a photograph of a series of oscilloscopic images which shows a number of superimposed action potentials during which a repetitive series of small negative currents were injected intracellularly. The intracellular pulses were injected randomly, so the superimposition of the action potentials results in a "band" of voltage deflections. Note that the band thickens during phase 2, becomes narrower during phase 3 and the beginning of phase 4. This fiber shows automaticity in that phase 4 progressively becomes less negative, and the "band" widens as the potential becomes less negative. Remembering that Ohm's Law is $V = IR = I/G$, where V is voltage, I is current, R is resistance, and G is conductance (the reciprocal of resistance that indicates the ease with which current can flow), a widening of the "band" indicates a great voltage response for the constant current input, therefore, membrane resistance must be increasing or conversely, membrane conductance is decreasing. Subsequently, more sophisticated analysis using voltage clamping has been performed, but the message is the same: Membrane resistance (i.e., conductance is lower is much higher) during the plateau than it is at the resting potential, so a small intracellularly applied current produces a larger change in potential during phase 2 than it does during phase 4.

Failed Repolarization. The repolarization process is exquisitely sensitive to small changes in electrophysiologic properties. Membrane conductance during the plateau, as mentioned, is low, and the depolarizing inward currents are almost equal to the repolarizing outward currents, which accounts for the gradual change in membrane potential. From time to time, repolarization can fail to occur normally. This is shown in Fig. 4 in which a cardiac Purkinje fiber was superfused with lysophosphatidylcholine (LPC), a putative toxic metabolite ischemia, before and after the application of lidocaine *(9)*. Figure 4A shows the control action potential. As shown in Fig. 4B, LPC superfusion resulted in the Purkinje fiber having two stable-steady states: One at a nearly normal resting potential and the other at the plateau. A very small injection of intracellular current

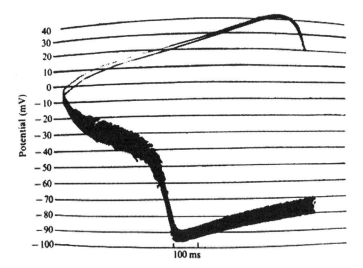

Fig. 3. Landmark recording from Sylvio Weidmann's 1951 paper on the effect of current flow on the membrane potential of a Purkinje fiber. The recording shows superimposed action potentials perturbed by the intracellular injection of small intracellular currents into the fiber. The injection was allowed to occur any time during the electrical cycle, which effectively scanned the entire normal action potential. The magnitude of the broadening of the voltage deflections caused by the intracellular current injection corresponds to the membrane resistance at various points during the electrical cycle. *See* text for discussion. From Weidmann *(8)*.

(18 na), could shift the preparation from the stable steady-state at the plateau to another at the resting potentia. Lidocaine normalized the action potential and made the resting potential more negative. With washout, the action potential duration increased progressively. Eventually, the situation characterized by two stable states recurred. The membrane potential would remain at this plateau potential indefinitely *(9)*. Phenytoin and propranolol also could facilitate the attainment of the repolarization "threshold" with normalization of the action potential *(10)*.

Failed Repolarization and Saltatory Conduction. Intuitively, one would think that an equilibrium at the plateau voltage would stop conduction because of inactivation of the sodium channels. This may occur, perhaps most of the time, but other things can result at such a membrane potential. We will consider two less obvious outcomes for which there is some basic evidence; namely, saltatory conduction which depends importantly on membrane resistance and then oscillatory activity and action potentials that depend on a current other than I_{Na}.

We recently have written extensively on the propagation of electrical activity through arrays of cells with emphasis on anisotropic and discontinuous propagation of the electrical impulse *(1,7)*. If action potentials cannot propagate through a region of tissue, the electronic currents must have decreased to the point where the liminal length requirements are no longer being met. The converse is not true in that electrotonic conduction through an inexcitable gap can support the propagation of action potentials. In an elegant experiment now two decades old, Antzelevitch and Moe put a Purkinje fiber into a three-compartment bath in which the central segment of the tissue, 1.5 mm long, was rendered inexcitable by superfusing it with a solution that had $[K^+]_o$ of 15 to 20 m*M (11)*. The experimental arrangement in shown in Fig. 5. Mechanically, hyperkalemia in the

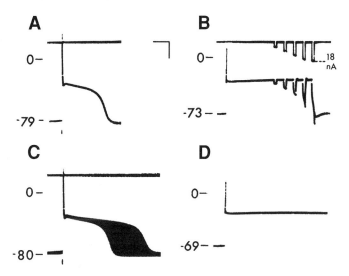

Fig. 4. Bistability as illustrated by failed repolarization that resulted in two stable quiescent equilibria. (**A**) Control with a V_r of –79 mV and an action potential duration of 290 ms. (**B**) After superfusion of the Purkinje fiber with lysophosphatidylcholine (LPC), one steady-state was observed at a V_r of –73 mV and a second at the plateau potential. Intracellularly applied hyperpolarizing constant current of increasing amplitude were applied with 18 nA finally causing attainment of the repolarization "threshold" and a return to V_r. If current was not applied, the membrane potential would have remained at the plateau indefinitely. (**C**) Superimposed action potentials. Lidocaine shortened the action potential duration to a normal value of 300 ms and somewhat hyperpolarized the resting cell with the V_r becoming –80 mV. With washout of lidocaine, the action potential duration progressively increased. (**D**) Eventually, during continued superfusion of the fiber with LPC, the cell depolarized with V_r becoming –69 mV and the return of two stable steady states. From Sawicki and Arnsdorf *(9)*.

central segment depolarizes that portion of the cell, and the relationship between the membrane potential and $[K^+]_o$ is closely approximated by the Nernst equation; that is, as $[K^+]_o$ increases V_r becomes less negative in a rather linear fashion. The less negative V_r inactivates the sodium channels, first partially, and then completely. At a $[K^+]_o$ of 15 to 20 mM, the segment in the central compartment has no sodium channels available for activation and, therefore, is inexcitable. As shown in Fig. 5, sufficient current could be made to flow from the proximal compartment through the gap junctions in the inexcitable segment and into the distal compartment to generate an electronically mediated depolarization which may evoke a regenerative action potential.

The more current that can flow electrotonically through the interior of the inexcitable segment, the more likely it becomes that the liminal length requirements in the distal segment can be met, thereby resulting in an action potential. Returning to the basic principles of cable analysis, the length or space constant (λ) is the distance over which V_m at the point of steady-state current application falls to about 37% of its value. λ is directly proportional to the square root of the resistance of the membrane, r_m, and is indirectly proportional to the square root of the longitudinal or inside resistance, r_i (determined largely by gap junctional resistances between cells) and the extracellular or outside resistances, r_o; that is: $\lambda = \sqrt{r_m / (r_i + r_o)}$. As mentioned, membrane resistance is much higher at the plateau voltage than at the resting potential. λ, then, would be greater

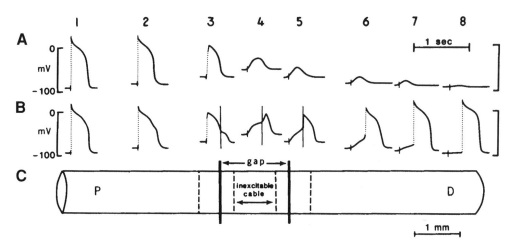

Fig. 5. An inexcitable gap preparation which demonstrates that electrotonic interactions can bridge an area of inexcitable cable and excite tissue in the distal segment. The experimental arrangement is shown in C in which the segment in the middle compartment was rendered inexcitable by depolarization with a high $[K^+]_o$ solution. The impulse is initiated in the proximal segment P, so propagation will be from left to right ($1\rightarrow8$). **(A)** The impulse propagates to the border of the block and stops there. The recording at 3 shows a diminished action potential, but 4 is only an electronically-induced subthreshold deflection. The electrotonic axial and local circuit current flow in the inexcitable gap was insufficient to bring the distal segment, D, to threshold. **(B)** In this case, the electrotonic axial and local circuit current flow was sufficient to meet the liminal length requirements in D to produce a propagated action potential. Adapted from Antzelevitch and Moe*(11)*.

at the plateau voltage than at the resting potential, so the distance over which electrotonic currents could affect neighboring cells also would be greater. This could facilitate saltatory conduction. The interested reader is referred to the classic papers by Sylvio Weidmann on the determination of electrical constants in Purkinje fibers and ventricular muscle *(12,13)* and to our recent discussion in the Appendix of a review which contains key equations relating to individual myocardial cells, one-dimensional cable theory, liminal length, uniformly anisotropic propagation, spatially discrete cable theories and functional properties of gap junctions *(1)*.

Failed Repolarization and Oscillatory Activity. Tissues that normally depend on i_{Na} for phase 0 depolarization have the sodium system partially or completely inactivated by depolarization. This is the experimental basis for determining the sodium current and the conductance of the sodium channel by voltage clamping before and after an intervention, say, after antiarrhythmic drug. A failure of repolarization at the plateau voltage effectively inactivates the sodium system. As a result, the tissue may be quiescent as in Fig. 4B, or the tissue may develop action potentials that are dependent on inward calcium currents. A striking example triggered sustained membrane activity following the failure of normal repolarization is shown in Fig. 6 *(14)*. In the control situation (Fig. 6A, B), an electrically provoked action potential arises from a resting membrane potential of –83 mV which then triggered slow oscillatory activity that developed into nondriven sustained action potentials. The triggered activity persisted for 45 min until a hyperpolarizing intracellular current of 7 nA (downward arrow) was applied which permitted attainment of the repolarization "threshold" and a return to the resting potential (Fig. 6B). Lidocaine caused an almost immediate attainment of the repolarization threshold and

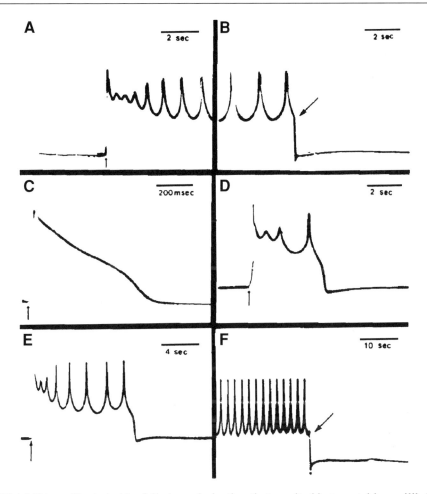

Fig. 6. Bistability as illustrated by failed repolarization that resulted in two stable equilibria, one quiescent and the other capable of triggering sustained rhythmic activity, in a Purkinje fiber injured by stretch. (**A**) From a normal V_r, an electrical stimulus induced a normal i_{Na}-dependent phase 0. The Purkinje fiber failed to repolarize normally, and the i_{Na}-dependent phase 0 triggered oscillatory activity at the plateau potential. The oscillatory activity increased in magnitude and resulted in nondriven sustained action potentials. Since sodium channels would be inactivated at this membrane potential, the oscillatory activity and subsequent sustained rhythmic activity must have depended on i_{Ca} for the inward current. (**B**) The triggered sustained rhythmic activity persisted indefinitely until terminated by a hyperpolarizing intracellular current that permitted attainment of the repolarization "threshold" and a return to V_r. (**C**) Lidocaine caused an almost immediate attainment of the repolarization threshold and a normalization of the action potential. (**D–F**) After the washout of lidocaine, triggered sustained rhythmic activity rapidly reappeared. From Arnsdorf *(14)*.

normalization of the stimulated action potential (Fig. 6C). After lidocaine was washed out, triggered sustained rhythmic activity rapidly reappeared (Fig. 6D-F). In this situation, the restoration of the normal action potential eliminated the triggered arrhythmia.

The oscillatory activity shown in Fig. 6 consists of early afterdepolarizations, so-called since they occur during phase 2, the plateau phase, of the action potential. The topic of afterdepolarizations and triggered activity has been reviewed recently *(15)* as well as in Chapter 8 of this book. Early afterdepolarizations have been reported following an increase in the depolarizing inward calcium current i_{Ca}; a decrease in the outward repolarizing potassium current i_{K1}, an increase in the Na/Ca exchange current; an increase in the late sodium current; or some combination of these. It is thought that such early afterdepolarizations are involved in the development of torsade de pointes in both congenital and acquired long QT syndrome (*see 15,16*).

Sustained Reentry. Rhythms that can be started or stopped by a single extrasystole or extrastimulus can also be considered an example of bistability. This would include a number of commonly encountered reentrant supraventricular and ventricular arrhythmias. Given the proper matrical configuration, the normal matrix would be a normal sinus rhythm, a timed extrastimuli would deform the matrix analogous to nudging the system from point A to B in Fig. 2, and a critically timed extrastimulus would cause the jump from point B to a new equilibrium, say point C, at which a sustained reentrant arrhythmia would arise.

An example would be the common variety of atrioventricular nodal reentrant tachycardia (AVNRT), the initiation of which depends importantly on the refractoriness of the slow and fast conduction pathways. Koch's triangle is the setting for this arrhythmia, and the environment consists of portions of the atrium which contain atrial tissue, relatively slowly conducting pathways (the so-called slow and fast pathways, both of which conduct slowly) and the AV node itself. Both the fast and slow pathways empty into a final common pathway. In this example, point A would be the situation during normal sinus rhythm. At point A in the bifurcation diagram in Fig. 2, the normal sinus beat enters this environment and travels down both the fast and slow pathways. The impulse traveling down the fast pathway reaches the His bundle first and creates a refractory wake. The impulse traveling down the slow pathway is extinguished when, in the area of the final common pathway, it runs into the refractory wake of the impulse that had traveled down the fast pathway. The faster pathway has a refractory period that is longer than that of the slow pathway. As a result, a critically time premature atrial beat may enter Koch's triangle, find the fast pathway refractory, and preferentially conduct down the slow pathway through the final common pathway to the bundle of His and finally the ventricles. In the event the fast pathway has recovered its excitability by the time impulse traveling down the slow pathway reaches the distal junction of the two pathways, the impulse may be able to conduct in a retrograde fashion up the fast pathway. The circuit may be capable of sustaining reentry with antegrade conduction down the slow pathway and retrograde conduction up the fast pathway resulting in the so-called slow-fast pathway type of AVNRT. The AVNRT would be a new stable equilibrium at point C.

Atrial premature beats that do not cause the jump from the fast to the slow pathway may strike the two pathways at times of varying partial refractoriness causing some oscillation, but the homeostatic feedback mechanisms would return the system to Point A. The jump to Point C may be very transient, as would occur in a single echo that cannot sustain itself.

The therapy of AVNRT would be directed toward returning the system from the equilibrium at Point C to that of point A by the use of drugs, extrastimuli, or ablation of one of the pathways.

HYSTERESIS

In hysteresis, the response after a stimulus has reached some fixed amplitude differs, depending on how fast and/or in what direction the stimulus had been changed previously in the course of reaching that amplitude. The response of a nonlinear system to a periodic input may include harmonic and/or subharmonic frequencies, or can fall in arbitrary ratios (N:M) of integers, with respect to the input period. Some intriguing experiments have been performed in the tissue bath that suggest that closed-loop or feedback control logic may use hysteresis in the logic (1,5).

CURRENT PERSPECTIVES ON THE ELECTROPHYSIOLOGIC MATRIX

Arnsdorf's Paradox

In 1990, as mentioned earlier, I laid claim to a Paradox. Let me quote myself:

"An intriguing, troublesome, and largely unconscious aspect of my career has been the creation of the Paradox. The Paradox was invisible to me for most of my career, but it recently materialized. I now seek its resolution. I dare lay claim to this Paradox for two reasons. First, it has become personal, immediate and disturbing in that the contradiction has arisen from my own entrenched scientific prejudices which are based, in large part, on my own experimental work . . . My own 20th Century Paradox has been perplexing and frustrating since it somehow arose from my misunderstanding of my own science and that of others. Second, no one else seems willing to claim this Paradox, at least recently—-so I will" (17).

The Paradox is that the multiplicities, discontinuities, dynamic interactions and other complexities that exist in and among the determinants of cardiac excitability should give rise to unpredictably complex behavior, yet electrophysiologic events usually are coordinated sufficiently to produce predictable outcomes. To put it another way, there must be some order in this seeming chaos. In the 1990 article, I traced the tracks of this paradox and found it venerable if not ancient, and the interested reader is referred to the article since not much has changed since the 18th century or perhaps earlier (17).

The solution to the Paradox, I believe, is that the electrophysiologic matrix changes as a *system* under arrhythmogenic influences and in the presence of antiarrhythmic drugs, a mechanism that causes this complex electrophysiologic universe to act predictably.

The Underlying Premises

The current iteration of the concept of the electrophysiologic matrix has three important premises or hypotheses and a couple of corollaries.

First, there is an electrophysiologic matrix of interacting active and passive cellular properties that determines normal cardiac excitability. This normal, stable electrophysiologic matrix represents a stable dynamic electrophysiologic equilibrium which is maintained by homeostatic feedback mechanisms. This has already been discussed in some detail.

Second, the normal matrix is altered by arrhythmogenic influences that affect one or more determinants of excitability producing a change in excitability that give rise to a proarrhythmic precursor state that may result in reentrant, automatic and triggered arrhythmias. In this situation, the previously stable normal dynamic equilibrium may give way under a variety of influences such as ischemia and autonomic surges, often explosively, to disequilibrium which, in turn, followed by self-organization into a new stable proarrhythmic or frankly arrhythmogenic equilibrium.

Third, the normal matrix or the matrix deformed by arrhythmogenic influences interacts with antiarrhythmic drugs or other interventions forming yet another self-organized matrix that may be antiarrhythmic, antifibrillatory or proarrhythmic. Moreover, the effects may be several, and the predominant effect depends on the type of matrix encountered.

Fourth, the electrophysiologic matrix changes as a system under arrhythmogenic influences, and, in the presence of antiarrhythmic drugs, a mechanism that causes this complex electrophysiologic universe to act predictably. This is the key to the resolution of the paradox.

Equilibrium, Disequilibrium, and Self-Organization

Consider the series of bifurcation diagrams depicted in Fig. 7 based on our work on flecainide *(18)*. Flecainide was of interest to use because of the proarrhythmic potential of the drug that was demonstrated in the Cardiac Arrhythmia Suppression Trial (CAST) *(19)*. Point A is the normal dynamic equilibrium shown as a normal, symmetrical matrix. At point B, flecainide is introduced into the medium, interacts with the normal matrix, and results in a new matrix at B^* which in this experiment is largely unchanged except for a slight decrease in sodium conductance, g_{Na}. Hyperkalemia alone ($[K]_o = 10$ mM) causes a number of alterations in the electrophysiologic matrix and moves the equilibrium from C to C^*. Hyperkalemia is responsible for an assisted bifurcation (see subheading Bifurcations and Assisted Bifurcations) that consistently will drive the system from point A to point C^*.

The electrophysiologic matrix resulting from hyperkalemia at C^* is then exposed to flecainide, and yet another bifurcation occurs is observed to the equilibrium at D^*. Further bifurcations occur that depend on the rate of stimulation resulting in a situation at point D^{**} in which the liminal length requirements are not met resulting in inexcitability or are met intermittently resulting in a 2:1 or some other response. Note the similarity between the matrices after the "arrhythmogenic" intervention of hyperkalemia and after the application of flecainide, suggesting a narrow toxic to therapeutic ratio. The dashed lines represent paths that might be taken were another drug used (B'), were $[K^+]_o$ lowered below 5.4 mM (C'), or were $[K^+]_o$ returned from 10 mM to 5.4 mM in the presence of flecainide (C^* to B^*).

CLINICAL IMPLICATIONS

The clinical implications of the hypothesis of altered excitability and the electrophysiologic matrix are many, and a detailed discussion can be found elsewhere *(1)*. I will touch on a few that seem particularly important to a discussion of cardiac repolarization.

Fixed and Transient Matrices

The electrophysiologic properties may be more or less fixed. Moreover, the anatomical substrate may also be fixed such as occurs with an accessory bypass tract or in the scar of infarcted heart muscle or at the rim of a ventricular aneurysm. Recently, we have considered in some detail the importance of integrated and fragmented wave fronts in impulse propagation and anisotropy in the context of the electrophysiologic matrix *(1)*. Constant functional pathways may also be important in arrhythmogenesis such as the "slow" and "fast" pathways involved in AVNRT. Such stable anatomical and functional pathways are likely to be associated with recurrent, chronic arrhythmias. Such pathways, moreover, are more likely to result in reproducible provocation by electrophysiological means in the clinical laboratory.

Many observations support the generalization that a decrease in cell membrane resistance, R_m, is a major change acutely after injury, whereas an increase of longitudinal resistance, R_i, is a major late or chronic effect *(1,20,21)*. The increased R_i is a consequence largely of gap junctional organization, distribution, and function after injury which results in a marked variation in conduction velocity as well as inhomogeneities in voltage distribution which may lead to late potentials and arrhythmias. So, orderly cardiac repolarization may be interrupted by abnormal conduction and repolarization during "diastole" when the normal integrative function of gap junctions is disrupted due to ischemia and injury. Perhaps the improved long-term outlook with open coronary arteries after myocardial infarction (the so-called "open artery hypothesis") has to do with improved perfusion, less fibrosis and, as a result, less disruption of the gap junctions. This, in turn, results in fewer lethal arrhythmias.

Transient or random modes of reentry or automaticity, although often associated with an event such as acute ischemia, may have no evident histological basis, and can be induced in anatomically normal tissue. Transient arrhythmias reflect nonstationarity in time and/or space of the altered refractoriness or conduction velocity that allows the initiation or maintenance of an arrhythmia. For example, fibrillation may be a random reentry phenomenon in which excitation progresses simultaneously along multiple wavefronts. A transient reentrant circuit may be very short and functional, or, as Allessie puts it, the head of the circulating waving front may be "biting on its own tail of relative refractoriness" called this smallest possible circuit where the wave length equals the pathway length, the "leading circle" *(22)*. This type of reentrant movement creates its own refractory center and does not require gross anatomical obstacles. Autonomic surges, hypoxia, drug effects, ischemic metabolites, and other determinants can cause transient arrhythmogenic deformations of the electrophysiologic matrix.

Predominant Drug Effect

The actions of antiarrhythmic drugs are complex and have been considered in great detail by the Task Force of the Working Group on Arrhythmias of the European Society of Cardiology *(23)*. The categorization proposed by the Task Force recognizes the multiple actions that drugs may have on ionic conductances and autonomic tone and is important because it underscores the complexity. The situation is further complicated by the fact that many of the studies were done in normal heart tissue. Clinicians, however, have used variations of the Vaughan-Williams classification of antiarrhythmic drugs *(24,25* among others) in which broad generalizations are made regarding predominant actions of the drugs. Class I drugs modulate sodium channels in some combination during the resting, active and/or inactive states. These drugs slow conduction in tissues that depend on the kinetically rapid sodium channel, but those of class IA (e.g., quinidine, procainamide, disopyramide) prolong refractoriness, those of class IB (e.g., lidocaine, mexilitine, phenytoin) shorten refractoriness, and those of class IC (e.g., flecainide, encainide, propafenone) leave refractoriness relatively unaffected. These drugs, however, differ fundamentally in structure and physical properties and must affect the sodium channel in different ways. The class II drugs are β-adrenoreceptor blockers. Class III drugs (e.g., amiodarone, sotalol) modulate potassium channels and often have reverse rate dependence, and class IV are calcium channel antagonists. The Vaughan Williams and similar classifications put apples of different varieties into one barrel, oranges into another, and even more exotic fruits into the remaining barrels.

And yet, these classifications are clinically useful. The reason they are useful is that the electrophysiologic universe moves as a system. The system, as discussed earlier, moves predictably for a given condition such as hyperkalemia or ischemia. Ischemia is common clinically, and the classification scheme has arisen in large part from the treatment of arrhythmias based on clinical ischemia.

It follows that the predominant drug effect depends on the matrix encountered. Ischemia predictably gives rise to the matrix at C^*, so flecainide will consistently create the matrix at D^* that is antiarrhythmic or at D^{**} that presumably is proarrhythmic. In the presence of a normal local $[K^+]_o$, the matrical configuration at B^* will obtain which may suppress premature ventricular beats but which has less proarrhythmic potential. Ischemia is more complicated than a simple increase in $[K^+]_o$, but a low pH, acidosis and the accumulation of active metabolites tend also to produce changes a reproducible matrix of some sort, likely similar to the matrix at C^*.

The Cardiac Arrhythmia Suppression Trial (CAST) *(19,26)* strongly suggests, in my view, bistabilities and a state-dependent duality of drug action. Enrollees in CAST had coronary artery disease and ventricular arrhythmias that could be suppressed effectively by flecainide and encainide. After the efficacy of suppression had been demonstrated, the patients were randomized either to placebo or to treatment with the drug that had suppressed the ventricular arrhythmia. More individuals died in the treatment group, suggesting that encainide and flecainide had a proarrhythmic effect, and the deaths were distributed equally through the period of drug treatment. It is interesting to speculate that the simple suppression of premature ventricular beats may have occurred with a matrical configuration such as that at B^* which has little proarrhythmic potential. The sudden deaths that were linearly distributed in time during the study may have occurred because of the coincidence of ischemia with the underlying drug effect, resulting in a proarrhythmic configuration such as at D^{**}. Proarrhythmia can represent either bifurcating chaotic or bistable system behavior. As discussed earlier, the similarity of the arrhythmogenic and the presumed antiarrhythmic matrices are apparent (*see* Fig. 7).

In summary, the Vaughan Williams and similar classifications are useful because disease, particularly a common condition such as ischemia, causes the matrix to change as a system. In ischemia, a rather predictable electrophysiologic matrix occurs. Because the predominant drug effect depends on the preexisting conditions or matrix encountered, a class I drug, for example, will have a reliable class I action under these conditions. If the initial conditions result from some other cause, such as hypokalemia, the actions of a class I drug may be quite different. Such a duality has been discussed above for quinidine (*see* Fig. 2).

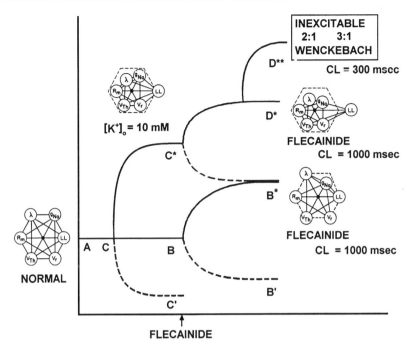

Fig. 7. Multiple bifurcations after the exposure of cardiac Purkinje fibers to flecainide. The legend is the same as for Fig. 2B. From Arnsdorf and Sawicki *(18)*.

THE ELECTROPHYSIOLOGIC UNIVERSE
AND THE ELECTROCARDIOGRAM: THE EXTRACELLULARLY
RECORDED POTENTIAL WITH EMPHASIS ON THE
DIASTOLIC ELECTROCARDIOGRAM

Solid Angle or Distributed Dipole Theory: General Considerations

As discussed, cardiac excitability suggests the ease with which cardiac cells undergo individual and sequential regenerative depolarization and repolarization, the manner in which cells communicate with each other, and the eventual propagation of the impulse. In considering the ECG, the electrophysiologic universe is detected by a lead system and is influenced by anatomy. All normal and abnormal recordings of extracellular potential depend on the interrelationship between several types of current flow including that across cell membranes, between groups of cells, and finally through the volume conductor containing an electrolyte solution that is the human thorax. The solid angle or distributed dipole theory is a useful intellectual framework to consider the implications of the relationship between the electrophysiologic universe, the anatomy which contains it, and the recording system that perceives the resulting electrical field.

The membrane acts as a capacitor and can be considered a dipole layer. Since the membrane has a relatively uniform dielectric constant and thickness, the amount of charge stored per unit of membrane surface area is proportional to the transmembrane voltage. The cell, of course, is enclosed by the dipole layer. At rest or at times of uniform activation such as the peak of the action potential, the dipole on one surface is balanced or canceled by an equal but oppositely directly dipole on the opposing surface and no extracellularly recordable potential results. The same principle holds for an aggregate of cells since the low resistance at the gap junctions facilitates intercellular electrotonic communication and, in effect, causes aggregates of cells to act as a single large cell. This situation changes when there is a difference in the transmembrane voltage (or more accurately charge) between two areas, as, for example, during the propagation of an action potential when resting and activated tissues are juxtaposed. The difference in V_m creates a boundary across which are unopposed positive and negative charges. This separation of charge creates a distributed dipole layer across the boundary composed of an infinite number of dipoles representing infinitely small portions of the boundary. This separation of charge is maintained by the passive and active cellular properties including the flow of currents across the membrane, within and between cells, and in the extracellular space of the tissues. The distributed dipole layer across the boundary established by the different transmembrane voltages is the source of current flow that is responsible for establishing the electrical field in the thorax detected by the electrocardiograph. In the tissue at a distance from the boundary, the dipoles on opposite sides of the cell will cancel each other out.

The solid angle, Ω, is defined as the area of spherical surface cut off a unit sphere inscribed about a point P by the cone formed by drawing lines from P to every point at a boundary of interest (*see* Fig. 8). The boundary is a source of current flow established by portions of the heart having different transmembrane voltages. The magnitude of the extracellularly recorded potential ($\in$) is determined both by spatial and nonspatial factors. Referring to Eq. 1 and Fig. 8, the spatial determinants include the geometry of the boundary separating areas with different it and the position of the extracellular recording electrode relative to this boundary. Nonspatial determinants include the polarity and magnitude of the difference in V_m across the boundary (transmembrane potential gradient, TPG) as well as tissue conductivities inside, between, and outside the cardiac cells (C_σ or sometimes K). These relationships can be described by the following:

$$\in = \underset{\substack{spatial \\ determinants}}{Sp} \times \underset{\substack{nonspatial \\ determinants}}{(V_{m_2} - V_{m_1}) \cdot C_\sigma} \qquad \text{[Eq. 1]}$$

SPATIAL DETERMINANTS

Spatial factors (Sp) are the distance between the boundary and the recording electrode as well as the geometry of the boundary. The spatial term is quantified by the solid angle (Ω) that includes both electrode position and a measurement of the apparent geometry of the boundary. Referring again to Fig. 8, the Ω is determined by drawing radii from the site of the electrode P to all points of the boundary thereby forming an irregular cone. A unit sphere is inscribed about P. The area of the unit sphere cut off or subtended by the cone is termed the solid angle or Ω. Remembering that a unit sphere has an area of 4π steradians, the maximum value of the solid angle, then, is 4π steradians. Equation 1 can be rewritten as:

$$\in = \underset{\substack{spatial \\ determinants}}{\frac{\Omega}{4\pi}} \times \underset{\substack{nonspatial \\ determinants}}{[TPG \cdot C_\sigma]} \qquad \text{[Eq. 2]}$$

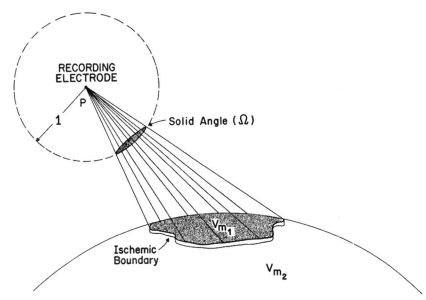

Fig. 8. Diagrammatic characterization of the solid angle theory. The solid angle (Ω) is defined as the area of spherical surface cut off a unit sphere, inscribed about the recording electrode, by a cone formed by drawing lines from the recording electrode o every point at the boundary of interest. The boundary is the source of current flow established by portions of the heart having different transmembrane voltages ($V_{m_2} - V_{m_1}$). Adapted from Holland and Arnsdorf *(53)*.

The solid angle is seen to vary directly with the radius of the boundary and inversely with the distance (*D*) between the electrode and the boundary. The term *proximity effect* refers to the inverse relationship between Ω and *D*. One of the major strengths of the solid angle model is that it mathematically accounts for boundary geometry and electrode position.

Let us now review our earlier discussion in terms of solid angle theory. In quiescent or uniformly depolarized tissue, the sum of solid angles for the entire closed boundary is zero since the electrode is faced by two oppositely and equally charged membranes that subtend identical solid angles, that is $\Omega_1 - \Omega_2 = 0$. As a result, no extracellular potential will be recorded. Only the distributed dipole layer that defines the boundary will give rise to unopposed solid angles. In the remainder of the tissue at a distance from the boundary, the sum of solid angles will again be zero. It is only the boundary, therefore, that is "seen" by the extracellular electrode.

Experiments in isolated hearts or the whole animal consider primarily changes in the spatial determinants of $\in$, such as the shape or size of ischemic or infarcted tissue *(27–29)*. When the effect of an intervention on ischemic injury is discussed in the literature, a frequent assumption is that the observed change in the TQ-ST segment results from an increase or decrease in the size of the ischemic area, that is, from a change in the spatial determinants. This, as will be discussed, may not be the case.

Nonspatial Determinants

The nonspatial determinants of $\in$ are those that depend neither on the geometry of the boundary nor on the position of the extracellular recording electrode. The nonspatial factors in Eqs. 1 and 2 are *TPG* and C_σ. *TPG* is the transmembrane potential gradient, that is, the difference between the V_m on both sides of the boundary $(V_{m_2} - V_{m_1})$. C_σ (or K) is a conductivity term which considers the ease with which intercellular, intracellular, and extracellular currents flow as a result of the distributed dipoles.

The Transmembrane Potential Gradient (TPG). Since the *TPG* equals the difference in V_m across the boundary Eq. 2 becomes:

$$\in = \frac{\Omega}{4\pi} \times (V_{m_2} - V_{m_1}) \cdot C_\sigma \qquad\qquad \text{[Eq. 3]}$$

The determinants of V_{m_1} and V_{m_2} in the *TPG* are those active and passive cellular properties and conductivities discussed earlier when considering the electrophysiologic matrix. Quite clearly, the *TPG* is independent of the spatial determinants.

Since charge separation defines the boundary, the change in the *TPG* can be temporal, configurational, or both. A *temporal* change results from a delay in the sequence of activation without a significant alteration in the resting potential or the shape of the action potential on one or both sides of the boundary. A *configurational* change results from an alteration in the resting potential or the shape of the action potential on one or both sides of the boundary. As will be discussed, both temporal and configurational changes can affect ST segments and their mapping as well as the types of measurements involved in QT dispersion. This is considered in more detail as part of a discussion on ischemia in Subheading "The Transmembrane Potential Gradient, TPG" and in Fig. 12 below.

A critically important point is that the *TPG* can be eliminated by making V_m identical on both sides of the boundary. The *TPG*, then, becomes zero as does $\in$ in Eq. 3 when either or both terms change so that V_{m_1} minus V_{m_2} equals zero.

The Conductivity Term (C_σ). The magnitude of the extracellular potential is also proportional to a conductivity term that considers the flow of ions inside, between, and outside the cell. As described by Plonsey (30), the conductivity term, C_σ can be described by the relationship:

$$C_\sigma = \left[1 + \frac{\sigma_o}{\sigma_i} \cdot \left(\frac{S}{A} - 1 \right) \right]^{-1} \qquad\qquad \text{[Eq. 4]}$$

where σ_i and σ_o are the respective intracellular and extracellular conductivities; A is the cross-sectional area of the cardiac fiber; and S is the area of the fiber plus its associated interstitial space. The conductivity term certainly changes in disease states. For example, the interventions that cause cellular uncoupling at the gap junction would influence C_σ and decrease $\in$.

Combining Eqs. 3 and 4 allows us to appreciate the number of variables that need be considered when attempting to correlate electrocardiographic changes with physiological, pharmacologic, and pathological alterations:

$$\in = \frac{\Omega}{4\pi} \times (V_{m_2} - V_{m_1}) \cdot \left[1 + \frac{\sigma_o}{\sigma_i} \cdot \left(\frac{S}{A} - 1 \right) \right]^{-1} \qquad\qquad \text{[Eq. 5]}$$

Each of the terms in Eq. 5, moreover, has itself several determinants. The amount of information included in the extracellularly recorded signal is immense and it has been a challenge to control these variables experimentally.

Application of the Solid Angle Theory to Ischemia, Injury, and Infarction

BACKGROUND

A decrease or interruption in the blood supply to the myocardium produces varying degrees of tissue damage. Traditionally, an area of tissue necrosis has been depicted as being surrounded by an area of "injury" and both these zones by yet another area of "ischemia." Many textbooks suggest that the zone of infarction is responsible for changes in the QRS morphology; the zone of "injury" in the ST segment change; and the zone of "ischemia" in T wave changes. The implication is that the myocardial damage is greatest in the zone of infarction; serious in the zone of "injury" where "leaky" membranes cause diastolic and systolic current flow; and least serious in the zone of "ischemia" where primarily alterations in repolarization occur. In this view, necrosis is irreversible, but both "injury" and "ischemia" are potentially reversible although both may proceed to tissue death. There is much interest in "preserving" the "injured" and "ischemic" myocardium from death and electrocardiographic measures have been suggested as indices of tissue "ischemia" and "injury."

Much of this is superstition based on the traditional literature. Anatomically, tissue death can be defined with reasonable accuracy although problems arise in the several hours immediately after infarction. Various states of irreversible injury cannot be clearly differentiated from each other, although ultrastructural studies may eventually permit such distinctions. Electrophysiologically, all the electrocardiographic deflections result from the normal or abnormal flow of currents during systole and diastole. Depolarization and repolarization are interdependent, and so are their electrocardiographic manifestations. Although it is attractive to relate three areas of supposedly differing degrees of cell damage to three different components of the electrocardiogram, little ultrastructural and electrophysiologic support can be mustered for such a separation. Ischemia is the actual deficiency of the blood supply to the myocardium with its resultant effects on pH, $[K^+]_o$, the buildup of ischemic metabolites, and the like. As such, it undoubtedly produces a spectrum of cellular damage, electrophysiologic change, and ultimately, electrocardiographic manifestations involving the QRS complex, the ST segment, the T wave, and, from time to time, other components of the electrocardiogram.

The current of injury was first described by Englemann in the 1870s *(31,32)* and associated with myocardial infarction in dogs by Fred Smith in 1918 *(33)* and in man by H.E.B. Pardee in 1920 *(34)*. Controversy still exists as to mechanisms involved and whether the electric events responsible for ST segment (or more properly, TQ-ST segment since as will be discussed diastole is involved) changes occur primarily in systole of diastole. Samson and Scher in 1960 presented experimental evidence that ST-segment elevation had both systolic and diastolic components *(35)*. Magnetocardiography indicates that in early ischemia, the deflection is primarily a diastolic event *(36)*. Experimentally, TQ-ST segment changes occur within seconds of coronary occlusion. The evidence that the agent producing these early changes is potassium is convincing *(27,37,38)*. A release of only one percent of the intracellular store would raise the extracellular K^+ concentration in the local extracellular space sufficiently to produce large diastolic and systolic electrical changes, including depolarization of the resting potential some 30 mV and shortening of the action potential duration. Smaller changes in $[K^+]_o$ would still have a profound influence on the resting potential (V_r). A less negative V_r would also increase the inactivation of the sodium channel resulting in a less rapid maximal rate of rise of phase 0, a lesser upstroke, and, generally, a slower conduction velocity. As a result, increased $[K^+]_o$ would change not only the TQ-ST segment, but the QRS and T waves as well. Many other factors common in ischemia and infarction may influence the transmembrane voltage in myocardial ischemia and infarction *(39)*.

Electrical activity may be lost because of tissue death. On the other hand, the loss of electrical influence may be owing to a tissue being electronically uncoupled from its neighbors. Such uncoupling has been observed after the intracellular concentration of calcium has been increased, in metabolic poisoning, after the tissue is exposed to high concentration of ouabain, after the intracellular application of antibodies specific to certain domains of the connexin protein, and other interventions *(40)*. Uncoupling may be reversible, so a decrease in the TQ-ST segment after infarction may be due to the recoupling of cells or, alternatively, to further tissue death. An electrophysiologically silent area does not necessarily imply tissue death since both reversible uncoupling and necrosis would result in such silence.

THE DETERMINANTS OF TQ-ST SEGMENT ($\in_{TQ\text{-}ST}$)

Ischemia, at its mildest, seems to first produce changes in the action potential duration and in the sequence of repolarization without much change in the resting potential, V_r. Alteration in the normal sequence of repolarization following ischemia affects the T wave in several ways: It makes the T wave more symmetrical; it may locally delay repolarization thereby increasing the QT duration; and it may affect the magnitude and/ or direction of the T wave. Myocardial ischemia, however, only unusually produces T wave changes in the absence of TQ-ST segment alterations; and, as will be discussed, TQ-ST segment changes rarely occur in the absence of changes in the QRS (R) complex. The more general topic of myocardial ischemia, therefore, will be considered in terms of the TQ-ST segment.

Normally, the TQ and ST segments are isoelectric. Cardiac injury may result in changes in the TQ and ST segments, producing an extracellular potential, $\in_{TQ\text{-}ST}$. The determinants of $\in_{TQ\text{-}ST}$ can be considered in terms of the distributed dipole theory, as expressed by the equations described earlier. To restate Eq. 5 in terms of $\in_{TQ\text{-}ST}$:

$$\in_{TQ\text{-}ST} = \frac{\Omega}{4\pi} \times (V_{m_2} - V_{m_1}) \cdot \left[1 + \frac{\sigma_o}{\sigma_i} \cdot \left(\frac{S}{A} - 1\right)\right]^{-1} \qquad [Eq.\ 6]$$

As compared to normal cardiac cells (Fig. 9, left panel), injured and ischemic cells have a less negative V_r, a slower rate of rise of phase 0, a less positive overshoot, and a shorter action potential duration. The transmembrane voltages, therefore, differ between the normal and injured cells during both diastole and systole (Fig. 9, right panel). The polarity of the distributed dipoles across the boundary, however, differs during systole and diastole, as do both the resultant current flow (positive to negative) and the extracellular electric field. Electrodes overlying the injured area would record a negative $\in_{TQ\text{-}ST}$ (ST depression) during diastole and a positive $\in_{TQ\text{-}ST}$ (ST elevation) during systole. The capacitative coupling circuitry of most electrocardiographs makes it difficult to recognize that the TQ segment may not be at the zero potential. Nevertheless, the so-called ST-segment elevation is actually a summation of a diastolic TQ depression and a systolic ST elevation. The relative contribution of the diastolic and systolic components to the total TQ-ST deflection has not been fully defined in different types of cardiac injury. As seen

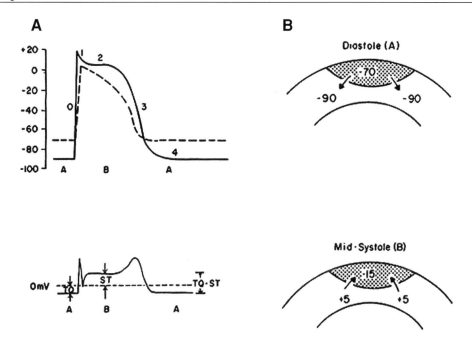

Fig. 9. Transmembrane events in the genesis of the TQ-ST segment deflection. Top Left: The transmembrane voltages of normal (solid curve) and ischemic (dashed curve) tissue. Phase 0 = initial rapid upstroke; phase 2 = plateau phase of slow repolarization; phase 3 = terminal phase of rapid repolarization; phase 4 = diastolic or resting transmembrane potential. Bottom left: Electrocardiogram recorded by an extracellular electrode overlying the ischemic tissue. The TQ segment is located below the isolectric line (dashed), and the ST segment is located above. Top right: Transmembrane potential gradients existing at a boundary between normal and ischemic tissue during electrical diastole. Bottom right: Transmembrane potential gradients existing during midsystole. In all panels, A = diastole and B = mid systole. Arrows indicate the direction of current flow (positive to negative) at the boundary. From Holland and Arnsdorf (53).

in Fig. 10, alterations in either the spatial (left panel) or nonspatial (right panel) determinants of the extracellular potential can produce identical changes in the TQ-ST segment.

SPATIAL DETERMINANTS

Geometry of the Boundary. Figure 11 depicts the manner in which the solid angle is influenced by the geometry of the boundary between normal and injured tissues. As recorded by a precordial electrode in midsystole (Fig. 11A), the boundary created by subepicardial injury subtends a positive solid angle (white disc, Ω_{ow} where ow represents the outside wall), and a TQ-ST segment elevation is recorded on the ECG. The boundary created by subendocardial injury (Fig. 11B) subtends a negative solid angle (black disc, Ω_{IW} where iw represents the inner wall), and a TQ-ST depression is recorded. The boundary produced by transmural injury (Fig. 11C) produces both positive (Ω_{ow}) and negative (Ω_{iw}) solid angles at the outer and inner walls, respectively. What is eventually perceived by the electrode is the *net* solid angle (Ω_T), which is the difference between Ω_{ow} and Ω_{iw}. A wedge-shaped injury of the type shown in Fig. 11C would result in a positive Ω_T and, therefore, in a TQ-ST-segment elevation at the site of the overlying electrode. Such wedge-shaped injury is common in transmural myocardial infarction and probably in angina pectoris caused by spasm of large coronary arteries, such as that of Prinzmetal. If

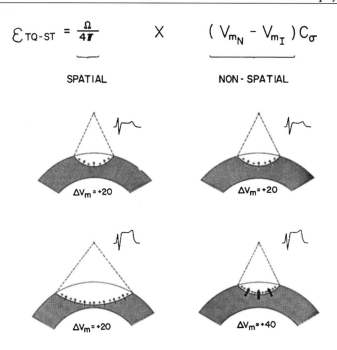

$$\mathcal{E}_{TQ\text{-}ST} = \underbrace{\frac{\Omega}{4\pi}}_{SPATIAL} \quad X \quad \underbrace{(V_{m_N} - V_{m_I})C_\sigma}_{NON\text{-}SPATIAL}$$

Fig. 10. Comparison of spatial (left) and nonspatial (right) influences on the ischemic TQ-ST segment deflection. In the example on the left, the solid angle subtending the boundary at a precordial position increases following an increase in ischemic area, and, so too must the TQ-ST segment deflection. In the example on the right, the electrode location, ischemic area, and solid angle are not changed. The potential difference between the transmembrane voltages in the normal and ischemic regions (ΔV_m) has widened and the current flow has intensified (bolder arrows). As a result, the magnitude of the TQ-ST deflection increases. From Holland and Arnsdorf *(53)*.

the ischemia is intramural, Ω_{ow} and Ω_{iw} may be equal and no net Ω_T subtended, resulting in no TQ-ST segment deflection despite ischemia.

Figure 11 makes the important point that although transmural injury may involve a greater volume of tissue (panel C) than, for example, subepicardial injury (panel A), the differences in polarity of the subtended solid angles contributing to Ω_{ow} and Ω_{iw} in transmural injury may result in a total solid angle and $\in_{TQ\text{-}ST}$ less than that for the smaller epicardial injury. Other factors that may influence boundary geometry are the existence of multiple areas of injury that require summation of their solid angles. Such summation may either increase or decrease $\in_{TQ\text{-}ST}$ depending on the polarity of the component solid angles. Similarly, wall thickness influences the extent of a boundary and may also influence its direction. Factors of this type must be considered in any study utilizing the TQ-ST segment as an index of myocardial ischemia.

Moreover, the solid angle increases as an electrode is moved closer to a boundary with a fixed geometry. If the size of the injured area increases, the solid angle and $\in_{TQ\text{-}ST}$ may increase at one recording site and decrease at another. The spatial relationship between the boundary or boundaries of interest and the site of the recording electrode determines the magnitude of the net solid angle and the TQ-ST segment or other components of the

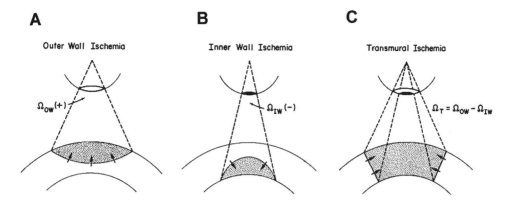

Fig. 11. Magnitude and polarity of the solid angle as a function of ischemic shape. When the region has a transmural shape (**C**), the resultant solid angle (Ω_T) is equal to the difference in the solid angle computed for ischemic regions localized to the outer (Ω_{OW}) (**A**) and inner (Ω_{IW}) (**B**) layers of the ventricular wall. The direction of current flow (positive to negative) across the ischemic boundary at midsystole is indicated by arrows. The polarity of the solid angle is then positive at electrode sites overlying outer wall and transmural ischemic regions and negative at sites overlying inner wall ischemic regions. From Holland and Arnsdorf *(53)*.

extracellularly recorded signal. The volume of infarcted, injured, or ischemic tissue is less important than its location, shape, and relationship to the electrode.

NONSPATIAL DETERMINANTS

The Transmembrane Potential Gradient (TPG). The TPG is the difference in the transmembrane potential (V_m) between the normal (N) and the ischemic (I) tissue, that is:

$$TPG = (V_{mN} - V_m) \qquad \text{[Eq. 7]}$$

For the sake of discussion and simplification, consider a single point in *diastole* when the TQ segment alteration is recorded on the ECG. In this situation, Eq. 3 can be written:

$$\in_{TQ} = \frac{\Omega}{4\pi} \quad \times \quad (V_{m_2} - V_{m_1}) \cdot C_\sigma \qquad \text{[Eq. 8]}$$

spatial   nonspatial
determinants   determinants

where $\in_{TQ}$ is the magnitude of the diastolic TQ-segment deflection.

Current flow originating at the border during diastole is dependent on the difference in V_m between normal and injured tissues. This current flow and the TQ-segment deflection it produces may be reduced by decreasing the difference between V_{mN} and V_{mI} in Eq. 8. Referring to Fig. 9 (diastole), the TPG could be reduced to 0 by repolarizing the depolarized area to equal that in the normal region, by depolarizing the normal region to the V_m in the ischemic region, or by making the V_m in both areas identical at some other value. A number of physiologic mechanisms have been verified experimentally *(41)*. Drugs could also affect the *TPG*. Lidocaine, for example, can "normalize" action potentials in injured tissue by making V_r more negative or by facilitating normal repolarization *(10,14,42–44*; Fig. 6). The possibilities by which either term in the *TPG* can be altered are numerous and must be understood by the clinician.

The systolic $\in_{ST}$ contribution to the total TQ-ST-segment change must also be considered. During phases 0 through 3 of the action potential, numerous changes occur in the membrane conductances for sodium, calcium, chloride and the components of the potassium current. Many physiologic and pharmacological influences affect these repolarization currents.

As mentioned earlier, the change in the *TPG* can be temporal, configurational, or both. A *temporal* change results from a delay in the sequence of activation without a significant alteration in the resting potential or the shape of the action potential on one or both sides of the boundary. A *configurational* change results from an alteration in the resting potential or the shape of the action potential on one or both sides of the boundary. This is depicted in Fig. 12. In experiments we performed a number of years ago, a strip of guinea pig ventricle was drawn through a hole in a latex diaphragm that separated two chambers (Left panel, Fig. 12) *(41)*. This arrangement rendered the spatial determinants of $\in$ constant since it created a constant and definable geometric boundary between the left and right portions of the tissue, allowed selective perfusion of each chamber, and intracellular potential recordings from each portion of the tissue. Extracellular electrodes were placed on opposite sides of the partition allowing recording of the electrogram. A temporal change in the TPG, in which there was an alternation in the sequence of activation without a significant change in the action potential configuration on either side of the partition, was produced by increasing the $[K]_o$ in both chambers to 12 m*M*. In Fig. 12A, hyperkalemia caused a conduction delay between the left and right portions of the preparation, but the action potential configuration remained virtually identical on both sides (V_{m_L} and V_{m_R}). The end of the QR interval is indicated by the arrow and is determined by the portion of the fiber that repolarized last. In the next beat (Fig. 12B), the conduction delay was less than in A, but the configurations of the action potentials remained similar. Note that the slight difference in conduction delay in panels A and B resulted in a different ST and T-wave morphology as well as a different QT duration. The experimental records in C were obtained 10 s later. Note that the action potential shape of V_{m_R} had changed with a slower rate of rise of phase 0 and a shorter action potential duration without much change in resting potential, while V_{m_L} remained much as it had been in panels A and B. The change in V_{m_R} imposed a significant configurational change on the underlying temporal determinant of the TQ-ST segment. The QT interval in panel C shortened further, and the QT duration was now determined entirely by the left half of the tissue. Note the reversal in the T wave polarity in panel C.

Following a physiologic or pharmacologic intervention, then, the possibility that a change in the ischemic TQ-ST segment can be reliably and exclusively attributed to a change in the extent of the injury (the spatial factor) and not to an influence on the TPG (a nonspatial factor) is unlikely.

The Conductivity Term (C_σ). Relatively little is known about the influence of the conductivity term on recorded potentials. In the 1870's, Engelmann *(31,32)* made a number of interesting observations concerning the extracellularly recorded potential following myocardial injury. He found that the current of injury rapidly decreased with time and that cells near a cut edge rapidly became inexcitable. When hearts were cut into small segments connected by narrow bridges of intact tissue, excitatory currents spread to all segments, regardless of which segment was stimulated. Microscopy revealed no neural connections, so apparently the spread was from cell to cell. The implications of these studies were that cells are normally electrically continuous but that injury or death

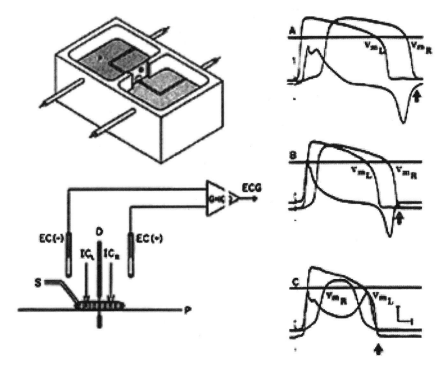

Fig. 12. (Left Panel) Diagrammatic representation of the experimental arrangement. In the upper panel, the tissue bath is partitioned with a latex diaphragm **(D)**. A strip of guinea pig ventricle was drawn through an aperture in the diaphragm. Inflow and outflow ports allowed independent changes in solution. In the lower panel, extracellular electrodes EC(–) and EC(+) were placed on opposite sides of the partition. I_{CL} and I_{CR} represent microelectrodes that recorded the intracellular potentials of the left and right portions of the ventricular strip, respectively. S is a teflon-coated extracellular bipolar stimulating electrode. G is a very low noise battery-powered preamplifier with a fixed gain of 100. P is a paraffin base in both panels. (Right Panel) Experimental records of the temporal and configurational origins of the TQ-ST segment deflection with a hyperkalemia-induced conduction delay in guinea pig ventricle. Both halves of the fiber were bathed in Tyrode solution containing $[K]_o$ of 12 mM. The arrows indicate the end of the QT intervals. A and B were recorded on consecutive beats and C within 10 s of B. Vertical calibration bar = –20 mV and 1 mV for the intracellular and extracellular potentials, respectively. Horizontal calibration bar = 100 ms. See text for discussion. Adapted with permission from Holland and Arnsdorf *(41)*.

seals that cell off from other cells leading to the dictum that "cells live together but die singly." Further, this "sealing-off" process affects the extracellularly recorded potential.

It is now thought that the major current interfered with in this situation is that through the gap junction *(40)*. Briefly, gap junctions are thought to be low resistance structures. The connexon channels connecting the interior of two adjacent cells are really hemichannels. The cardiac gap junctional protein, connexin-43 (Cx43) has sites on the cytoplasmic side of the junction, on the amino terminus, the cytoplasmic loop, the carboxy tail, and the carboxy tip that inhibit junctional conductance with changes in pH, Ca^{2+}, and perhaps other influences. After a cut or other injury, the cell heals-over in the region of injury, becoming very resistive to current flow. Evidence suggests that healing-over is owing to cellular uncoupling rather than to the formation of a new membrane.

The uncoupling process would have the following benefits: It would prevent the high intracellular calcium and hydrogen ions in injured cells from spreading to uninjured cells; it would prevent the loss of ions and molecules from uninjured cells to the extracellular space via their junction with the injured cell; and it would eliminate a low-resistance electrical shunt between the cytoplasm of the uninjured cells and the extracellular compartment.

Referring to Eq. 7 and assuming that the spatial term remains constant, a decrease in C_σ because of cellular uncoupling, without an associated change in action potentials on either side of the boundary (i.e., the transmembrane potential gradient remains constant) would result in an overall decrease in the amplitude of all ECG signals including the QRS, TQ-ST, and the T wave, but their magnitude relative to each other would not change. Using the experimental arrangement shown in Fig. 12, we tested this hypothesis experimentally in hypoxic ventricular muscle exposed to a metabolic poison and found a good correlation between theoretical prediction and observation *(41)*.

Interrelationships Between $\in_R$, $\in_{TQ\text{-}ST}$, and $\in_T$

There is a tendency to consider each deflection on the electrocardiogram as being an isolated event. Little attention has been paid to the interrelationships between these deflections, for example, as between the R amplitude and the $\in_{TQ\text{-}ST}$, or, more precisely, the individual diastolic $\in_{TQ}$ and systolic $\in_{ST}$ contributions to the total TQ-ST deflection. The manner in which the apparent total amplitude of the QRS may be quantitatively influenced by $\in_{TQ}$ is shown in Fig. 12. The peak T wave potential can also be influenced by the same types of configurational and temporal components of the nonspatial determinants included in these equations. Suffice it to emphasize that any analysis of R, TQ-ST, and T deflections as well as QT durations during a disease state such as ischemia must consider such interrelationships (Fig. 13).

Another Form of Arnsdorf's Paradox?: QT Dispersion, T-Wave Loop Variables, T wave Alternans, and the Signal Averaged Electrocardiogram

Each of these issues is a topic in itself. The unifying theme, however, is that all three are body surface analyses of events that are considered to be primarily diastolic.

The dispersion of ventricular repolarization experimentally has been found to be associated with the development of ventricular arrhythmias. The measured QTd from the ECG correlates with the dispersion of repolarization measured from the myocardium *(45)*. The QTd measured from the 12-lead surface ECG was developed by the late Ronald W. F. Campbell's group as a marker of the dispersion of ventricular repolarization *(46)*, and its simplicity and ease of measurement has held great appeal for clinicians. But even today, the electrophysiologic basis is not well understood. Some critics have been quite vocal, such as P.M. Rautharju, who published an article in *Circulation* in 1999 entitled "QT and Dispersion of Ventricular Repolarization: The Greatest Fallacy in Electrocardiography in the 1990s" *(47)*. On balance, however, there seems to be clinical usefulness in this approach *(48)*.

The calculation of various types of T-wave vector loop variables is also being looked at in risk stratification *(45)*. As considered in our earlier discussion of the T wave, the T wave vector is inextricably tied into the determinants of the TQ-ST segment. Some variables, such as the total cosine R-to-T variable mathematically reflects the difference in the angles between the wavefronts of activation and repolarization *(49)* which, as

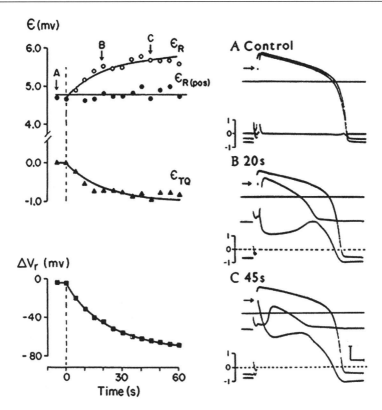

Fig. 13. Interrelationship between TQ segment deflection and R (QRS) wave amplitude in guinea pig ventricle. The experimental arrangement was the same as in Fig. 12. The effects of a sudden infusion of 1.0 M KCl into the right chamber on the diastolic transmembrane potential gradient (ΔV_r), the TQ-segment ($\in_{TQ}$) and components of the R wave are shown graphically (left) and by experimental tracings (right). (**A**), control period. Action potentials on both side of the partition are virtually superimposable and no TQ-ST segment deflection is seen. The arrow indicates the peak of the R wave. (**B** and **C**), B and C were recorded at 20 and 45 s, respectively after KCl infusion. Both V_r and $\in_{TQ}$ are seen to increase. The experimental records show that the positive portion of the R wave, $\in_{Rpos}$, as measured from the isoelectric (dashed line) to peak of R (arrow) did not change at 20 and 45 after KCl infusion. The total R-wave amplitude, $\in_R$, as measured from the TQ-segment to the peak of the R (arrow), however, increased. As shown graphically (left), the increase in $\in_R$ was identical to the change in $\in_{TQ}$, which, in turn, paralleled V_r. Vertical calibration bar = 20 mV; horizontal calibration bar = 100 ms; extracellular voltage scale in mV is left of experimental records. From Holland and Arnsdorf *(41)*.

discussed by Franz and Zabel *(45)* brings to mind the older concepts of the ventricular gradient and the calculation of the QRST areas from body surface maps.

Electrical alternans of the ST segment and the T wave on the surface ECG has also been used as a noninvasive approach to identifying the patient at risk for ventricular arrhythmias, and T wave alternans is thought to reflect the dispersion and heterogeneity of repolarization *(50)*. Evidence has been presented in the guinea pig heart using voltage-sensitive dyes to record action potentials, that discordant alternans produces spatial gradients of repolarization of sufficient magnitude to cause unidirectional block and reentrant ventricular fibrillation *(51)*. Years ago, while using the model shown in Fig. 12, we observed 2:1 TQ-ST segment alternans owing to the development of 2:1 conduction block between the portions of the guinea pig ventricular strips (*see* Fig. 14B, marked alternans). Note also the "action potential" shape of the TQ-ST segment in complexes 1 and 3, a common clinical observation, which I believe denotes ischemia sufficiently intense to produce a conduction delay in the ischemic tissue but insufficient to close the gap junctions.

The signal-averaged electrocardiogram has been used to obtain information about electrophysiologic events *(52)*. It has fallen somewhat out of favor, and perhaps the reason is that the signal-averaging eliminates transient diastolic events which likely are more important than the recorded fixed potentials.

Again, the determinants of the events of repolarization reflected in these electrocardiographic measures are incredibly complex and susceptible to many possible combinations and permutations; seemingly a variant of Arnsdorf's Paradox. I believe that the likely empirical usefulness of these measurements may be analogous to the empirical usefulness of traditional antiarrhythmic drug classifications which have little to commend them scientifically. The solution to that paradox was that the electrophysiologic universe moves as a system, so, for example, given the relatively reproducible ischemic matrix, class I antiarrhythmic drugs have a consistent effect on this matrix, and the drug effect becomes predictable. I would suggest that noninvasive electrocardiographic indices that can assess transients, such as the measurement of ST segments, QTd, T-wave variables, and T-wave alternans are useful because they are recording consistently reproducible shifts in the diastolic universe which occur during common disease states, particularly ischemia.

RECOMMENDATIONS FOR FUTURE RESEARCH

As I mentioned in the Introduction, the editors urged me to revisit Arnsdorf's Paradox. The Paradox, once again, was that the multiplicities, discontinuities, dynamic interactions and other complexities that exist in and among the determinants of cardiac excitability should result in unpredictably complex behavior, yet, electrophysiologic events usually are coordinated sufficiently to produce predictable outcomes. In other words, there is order in this seeming chaos. The original concern of the Paradox considered the self-organization and ordering of electrophysiologic matrices after exposure to arrhythmogenic influences. This was extended to the consideration of the predominant effects of antiarrhythmic drugs. In this chapter, I have commented upon the use of electrocardiographic measures such as the TQ-ST segment, QTd, T wave loop variables, and ST-T wave alternans as perhaps another example of the Paradox.

I believe that the resolution of the paradox, for the reasons discussed in this chapter and elsewhere, resides in the self-organization of the electrophysiologic universe which moves as a system in response to normal, pathophysiologic, and pharmacologic influences. This results in some reproducible change in the system and, therefore, some predictability of the type of change expected. The movement of the system, as discussed previously, explains predominant drug actions and the resulting empirical usefulness of scientifically shaky clinical classifications of antiarrhythmic agents as well as the seeming empirical usefulness of hopelessly simplified electrocardiographic measurements during electrical diastole.

Electrophysiologic research has become reductionist. Virtually no integrative work is being done at the tissue level, and little is being conducted at the organ level to study

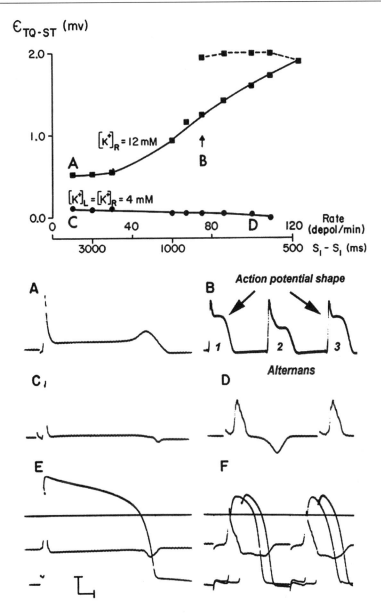

Fig. 14. The effect of increasing the stimulation rate on $\epsilon_{TQ\text{-}ST}$. The experimental arrangement was the same as in Fig. 12. Top: With $[K]_L$ and $[K]_R$ at 4 and 12 mM, respectively, $\epsilon_{TQ\text{-}ST}$ steadily increased with increasing stimulation rate (S_1–S_1). A decrease in the cycle length to 800 ms resulted in development of 2:1 conduction block and TQ-ST segment alternans (1:1 at A; 2:1 with alternans in at B). When both sides of the same fiber were bathed at $[K]_o = 4.0$ mM, $\epsilon_{TQ\text{-}ST}$ decreased slightly in magnitude (**C** and **D**). **A-D** taken at times indicated in top panel. (**E** and **F**) are from another experiment in which a TQ-ST deflection developed at a short cycle length even though both sides of the fiber were bathed at $[K]_o = 4.0$ mM. Vertical calibration bar = 20 mV and 1 mV for intracellular and extracellular recordings, respectively. Horizontal calibration bar – 100 ms for A and C-F and 200 ms for B. From Holland and Arnsdorf (*41*).

issues of cardiac excitability. In my view, since the perturbations in the matrices that form the electrophysiologic universe determines cardiac excitability, and since these perturbations reflect the interaction of many parameters of excitability which in turn are fundamentally nonlinear, integrative research needs to be revived. I would suggest that cell-cell communication, interventions that can either close or open gap junctions, and the relationship of such manipulations to arrhythmias, antiarrhythmic strategies, and proarrhythmias should be emphasized. I look forward to further tissue level studies on anisotropy and discontinuous propagation. As has already been demonstrated, there is a great deal of information in the electrocardiographically recorded signal that is of great clinical significance. Of importance, a number of investigators who understand nonlinearities and chaos theory are involved in investigating the clinical secrets contained in such signals.

REFERENCES

1. Arnsdorf MF, Makielski JC. Excitability and impulse propagation. In: Sperelakis N, Kurachi Y, Terzic A, Cohen MV, eds. Heart Physiology and Pathophysiology. 4th ed. New York: Academic Press, 2000: 99–132.
2. Fozzard HA, Schoenberg M. Strength-duration curves in cardiac Purkinje fibres: Effects of liminal length and charge distribution. J Physiol (Lond) 1972;226:593–618.
3. Prigogine I, Stengers I. Order Out of Chaos: Man's New Dialogue with Nature. Boulder, CO: New Science Library, 1984.
4. Arnsdorf MF, Sawicki GJ. The effects of quinidine sulfate on the balance among active and passive cellular properties which comprise the electrophysiologic matrix and determine excitability in sheep Purkinje fibers. Circ Res 1987;61:244–255.
5. Ginsburg K, Arnsdorf MF. Cardiac excitability, gap junctions, cable properties and impulse propagation. In: Sperelakis N, ed. Physiology and Pathophysiology of the Heart. 3rd ed. Boston: M. Nijhoff, 1995:153–199.
6. Ginsburg KS, Arnsdorf MF. Interaction of transient ischemia with antiarrhythmic drugs. In: Breithardt G, ed. Modulation of Antiarrhythmic Drug Action by Disease and Injury. Berlin: Springer GmbH & Co, 1995:109–121.
7. Arnsdorf MF, Dudley S. Gap junctions, cardiac excitability and clinical arrhythmias. In: DeMello W, ed. Heart Cell Communication in Health and Disease. 1st ed. Philadelphia: Kluwer Academic Publishers, 1998:217–288.
8. Weidmann S. Effect of current flow on the membrane potential of cardiac muscle. J Physiol 1951;115:227–236.
9. Sawicki GJ, Arnsdorf MF. Electrophysiologic actions and interactions between lysophosphatidylcholine and lidocaine in the non-steady state: The match between multiphasic arrhythmogenic mechanisms and multiple drug effects in cardiac Purkinje fibers. J Pharmacol Exp Ther 1985;235:829–838.
10. Arnsdorf MF, Mehlman DJ. Observations on the effects of selected antiarrhythmic drugs on mammalian cardiac Purkinje fibers with two levels of steady-state potential: influences of lidocaine, phenytoin, propranolol, disopyramide, and procainamide on repolarization, action potential shape and conduction. J Pharmacol Exp Ther 1977;207:983–991.
11. Antzelevitch C, Moe GK. Electrotonically mediated delayed conduction and reentry in relation to ventricular conducting tissue. Circ Res 1981;49:1129–1139.
12. Weidmann S. The electrical constants of Purkinje fibres. J Physiol (Lond) 1952;118:348–360.
13. Weidmann S. Electrical constants of trabecular muscle from mammalian heart. J Physiol 1970;210: 1041–1054.
14. Arnsdorf MF. The effect of antiarrhythmic drugs on triggered sustained rhythmic activity in cardiac Purkinje fibers. J Pharmacol Exp Ther 1977;201:689–700.
15. Antzelevitch C, Burashnikov A. Cardiac arrhythmias: Reentry and triggered activity. In: Sperelakis N, Kurachi Y, Terzic A, Cohen MV, eds. Heart Physiology and Pathophysiology. 4th ed. New York: Academic Press, 2000:1153–1179.
16. Roden DM, Lazzara R, Rosen MR, et al. Multiple mechanisms in the long-QT syndrome: Current knowledge, gaps, and future directions. Circulation 1996;47:681–689.

17. Arnsdorf MF. Arnsdorf's Paradox. J Cardiovas Electrophys 1990;1:42–52.
18. Arnsdorf MF, Sawicki GJ. Flecainide and the electrophysiologic matrix: The effects of flecainide acetate on the determinants of cardiac excitability in sheep Purkinje fibers. J Cardiovasc Electrophysiol 1996;7:1172–1182.
19. Cardiac Arrhythmia Suppression Trial (CAST) Investigators. Increased mortality due to encainide or flecainide in a randomized trial of arrhythmia suppression after myocardial infarction. N Engl J Med 1989;321:406–412.
20. Janse MJ, Wit AL. Electrophysiological mechanisms of ventricular arrhythmias resulting from myocardial ischemia and infarction. Physiol Rev 1989;69:1049–1169.
21. Kleber AG, Janse MJ. Impulse propagation in myocardial ischemia. In: Zipes DP, Jalife J, eds. Cardiac Electrophysiology: From Cell to Bedside. 1st ed. Philadelphia: W. B. Saunders, 1990:156–161.
22. Allessie MA, Bonke FIM, Schopman FJG. Circus movement in rabbit atrial muscle as a mechanism of tachycardia. III. The "leading circle" concept: A new model of circus movement in cardiac tissue without the involvement of an anatomic obstacle. Circ Res 1977;41:9–18.
23. Task Force of the Working Group on Arrhythmias of the European Society of Cardiology. The Sicilian Gambit: A new approach to the classification of antiarrhythmic drugs based on their actions on arrhythmogenic mechanisms. Circulation 1991;84:1831–1851.
24. Vaughan Williams EM. Classification of antiarrhythmic drugs. In: Sandoe E, Flensted-Jensen E, Olesen KH, eds. Symposium on Cardiac Arrhythmias. Sodertalje, Sweden: Astra, 1970:449–472.
25. Vaughan Williams EM. A classification of antiarrhythmic actions reassessed after a decade of new drugs. J Clin Pharmacol 1984;24:129–147.
26. Cardiac Arrhythmia Suppression Trial II (CAST-II) Investigators. Effect of the antiarrhythmic agent moricizine on survival after acute myocardial infarction. N Engl J Med 1992;327:227–233.
27. Holland RP, Brooks H. TQ-ST segment mapping: critical review and analysis of current concepts. Am J Cardiol 1977;40:110–128.
28. Holland RP, Brooks H, Lidl B. Spatial and non-spatial influences on the TQ-ST segment deflection in ischemia: A theoretical and experimental analysis in the pig. J Clin Invest 1977;60:197–214.
29. Richeson F, Akiyama T, Schek E. A solid angle analysis of the epicardial ischemic TQ-ST deflection in the pig: A theoretical and experimental study. Circ Res 1978;43:879–888.
30. Plonsey R. An evaluation of several cardiac activation models. J Electrocardiol 1974;7:237–244.
31. Engelmann TW. Ueber die Leitung der Erregung im Herzmuskel. Pfluegers Arch Physiol 1875;11:465–480.
32. Engelmann TW. Vergleichende Untersuchungen zur Lehre von der Muskel-und Nervenelectricitat. Pfluegers Arch Physiol 1877;15:116–148.
33. Smith F. The ligation of coronary arteries with electrocardiographic study. Arch Int Med 1918;22:8.
34. Pardee HEB. An electrocardiographic sign of coronary artery obstruction. Arch Int Med 1920;26:244.
35. Samson WE, Scher AM. Mechanism of ST segment alteration during acute myocardial injury. Circ Res 1960;8:780–787.
36. Cohen D, Kaufman LA. Magnetic determination of the relationship between the ST segment shift and the injury current produced by coronary artery occlusion. Circ Res 1975;36:414–424.
37. Holland RP, Brooks H. Precordial and epicardial surface potentials during myocardial ischemia in the pig: A theoretical and experimental analysis of the TQ and ST segment. Circ Res 1975;37:471–480.
38. Kleber AG, Fleischhauer J, Cascio WE. Ischemia-induced propagation failure in the heart. In: Zipes DP, Jalife J, eds. Cardiac Electrophysiology: From Cell to Bedside. 2nd ed. Philadelphia: W. B. Saunders Company, 1995:174–181.
39. Boyden PA. Cellular electrophysiology of ischemic and infarcted tissues. In: Rosen MR, Janse MJ, Wit AL, eds. Cardiac Electrophysiology: A Textbook. 1st ed. Mt. Kisco, NY: Futura Publishing Co, 1990:673–694.
40. DeMello WC. On the control of junctional conductance. In: DeMello WC, Janse MJ, eds. Heart Cell Communication in Health and Disease. Boston: Kluwer Academic Publishers, 1998:105–124.
41. Holland RP, Arnsdorf MF. Nonspatial determinants of electrograms in guinea pig ventricle. Am J Physiol 1981;240:C148–C160.
42. Arnsdorf MF, Bigger JT Jr. Effect of lidocaine hydrochloride on membrane conductance in mammalian cardiac Purkinje fibers. J Clin Invest 1972;51:2252–2263.
43. Arnsdorf MF, Bigger JT Jr. The effect of lidocaine on components of excitability in long mammalian cardiac Purkinje fibers. J Pharmacol Exp Ther 1975;195:206–215.
44. Arnsdorf MF. The effect of antiarrhythmmic drugs on sustained rhythmic activity in cardiac Purkinje fibers. J Pharmacol Exp Ther 1977;201:689 700.

45. Franz MR, Zabel M. Electrophysiologic basis of QT dispersion measurements. Progr Cardiovasc Dis 2000;42:311–324.
46. Day CP, McComb JM, Campbell RW. QT dispersion: An indication of arrhythmia risk in patients with long QT intervals. Brit Heart J 1990;63:342–344.
47. Rautaharju PM. QT dispersion of ventricular repolarization: The greatest fallacy in electrocardiography in the 1990's. Circulation 1999;18:2477–2478.
48. Steinberg J, ed. QT Dispersion. Progr Cardiovasc Dis 2000;42:311–396.
49. Acar B, Yi G, Hnatkova K, Malik M. Spatial, temporal and wavefront direction characteristics of 12 lead T-wave morphology. Med Biol Eng Comput 1999;37:574–584.
50. Murda'h MA, McKenna WJ, Camm AJ. Repolarization alternans: Techniques, mechanisms and cardiac vulnerability. PACE 1997;20:2641–2657.
51. Pastore JM, Girouard SD, Laurita KR, Akar FG, Rosenbaum DS. Mechanism linking T wave alternans to the genesis of cardiac fibrillation. Circulation 1999;99:1385–1394.
52. Breithardt G, Cain ME, El-Sherif N, et al. Standards for analysis of ventricular late potentials using high resolution or signal-averaged electrocardiography: A statement by a task force committee of the European Society of Cardiology, the American Heart Association, and the American College of Cardiology. J Am Coll Cardiol 1991;999–1006.
53. Holland R, Arnsdorf MF. Solid angle theory and the electrocardiogram. Progr Cardiovasc Dis 1977;19:431–457.

17 Antiarrhythmic Drugs and Future Direction

Arshad Jahangir, MD, Andre Terzic, MD, PhD, and Win-Kuang Shen, MD

CONTENTS

INTRODUCTION
TARGET FOR ANTIARRHYTHMIC DEVELOPMENT
GENOMICS AND ANTIARRHYTHMIC THERAPY: THE NEW FRONTIER
CARDIAC ELECTRICAL REMODELING AND ANTIARRHYTHMICS
FUTURE DIRECTIONS: THE SEARCH FOR THE IDEAL ANTIARRHYTHMICS
ACKNOWLEDGMENTS
REFERENCES

INTRODUCTION

Antiarrhythmic agents play an important role in the termination and suppression of both atrial and ventricular arrhythmias as primary or adjunctive therapy. The use of hybrid treatment, combining drugs with radiofrequency ablation or ICD implantation, is expected to rise as the number of patients with complex arrhythmias continues to increase *(1,2)*. In this evolving management scenario, selection of an effective yet safe pharmacologic agent is challenging. The challenge arises from factors intrinsic to the patient, disease condition or the drug itself. These factors primarily include variability in the pathophysiologic substrate, diverse arrhythmia mechanisms, multiple clinical presentation with differing prognostic implications, along with variability in drug disposition and/or response in a highly heterogeneous patient population. Moreover, the availability of multiple therapeutic options and the narrow therapeutic index with limited ability to determine satisfactory endpoints further emphasize the need for better understanding of interactions between drug, end target, and disease condition.

In fact, clinical trials, such as the Cardiac Arrhythmia Suppression Trial (CAST) *(3)* and the Survival With Oral D-Sotalol (SWORD) Trial *(4)*, which demonstrated increased mortality in patients treated with antiarrhythmic agents compared to placebo have increased the awareness of the proarrhythmic potential of antiarrhythmic agents and emphasized the need to better understand the mechanism of arrhythmogenesis and drug action. Treating arrhythmias regardless of its prognostic significance or consideration of

From: Contemporary Cardiology: Cardiac Repolarization: Bridging Basic and Clinical Science
Edited by: I. Gussak et al. © Humana Press Inc., Totowa, NJ

387

the underlying substrate and choosing antiarrhythmic agents by trial and error are no longer acceptable practices. Understanding the concepts related to arrhythmogenesis and antiarrhythmic mechanisms, improved selection of patients based on risk stratification as well as knowledge of the pharmacokinetics and pharmacodynamics of the drug in an individual are crucial to safer and more effective therapy.

Progress has been made in all these areas. In particular, insight into arrhythmia mechanism based on the underlying macroscopic or microscopic substrate and knowledge of the electrophysiological effect of drugs in physiologic and pathologic states have increased our understanding of antiarrhythmic mechanisms (5,6). Available antiarrhythmic agents are rarely selective for a single target (7) and the interactions with the primary or other targets may change with the pathophysiologic state and may thus, result in either increased antiarrhythmic effect or worsening of proarrhythmic potential (8). Experimental models with progression of disease and changing electrical substrate have provided insight into such dynamic nature of drug action (9). The requirement for drug dosage adjustment to achieve therapeutic effect increases with decreased effectiveness in terminating arrhythmias, such as atrial fibrillation (10). These models have also provided information on different effects of the same drug depending upon the underlying substrate, e.g., presence of ischemia or not (11), or tachycardia-induced vs heart failure-mediated atrial myopathy (12). The underlying basis for these differences are not fully understood, but are related to ionic and structural remodeling that occurs with persistence of abnormal excitability (13).

Recognition of triggers and substrate as critical component of the arrhythmia and identification of vulnerable parameters and the cellular and subcellular structures central to the pathogenesis provides potential target(s) for antiarrhythmic development (6,7). With the concern that conduction slowing Class I antiarrhythmics may have an excessive proarrhythmic effect with an increase in overall mortality in patients with structural heart disease (3), emphasis has been placed on the development of repolarization prolonging agents (14), resulting in release of several new Class III antiarrhythmic drugs, both for the management of supraventricular and ventricular arrhythmias (15).

Overall, recent determination of the structure of ion channels and the molecular determinants of antiarrhythmic drug action on specific ion channels, pumps, and receptors and its modulation by disease process and other factors have opened new avenues for drug development (16). In addition, channelopathies associated with the uncommon inherited arrhythmic syndromes have provided further insight not only in the arrhythmogenic mechanisms underlying the familial disorders of electrical instability, such as the long QT or the Brugada syndrome, but also provided insight into the cellular basis for electrophysiologic changes in the more common acquired disorders (17). Repolarization abnormalities and altered expression of both depolarizing and repolarizing membrane currents occur with atrial fibrillation, heart failure, cardiac hypertrophy and after myocardial infarction (9,17–21). Even though, these abnormalities have been recognized, molecular target-based strategies for the management of these disorders or discovery of new antiarrhythmic agents have not yet been successfully implemented. Since alteration of repolarization appears to be a common theme in both familial and acquired diseases associated with high risk of cardiac arrhythmias and sudden death (17), targeting K^+ channels, which plays a major role in repolarization (22), may provide a basis for the development of effective antiarrhythmic strategy (23–25). In this chapter, we will focus on various K^+ channels in the heart as potential targets for antiarrhythmic agents. Furthermore, knowledge of an individual's genotype as basis for tailoring therapy for the substrate for arrhythmogenesis, as well as drug metabolism affecting susceptibility of an individual to beneficial and harmful effects of antiarrhythmic agents will be discussed.

TARGET FOR ANTIARRHYTHMIC DEVELOPMENT

Delayed Rectifier K^+ Currents

The major antiarrhythmic effect of the Singh-Vaughn Williams Class III agents is mediated through blockade of the delayed rectifier potassium channels, which normally repolarizes the heart (Table 1) *(26,27)*. Potassium channel blockade results in prolongation of the action potential duration and an increase in refractoriness of the atria and ventricles, without concomitant reduction in conduction velocity. This, in turn, increases the wavelength for reentry, which determines the number of reentry circuits during fibrillation and the stability of the arrhythmic event *(28,29)*. The current source-sink relationship is also affected by the class III antiarrhythmics, especially at the "turning points" in the circuit with high wavefront curvature, resulting in conduction slowing or block, failure of wavefront propagation and an increased likelihood of termination of reentry *(30,31)*. Most of the clinically available Class III agents (dofetilide, sotalol) block the rapidly activating delayed rectifier potassium (I_{Kr}) channel (derived from KCNH2/KCNE2, previously known as HERG/MiRP) but other potassium channels, including the slowly activating delayed rectified potassium (I_{Ks}) channel (derived from KCNQ1/KCNE1, previously known as KVLQT1/MinK) are targets for drugs such as azimilide and amiodarone *(15,32,33)*. Since I_{Ks} contributes relatively more to repolarization than I_{Kr} at faster heart rates *(34–36)*, inhibition of I_{Kr} alone, with a pure I_{Kr} blocker does not maintain the increased refractoriness at faster heart rate, thereby limiting its antiarrhythmic efficacy *(35)*. Moreover, because of the greater prolongation of the action potential at slower heart rates (reverse use dependence) QT interval is more prolonged with bradycardia and following pauses after ectopic beats, resulting in electrophysiological instability and risk of torsade de pointes *(36,37)*. Therefore, blockade of I_{Ks} is in principle more advantageous than blockade of I_{Kr} with a more homogenous and persistent prolongation of the action potential independent of the heart rate, thus maintaining antiarrhythmic efficacy at faster heart rate *(26,38,39)*. An ideal class III agent would be one that prolongs action potential duration only with increase in the heart rate (use-dependently), increasing the refractoriness more than the cycle length of the tachycardia, thus effectively terminating the arrhythmia, acting in essence like a chemical defibrillator *(40)*.

The structural basis for the higher susceptibility of I_{Kr} to block by diverse compounds was recently discovered and provide further insight into "smart," structure-based, drug development *(41–43)*. The binding site for drugs that prolong QT interval on the S6 transmembrane domain of the I_{Kr} channel protein has two aromatic residues (Tyr652, Phe656) facing the inner cavity that is unique to the HERG channel and absent from other voltage-gated K^+ channels. These aromatic residues form a receptor site in the I_{Kr} channel that can accommodate drugs, which will not interact with other channels. Furthermore, the inner cavity of the I_{Kr} channel appears to be much larger than other voltage-gated K^+ channels because of the absence of the proline residues in the S6 domains present in almost all other voltage-gated K^+ channels *(44)*. These proline residues cause a kink in the S6 segment with reduction in the volume of the inner cavity of the channel *(44)*. The larger inner cavity of the I_{Kr} channel, thus can trap and lodge larger drugs that other K^+

Table 1
Specificity of K$^+$ Channel Blocking Drugs

	I_{Kr}	I_{KS}	I_{K1}	I_{to}
Class IA				
Quinidine	+		+	+
Disopyramide	+		+	+
Procainamide	+		−	−
Class IC				
Flecainide	+		−	−
Encainide	+		−	−
Class III				
Sotalol	+		+	+
Amiodarone	+	+	+	−
Bretylium	+		−	+
Dofetilide	+		−	−
Tedisamil	+		−	+
Azimilide	+	+		

channels cannot trap *(42)*. These findings provide a possible structural basis for the increased sensitivity of block of I_{Kr} (and not other voltage-gated K$^+$ channels) by medications causing acquired long QT syndrome. Further information on the structural basis of high affinity binding may help improve our ability to predict drugs that are likely to cause a significant risk of torsade de pointes and facilitate the design and development of drugs devoid of enhanced I_{Kr} channel binding, and therefore reduce proarrhythmic potential. With recent advances in understanding of the crystal structure of ion channels it is further anticipated that more selective drugs could be developed *(45,46)*.

Another target for antiarrhythmic therapy is the ultra rapidly activating delayed rectifier current (IK$_{ur}$). The Kv1.5 is the major component of the cardiac ultrarapid delayed rectifier in human atria *(47)*. Since, Kv1.5 is mainly expressed in the atria (Table 2), selective blockers of IK$_{ur}$ by prolonging refractoriness in the atrium could be useful for the treatment of atrial arrhythmias with minimum effect on ventricular repolarization and therefore ventricular proarrhythmia *(39)*.

Targeting auxiliary channel subunits (KCNE1 and KCNE2) or modulating the interactions of auxiliary subunits with thc porc-forming delayed rectifier subunit (KCNH2 and the KCNQ1) may also provide alternate avenues for identifying selective regulators of ion channel function, such as modulation of gating (inactivation), expression, and/or trafficking of the ion channel complex or binding with endogenous or exogenous ligands *(48)*.

In addition to the traditional pharmacological strategies, gene therapy with transfer of genes coding for specific ion channel subunits or regulatory proteins has recently emerged as novel antiarrhythmic approaches under investigation. Gene delivery and overexpression of K$^+$ channels could be a strategy for prevention of arrhythmias triggered by altered cardiac repolarization. Overexpression of voltage-gated K$^+$ channel or KCNH2 encoded I_{Kr} in ventricular myocytes by recombinant adenovirus can reverse action potential prolongation in the failing ventricular myocytes *(49)* and suppress early-after

Table 2
K$^+$ Channels in the Heart: Atrial vs Ventricular Selectivity

Channel	Atrium	Ventricle
HERG	+++	+++
Kv4.x	+++	+++
Kv1.5	+++	+
Kv1.4	+++	+
Kv2.1	+++	–
KvLQT1	++	++

depolarization *(50)*. More recently, the feasibility of atrioventricular nodal modification and slowing of ventricular rate response by locally overexpressing an inhibitory G protein (G$_i$) subunit gene was also shown in atrial fibrillation *(51)*. Modification of cardiac excitability and contractility using dual gene therapy is also being explored as a way to exploit opposing or synergistic therapeutic principles to achieve a tailored phenotype, for example increased myocardial contractility without increasing propensity toward arrhythmia in failing hearts *(52)*. Advances in molecular genetics and improvement in techniques to deliver and control the level and distribution of gene expression in diseased tissues *(53)* may open additional approaches to treat arrhythmias and develop novel therapeutic strategies.

Transient Outward K$^+$ Current

The major portion of the cardiac transient outward current (I$_{to}$) current is formed by Kv4.3 channel, with Kv1.4 and Kv4.2 channels representing a minor fraction with distinct kinetics in different regions of the heart *(16,54)*. The density of the I$_{to}$ varies across the myocardial wall and in different regions of the heart *(18,55)*. An alteration in the expression and distribution of I$_{to}$ is observed in various pathophysiologic conditions. A regional alteration and reduction in the I$_{to}$ density occurs in patients with left ventricular hypertrophy *(56)*, dilated cardiomyopathy and heart failure *(12,18–20)*, postmyocardial infarction *(21)* and with atrial fibrillation *(13)*. The reduction in I$_{to}$ results in attenuation of early repolarization (phase 1), especially in the epicardium and affects the level of plateau (phase 2) of the action potential and other currents involved in delayed repolarization (phase 3) resulting in prolongation and increased heterogeneity of action potential duration *(16,57)*. The regional heterogeneity in the expression of I$_{to}$ and action potential prolongation as seen in cardiac hypertrophy and heart failure, may underlie the increased predisposition to ventricular arrhythmias and sudden death *(58)*. A possible means to reduce the heterogeneity of repolarization owing to heterogeneous expression of the I$_{to}$ in hypertrophy or heart failure would be to normalize I$_{to}$ by pharmacologic modulation or channel gene expression. An I$_{to}$ opener or gene expression enhancement, as for example by thyroid hormone treatment or gene transfer would be clinically beneficial *(57,59)*. Currently, a cardioselective and channel-specific I$_{to}$ opener or blocker is not available for clinical use. Development of an I$_{to}$-selective drug capable of targeting channel function and/or expression will be expected to be beneficial in patients with primary abnormality in the I$_{to}$ or in other channels, such as the Brugada syndrome where the heterogeneity in the expression of I$_{to}$ between epicardium and endocardium in the right ventricles results in the substrate responsible for reentry and ventricular arrhythmias *(55,58)*.

Adenosine Triphosphate-Sensitive K^+ Current

Adenosine triphosphate-sensitive potassium (K_{ATP}) channels, couple cellular metabolism with membrane excitability *(60–63)*. A member of the inward rectifier K^+ channel family, the K_{ATP} channel is a heteromultimeric complex composed in the myocardium of a potassium conducting subunit, Kir6.2, and a sulfonylurea receptor, SUR2A *(64)*. Opening of K_{ATP} channels leads to shortening of the action potential and membrane hyperpolarization, which in turn reduces Ca^{2+} influx through voltage-dependent Ca^{2+} channels resulting in a decrease in cellular excitability and protection of the heart under metabolic stress and ischemia-reperfusion injury *(61,65–73)*. Potassium channel openers, which target K_{ATP} channels and act through the SUR subunit to promote K^+ efflux through the Kir subunit have emerged as a unique class of agents capable of enhancing cellular tolerance to metabolic injury *(25,74–76)*. Potassium channel openers by shortening the cardiac action potential may prevent arrhythmias related to triggered activity resulting from abnormal repolarization and early or delayed afterdepolarization *(77–79)*. In models of prolonged QT syndrome and drug-induced ventricular arrhythmias, pinacidil and nicorandil were effective in suppressing abnormal automaticity, triggered activity and torsade de pointes *(78–81)*. In patients with congenital long QT syndrome and history of syncope, nicorandil improved repolarization abnormalities, abolished early afterdepolarization and prevented recurrence of syncope *(82,83)*. Potassium channel openers, are therefore attractive therapeutic agents in conditions with congenital and acquired prolongation of repolarization. Because of their heterogeneous effect on shortening of refractoriness in the epicardium vs endocardium and ischemic vs nonischemic areas, concerns have been raised that potassium channel openers may further increase dispersion of refractoriness and facilitate reentrant arrhythmias by increasing electrical inhomogeneity *(84)*. However, in clinical trials in patients with ischemic heart disease, arrhythmia aggravation or induction of life-threatening arrhythmias has not been documented for any of the potassium channel openers tested *(85–87)*. In fact, a recent study in patients with acute myocardial infarction showed a reduction in malignant ventricular arrhythmia when treated with intravenous nicorandil at the time of coronary angioplasty *(88)*. Yet, the clinical experience with potassium channel openers and its effect on life-threatening arrhythmias is still limited.

Extensive experimental studies and limited clinical experience point toward the safety and efficacy of potassium channel openers as a class *(87,89)*, yet large-scale clinical trials are necessary before these novel ion channel modulators are accepted in clinical medicine. Improved tissue selectivity and condition specificity are prerequisites for the full exploitation of potassium channel openers in clinical practice. Indeed, the clinical utility of potassium channel openers has been limited by the lack of selectivity of available agents *(90)*. Cloning of K_{ATP} channel subunit isoforms and tissue-specific distribution of the channel subunits with distinct biophysical properties and pharmacological responsiveness *(64,75)* provides a molecular framework to develop new generations of potassium channel opening drugs to target specific tissues with selective openers. Although most currently available potassium channel openers are not tissue-selective, newer generations of drugs are being developed to preferentially target a specific tissue *(91)*. Moreover, with further understanding of the pathogenesis of disease conditions associated with altered function of potassium channels, including channelopathies *(17,90)*, a rational design of potassium channel openers with selectivity for specific pathological states could be envisioned.

G-Protein-Gated Inwardly Rectifying K^+ Current

Related to K_{ATP} channels is the inwardly rectifying G-protein gated K^+ channel, formed by association of two K^+-channel proteins GIRK1 (Kir2.1) and GIRK4 (Kir2.4) in the heart *(92)*. These channels, mainly expressed in the pacemaker tissue (sinoatrial and atrioventricular [AV] node and Purkinje fibers) and the atria *(93,94)* are involved in the parasympathetic modulation of heart rate and are the target for modulation by the autonomic nervous system and adenosine *(95–97)*. Enhanced activation of the channel results in hyperpolarization of the sinoatrial and AV nodal cells and shortening of action potential in the atria, resulting in a negative chronotropic and dromotropic response and an increased propensity toward atrial fibrillation *(96,97)*. Disruption of the channel results in loss of spontaneous beat-to-beat fluctuations in heart rate and the loss of the negative chronotropic effects of vagal stimulation and adenosine *(95)*. With hypervagotonia, such as seen during early inferior wall myocardial infarction, the AV conduction could be severely impaired causing high grade AV block requiring temporary artificial pacemaker. A selective blocker of the GIRK channel, in principle could be beneficial in such emergency settings enhancing AV conduction, thus avoiding the need for emergency pacing *(97,98)*. Enhanced vagal stimulation or excessive adenosine by activation of the GIRK channel and heterogeneous shortening of the atrial action potential could also be proarrhythmic promoting reentry and atrial fibrillation *(99–101)*. Specific blockers of the channel might be useful in these circumstances, as for example for the treatment of vagally-mediated atrial fibrillation without significant adverse effects in the ventricles *(101)*. Further investigation of channel function and its pharmacology in the sinoatrial node may also provide insight for management of patients with inappropriate sinus tachycardia.

GENOMICS AND ANTIARRHYTHMIC THERAPY: THE NEW FRONTIER

Molecular Diagnosis Dictating Therapy

Advances in basic electrophysiology and genetics have greatly facilitated identification of "cardiac channelopathies" with altered ion channel function as underlying mechanism for both inherited and acquired arrhythmia syndromes *(17,90,102,103)*. Insight into the structure, function, and regulation of ion channel proteins and the knowledge of genetic and disease-induced alteration in channel function has helped improve molecular diagnosis of the arrhythmogenic syndromes and identification of potential targets for the development of novel therapies *(104,105)*. Repolarization abnormalities underlie the ventricular arrhythmias characteristic of many cardiac channelopathies. Mutations in genes encoding for the KCNQ1 or KCNE1 subunits of I_{Ks} or KCNH2 or KCNE2 subunits of I_{Kr} form the molecular basis of the LQT syndromes 1, 5, 2 and 6, respectively *(102,106–111)*. A reduction in the repolarizing K^+ current prolongs the QT interval and sets the background for the development of torsade de pointes. Therefore, drugs or interventions that can restore the function of defective K^+ channels or increase K^+ conductance through other normal K^+ channels may prove useful in the treatment of long QT syndromes. In this regard it was recently shown that stilbenes and fenamates (I_{Ks} channel activators) by binding to KCNE1 subunit of the I_{Ks} channel restored I_{Ks} channel function in otherwise inactive KCNE1 C-terminal mutants *(48)*. Pharmacological chaperones that can correct folding defects in mutated protein causing abnormal protein trafficking were also shown to restore normal channel function by rescuing the "trapped" otherwise functional channel proteins and represent another novel approach in the treatment of inherited arrhythmia syndromes *(112,113)*. Understanding mechanisms of loss of normal ion channel function has helped identify novel targets for drug design that can pharmacologically repair the functional defect responsible for the long QT syndrome. With further insight into the molecular basis for various arrhythmias, these approaches may extend to rescue function of the suppressed channel by selectively modifying regulation or expression of the abnormal or other normal channels correcting or compensating the functional defects, thus restoring normal function. For example, repolarization can be maintained pharmacologically or genetically by increasing K^+ efflux through other K^+ channels, such as the K_{ATP} channel *(78,81)*, or by increasing extracellular K^+ and thereby decreasing KCNH2 inactivation *(114,115)*.

Long QT 3 syndrome caused by mutations in the sodium channel (SCN5A), which results in noninactivating sodium current and a gain of function of the Na^+ channel *(116)* can be treated using Na^+ channel blockers, such as mexiletine which preferentially blocks the late Na^+ current *(104,117)*. In the Brugada syndrome, on the other hand a loss of function of the Na^+ channel occurs *(118)*, which results in an outward shift of the net current active at the end of phase 1 of the right ventricular action potential owing to an unopposed I_{to} current *(58)*. Because of the transmyocardial heterogeneity in the expression of I_{to}, loss of action potential dome and abbreviation of the right ventricular epicardial but not endocardial action potential occurs with increased transmural dispersion of refractoriness, resulting in a substrate that predisposes phase 2 reentry and ventricular arrhythmia *(58,119)*. Because a prominent I_{to} is responsible for the phase 2 reentry, antiarrhythmics that inhibit I_{to} (such as tedisamil, quinidine, or 4-aminopyridine) could restore electrical homogeneity and suppress arrhythmia *(58,120–122)*. Similarly, class III antiarrhythmic agents by prolonging repolarization may also prevent phase 2 reentry and arrhythmias in the Brugada syndrome *(58)*. The Na^+ channel blockers, on the other hand can unmask and aggravate the electrical heterogeneity and be proarrhythmic *(123,124)*. Thus, understanding specific cardiac substrate underlying the arrhythmia syndrome is a prerequisite for selecting the optimum therapy and guiding future discovery of novel antiarrhythmic agents for specific conditions. Further insight into the molecular basis for various arrhythmias and mechanisms underlying abnormal ion channel function will help in identification of additional targets for drug design that can repair the functional defect responsible for the arrhythmia substrate.

Genetic Susceptibility to Drug-Induced Adverse Effects

Majority of abnormal drug reactions is because of inappropriate formulations and excessive exposure, but adverse effects may occur even at normal doses. This may be owing to differences in drug absorption, distribution, metabolism or excretion. Genetic differences in metabolic pathways and/or drug targets may explain some of the idiosyncratic drug reactions. The cytochrome P450 family of enzymes, located in the liver and gastrointestinal tract, is responsible for majority of drug oxidation *(125)*. Several polymorphisms that affect genes encoding these enzymes result in variability in drug metabolism and have been implicated in adverse drug reactions and proarrhythmia *(125,126)*. Individuals with absent or reduced CYP2D6 activity (six percent of Caucasians) have reduced first pass metabolism of metoprolol and can experience excessive bradycardia *(127)*. Similarly, "slow metabolizers" of propafenone, a sodium channel blocker with additional β-adrenergic receptor blocking effect can exhibit markedly greater β-adrenoceptor blockade with central nervous system and bradycardiac side effects than patients with high enzyme activity *(128)*. Even with a normal genotype, drug interactions, with coadministration of an agent which is a potent inhibitor of the enzyme system that normally degrades the drug modulating ion channel function can result in life threatening arrhythmias *(129,130)*. Because of the narrow therapeutic index, these pharmacokinetic interactions are of extreme importance and are a major safety concern in antiarrhythmic drug development and use. A better understanding of the way in which individuals with a particular genotype respond to a drug allows identification of population subgroups that will benefit most from a particular drug with minimum adverse effects *(126)*.

Adverse drug response, in addition to the pharmacokinetic factors, may also result from genetic variation in drug targets (pharmacodynamic factors). Recently, the use of several "noncardiac" drugs (Table 3), including long-term antihistamines (terfenadine), gastrointestinal motility promoting drugs (cisapride) and antipsychotics (thioridazine) has been restricted because of the occurrence of QT-interval prolongation and lethal arrhythmias *(126,131)*. Genetic variations in various ion channels responsible for the normal ventricular repolarization and known to cause inherited long QT syndromes have been hypothesized as a cause of the acquired or drug-induced long QT syndrome *(16,126,132)*. Mutations or polymorphisms in these ion channels could result in a "silent" reduction in the "cardiac repolarization reserve" and therefore, an increase sensitivity of the channel to inhibition which manifest only after exposure to a K^+ channel blocker or factors that can prolong repolarization *(5,126)*. In this regard, a missense mutation in KCNE2 subunit of the I_{Kr} channel was recently identified as the basis for clarithromycin-induced torsade de pointes *(111)*. This mutation decreases activation of the K^+ channel, resulting in a threefold increased sensitivity to drug inhibition compared to the wild-type channel *(111)*. Also, a common polymorphism in the KCNE2 gene results in QT interval prolongation following sulfamethoxazole-trimethoprim administration *(133)*. It is expected that advances in pharmacogenomics and development of inexpensive, high-throughput technologies for screening large number of polymorphisms will facilitate discovery of molecular basis for other occult arrhythmogenic substrate and in identification of additional targets for the development of novel therapies. A more rapid and inexpensive screening of patients who are likely to experience efficacy or adverse events, will also help in individualizing therapy with optimum selection and dosage of "older" drugs based on an individual's genetic constitution of the metabolizing enzymes, transporters, and drug receptors. This will also accelerate drug development and assessment by making clinical trials smaller, faster and more efficient *(134,135)*. Thus, a safer and more efficient pharmacotherapy could be developed and selected decreasing the number of adverse reactions and associated morbidity and mortality, which will have an enormous impact on health care cost *(136,137)*.

Table 3
Repolarization Prolonging Cardiac and Noncardiac Drugs

Antiarrhythmics
    IA: Quinidine, procainamide, disopyramide
    III: Sotalol, NAPA, ibutilde, dofetilide, azimilide, amiodarone,
    IV: Bepridil
Antimicrobials
    antibiotics: Macrolides (erythromycin), TMP/SMX
    antifungals: Itraconazole, ketoconazole
    antimalarials: Chloroquine
    antiparasitic: Pentamidine
    antivirals: Amantadine
Antihistamine: Terfenadine, asetmizole,
Antidepressants: Tricyclics (amitriptyline, tetracyclics
Psychotropics: Holaperidol, droperidol, Phenothiazines
Miscellaneous
    Cisapride, metoclopramide
    Probucol
    Ketanserin,
    Vasopressin,
    Organophosphate poisoning, chloarl hydrate overdose

CARDIAC ELECTRICAL REMODELING AND ANTIARRHYTHMICS

Progression of the underlying disease and cardiac adaptation or remodeling that occurs with disease and rapid heart rate can also modify the electrophysiologic drug actions *(10)*. This can occur because of alteration in ion channels *(9,56,138)*, signaling or Ca^{2+} handling proteins, structural changes in the myocytes or extracellular matrix *(139)*, or the activity of the neurohumoral system *(6,140)*. The drug which targets an ionic current reduced by remodeling may lose its effect because of the reduction in the contribution of that current to overall action potential and changes in the density of other currents that may counteract the effect of the drug *(141)*. On the other hand, ionic remodeling can enhance the effect of drugs, increasing the risk of proarrhythmia. This could be owing to reduction in ionic current, normally not blocked by the drug with increased dependence of repolarization on the ionic current blocked by the drug. This is seen in congestive heart failure, where a reduction in I_{Ks} occurs in the ventricles *(9)*, with increased dependence of repolarization on I_{Kr}, and hence increased sensitivity to I_{Kr} blockade and risk of proarrhythmia. In atrial fibrillation with rapid atrial rates, electrical remodeling of the atria also occurs, with a decrease in atrial refractoriness, a reduction in the rate adaptation of refractoriness and an increase in the dispersion of refractoriness *(13,139)*. There is significant reduction in I_{to}, L-type Ca^{2+} and voltage-gated sodium current *(13)*, associated with decreased transcription and protein expression of the Kv4.3, the $\alpha1$-subunit of L-type Ca^{2+}, and the cardiac Na^+ channels *(12,13,142)*. Depending on the underlying substrate, the electrophysiologic and ionic changes in the heart may vary *(143)*, and provide basis for the differences in the pathophysiology of the arrhythmia and variability in response to treatment *(13)*. Further insights into mechanisms of changes in ionic homeostasis, signal transduction, and structural remodeling may also allow improved approaches to alter molecular pathophysiology with possibility of therapeutic interventions at the molecular and genetic level *(144)*. These approaches include use of drugs not normally considered as antiarrhythmic agents, such as angiotensin converting enzyme inhibitors *(145,146)*, angiotensin II receptor antagonists *(140)*, spironolactone *(147)*, statins, and others that limit the progression of underlying heart disease and therefore, modify the electrophysiological and mechanical substrate that can predispose to arrhythmogenesis *(6,139–147)*.

FUTURE DIRECTIONS: THE SEARCH FOR THE IDEAL ANTIARRHYTHMICS

Several strategies have been followed to improve efficacy and safety of class III antiarrhythmic agents *(27)*. These include development of drugs that target a single (dofetilide) or multiple K^+ channels (azimilide, amiodarone) or increase refractoriness by other measures, such as increasing the slow inward Na^+ current (ibutilide) *(14,15,36,148)*. Existing drugs are also being modified to reduce adverse effects (dronedarone) *(149)*. Efforts are on going for making drugs less reverse-use dependent (thus decreasing the risk of torsade de pointes with sudden changes in heart rate), and less susceptible to reversal with adrenergic agents (amiodarone, azimilide) *(14,39)*. Besides the I_{Kr} and I_{Ks}, other potassium channels such as I_{to} are under consideration as targets for the development of condition-specific antiarrhythmic agents with utility in specific arrhythmogenic conditions, such as the Brugada syndrome *(58)*. Tissue-selective antiarrhythmics targeting ion channels, such as the GIRK channel predominantly expressed in the conduction system *(93,96)* and I_{Kur} in the atrium *(39,47)* may be more effective for managing supraventricular arrhythmias without the risk for ventricular proarrhythmia. Furthermore, targeting of channels that become active mainly during pathological states, such as the K_{ATP} or stretch-activated channels may allow development of condition-specific drugs, selective for the abnormal substrate without affecting the normal tissue *(25,65)*. Further identification of other channel isoforms, auxiliary subunits and regulatory proteins, specifically expressed in the affected tissue, may allow substrate-specific therapy to achieve the desirable therapeutic effect without the undesirable systemic side effects. Information about the three-dimensional arrangement of amino acid residues on the target protein forming the binding site for the drug is also expected to provide further insight into drug-receptor interactions and development of structure-based drugs to optimize affinity and specificity for the selected molecule in the target tissue *(45,46,150)*.

With the development of new genetic diagnostic and prognostic capabilities it may be possible to specifically tailor an individual's therapy based on information about drug targets or metabolic pathway. Recognition of biochemical intermediaries and modulation of molecular and genetic substrate involved in arrhythmogenesis may form the basis of future development of antiarrhythmics with selectivity for the pathological substrate. Newer targets include gap junction *(151)*, ion transporters (such as sodium-calcium exchanger, sodium-hydrogen exchanger or Ca ATPase) *(152–155)*, intracellular channels (such as, sarcoplasmic reticulum Ca^{2+} release channel or mitochondrial K_{ATP} channel) *(65,156,157)*, cytoskeletal proteins *(158)* and proteins involved in signal transduction or intracellular Ca^{2+} homeostasis (calmodulin or phospholamban) *(6,159,160)*. Furthermore, identification of critical steps in posttranslational processing of proteins involved in cardiac excitability may allow development of pharmacological chaperones that can modify an abnormal protein, therefore, restore its function or change the density of the normal proteins, such as the number of ion channels on cell membrane to correct the electrophysiologic defect *(161)*. Gene therapy with transfer of genes encoding for ion channel subunits *(49,50,52)* or their regulatory proteins *(51)* or modulation of gene expression at the transcriptional level *(59,144)* to alter the myocardial arrhythmogenic substrate are other novel strategies currently under investigation *(17)*. Furthermore, the availability of cost-effective genotyping technologies may allow substrate-based tailoring of the drug therapy based on the genetic make up affecting pharmacokinetic and pharmacodynamic profile, thus limiting the incidence of proarrhythmia or other adverse effects.

Future research should focus on further elucidation of the structure, function, and regulation of various proteins involved in action potential, signal transduction, and maintenance of ionic homeostasis and in understanding the mechanism of drug actions at the cellular and the organism level and how it is affected by the disease process and changes in the arrhythmogenic substrate *(162)*. New perspectives about the mechanisms underlying various arryhthmias and modalities to prevent structural and functional abnormalities that leads to arrhythmogenesis open the opportunity for novel antiarrhythmic strategies *(6,17)*. It is to be anticipated that these efforts could collectively enhance the development of cardiac selective compounds that modulate the arrhythmogenic substrate with promising therapeutic and prophylactic utility.

ACKNOWLEDGMENTS

Arshad Jahangir is a recipient of the CR75 Award from the Mayo Foundation, the Merck Award in Basic Sciences from the Society of Geriatric Cardiology and Scientist Development Grant from the National American Heart Association. Andre Terzic is an Established Investigator of the American Heart Association. Work in the authors laboratory was supported, in part, by the National Institutes of Health, American Heart Association, Miami Heart Research Institute, the Bruce and Ruth Rappaport Program in Vascular Biology and Gene Delivery, and the Marriott Foundation.

REFERENCES

1. Murgatroyd FD. "Pills and pulses": hybrid therapy for atrial fibrillation. J Cardiovasc Electrophysiol 2002;13:S40–S46.
2. Ozcan C, Jahangir A, Friedman PA, et al. Long-term survival after ablation of the atrioventricular node and implantation of a permanent pacemaker in patients with atrial fibrillation. N Engl J Med 2001;344:1043–1051.
3. Echt DS, Liebson PR, Mitchell LB, et al. Mortality and morbidity in patients receiving encainide, flecainide or placebo. The Cardiac Arrhythmia Suppression Trial (CAST). N Engl J Med 1991;324: 781–788.
4. Waldo AL, Camm AJ, Deruyter H, et al. Effect of d-sotalol on mortality in patients with left ventricular dysfunction after recent and remote myocardial infarction. Lancet 1996;348:7–12.
5. Roden DM, Spooner PM. Inherited long QT syndromes: a paradigm for understanding arrhythmogenesis. J Cardiovasc Electrophysiol 1999;10:1664–1683.
6. Members of the Sicilian Gambit. New approaches to antiarrhythmic therapy—Emerging therapeutic applications of the cell biology of cardiac arrhythmias. Eur Heart J 2001;22:2148–2163.
7. Task Force of the Working Group on Arrhythmias of the European Society of Cardiology: The Sicilian Gambit: A new approach to the classification of antiarrhythmic drugs based on their actions on arrhythmogenic mechanisms. Circulation 1991;84:1831–1851.

8. Greenberg HM, Dwyer EM Jr, Hochman JS, Steinberg JS, Echt DS, Peters RW. Interaction of ischaemia and encainide/flecainide treatment: a proposed mechanism for the increased mortality in CAST I. Br Heart J 1995;74:631–635.

9. Nattel S, Li DS. Ionic remodeling in the heart—Pathophysiological significance and new therapeutic opportunities for atrial fibrillation. Circ Res 2000;87:440–447.

10. Nattel S. Effects of ionic remodeling on cardiac antiarrhythmic drug actions. J Cardiovasc Pharmacol 2001;38:809–811.

11. Aupetit JF, Loufouamoundanga J, Faucon G, Timour Q. Ischaemia-induced loss or reversal of the effects of the class I antiarrhythmic drugs on vulnerability to fibrillation. Br J Pharmacol 1997;120: 523–529.

12. Li D, Melnyk P, Feng J, Wang Z, Petrecca K, Shrier A, Nattel S. Effects of experimental heart failure on atrial cellular and ionic electrophysiology. Circulation 2000;101:2631–2638.

13. Nattel S. New ideas about atrial fibrillation 50 years on. Nature 2002;415:219–226.

14. Singh BN. Current antiarrhythmic drugs: An overview of mechanisms of action and potential clinical utility. J Cardiovasc Electrophysiol 1999;10:283–301.

15. Sager PT. New advances in class III antiarrhythmic drug therapy. Curr Opin Cardiol 2000;15:41–53.

16. Roden DM, Balser JR, George AL, Anderson ME. Cardiac ion channels. Annu Rev Physiol 2002;64:431–475.

17. Marbán E. Cardiac channelopathies. Nature 2002;415:213–218.

18. Kaab S, Dixon J, Duc J, et al. Molecular basis of transient outward potassium current downregulation in human heart failure: A decrease in Kv4.3 mRNA correlates with a reduction in current density. Circulation 1998;98:1383–1393.

19. Wickenden AD, Kaprielian R, Kassiri Z, et al. The role of action potential prolongation and altered intracellular calcium handling in the pathogenesis of heart failure. Cardiovasc Res 1998;37:312–323.

20. Tomaselli GF, Marban E. Electrophysiological remodeling in hypertrophy and heart failure. Cardiovasc Res 1999;42:270–283.

21. Pinto JM, Boyden PA. Electrical remodeling in ischemia and infarction. Cardiovasc Res 1999;42: 284–297.

22. Colatsky TJ. Controlling cardiac arrhythmias: New drugs in development and insights from molecular biology. J Cardiovasc Pharmacol Ther 1998;3:337–342.

23. Curran ME. Potassium ion channels and human disease: Phenotypes to drug targets? Curr Opin Biotechnol 1998;9:565–572.

24. Shieh CC, Coghlan M, Sullivan JP, Gopalakrishnan M. Potassium channels: molecular defects, diseases, and therapeutic opportunities. Pharmacol Rev 2000;52:557–594.

25. Jahangir A, Terzic A, Shen WK. Potassium channel openers: therapeutic potential in cardiology and medicine. Exp Opin Pharmacother 2001;2:1995–2010.

26. Nair LA, Grant AO. Emerging class III antiarrhythmic agents: Mechanism of action and proarrhythmic potential. Cardiovasc Drugs Ther 1997;11:149–167.

27. Nattel S, Singh BN. Evolution, mechanisms, and classification of antiarrhythmic drugs: Focus on class III actions. Am J Cardiol 1999;84:11R-19R.

28. Rensma PL, Allessie MA, Lammers WJ, Bonke FI, Schalij MJ. Length of excitation wave and susceptibility to reentrant atrial arrhythmias in normal conscious dogs. Circ Res 1988;62:395–410.

29. Wang J, Bourne GW, Wang Z, Villemaire C, Talajic M, Nattel S. Comparative mechanisms of antiarrhythmic drug action in experimental atrial fibrillation. Circulation 1993;88:1030–1044.

30. Wijffels MC, Dorland R, Mast F. Widening of the excitable gap during pharmacological cardioversion of atrial fibrillation in the goat: effects of cibenzoline, hydroquinidine, flecainide, and d-sotalol. Circulation 2000;102:260–267.

31. Tai CT, Chen SA, Feng AN, Yu, WC, Chen YJ, Chang MS. Electropharmacologic effects of class I and class III antiarrhythmic drugs on typical atrial flutter: Insights into the mechanism of termination. Circulation 1998;97:1935–1945.

32. Weerapura M, Hebert TE, Nattel S. Dofetilide block involves interactions with open and inactivated states of HERG channels. Pflugers Arch 2002;443:520–531.

33. Singh BN, Sarma JS. What niche will newer class III antiarrhythmic drugs occupy? Curr Cardiol Rep 2001;3:314–323.

34. Viswanathan PC, Shaw RM, Rudy Y. Effects of I_{Kr} and I_{Ks} heterogeneity on action potential duration and its rate dependence: a simulation study. Circulation 1999;99:2466–2474.

35. Jurkiewicz NK, Sanguinetti MC. Rate-dependent prolongation of cardiac action potentials by a methanesulfonanilide class III antiarrhythmic agent: specific block of rapidly activating delayed rectifier K$^+$ current by dofetilide. Circ Res 1993;72:75–83.

36. Carmeliet E. Use-dependent block of the delayed K$^+$ current in rabbit ventricular myocytes. Cardiovasc Drugs Ther 1993;3:599–604.

37. Hondeghem LM. Classification of antiarrhythmic agents and the two laws of pharmacology. Cardiovasc Res 2000;45:57–60.

38. Bauer A, Becker R, Freigang KD, et al. Electrophysiologic effects of the new I-Ks-blocking agent chromanol 293b in the postinfarction canine heart—Preserved positive use-dependence and preferential prolongation of refractoriness in the infarct zone. Bas Res Cardiol 2000;95:324–332.

39. Nattel S. The molecular and ionic specificity of antiarrhythmic drug actions. J Cardiovasc Electrophysiol 1999;10:272–282.

40. Hondeghem LM. Computer aided development of antiarrhythmic agents with class IIIa properties. J Cardiovasc Electrophysiol 1994;5:711–721.

41. Mitcheson JS, Chen J, Lin M, Culberson C, Sanguinetti MC. A structural basis for drug-induced long QT syndrome. Proc Natl Acad Sci 2000;97:12329–12333.

42. Mitcheson JS, Chen J, Sanguinetti MC. Trapping of a methanesulfonanilide by closure of the HERG potassium channel activation gate. J Gen Physiol 2000b;115:229–239.

43. Lees-Miller JP, Duan Y, Teng GQ, Duff HJ. Molecular determinant of high-affinity dofetilide binding to HERG1 expressed in Xenopus oocytes: involvement of S6 sites. Mol Pharmacol 2000;57:367–374.

44. del Camino D, Holmgren M, Liu Y, Yellen G. Blocker protection in the pore of a voltage-gated K$^+$ channel and its structural implications. Nature 2000;403:321–325.

45. Doyle DA, Morais Cabral J, Pfuetzner RA, et al. The structure of the potassium channel: Molecular basis of K$^+$ conduction and selectivity. Science 1998;280:69–77.

46. Dutzler R, Campbell EB, Cadene M, Chait BT, MacKinnon R. X-ray structure of a ClC chloride channel at 3.0 angstrom reveals the molecular basis of anion selectivity. Nature 2002;415:287–294.

47. Feng J, Wible B, Li GR, Wang Z, Nattel S. Antisense oligodeoxynucleotides directed against Kv1.5 mRNA specifically inhibit ultrarapid delayed rectifier K$^+$ current in cultured adult human atrial myocytes. Circ Res 1997;80:572–579.

48. Abitbol I, Peretz A, Lerche C, Busch AE, Attali B. Stilbenes and fenamates rescue the loss of I$_{KS}$ channel function induced by an LQT5 mutation and other IsK mutants. EMBO J 1999;18:4137–4148.

49. Nuss HB, Johns DC, Kaab S, et al. Reversal of potassium channel deficiency in cells from failing hearts by adenoviral gene transfer: a prototype for gene therapy for disorders of cardiac excitability and contractility. Gene Ther 1996;3:900–912.

50. Nuss HB, Marban E, Johns DC. Overexpression of a human potassium channel suppresses cardiac hyperexcitability in rabbit ventricular myocytes. J Clin Invest 1999;103:889–896.

51. Donahue JK. Focal modification of electrical conduction in the heart by viral gene transfer. Nature Med 2000;6:1395–1398.

52. Ennis IL, Li RA, Murphy AM, Marban E, Nuss HB. Dual gene therapy with SERCA1 and Kir2.1 abbreviates excitation without suppressing contractility. J Clin Invest 2002;109:393–400.

53. Neyroud N, Nuss HB, Leppo MK, Marban E, Donahue JK. Gene delivery to cardiac muscle. Methods Enzymol 2002;346:323–334.

54. Dixon JE, Shi W, Wang HS, McDonald C, Yu H, Wymore RS, Cohen IS, McKinnon D. Role of the Kv4.3 K$^+$ channel in ventricular muscle. A molecular correlate for the transient outward current. Circ Res 1996;79:659–668.

55. Di Diego JM, Sun ZQ, Antzelevitch C. I$_{TO}$ and action potential notch are smaller in left vs. right canine ventricular epicardium. Am J Physiol 1996;271:H548–H561.

56. Bailly P, Benitah JP, Mouchoniere M, Vassort G, Lorente P. Regional alteration of the transient outward current in human left ventricular septum during compensated hypertrophy. Circulation 1997;96:1266–1274.

57. Hoppe UC, Marban E, Johns DC. Molecular dissection of cardiac repolarization by in vivo Kv4.3 gene transfer. J Clin Invest 2000;105:1077–1084.

58. Antzelevitch C, Fish J. Electrical heterogeneity within the ventricular wall. Bas Res Cardiol 2001;96:517–527.

59. Shimoni Y. Hormonal control of cardiac ion channels and transporters. Prog Biophy Mol Biol 1999;72:67–108.

60. Noma A. ATP-regulated K$^+$ channels in cardiac muscle. Nature 1983;305:147–148.

61. Yamada K, Ji JJ, Yuan HJ, et al. Protective role of ATP-sensitive potassium channels in hypoxia-induced generalized seizure. Science 2001;292:1543–1546.
62. Zingman LV, Alekseev AE, Bienengraeber M, et al. Signaling in channel/enzyme multimers. ATPase transitions in SUR module gate ATP-sensitive K⁺ conductance. Neuron 2001;31:233–245.
63. Carrasco AJ, Dzeja PP, Alekseev AE, et al. Adenylate kinase phosphotransfer communicates cellular energetic signals to ATP-sensitive potassium channels. Proc Natl Acad Sci 2001;98:7623–7628.
64. Inagaki N, Gonoi T, Clement JP, et al. Reconstitution of IK$_{ATP}$: An inward rectifier subunit plus the sulfonylurea receptor. Science 1995;270:1166–1170.
65. Gross GJ, Fryer RM. Sarcolemmal versus mitochondrial ATP-sensitive K⁺ channels and myocardial preconditioning. Circ Res 1999;84:973–979.
66. Grover GJ, Garlid KD. ATP-Sensitive potassium channels: a review of their cardioprotective pharmacology. J Mol Cell Cardiol 2000;32:677–695.
67. Terzic A, Jahangir A, Kurachi Y. Cardiac ATP-sensitive K⁺ channels: regulation by intracellular nucleotides and K⁺ channel-opening drugs. Am J Physiol 1995;269:C525–C545.
68. Jovanovic N, Jovanovic S, Jovanovic A, Terzic A. Gene delivery of Kir6.2/SUR2A in conjunction with pinacidil handles intracellular Ca²⁺ homeostasis under metabolic stress. FASEB J 1999;13:923–929.
69. Suzuki M, Sasaki N, Miki T, et al. Role of sarcolemmal K$_{ATP}$ channels in cardioprotection against ischemia/reperfusion injury in mice. J Clin Invest 2002;109:509–516.
70. Lopez JR, Jahangir R, Jahangir A, Shen WK, Terzic A. Potassium channel openers prevent potassium-induced calcium loading of cardiac cells: Possible implications in cardioplegia. J Thorac Cardiovasc Surg 1996;112:820–831.
71. Ozcan C, Holmuhamedov EL, Jahangir A, Terzic A. Diazoxide protects mitochondria from anoxic injury: Implications for myopreservation. J Thorac Cardiovasc Surg 2001;121:298–306.
72. Jahangir A, Ozcan C, Holmuhamedov EL, Terzic A. Increased calcium vulnerability of senescent cardiac mitochondria: protective role for a mitochondrial potassium channel opener. Mech Ageing Dev 2001;122:1073–1086.
73. Holmuhamedov EL, Ozcan C, Jahangir A, Terzic A. Restoration of Ca²⁺-inhibited oxidative phosphorylation in cardiac mitochondria by mitochondrial Ca²⁺ unloading. Mol Cell Biochem 2001;220:135–140.
74. Ashcroft FM, Gribble FM. New windows on the mechanism of action of K-ATP channel openers. Trends Pharmacol Sci 2000;21:439–445.
75. Terzic A, Vivaudou M. Molecular pharmacology of ATP-sensitive K⁺ channels: How and why? In Potassium Channels in Cardiovascular Biology. Archer SL, Rusch NJ, eds. San Diego: Academic Press, 2001;257–277.
76. Seino S. ATP-sensitive potassium channels: A model of heteromultimeric potassium channel/receptor assemblies. Annu Rev Physiol 1999;61:337–362.
77. Haverkamp W, Borggrefe M, Breithardt G. Electrophysiologic effects of potassium channel openers. Cardiovasc Drug Ther 1995;9:195–202.
78. Kondo M, Tsutsumi T, Mashima S. Potassium channel openers antagonize the effects of class iii antiarrhythmic agents in canine purkinje fiber action potentials—implications for prevention of proarrhythmia induced by class III agents. Jpn Heart J 1999;40:609–619.
79. Vegh A, Gyorgyi K, Papp JG, Sakai K, Parratt JR. Nicorandil suppressed ventricular arrhythmias in a canine model of myocardial ischaemia. Eur J Pharmacol 1996;305:163–168.
80. Carlsson L, Abrahamsson C, Drews L, Duker G. Antiarrhythmic effects of potassium channel openers in rhythm abnormalities related to delayed repolarization. Circulation 1992;85:1491–1500.
81. Shimizu W, Antzelevitch C. Effects of a K⁺ channel opener to reduce transmural dispersion of repolarization and prevent torsade de pointes in LQT1, LQT2, and LQT3 models of the long-QT syndrome. Circulation 2000;102:706–712.
82. Shimizu W, Kurita T, Matsuo K, et al. Improvement of repolarization abnormalities by a K⁺ channel opener in the LQT1 form of congenital long-QT syndrome. Circulation 1998;97:1581–1588.
83. Sato T, Hata Y, Yamamoto M, et al. Early afterdepolarization abolished by potassium channel opener in a patient with idiopathic long QT syndrome. J Cardiovasc Electrophysiol 1995;6:279–282.
84. Wilde AA, Janse MJ. Electrophysiological effects of ATP sensitive potassium channel modulation: implications for arrhythmogenesis. Cardiovasc Res 1994;28:16–24.
85. Miyazaki T, Moritani K, Miyoshi S, et al. Nicorandil augments regional ischemia-induced monophasic action potential shortening and potassium accumulation without serious proarrhythmia. J Cardiovasc Pharmacol 1995;26:949–956.

86. The IONA Study Group. Trial to show the impact of nicorandil in angina (IONA): design, methodology and management. Heart 2001;85:e9.

87. Markham A, Plosker GL, Goa KL. Nicorandil - An updated review of its use in ischaemic heart disease with emphasis on its cardioprotective effects. Drugs 2000;60:955–974.

88. Ito H, Taniyama Y, Iwakura K, et al. Intravenous nicorandil can preserve microvascular integrity and myocardial viability in patients with reperfused anterior wall myocardial infarction. J Am Coll Cardiol 1999;33:654–660.

89. Gumina RJ, Jahangir A, Gross GJ, Terzic A. Cardioprotection: Emerging pharmacotherapy. Exp Opin Pharmacother 2001;2:739–752.

90. Lawson K, Dunne MJ. Peripheral channelopathies as targets for potassium channel openers. Exp Opin Investig Drug 2001;10:1345–1359.

91. Atwal KS, Grover GJ, Lodge NJ, et al. Binding of ATP-sensitive potassium channel K_{ATP} openers to cardiac membranes: correlation of binding affinities with cardioprotective and smooth muscle relaxing potencies. J Med Chem 1998;41:271–275.

92. Krapivinsky G, Gordon EA, Wickman K, Velimirovic B, Krapivinsky L, Clapham DE. The G-protein-gated atrial K+ channel IKACh is a heteromultimer of two inwardly rectifying K+-channel proteins. Nature 1995;374:135–141.

93. Kurachi Y, Tung R, Ito H, Nakajima T. G protein activation of cardiac muscarinic K+ channels. Prog Neurobiol 1992;39:226–246.

94. Yamada M, Jahangir A, Hosoya Y, Inanobe A, Katada T, Kurachi Y. GK and brain G beta gamma activate muscarinic K+ channel through the same mechanism. J Biol Chem 1993;268:24551–24554.

95. Wickman K, Nemec J, Gendler SJ, Clapham DE. Abnormal heart rate regulation in GIRK4 knockout mice. Neuron 1998;20:103–114.

96. Yamada M. The role of muscarinic K+ channels in the negative chronotropic effect of a muscarinic agonist. J Pharmacol Exp Ther 2002;300:681–687.

97. Srinivas M, Song YJ, Shryock JC, Belardinelli L. Cardiac electrophysiological actions of adenosine. Drug Develop Res 1998;45:420–426.

98. Drici MD, Diochot S, Terrenoire C, Romey G, Lazdunski M. The bee venom peptide tertiapin underlines the role of I(KACh) in acetylcholine-induced atrioventricular blocks. Br J Pharmacol 2000;131:569–577.

99. Jahangir A, Munger TM, Packer DL, Crijns H. Atrial fibrillation. In: Podrid PJ, Kowey PR, eds. Cardiac arrhythmia: mechanisms, diagnosis, and management. 2nd edition. Philadelphia: Lippincott Williams & Wilkins, 2001:457–499.

100. Kabell G, Buchanan LV, Gibson JK, Belardinelli L. Effects of adenosine on atrial refractoriness and arrhythmias. Cardiovasc Res 1994;28:1385–1389.

101. Kovoor P, Wickman K, Maguire CT, et al. Evaluation of the role of I-KACh in atrial fibrillation using a mouse knockout model. J Am Coll Cardiol 2001;37:2136–2143.

102. Ackerman MJ, Schroeder JJ, Berry R, et al. A novel mutation in KVLQT1 is the molecular basis of inherited long QT syndrome in a near-drowning patient's family. Pediatr Res 1998;44:148–153.

103. Abraham MR, Jahangir A, Alekseev AE, Terzic A. Channelopathies of inwardly rectifying potassium channels. FASEB J 1999;13:1901–1910.

104. Priori SG, Napolitano C, Paganini V, Cantu F, Schwartz PJ. Molecular biology of the long QT syndrome: impact on management. Pacing Clin Electrophysiol 1997;20:2052–2057.

105. Priori SG, Aliot E, Blomstrom-Lundqvist C, et al. Task Force on Sudden Cardiac Death of the European Society of Cardiology. Eur Heart J 2001;22:1374–1450.

106. Sanguinetti MC, Jiang C, Curran ME, Keating MT. A mechanistic link between an inherited and an acquired cardiac arrhythmia: HERG encodes the I_{Kr} potassium channel. Cell 1995;81:299–307.

107. Curran ME, Splawski I, Timothy KW, Vincent GM, Green ED, Keating MT. A molecular basis for cardiac arrhythmia: HERG mutations cause long QT syndrome. Cell 1995;80:795–803.

108. Wang Q, Curran ME, Splawski I, et al. Positional cloning of a novel potassium channel gene: KVLQT1 mutations cause cardiac arrhythmias. Nat Genet 1996;12:17–23.

109. Neyroud N, Tesson F, Denjoy I, et al. A novel mutation in the potassium channel gene KVLQT1 causes the Jervell and Lange-Nielsen cardioauditory syndrome. Nat Genet 1997;15:186–189.

110. Splawski I, Tristani-Firouzi M, Lehmann MH, Sanguinetti MC, Keating MT. Mutations in the hminK gene cause long QT syndrome and suppress I_{Ks} function. Nat Genet 1997;17:338–340.

111. Abbott GW, Sesti F, Splawski I, et al. MiRP1 forms I_{Kr} potassium channels with HERG and is associated with cardiac arrhythmia. Cell 1999;97:175–187.

112. Zhou Z, Gong Q, January CT. Correction of defective protein trafficking of a mutant herg potassium channel in human long QT syndrome. J Biol Chem 1999;274:31123–31126.

113. Ficker E, Obejero-Paz CA, Zhao S, Brown AM. The binding site for channel blockers that rescue misprocessed human long QT Syndrome type 2 ether-a-gogo-related gene (HERG) mutations. J Biol Chem 2002;277:4989–4998.

114. Compton SJ, Lux RL, Ramsey MR, et al. Genetically defined therapy of inherited long-QT syndrome. Correction of abnormal repolarization by potassium. Circulation 1996;94:1018–1022.

115. Numaguchi H, Johnson JP, Petersen CI, Balser JR. A sensitive mechanism for cation modulation of potassium current. Nature Neurosci 2000;3:429–430.

116. Balser JR. The cardiac sodium channel: gating function and molecular pharmacology. J Mol Cell Cardiol 2001;33:599–613.

117. Schwartz PJ, Priori SG, Locati EH, et al. Long QT syndrome patients with mutations of the SCN5A and HERG genes have differential responses to Na$^+$ channel blockade and to increases in heart rate. Implications for gene-specific therapy. Circulation 1995;92:3381–3386.

118. Chen Q, Kirsch GE, Zhang D, et al. Genetic basis and molecular mechanisms for idiopathic ventricular fibrillation. Nature 1998;392:293–296.

119. Yan GX, Antzelevitch C. Cellular basis for the Brugada syndrome and other mechanisms of arrhythmogenesis associated with ST segment elevation. Circulation 1999;100:1660–1666.

120. Belhassen B, Viskin S, Fish R, Glick A, Setbon I, Eldar M. Effects of electrophysiologic-guided therapy with Class IA antiarrhythmic drugs on the long-term outcome of patients with idiopathic ventricular fibrillation with or without the Brugada syndrome. J Cardiovasc Electrophysiol 1999;10:1301–1312.

121. Alings M, Dekker L, Sadee A, Wilde A. Quinidine induced electrocardiographic normalization in two patients with Brugada syndrome. PACE 2001;24:1420–1422.

122. Suzuki H, Torigoe K, Numata O, Yazaki S. Infant case with a malignant form of Brugada syndrome. J Cardiovasc Electrophysiol 2000;11:1277–1280.

123. Brugada R, Brugada J, Antzelevitch C, et al. Sodium channel blockers identify risk for sudden death in patients with ST-Segment elevation and right bundle branch block but structurally normal hearts. Circulation 2000;101:510–515.

124. Priori SG, Napolitano C, Schwartz PJ, Bloise R, Crotti L, Ronchetti E. The elusive link between LQT3 and Brugada syndrome: the role of flecainide challenge. Circulation 2000;102:945–947.

125. Abernethy DR, Flockhart DA. Molecular basis of cardiovascular drug metabolism implications for predicting clinically important drug interactions. Circulation 2000;101:1749–1753.

126. Roden DM. Pharmacogenetics and drug-induced arrhythmias. Cardiovasc Res 2001;50:224–231.

127. Ingelman-Sundberg, M. Polymorphic human cytochrome P450 enzymes: an opportunity for individualized drug treatment. Trends Pharmacol Sci 1999;20:342–349.

128. Siddoway LA, Thompson KA, McAllister BC, et al. Polymorphism of propafenone metabolism and disposition in man: clinical and pharmacokinetic consequences. Circulation 1987;75:785–791.

129. Legebrve RA, Van Peer A, Woestenborghs R. Influence of itraconazole on the pharmacokinetics and electrocardiographic effect of astemizole. Br J Clin Pharmacol 1997;43:319–322.

130. Neuvonen PJ, Kantola T, Kivisto KT. Simvastatin but not pravastatin is very susceptible to interaction with the CYP3A4 inhibitor itraconazole. Clin Pharmacol Ther 1998;63:332–341.

131. Escande D. Pharmacogenetics of cardiac K$^+$ channels. Eur J Pharmacol 2000;410:281–287.

132. Napolitano C, Schwartz PJ, Brown AM, et al. Evidence for a cardiac ion channel mutation underlying drug-induced QT prolongation and life-threatening arrhythmias. J Cardiovasc Electrophysiol 2000;11:691–696.

133. Sesti F, Abbott GW, Wei J, et al. A common polymorphism associated with antibiotic-induced cardiac arrhythmia. Proc Natl Acad Sci 2000;97:10613–10618.

134. Bonnie A, Fijal MS, Hall JM, Witte JS. Clinical trials in the genomic era. Effects of protective genotypes on sample size and duration of trial 2000. Controlled Clin Trials 2000;21:7–20.

135. Roses AD. Pharmacogenetics and the practice of medicine. Nature 2000;405:857–865.

136. Bates DW, Spell N, Cullen DJ, et al. The costs of adverse drug events in hospitalized patients. J Am Med Assoc 1997;277:307–311.

137. Lazarou J, Pomeranz BH, Corey PN. Incidence of adverse drug reactions in hospitalized patients—a meta-analysis of prospective studies. J Am Med Assoc 1998;279:1200–1205.

138. Yao JA, Jiang M, Fan JS, Zhou YY, Tseng GN. Heterogeneous changes in K currents in rat ventricles three days after myocardial infarction. Cardiovasc Res 1999;44:132–145.

139. Allessie MA, Boyden PA, Camm AJ, et al. Pathophysiology and prevention of atrial fibrillation. Circulation 2001;103:769–777.

140. Yu H, Gao J, Wang H. Effects of the renin-angiotensin system on the current I_{to} in epicardial and endocardial ventricular myocytes from the canine heart Circ Res 2000;86:1062–1068.

141. Courtemanche M, Ramirez RJ, Nattel S. Ionic targets for drug therapy and atrial fibrillation-induced electrical remodeling: insights from a mathematical model. Cardiovasc Res 1999;42:477–489.

142. Van Wagoner DR, Pond AL, Lamorgese M, Rossie SS, McCarthy PM, Nerbonne JM. Atrial L-type Ca^{2+} currents and human atrial fibrillation. Circ Res 1999;85:428–436.

143. Shinagawa K, Li DS, Leung TK, Nattel S. Consequences of atrial tachycardia-induced remodeling depend on the preexisting atrial substrate. Circulation 2002;105:251–257.

144. Shimoni Y. Inhibition of the formation or action of angiotensin II reverses attenuated K^+ currents in type 1 and type 2 diabetes. J Physiol 2001;537:83–92.

145. Li DS, Shinagawa K, Pang L, et al. Effects of angiotensin-converting enzyme inhibition on the development of the atrial fibrillation substrate in dogs with ventricular tachypacing-induced congestive heart failure. Circulation 2001;104:2608–2614.

146. Pedersen OD, Bagger H, Kober L, Torp-Pedersen C. Trandolapril reducs the incidence of atrial fibrilation after myocardial infarction in patients with left ventricular dysfunction. Circulation 1999;100:376–380.

147. Pitt B, Zannad F, Remme WJ, et al. The effect of spironolactone on morbidity and mortality in patients with severe heart failure. N Engl J Med 1999;341:709–717.

148. Abrol R, Page RL. Azimilide dihydrochloride: a new class III antiarrhythmic agent. Exp Opin Investigat Drug 2000;9:2705–2715.

149. Sun W, Sarma JSM, Singh BN. Electrophysiological effects of dronedarone (SR33589), a noniodinated benzofuran derivative, in the rabbit heart—Comparison with amiodarone. Circulation 1999;100:2276–2281.

150. Pattabiraman N. Analysis of ligand-macromolecule contacts: computational methods. Curr Med Chem 2002;9:609–621.

151. Kanno S, Saffitz JE. The role of myocardial gap junctions in electrical conduction and arrhythmogenesis. Cardiovasc Pathol 2001;10:169–177.

152. Pogwizd SM, Schlotthauer K, Li L, Yuan W, Bers DM. Arrhythmogenesis and contractile dysfunction in heart failure: roles of sodium-calcium exchange, inward rectifier potassium current, and residual [beta]-adrenergic responsiveness. Circ Res 2001;88:1159–1167.

153. Adachi-Akahane S, Kurachi Y. New era for translational research in cardiac arrhythmias. Circ Res 2001;88:1095–1096.

154. Elias CL, Lukas A, Shurraw S, et al. Inhibition of Na^+/Ca^{2+} exchange by KB-R7943: transport mode selectivity and antiarrhythmic consequences. Am J Physiol 2001;281:H1334–H1345.

155. Gazmuri RJ, Ayoub IM, Hoffner E, Kolarova JD. Successful ventricular defibrillation by the selective sodium-hydrogen exchanger isoform-1 inhibitor cariporide. Circulation 2001;104:234–239.

156. Priori SG, Napolitano C, Tiso N, et al. Mutations in the cardiac ryanodine receptor gene (hRyR2) underlie catecholaminergic polymorphic ventricular tachycardia. Circulation 2001;103:196–200.

157. Dzeja PP, Holmuhamedov EL, Ozcan C, Pucar D, Jahangir A, Terzic A. Mitochondria: gateway for cytoprotection. Circ Res 2001;89:744–746.

158. Terzic A, Kurachi Y. Actin microfilament disrupters enhance K(ATP) channel opening in patches from guinea-pig cardiomyocytes. J Physiol 1996;492:395–404.

159. Dzhura I, Wu YJ, Colbran RJ, Balser JR, Anderson ME. Calmodulin kinase determines calcium dependent facilitation of L-type calcium channels. Nat Cell Biol 2000;2:173–177.

160. Anderson ME. Calmodulin and the philosopher's stone: Changing Ca^{2+} into arrhythmias. J Cardiovasc Electrophysiol 2002;13:195–197.

161. January CT, Gong QM, Zhou ZF. Long QT syndrome: Cellular basis and arrhythmia mechanism in LQT2. J Cardiovasc Electrophysiol 2000;11:1413–1418.

162. Keating MT, Sanguinetti MC. Molecular and cellular mechanisms of cardiac arrhythmias. Cell 2001;104:569–580.

PART IV

SPECIFIC ELECTROCARDIOGRAPHIC PHENOMENA AND CLINICAL SYNDROMES OF VENTRICULAR REPOLARIZATION

Edited by Ihor Gussak,
Charles Antzelevitch,
and Preben Bjerregaard

18 ECG Phenomena of the Early Ventricular Repolarization
Early Repolarization Syndrome

Ihor Gussak, MD, PhD,
Charles Antzelevitch, PhD,
and Preben Bjerregaard, MD, DMsc

CONTENTS

ECG PHENOMENA OF THE EARLY VENTRICULAR REPOLARIZATION: INTRODUCTION AND TERMINOLOGY

ECG phenomena of the early ventricular repolarization have in the past often been misdiagnosed or misinterpreted. This happened mainly because of prevailing opinion of the "benign" or "innocent" nature of the early repolarization syndrome (ERS) *(1,2)*. As an example, early repolarization changes consistent with Brugada syndrome were overlooked for decades. Clinical interest in ERS has been rekindled recently because of its similarities with the electrocardiographic manifestations of the highly arrhythmogenic Brugada syndrome and the potential for misdiagnosis *(3–8)*.

From: *Contemporary Cardiology: Cardiac Repolarization: Bridging Basic and Clinical Science*
Edited by: I. Gussak et al. © Humana Press Inc., Totowa, NJ

Table 1
Major Factors that Can Attribute to the ECG Contour Corresponding
to the Early Ventricular Repolarization

- An intrinsic configuration of the early phase of the actions potentials in different ventricular layers (endomyocardium, midmyocardium and epicardium)
- A modification of the time-course of repolarization across the ventricular wall (transventricular vector gradient)
- A temporal overlap between the end of depolarization and the beginning of repolarization

Ventricular repolarization begins when ventricular depolarization ends. In the normal heart, the evolution of depolarization into repolarization is a relatively short process, and the magnitude of the overlap between the latest depolarization and the earliest repolarization is approx 10 msec *(9)*. The duration of this time-interval is greatly influenced by any abnormal conditions that affect either propagation of the excitation wave through ventricular wall or recovery of its excitability, or both (Table 1).

In a normal ECG, the transition of depolarization into repolarization corresponds on the surface ECG to the *J point*. The J point defined as the point at which there is abrupt transition from the QRS complex to the ST-segment. Deviation of the J point from the isoelectric line leads to the presence of a *J deflection*, which is a common ECG feature of early repolarization syndrome, but also seen in acute myocardial ischemia, hypercalemia, and various intraventricular conduction disturbances. If a J deflection takes the shape of a dome or a hump, it is usually referred to as a *J wave (9)*.

However, a clear distinction between the delayed conduction and the early ventricular repolarization cannot always be made on the basis of an ECG alone. Although, the differentiation of these processes is important since an abnormal early ventricular repolarization is often accompanied by electrical instability, whereas an arrhythmogenic potential of the delayed intraventricular conduction is much more benign, especially in otherwise healthy individuals. The signal-averaged ECG could be a helpful diagnostic tool but of limited clinical value in some cases *(10)*. Nevertheless, depolarization and repolarization processes can be differentiated (to some extent) by their differences with respect to the heart rate, different drugs and neurotransmitters (*see* Chapters 4 and 6).

J WAVES

Different names have been used at different time for the J wave. They include camel hump sign, hathook junction, K wave, H wave, late delta wave, current of injury, J point wave, hypothermic wave, hypothermic hump, and Osborn wave *(9)*. J waves can be classified as:

1. Hypothermic.
2. Nonhypothermic.
3. Idiopathic.

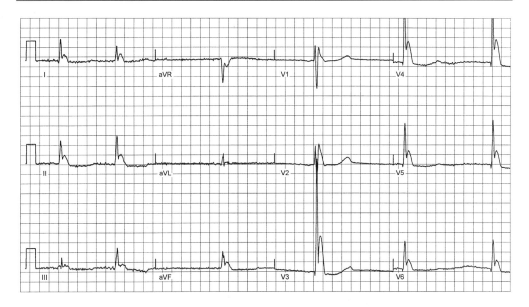

Fig. 1. Prominent J (Osborn) wave on the 12-lead ECG obtained from an accidentally frozen patient.

HYPOTHERMIC J WAVE

History and Pathophysiology

Historically, an accentuated J wave in the human ECG has been considered as a pathognomonic sign of hypothermia (Osborn wave) (Fig. 1) and most recently—its idiopathic appearance was ascribed as an ECG marker of the Brugada syndrome. The hypothermic J wave was first reported in 1938 when Tomashewski described as extra slowly inscribed deflection between the QRS complex and the earliest part of the ST-segment on the ECG obtained from an accidentally frozen man. Since 1943, the ECG changes identical to the J wave were produced in variety of experiments with a lowering of body temperature. In 1953, Osborn brought attention to the possible link between the degree of hypothermia, prominence of the J wave, which he called "current of injury" (later named Osborn wave), and ventricular fibrillation. Emslie-Smith et al. (1958) established the differences in the endocardial and epicardial responses of the ventricular myocardium to cold; J wave was found to be more prominent in epicardial than endocardial leads. West et al. (1989) found that "spike and dome" pattern in the epicardial action potential markedly accentuated under hypothermic conditions and resulting "notch" was rate-sensitive (inverse correlation) *(9)*.

These findings were confirmed later and further investigated in open-chest and arterially perfused wedge-preparation experiments.

In Open-Chest Experiments with Dogs

1. Hypothermic J wave was found to be:

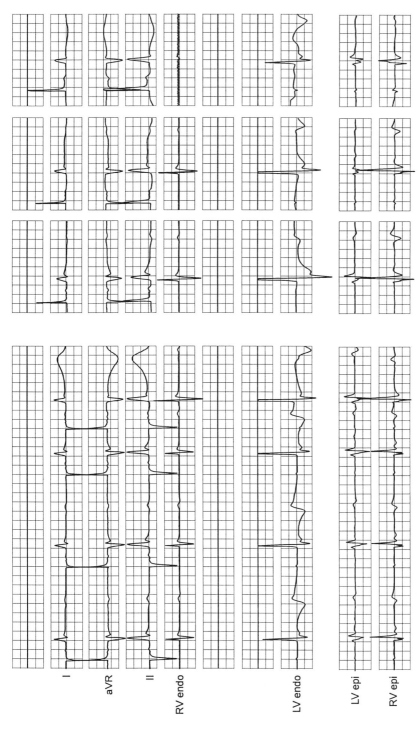

Fig. 2. The effects of the cardiocycle length, 4-aminopyridine and isoproterenol on the magnitude of the hypothermia-induced J wave. Temperature: 22.4°C. Leads I, aVR, II, RV*endo* (right ventricle endocardium), LV*endo* (left ventricle endocardium), LV*epi* (left ventricle epicardium), and RV*epi* (right ventricle epicardium). Basic cardiocycle length = 1000 ms. Left Panel (programmed atrial pacing): (**A**) Reduction in the magnitude of the J wave (best seen in leads II, I, and RV*epi*) due to abrupt shortening of the cardiocycle length to 500 msec (deceleration-dependence) and (**B**) Hypothermic J wave is more prominent in right than left ventricular epicardium, less prominent in left ventricular epicardium, and absent in endocardium in both ventricles. Right Panel (atrial pacing): At the same degree of hypothermia and heart rate, the prominence of the J wave was: (**A**) significantly reduced after administration of 4-aminopyridine (middle section) and (**B**) completely eliminated after infusion of the isoproterenol (right section). Left section—baseline (temperature—22.4°C, cardiocycle length—1000 ms).

410

   a. More prominent in right than left ventricular epicardium.
   b. Less prominent in left ventricular epicardium.
   c. Absent in endocardium in both ventricles (Fig. 2).
2. Abrupt shortening of the cardiocycle length by programmed electrical stimulation revealed definite deceleration-dependent behavior (Fig. 2, left panel).
3. At the same degree of hypothermia and heart rate, the prominence of the J waves were significantly reduced after administration of 4-aminopyridine (4-AP) and J waves were completely eliminated after infusion of the isoproterenol (Fig. 2, right panel).

These findings provided an evidence that appearance of the J wave on a surface ECG during hypothermia is modulated by changes of the early ventricular repolarization in epicardial tissue and involved primarily 4-AP sensitive transient outward current (I_{to}) and possibly inward calcium current. The possible similarities in the pathophysiologic mechanisms between hypothermic J wave and ECG marker of Brugada syndrome have been pointed out (11).

Studies Involving the Arterially Perfused Ventricular Wedge Preparation

Provided direct evidence in support of the hypothesis that accentuation of the action potential notch leading to loss or depression of the action potential dome in epicardium but not endocardium underlie the development of prominent J waves and ST segment elevation in hypothermia as well as in Brugada syndrome.

As discussed in more detail below and in Chapters 8 and 11, the presence of a prominent action potential notch in ventricular epicardium, but not endocardium, creates a transmural voltage gradient responsible for the inscription of the J deflections and J waves. Accentuation of the epicardial action potential notch secondary to a rebalancing of the currents that contribute to the early phases of the action potential gives rise to abnormally large J waves in the wedge preparation. A further shift in the balance of currents leads to either depression or loss of the action potential dome at the end of phase 1 of the epicardial action potential. Depression of the dome gives rise to J point and ST segment elevation consistent with that observed in clinical cases of early repolarization syndrome, whereas loss of the action potential dome gives rise to either a coved ST segment elevation consistent with that observed in patients with the Brugada syndrome (12,13–17).

ARRHYTHMOGENIC POTENTIAL

Clinical as well as experimental data linking hypothermic J waves and cardiac arrhythmias remain sparse and somewhat contradictory; the occurrence of ventricular tachyarrhythmias associated with hypothermic J wave varies from none to almost 100% (9). Noteworthy, sodium channel blockers, such as procainamide and lidocaine, are proarrhythmogenic rather than effective in both prevention and treatment of the malignant ventricular tachyarrhythmias in hypothermic patients during their rewarming.

Nonhypothermic J Waves

ECG changes resembling those in hypothermia-induced J waves have been observed in various clinical and experimental settings with normal body temperature, such as myocardial ischemia, acute pulmonary thromboembolism or right ventricular infarction, electrolyte or metabolic disorders, pulmonary or inflammatory diseases or abnormalities of central or peripheral nervous system, intoxication by heterocyclic antidepressant or

Table 2
Abnormalities that Can Lead to ST Segment Elevation in the Right Precordial Leads

In the Clinic:
  Right or left bundle branch block, left ventricular hypertrophy
  Acute myocardial infarction
  Left ventricular aneurysm
  Exercise test—induced
  Acute myocarditis
  Right ventricular infarction
  Dissecting aortic aneurysm
  Acute pulmonary thromboemboli
  Various central and autonomic nervous system abnormalities
  Heterocyclic antidepressant overdose
  Duchenne muscular dystrophy
  Frederic's s ataxia
  Thiamine deficiency
  Hypercalcemia
  Hyperkalemia
  Compression of the right ventricular outflow tract by metastatic tumor
  Cocaine intoxication

In Experimental Models:
  Isolated sheets of canine ventricular epicardium exposed to potassium channel openers, sodium
      and calcium channel blockers, acetylcholine, metabolic inhibition, and ischemia
  Injection of potassium salts into blood perfusing the coronary arteries or into subepicardium
  Potassium chloride application on the pericardial surface
  Right ventricular infarction

cocaine (Table 2). Among those clinical situations, prominent J waves most frequently are observed in acute myocardial ischemia (Fig. 3) and hyperkalemia (Fig. 4).

A link between the nonhypothermic J waves and electrical instability has not been established yet. It is the prevailing opinion that in most clinical settings associated with this ECG phenomenon, the propensity to malignant ventricular arrhythmias is chiefly dependent upon the underlying disease.

Idiopathic J Waves

In the absence of any structural cardiac abnormalities or extracardiac diseases, changes of early ventricular repolarization can be classified as primary or *idiopathic*. The J waves have been described in the ECG of many species, including men, under normal and abnormal conditions.

IN ANIMALS

Both the shape and the duration of ventricular repolarization in small rodents, including rats and mice (but not guinea pigs), are very striking *(18)*. The characteristic features in ECG recordings from these rodents, are consistent with:
  1. Absence of a distinct isoelectric interval between the QRS complex and the T wave.
  2. Short QT interval.

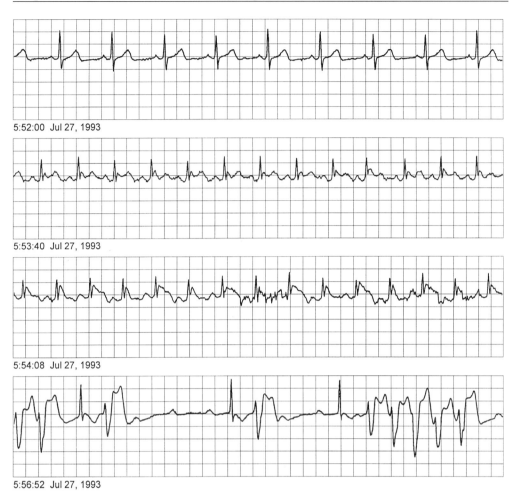

5:52:00 Jul 27, 1993

5:53:40 Jul 27, 1993

5:54:08 Jul 27, 1993

5:56:52 Jul 27, 1993

Fig. 3. Appearance of the J-wave, ST-T segment and QT interval alternans, and development of the complete atrioventricular block and ectopic ventricular activity in patient with a documented coronary artery spasm (Holter monitoring).

HISTORY AND TERMINOLOGY

Confusion and inconsistency have surrounded the ECG interpretation of such unusual manifestation of the ventricular repolarization in small mammals since 1929, when the first murine ECG was recorded. Agduhr and Stenström reported that they were unable to find "discernible T waves" in ECG recordings from mice obtained using a string galvanometer. Although O'Bryant and colleagues identified R and T waves in mice 20 yr later, a report by Lombard in 1952 described the putative "R and T waves" as a "notch at the end of the QRS complex," and again suggested that T waves are absent in mice. Similarly, Richards and coworkers reported in 1953 that a distinct T wave could not be detected in murine ECGs, whereas the T wave was clearly visible in ECGs from guinea pigs. They also mentioned that the "notch" between the two peaks of the QRS complex was deepened and the amplitudes of the separated waves were increased in ECG recordings from hypothermic mice. Subsequently, Goldbarg and colleagues suggested that this reflected

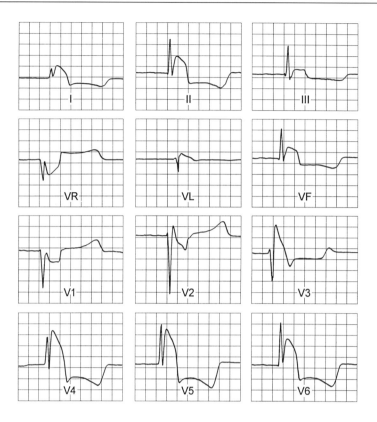

Fig. 4. Prominent J wave in the patients with a severe hyperkalemia.

"erroneously ascribed T wave." This recurring confusion led subsequent investigators to use such terms as "no measurable ST segment," "merging QRS with the T wave," or "lack of distinct ST segment" to describe the presence of a distinct J wave *(18)*.

Although, the unique features of these rodent ECGs, particularly the prominent J wave, are not typically seen in larger animals (except a kangaroo) or in humans, they do bear some resemblance to ECG abnormalities seen in patients with Brugada syndrome and in several pathophysiologic conditions, including hypothermia and ischemia *(18)*.

Considerable experimental evidence suggests the murine ECG morphology is apparently attributable to the presence of large-amplitude repolarizing K^+ currents, specifically the transient outward K^+ current, I_{to} that dominate the early phase of ventricular repolarization. In rats and mice, the predominant current underlying the early phase of repolarization appears to be the rapidly activating and inactivating 4-aminopyridine-sensitive transient outward current (i.e., I_{to}). Importantly, the density of I_{to} in rats and mice is high, whereas this current is not evident in the ventricular myocytes of guinea pigs. The high density of I_{to} appears to underlie the prominent J wave seen in rats and mice, whereas the ST segment is isoelectric in guinea pigs *(see* Chapter 3).

These observations suggest that:

1. Alterations in the contribution of I_{to} to ventricular repolarization may be an important factor in the ECG abnormalities seen in humans under certain pathophysiological conditions.
2. The prominent J waves in murine ECGs might therefore serve as an experimental model for idiopathic J wave *(18)*.

IN HUMAN

Several forms of idiopathic appearances of a J wave with or without accompanying ST segment elevation have been described. Idiopathic J wave followed by downsloping ST segment elevation with inverted T wave in the right chest leads is an ECG hallmark of the *Brugada syndrome* (*see* Chapter 19). Clinically noteworthy, J wave-like ECG abnormalities have been recently described as case reports in otherwise healthy individuals prone to paroxysmal ventricular tachycardia/fibrillation:

1. Aizawa and his colleagues *(19)* described several patients with idiopathic ventricular fibrillation in whom they found bradycardia-dependent intraventricular block (Fig. 5). The common ECG features of these patients included:
   a. Incomplete right bundle branch block.
   b. Prominent "notch" on downsloping limb of the QRS complex in leads V_3–V_5, II, III, and aVF.
   c. Elevated ST segment with positive T waves leads V_2–V_3.
   d. Rate (deceleration)—dependent accentuation of the prominence of the "notch."
2. Garg and his associates *(20)* reported a case of "familial sudden cardiac death associated with a terminal QRS abnormality on surface 12-lead electrocardiogram" (Fig. 6A). The abnormal low-amplitude deflections in the downsloping limp of the QRS complex (J wave) in leads II, III, aVF and I, aVL and V6 were coincident with the late potential on the signal-averaged ECG (Fig. 6B). Noteworthy:
   a. Both surface ECG and signal-averaged ECG were normalized by quinidine but not by procainamide or beta-blockers (Fig. 6C).
   b. J wave appeared to be more prominent after procainamide compared to baseline (Fig. 6D).
   c. Sustained polymorphic ventricular tachycardia, which degenerated to ventricular fibrillation was easily inducible during programmed stimulation from the right ventricular apex, despite administration of procainamide or atenolol.

The clinical significance of these ECG findings is not fully understood at present and further investigations are warranted.

EARLY REPOLARIZATION SYNDROME: INTRODUCTION AND TERMINOLOGY

Early repolarization (ERS) is an ECG diagnosis that is commonly regarded so far as a benign abnormality. The prevalence of ERS varies between 1% *(21)* and 2% *(22)*. It is more commonly seen in young individuals (27.5%) *(23)*, especially those predisposed to vagotonia, and shows a male preponderance (77%) *(21)*. The syndrome is also often observed in:

1. Athletes *(24)*.
2. Cocaine users *(25)*.

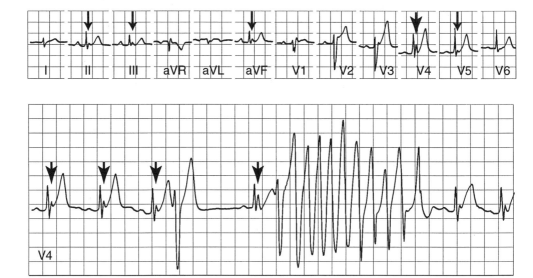

Fig. 5. Twelve-lead ECG of a patient with idiopathic ventricular fibrillation. Upper Panel: Note: **(A)** incomplete right bundle branch block, **(B)** elevated ST segment in leads V_2–V_3, and **(C)** prominent "notch" on downsloping limb of the QRS complex in leads V_3–V_5 and inferior leads. Lower Panel: rate (deceleration)—dependent accentuation of the prominence of the "notch" is followed by a short episode of nonsustained ventricular tachycardia. Adapted from *19*, with permission.

3. Obstructive hypertrophic cardiomyopathy *(26)*.
4. Defects and/or hypertrophy of the interventricular septum *(26)*.

The electrocardiographic signature of ERS is often dependent on heart rate, normalizing during exercise or with rapid pacing, as well as with advancing age *(27)*. Familial occurrence of the syndrome has been suggested *(28,29)*. Although early studies were interpreted to suggest that the syndrome is more prevalent in the Black population, more-recent studies challenge this notion *(21,30)*.

Thus far, its clinical significance has been largely limited to its contribution to the differential diagnosis of acute myocardial infarction *(31)*, pericarditis *(32,33)*, intraventricular conduction defects *(34)*, and electrical alternans *(26)*.

The term, early repolarizations syndrome, was introduced nearly half a century ago and has traditionally been regarded as idiopathic, benign or innocent *(1)* or misleading *(2)* ECG pattern of ventricular repolarization. The ERS has been ascribed a number of names, including early repolarization, early ventricular repolarization, benign early repolarization, benign J wave, aspecific changes of ventricular repolarization, repolarization variant, normal variant RS-T segment elevation, and juvenile or unconventional ST-T pattern, etc. to describe the characteristic ECG pattern of J deflection followed by horizontal ST-T segment elevation *(16)*.

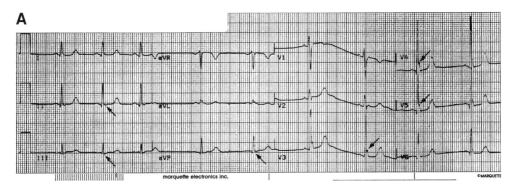

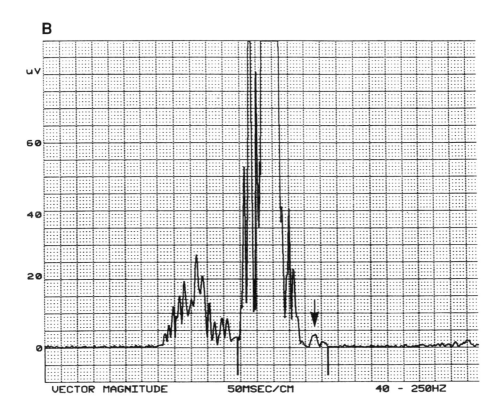

Fig. 6. 12-lead ECG and the signal-averaged ECG from a patient with familial sudden cardiac death (Courtesy by Dr. Gregory K. Feld). **(A)** The abnormal low-amplitude deflections in the downsloping limp of the QRS complex (J wave) in leads II, III, aVF and I, aVL and V6. **(B)** Late potential on the baseline signal-averaged ECG coincident with the abnormal low-amplitude deflections in the downsloping limp of the QRS complex on the 12-lead ECG. **(C)** Both surface ECG (left) and signal-averaged ECG (right) were normalized by quinidine. **(D)** J wave appeared to be more prominent after procainamide compared to baseline.

C

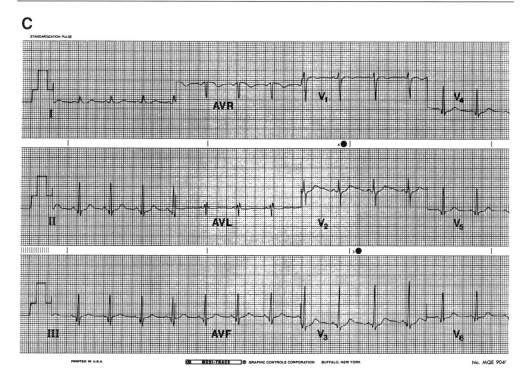

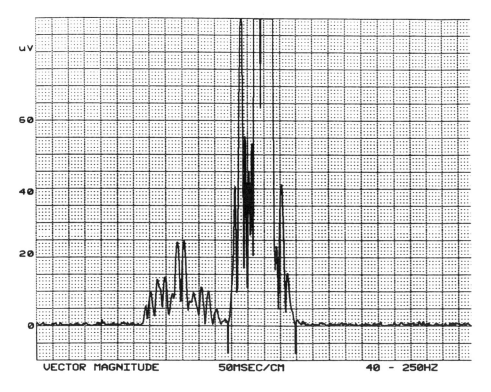

Fig. 6. *(Continued)*

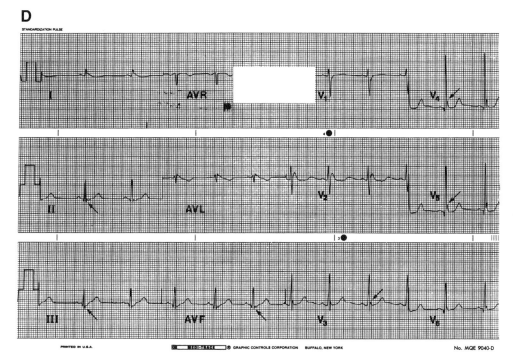

Fig. 6. *(Continued)*

ELECTROCARDIOGRAPHIC FEATURES

The classical ECG pattern of ERS consists of:

1. Prominent *notch* or slur on the downslopping portion of the QRS complex, followed by,
2. *J deflection*, followed by,
3. Diffuse upward *ST segment* concavity concordant with the QRS,
4. Positive T wave in the same lead.

Additional electrocardiographic feature that defines this ECG phenomenon include:

1. Localization of the ECG pattern of ERS in scalar ECG. Mid-to-lateral precordial leads V_2–V_4 *(5)* have been recognized as showing the most prominent repolarization changes consistent with ERS. Noteworthy, similar changes might appear in other leads but to a lesser extent (Fig. 7).
2. Reciprocal ST segment depression in aVR.
3. Waxing and waning of the ST-T segment over time.

Nevertheless, in some clinical instances, it is still difficult to distinguish subjects with ERS from those with the Brugada syndrome or various intraventricular conduction blocks, based solely on a resting ECG *(10,16,35)*. Moreover, the ECG alterations in response to changes in heart rate, drug effects and autonomic tone observed in ERS are similar to those observed under hypothermic conditions and the Brugada syndrome.

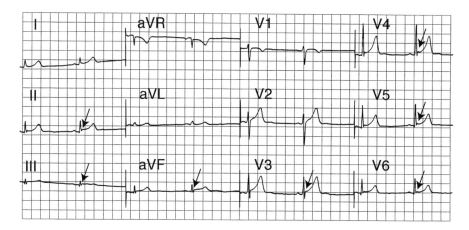

Fig. 7. 12-lead ECG in apparently healthy individual with an early repolarization syndrome. Note: An elevated "notch" is apparent on the downsloping limb of the QRS complex and is followed by an upsloping ST-segment elevation that is most prominent in leads V_3–V_6. These changes are also seen in the inferior leads, but to a lesser extent. Reciprocal ST segment depression in aVR are also evident

POSSIBLE CELLULAR AND IONIC MECHANISMS

Concordant with the QRS complex, ST segment elevation is most commonly recognized as a sign of acute myocardial damage, often associated with the development of cardiac arrhythmias. The electrophysiological nature of the ST-segment elevation in ERS, whether idiopathic or owing to so-called current of injury, has been investigated by means of a direct-current magnetocardiogram, which, in contrast to conventional 12-lead ECG, is capable of determining TQ interval shifts. The results showed clearly that ST shifts in subjects with ERS are unrelated to ischemic injury *(36)*. However, the cellular and ionic mechanisms that determine the ECG contour in the ERS are not well defined and are suggestive rather than conclusive *(16)*.

The appearance of a prominent I_{to}-mediated action potential notch in epicardium but not endocardium leads to the development of a transmural voltage gradient during ventricular activation that manifests on the ECG as prominent J deflection or J wave. Under the conditions, when an outward shift of the currents active at the end of phase 1 can dramatically augment the action potential notch in ventricular epicardium and thus increase the magnitude of the J wave. A further outward shift of the currents active at the end of phase 1 of the action potential can cause additionally the depression of the plateau of the AP that was thought to be corresponding to the elevation of the ST segment on ECG. Regions where the I_{to}-mediated notch is relatively small (e.g., left ventricle) are more likely to manifest as a depression of the epicardial action potential plateau in response to an outward shift of net plateau current. In contrast, regions displaying a prominent I_{to} are more likely to lose the dome under these conditions. This observation may account for why ERS also manifests in the inferior and left precordial ECG leads, where the I_{to} is generally less intense. Because ST segment elevation in ERS is apparent in mid-to-left precordial leads, the ECG morphology is likely to involve widespread augmentation of net repolarizing forces within right and left ventricular epicardium, particularly near the apical region of the heart.

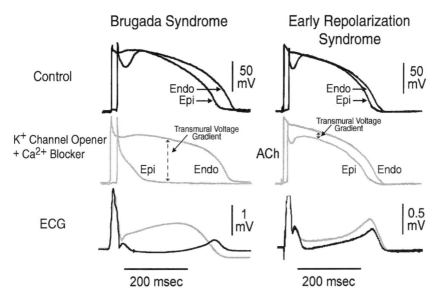

Fig. 8. Electrocardiographic phenotype of the Brugada and Early Repolarization Syndromes (Proposed mechanisms). Transmembrane action potentials from epicardium (Epi) and endocardium (Endo) and an ECG were simultaneously recorded from two different canine arterially perfused right ventricular wedge preparation. Left Panel: Brugada Syndrome. Combined K+ channel opener and calcium channel blocker cause loss of the action potential, leading to the development of a large transmural voltage gradient, which is responsible for the marked ST segment elevation. A marked transmural dispersion of repolarization gives rise to a large vulnerable window for the precipitation of reentry. Because not all epicardial sites display a loss of the action potential dome, a transepicardial dispersion of repolarization develops as well. Right Panel: Early Repolarization syndrome. Acetylcholine (Ach, 3 μ*M*)- depresses of the epicardial action potential plateau, thus leading to the development of a transmural voltage gradient, responsible for a relatively smaller ST segment elevation. This mechanism does not create an arrhythmogenic substrate; neither transmural nor transepicardial dispersion of repolarization develop under these conditions.

Thus, transmural and interventricular differences in the density of I_{to} are thought to contribute to the manifestation of the electrocardiographic J wave, to the differential response of epicardium and endocardium to a variety of drugs and pathophysiologic states, and to the development of an elevation of the J point (J deflection) and ST segment in the ERS, as well as in Brugada syndrome.

The elevated J point and ST segment observed in subjects with the ERS may be owing to mechanisms similar to those described for the Brugada syndrome. Although the ST segment elevation in the Brugada syndrome may be secondary to loss of the action potential dome in epicardium but not endocardium, that attending ERS is more likely to be because of depression rather than loss of the epicardial action potential plateau, as illustrated in Fig. 8 *(16)*. The principal difference between the two mechanisms is that loss of the action potential dome is accompanied by the development of a very significant transmural as well as epicardial dispersion of repolarization and refractoriness, setting the stage for both phase 2 and circus movement reentry, whereas mere depression of the epicardial action potential dome is not. Therein, lies a possible explanation for why the Brugada syndrome is highly arrhythmogenic whereas ERS is not.

Table 3
Autonomic and Pharmacologic Modulation of the J Wave Magnitude Under Hypothermic
Conditions, in the Early Repolarization (ERS) and Brugada Syndromes (BS)

	Sodium blockers	Isoproterenol	β-blockers	Exercise	Nitroglycerine
Hypothermic J Wave	↑	↓	↑	↓	not determined
ERS	↑	↓	↑	↓	no effect
BS	↑	↓	↑	↓	no effect

ECG MARKERS OF EARLY REPOLARIZATION SYNDROME AND BRUGADA SYNDROMES: SIMILARITIES AND DIFFERENCES

Like the Brugada syndrome,

1. ERS has been identified predominantly in young otherwise healthy males.
2. ERS is characterized by predisposition to familial occurrence.
3. The ECG manifestation of ERS shows transient normalization in many individuals.
4. ERS shows a similar response to drugs and autonomic modulation (Table 3).

Two major features permit differentiation of the ECG signatures of ERS and the Brugada syndrome:

1. Pattern.
2. Leads specificity.

The elevated ST segment in ERS is usually localized in leads V_2–V_4 (or 5) and has an upward concavity with positive T wave polarity accompanied by a notched J point. In contrast, the ECG of Brugada patients generally displays a prominent J point elevation, followed by a downslopping ST segments and negative T wave in the right precordial leads (V_1–V_3) only.

It is sometimes difficult to distinguish subjects with ERS from those with the Brugada syndrome, especially when the latter also display intraventricular conduction slowing or block. The dynamicity of ECG changes in both syndromes is also confounding. When the clinical history is malignant, an invasive electrophysiological study examining the inducibility of ventricular tachycardia/fibrillation may be useful in assessing arrhythmogenic risk.

Interestingly enough, ECG changes consistent with the Brugada syndrome have also been referred to as a benign repolarization variant or Ideiken phenomenon for more than three decades and some patients having such ECG abnormalities have been described as unwitting victims of electrocardiography (16).

MODULATION BY DRUGS, RATE, AND NEUROTRANSMITTERS

The changes in the magnitude of the early repolarization abnormalities in ERS and Brugada syndrome, like a hypothermic J wave, display qualitatively similar responses to a variety of drugs as well as to changes in rate and autonomic tone (Table 3) (16):

1. *Slowing of heart rate* exaggerates J waves and ST segment.
2. *Increase in heart rate* elevation during *exercise* or following *isoproterenol* reduces or even eliminates these ECG abnormalities.
3. *Sodium channel blockers* (known to unmask the Brugada syndrome) increase ST segment elevation in ERS subjects and hypothermic J waves.
4. *Sympathetic stimulation* and *β-adrenergic agonists* normalize the ST segment in both syndromes, whereas *β-adrenergic blockers* augment ST segment elevation in both, *propranolol* increases its magnitude and its toxicity may even induce classical pattern of ERS.

THE ROLE OF NERVOUS SYSTEM

Clinical and experimental studies point to high spinal cord injury as a cause of ERS-like changes in the ECG. High cervical spinal chord injury can lead to significant deterioration or even complete disruption of the cardiac sympathetic activity, leaving parasympathetic activity unopposed *(37)*. Parasympathetic activation has an opposite effect in both syndromes, causing ST segment elevation because of depression or loss of the action potential plateau (see below). ECG patterns wax and wane in both syndromes, possibly owing to variations of autonomic activity *(16)*.

ARRHYTHMOGENIC POTENTIAL

ERS is not malignant *per se*. However, the similarities between the Brugada syndrome and ERS in response to rate, neuromodulation, and pharmacologic agents suggest a parallelism of mechanisms. Recent experimental studies also suggest a cellular basis for the electrocardiographic signature of ERS. The hypothesis presumes that depression of the epicardial, but not endocardial, action potential plateau creates a transmural gradient that manifests on the scalar ECG as a complex ST segment elevation with a positive T wave. As such the cellular substrate is not arrhythmogenic, but in case of further increase in net repolarizing current as a result of complete loss of the epicardial action potential dome and the attendant development of a large transmural dispersion of repolarization could become arrhythmogenic. These proposed mechanisms also explain the highly arrhythmogenic character of the Brugada syndrome and apparently benign exceptions.

Although ERS has long been considered to be benign, it is noteworthy that in experimental models, the ECG signature of ERS can be *converted* to that of the Brugada syndrome *(13,14,16)*. This raises the possibility that ERS may not be as benign as generally believed, and that under certain conditions known to cause predisposition to ST-segment elevation, ERS subjects may be at increased risk. In considering these possibilities, it is instructive to remember that the Brugada syndrome was considered benign for more than three decades, and that one syndrome can be readily converted to the other in experimental models involving the wedge preparation.

It is important to emphasize that these hypotheses remain to be more rigorously tested and that the distinct nosologic entity that is referred to as the early repolarization syndrome needs to be more fully delineated within the framework of what we have learned about the Brugada syndrome in recent years. A careful clinical history and invasive electrophysiological studies may be required to determine whether or not the early ventricular repolarization abnormalities in a given patient are benign or malignant.

SUMMARY AND CONCLUSIONS

The available clinical data suggest that the different ECG phenomena of the early ventricular repolarization syndromes often share similar mechanisms with wide range of their arrhythmogenic potentials. Although, the ECG similarities between these phenomena raises some concerns for their misdiagnosis. Therefore:

1. ERS should be regarded as benign until otherwise proven.
2. ECG as a diagnostic tool to identify patients at risk is often of limited value. Detailed medical history and further diagnostic work-up, including the signal-averaged ECG, drug testing, and invasive electrophysiologic studies may be required for further risk stratification.
3. There could be a potential risk that ERS subjects could be more easily predisposed to the drug-induced ventricular arrhythmias.

REFERENCES

1. Martinez-Lopez JI. ECG of the month. Innocent abnormality. Early repolarization pattern. J La State Med Soc 1991:143(11);7,9.
2. Netter FH. Misleading electrocardiographic findings. In: Heart. The CIBA collection of medical illustrations. V. 5., Section II - Plate 32. Yonkman FF, ed. Ciba Pharmaceutical Company, USA, 1987.
3. Martini B, Nava A, Thiene G, Buja GF, Canciani B, Scognamiglio R, Daliento L, Dalla Volta S. Ventricular fibrillation without apparent heart disease. Description of six cases. Am Heart J 1989;118:1203.
4. Fontaine G, Aouate P, Fontaliran F. Arrhythmogenic right ventricular dysplasia, torsades de pointes and sudden death. New concepts. Ann Cardiol Angeiol (Paris). 1997;46(8):531.
5. Sgarbossa EB, Wagner G. Electrocardiography. In: Textbook of Cardiovascular Medicine. Topol EJ, Califf RM, eds. Philadelphia, PA: Lippincott-Raven Publishers, 1998;1545.
6. Brugada P, Brugada J, Brugada R. Brugada syndrome: relation with "early repolarization." Available at: http://www.brugada.crtia.be/. Accessed October 21, 1999.
7. Gussak I, Bjerregaard P, Antzelevitch C, Towbin J, Chaitman BR. The Brugada syndrome: clinical, electrophysiological and genetic aspects. J Am Coll Cardiol 1999;3(1):5.
8. Antzelevitch C, Brugada P, Brugada J, Brugada P, Nademanee K, Towbin JA. The Brugada Syndrome. Armonk, NY: Futura Publishing Co., 1999.
9. Gussak I, Bjerregaard P, Egan TM, Chaitman BR. ECG phenomenon called J wave. J Electrocardiol 1995;28(1):49–58.
10. Gussak I, Bjerregaard P, Hammill SC. Clinical Diagnosis and Risk Stratification in Patients with Brugada Syndrome. Editorial Comments. J Am Coll Cardiol 2001;37(6):1635–1638.
11. Gussak I, Bjerregaard P, Greenwalt T, Chaitman BR. Electrophysiological peculiarities of the ECG J wave: from hypothermia to Brugada syndrome. In: Electrocardiology 96: From the Cell to the Body Surface. J. Liebman, ed. Singapore, World Scientific Co. Pte. Ltd., 1997;261–264.
12. Yan GX, Antzelevitch C. Cellular basis for the electrocardiographic J wave. Circulation 1996;93: 372–379.
13. Yan GX, Antzelevitch C. Cellular basis for the Brugada Syndrome and other mechanisms of arrhythmogenesis associated with ST segment elevation. Circulation 1999;100:1660–1666.
14. Antzelevitch C, Dumaine R. Electrical heterogeneity in the heart: Physiological, pharmacological and clinical implications. In: Page E, Fozzard HA, Solaro RJ, eds. Handbook of Physiology. The Heart. New York: Oxford University Press, 2002:654–692.
15. Antzelevitch C. The Brugada syndrome: Ionic basis and arrhythmia mechanisms. J Cardiovasc Electrophysiol 2001;12:268–272.
16. Gussak I, Antzelevitch C. Early repolarization syndrome: Clinical characteristics and possible cellular and ionic mechanisms. J Electrocardiol 2000;33(4):299–309.
17. Naccarelli GV, Antzelevitch C, Wolbrette DL, Luck JC. The Brugada syndrome. Curr Opin Cardiol 2002;17(1):19–23

18. Gussak I, Chaitman BR, Kopecky SL, Nerbonne JM. Rapid ventricular repolarization in rodents: electrocardiographic manifestations, molecular mechanisms, and clinical insights. J Electrocardiol 2000;33(2):159–170.
19. Aizawa Y, Tamura M, Chinushi M, et al. Idiopathic ventricular fibrillation and bradycardia-dependent intraventricular block. Am Heart J 1993;126(6):1473.
20. Garg A, Finneran W, Feld GK. Familial sudden cardiac death associated with a terminal QRS abnormality on surface 12-lead electrocardiogram in the index case. J Cardiovasc Electrophysiol 1998;9(6): 642–647.
21. Mehta MC, Jain AC. Early repolarization on scalar electrocardiogram. Am J Med Sci 1995;309:305.
22. Mehta M, Jain AC, Mehta A. Early repolarization. Clin Cardiol 1999;22:59.
23. Lazzoli JK, Annarumma M de O, de Araujo CG. Criteria for electrocardiographic diagnosis of vagotonia. Is there a consensus in the opinion of specialists? Arq Bras Cardiol 1994;63(5):377.
24. Bjørnstad H, Storstein L, Meen HD, Hals O. Electrocardiographic findings according to level of fitness and sport activity. Cardiology 1993;83:268.
25. Hollander JE, Lozano M, Fairweather P, et al. "Abnormal" electrocardiograms in patients with cocaine-associated chest pain are due to "normal" variants. J Emerg Med 1994;12(2):199.
26. Vorob'ev LP, Gribkova IN, Petrusenko NM, Trofimenko NB. The clinico-electrocardiographic classification of the early ventricular repolarization syndrome. Ter Arkh 1992;64(3):93.
27. Huston TP, Puffer JC, Rodney WM. The athletic heart syndrome. N Engl J Med 1985;313:24.
28. Gritsenko ET. Several aspects of early ventricular repolarization syndrome. Kardiologiia 1990;30(6):81.
29. Beliaeva LM, Rostovtsev VN, Novik II. The role of genetic factors in determining the ECG indicators. Kardiologiia 1991;31(3):54.
30. Vitelli LL, Crow RS, Shahar E, Hutchinson RG, Rautaharju PM, Folsom AR. Electrocardiographic findings in a healthy biracial population. Atherosclerosis Risk in Communities (ARIC) Study Investigators. Am J Cardiol 1998;81(4):453.
31. Eastaugh JA. The early repolarization syndrome. J Emerg Med 1989;7(3):257–262.
32. Wanner WR, Schaal SF, Bashore TM, Norton VJ, Lewis RP, Fulkerson PK. Repolarization variant vs acute pericarditis. A prospective electrocardiographic and echocardiographic evaluation. Chest 1983;83(2):180.
33. Saviolo R, Spodick DH. Electrocardiographic responses to maximal exercise during acute pericarditis and early repolarization. Chest 1986;90(3):460.
34. Kambara H, Phillips J. Long-term evaluation of early repolarization syndrome (normal variant RS-T segment elevation). Am J Cardiol 1976;38(2):157.
35. Bjerregaard P, Gussak I, Antzelevitch C. The enigmatic ECG manifestation of the Brugada Syndrome. J Cardiovasc Electrophysiol 1998;9:109–111.
36. Mirvis DM. Evaluation of normal variations in ST segment pattern by body surface mapping: ST segment elevation in absence of heart disease. Am J Cardiol 1982;50:122.
37. Lehman KG, Shandling AH, Yusi AU, Froulicher VF. Altered ventricular repolarization in central sympathetic dysfunction associated with spinal cord injury. Am J Cardiol 1989;63:1498.

19   The Brugada Syndrome

Pedro Brugada, MD, PhD, Ramon Brugada, MD,
Charles Antzelevitch, PhD,
Koonlawee Nademanee, MD,
Jeffrey Towbin, MD, PhD,
and Josep Brugada, MD, PhD

CONTENTS

INTRODUCTION

In 1992 a syndrome consisting of syncope episodes and/or sudden death in patients with a structurally normal heart and a characteristic electrocardiogram (ECG) displaying a pattern resembling right bundle branch block with ST segment elevation in leads V1 to V3 was described. The disease is genetically determined with an autosomal dominant pattern of transmission in 50% of the familial cases. Several different mutations have been identified affecting the structure and the function of the sodium channel gene SCN5A. These mutations result in loss of function of the sodium channel. The syndrome appears ubiquitous. The incidence of the disease is difficult to estimate worldwide, but

From: *Contemporary Cardiology: Cardiac Repolarization: Bridging Basic and Clinical Science*
Edited by: I. Gussak et al. © Humana Press Inc., Totowa, NJ

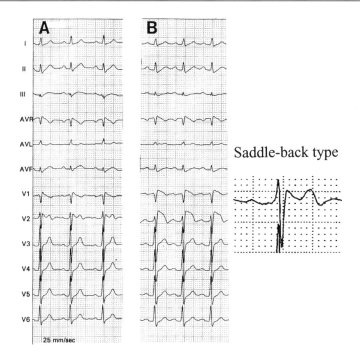

Saddle-back type

Fig. 1. Typical ECG of the syndrome. In panel B the "coved" type is shown. Please note the pattern resembling a right bundle branch block in lead V1 and the ST segment elevation in leads V1 to V3. There is also slight prolongation of the P-R interval. Paper speed 25 mm/s. (**A**) shows the "saddle-back" type. This last should not be considered diagnostic unless changed to a "coved" type by the administration of a class I drug.

it may cause 4 to 10 sudden deaths per 10,000 inhabitants per year in areas like Thailand and Laos. In these countries, the disease represents the most frequent cause of natural death in young adults. It is estimated that 20 to 50% of sudden deaths in patients with a normal heart result from this syndrome. The disease has been linked to the sudden infant death syndrome and to the sudden unexpected death syndrome by showing that the electrocardiogram and mutations are the same as in Brugada syndrome. The diagnosis is easily made by means of the ECG when it is typical. There exist, however, patients with conccalcd and intermittent electrocardiographic forms that make the diagnosis difficult. The ECG can be modulated by changes in autonomic balance, body temperature, glucose level, and the administration of drugs like antiarrhythmics, but also neuroleptic and antimalaria drugs. Beta adrenergic stimulation normalizes the ECG, whereas intravenous ajmaline, flecainide or procainamide accentuate the ST segment elevation and are capable of unmasking concealed and intermittent forms of the disease. Loss of the action potential dome in right ventricular epicardium but not in endocardium underlies the ST segment elevation. Electrical heterogeneity within right ventricular epicardium leads to the development of closely coupled extrasystoles via phase 2 reentry that precipitate ventricular fibrillation. Implantation of an automatic cardioverter-defibrillator is the only currently proven effective therapy. Patients with frequent electrical storms may require cardiac transplantation.

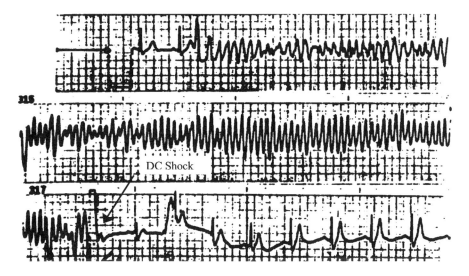

Fig. 2. Polymorphic ventricular arrhythmias documented during electrocardiographic monitoring. The arrhythmia was sustained and required external DC shock to be terminated.

DEFINITION

The syndrome of right bundle branch block, ST segment elevation in V1 to V3, and sudden death is a clinical-electrocardiographic diagnosis combining syncopal or sudden death episodes in patients with a structurally normal heart with a characteristic electrocardiographic pattern *(1)*: The electrocardiogram (ECG) shows ST segment elevation in the precordial leads V1 to V3, with a morphology of the QRS complex resembling a right bundle branch block (Fig. 1B). This pattern of right bundle branch block has also been called J point elevation *(2–3)*. Some patients do not present right bundle branch block at all. There is no prolongation of the QT interval during sinus rhythm in the typical cases. It is not infrequent to observe elevation of the ST segment in lead aVL. There are variants of the syndrome with ST segment elevation in the inferior leads. When ST elevation is the most prominent feature the pattern is called "coved-type" (Fig. 1B). When the most prominent feature is J point elevation without ST elevation the pattern is called "saddle-type" (Fig. 1A). It is important to exclude other causes of ST segment elevation before making the diagnosis of Brugada syndrome. These other causes include ischemia, mediastinal tumors, hypothermia, and right ventricular disease. Brugada syndrome and right ventricular dysplasia appear not to be related genetically (see below). Most publications suggesting right ventricular dysplasia as a cause of Brugada syndrome have reported only nonspecific findings.

The episodes of syncope and sudden death (aborted or not) are caused by fast polymorphic ventricular tachycardias (VT) or ventricular fibrillation (VF) (Fig. 2). These arrhythmias appear with no warning. Only in very few cases is there alternation of long-short sequences before the onset of polymorphic VT, a finding common in other arrhythmias, like "torsade de pointes" in the long QT syndrome *(4)*. There is no preceding acceleration of the heart rate as is the case of cathecolamine-dependent polymorphic VT *(5)*, an arrhythmia caused by mutations in the ryanodine receptor.

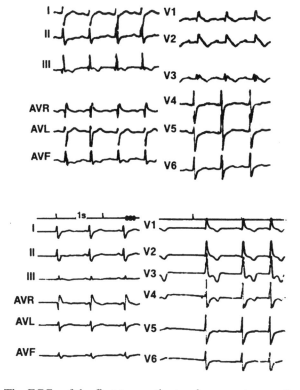

Fig. 3. The ECGs of the first two patients who came to our attention.

HISTORY

We saw the first patient with this syndrome in 1986. The patient was a three-year-old Polish boy. He had presented multiple episodes of loss of consciousness and had been resuscitated multiple times by his father. Interestingly, many of the episodes occurred during febrile illnesses. The child's sister had died suddenly at age two after multiple episodes of aborted sudden death. She was receiving amiodarone and had a permanent ventricular pacemaker implanted before dying. The ECGs of the two siblings were very similar and abnormal (Fig. 3). The identification of two additional patients allowed presentation of the preliminary data at the meeting of the North American Society of Pacing and Electrophysiology (NASPE) in 1991 *(6)*. The first paper including eight patients was published in 1992 *(1)*. Since then, there has been an exponential increase in the number of patients recognized all over the world. The database of our Working Group contains over 1000 carriers of the disease at present. The discovery of the genetic abnormalities linked to this syndrome, points to it being a primary electrical disease, providing an important first step in the prevention and effective treatment of this form of sudden death in individuals with a structurally normal heart.

Several authors have previously reported ECGs similar to the one presented in Fig. 1 *(7–12)*. For the most part, these were considered variants of the normal ECG and no definitive link to sudden death was established.

In the 1980s the CDC (Center for Disease Control) in Atlanta, reported an abnormally high incidence of sudden death in young immigrants from Southeast Asia *(13)*. The striking pattern of unexpected death usually occurred at night when the victims, who were predominantly young men in apparently good health, were asleep. Death occurred within minutes after the onset of agonal respiration. A few patients who were successfully resuscitated were found to have VF and inducible polymorphic VT/VF in the electrophysiology laboratory.

It is worth noting that the natives in Asia knew about the problem for many decades. In the Philippines it was known as Bangungut (scream followed by sudden death during sleep) and in Japan as Pokkuri (unexpected sudden death at night). In Thailand, this form of death is known as Lai Tai (death during sleep). The sudden unexplained death syndrome is known as SUDS (13). The incidence of this form of sudden death has been estimated between 26 and 38 cases per 100,000 inhabitants per year. In Laos it may cause 1 sudden death per 1000 inhabitants per year. Sudden death is the most common cause of natural death in young Thai men. In 1997 it was discovered that these patients suffer the syndrome of right bundle branch block, ST segment elevation in V1 to V3, and sudden death (13). Recently we have shown that the mutations of Thai men with SUDS produce ion channel dysfunction similar to that observed in patients with the Brugada syndrome (14).

ETIOLOGY AND GENETICS

The formation of the cardiac action potential is based on the perfect interaction of multiple ion channels with the surrounding structures. This balance is kept throughout life, with adaptation to the minimal environment changes occurring to prevent arrhythmogenesis. An alteration in this ionic balance by an external factor (i.e., ischemia), or a defect in the gene that encodes the channel can be sufficient to tilt the balance toward a devastating outcome, i.e., malignant arrhythmia. In many of these diseases, gene identification will be difficult because the families are not extensive enough to allow linkage analysis owing to the high degree of sudden death. The identification of the genes in these families will depend on the analysis of candidate genes already identified.

Brugada syndrome is usually identified as a sporadic case. However, the majority of individuals who present with this syndrome have a family history of sudden death or malignant arrhythmia, if properly questioned. This has led to the understanding that there are strong genetic factors leading to the disease. The higher prevalence of this disease in some areas of Southeast Asia is also suggestive of an underlying genetic defect causing the disease.

Controversy exists as to whether the Brugada syndrome is a form frusta of arrhythmogenic right ventricular dysplasia (ARVD) which may present with ventricular arrhythmias and typically is associated with fatty infiltration of the right ventricular myocardium. Although no genes have been identified for true ARVD, linkage analysis has identified five genetic loci including ARVD 1 (14q23) (15), ARVD 2 (1q42) (16), ARVD 3 (14q12) (17), and ARVD 4 (2q32) (18). Evaluation of families with Brugada syndrome for genetic mutations has clarified this picture somewhat.

The genetic abnormalities causing Brugada syndrome have been linked to mutations in the ion channel gene SCN5A which encodes for the cardiac sodium channel. Mutations in this gene result in a loss in function of the channels or alterateration in the kinetics and/or voltage dependence of activation and inactivation. SCN5A was previously shown to be the cause of LQT3, a form of Romano-Ward long QT syndrome (19). The differences in the clinical findings between LQT3 and Brugada syndrome occur because of the different biophysical results based on the position of the mutations within the gene. Unlike the Brugada syndrome, LQT3 occurs owing to an augmentation of late INa.

Despite the differences between LQTS and Brugada syndrome, important similarities should be noted. In particular, both of these disorders in which life-threatening ventricular tachyarrhythmias occur are owing to mutations in genes encoding ion channels. This similarity is somewhat akin to what has previously been described in familial hypertrophic cardiomyopathy (FHCM) where mutations in genes encoding for sarcomeric proteins have been identified *(20–25)*. Here, seven genes (β-myosin heavy chain, α-tropomyosin, cardiac troponin T, myosin binding protein-C, myosin essential light chain, myosin regulatory light chain, and troponin I), all encoding members of the sarcomeric unit have been found mutated in patients with FHCM. The clinical phenotype, including outcome, appears to differ based on the gene mutated and the specific mutation *(26,27)*. Similar findings are emerging in familial dilated cardiomyopathy (FDCM) as well. Thus, it appears that affecting a particular cascade at any point within the final common pathway leading to a specific cardiac function (i.e., contractile apparatus resulting in cardiac function; ion channels resulting in cardiac rhythm; cytoskeletal proteins resulting in cardiac structural support) results in a spectrum of similar disease (i.e., contractile apparatus mutations causes HCM; ion channel mutations result in LQTS, Brugada syndrome; mutations in cytoskeletal protein genes result in FDCM). This "Final Common Pathway" hypothesis *(28)* is being used in Brugada syndrome to identify the remaining genes responsible for this disorder.

INCIDENCE AND DISTRIBUTION

Because the syndrome has been identified only recently, it is difficult to ascertain its incidence and distribution in the world. When we analyze the data from the different published studies, the disease is responsible for 4 to 12% of unexpected sudden deaths, and for 20 to 50% of all sudden death in patients with an apparently normal heart. The incidence may even be larger in the younger population. Indeed, this syndrome is the most common cause of sudden death in individuals younger than 50 in South Asia with no underlying cardiac disease *(13)*. Based on a database of 48 Thai individuals who died suddenly without evidence of structural heart disease, 57% had the right bundle branch block pattern with ST elevation in leads V1 to V3. It is striking that all patients who had this pattern were male. Ten of the 48 patients were female, six of whom had idiopathic VF, yet they had no evidence of an abnormal ECG pattern. Therefore, it should be emphasized that the syndrome affects almost exclusively male patients. It should also be stressed that the physician plays an important role in identifying this syndrome to estimate its real prevalence. This syndrome may possibly be more prevalent, but the magnitude of it has yet to be determined. The difficulty in estimating the incidence and prevalence of the disease becomes even more complicated as we unravel the syndrome and some of its peculiar characteristics. It is a syndrome that in some cases presents with a typical ECG, but in other cases the concealed or intermittent forms—meaning that the ECG is normal at certain times. Several studies have provided important clues in identifying these concealed forms: Ajmaline continues to be the best agent to unmask them. Procainamide and flecainide although useful, are less sensitive. This is one of the reasons why the prevalence of the disease may be underestimated. Only prospective studies will be able to give an exact answer.

With present data, the disease appears to exist throughout the world, not surprising given the high mobility of the population and the genetic basis of the disease. In the future we might expect a sizeable increase in the number of identified cases, as the recognition of the disease grows. A prospective study of an adult Japanese population (22,027 subjects) showed an incidence of 0.05% of ECG's compatible with the syndrome (12 subjects) *(29)*. A second study of adults in Awa (Japan) showed an incidence of 0.6% (66 cases out of 10,420) *(30)*. However, a third study in children from Japan showed an incidence of ECG's compatible with the syndrome of only 0.0006% (1 case in 163,110) *(31)*. These results suggest that the syndrome manifests primarily during adulthood, which is in concordance with the mean age of sudden death victims (35 to 40 yr). The youngest patient in our database was two years old at the time of sudden death, whereas the oldest *74*. We are aware of a baby with Brugada syndrome who was two days old at the time of his first ventricular fibrillation (unpublished observations). The ECG is very variable over time, with periods in which it is clearly normal. This fact makes it very difficult to estimate the incidence of the disease in the general population.

To illustrate this problem, one has to realize that, so far, 67 families with the syndrome have been identified in the Flemish area of Belgium (6 million inhabitants). These 67 families with more than 600 members have 126 members affected with the disease (about 25%) giving an incidence of the disease of almost 1 in 50,000 in the Flemish area.

ELECTROPHYSIOLOGIC SUBSTRATE

Patients with this ECG pattern clearly have a proclivity to develop rapid polymorphic VT/VF. Before the episode, the patients present with a regular sinus rhythm, with no changes in the QT interval (Fig. 2). In some rare cases it seems that the ST segment elevation increases just prior to the onset of polymorphic VT. We have observed the triggering of the arrhythmia after a short-long-short cycle in only two cases (Fig. 4). It is clear that these patients have an electrophysiologic substrate for VT/VF as evidenced by the fact that the majority of patients who have the syndrome have inducible polymorphic VT/VF and frequently a positive signal averaged ECG. This is despite their normal cardiac function and lack of gross structural cardiac abnormalities. When comparing patients with abnormal ECG patterns to those with normal ECGs in the SUDS study *(13)*, VF could be induced in 93% of patients with the Brugada pattern, but only in 11% of those with a normal ECG. Patients with the syndrome also had a prolonged His-Purkinje conduction time (H-V interval), something that has also been shown in several other studies *(32)*. Whether this abnormality contributed to VF occurrence is unclear. But there is a correlation between the duration of the H-V interval and the degree of ST segment elevation *(32,33)*.

TRIGGERING MECHANISMS

It has been shown that in some cases the development of the arrhythmia is clearly bradycardia-dependent *(34)*. This fact could explain the higher incidence of sudden death at night in individuals with the syndrome. Proclemer et al. published one case of a patient in whom the episodes of ventricular arrhythmias could only be controlled during fast

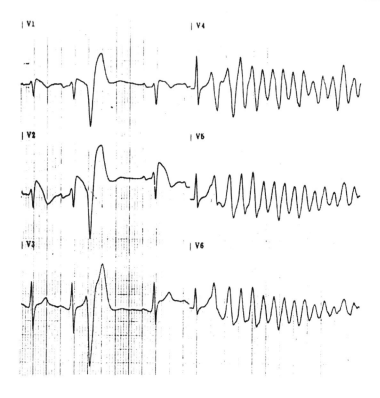

Fig. 4. An exceptional case of initiation of the polymorphic VT after short-long sequences caused by ventricular extrasystoles.

ventricular pacing *(35)*. However, not all the patients die at night and not all the cases are controlled with fast ventricular pacing. Patients from South Asia who have the ECG pattern usually develop VT/VF during sleep at night. The episodes that were detected by the implanted cardioverter-defibrillator in these patients show no evidence of bradycardia-dependence and in many cases the rate preceding the VF episode was relatively fast.

SPONTANEOUS TERMINATION OF VF

Bjerregaard et al. were the first to report a patient with the Brugada syndrome who developed a spontaneously terminating episode detected by ECG monitoring *(2)*. This patient had a typical ECG pattern with the right bundle branch block-like QRS and ST elevation from V1 to V3. In patients with the syndrome implanted with an automatic cardioverter-defibrillator with electrogram storage many spontaneous episodes of VT/ VF have now become available. Many of the episodes are self-terminating. This explains why patients present with syncope or wake up at night after episodes of agonal respiration or seizure caused by the arrhythmia. One also needs to understand why some episodes self terminate and why others are sustained and lead to cardiac arrest or even sudden death. Whether certain modulating factors such as drugs, hypokalemia, sleep-related factors (sleep apnea?) make the episode sustained remains unclear.

Table 1
Brugada Syndrome: Clinical Manifestations

a. Complete syndrome (symptomatic individuals)

- Typical ECG with symptoms consisting of recurrent syncope or sudden death (aborted or not) caused by polymorphic VT

b. Clinical variants

- Typical ECG in asymptomatic individual without family history of sudden death or Brugada syndrome.
- Typical ECG in asymptomatic individual, family member of a symptomatic individual with the syndrome.
- Typical ECG after administration of a drug in an asymptomatic individual without family history of sudden death or Brugada syndrome.
- Typical ECG after administration of a drug in an asymptomatic individual family member of a symptomatic individual with the syndrome.
- Typical ECG after administration of a drug in a patient with recurrent syncope or resuscitated sudden death (ventricular fibrillation diagnosed as idiopathic).

c. Electrocardiographic variants

- Typical ECG with clear right bundle branch block, ST elevation and P-R prolongation
- Typical ECG with ST elevation but no right bundle branch block, nor P-R prolongation
- Incomplete right bundle branch block with saddle-type ST segment elevation
- Incomplete right bundle branch block without ST segment elevation
- Isolated P-R interval prolongation

ROLE OF THE AUTONOMIC NERVOUS SYSTEM

The role of the autonomic nervous system in this syndrome is still not fully understood. Vagal stimulation is believed to trigger the arrhythmia in some patients because many episodes occur at night and sympathetic stimulation normalizes the abnormal ECG pattern. There was a report from Japan on a few patients *(34)* in whom VT/VF induction was facilitated by vagal stimulation or sympathetic blockade. On the other hand, there are patients who suffer the arrhythmia during adrenergic stimulation and still others present the arrhythmias with no apparent correlation with changes in the autonomic balance.

One of the observations in patients with the Brugada syndrome that may compel physicians to think that sympathetic blockade and vagal stimulation can enhance the induction or spontaneous occurrence of VT/VF is that the abnormal ECG pattern normalizes B adrenergic stimulation, whereas vagal stimulation enhances the abnormal pattern. However, at present we do not have sufficient data to support the concept that normalization of the ECG correlates with a decreased occurrence of VT/VF.

CLINICAL MANIFESTATIONS (TABLE 1)

The complete syndrome is characterized by episodes of rapid polymorphic VT (Fig. 2) in patients with an ECG pattern of right bundle branch block and ST segment elevation in leads V1 to V3 (Fig. 1B). The manifestations of the syndrome are caused by episodes

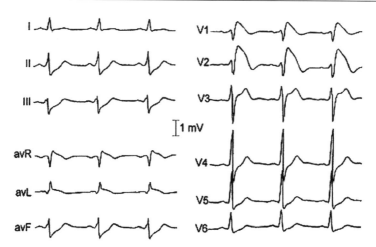

Fig. 5. ECG of an asymptomatic patient. This patient had polymorphic VT induced during programmed electrical stimulation of the heart and received an implantable cardioverter-defibrillator. Two and a half years after implant the patient received an appropriate shock because of polymorphic VT. The ECG of this asymptomatic patient cannot be distinguished from the one in Fig. 1A.

of polymorphic VT/VF. When the episodes terminate spontaneously the patient develops syncopal attacks. When the episodes are sustained full blown cardiac arrest and eventually sudden death occur. Thus, these manifestations can range widely: At the one end of the spectrum we have asymptomatic individuals and at the other end of the spectrum those who die suddenly. Other symptoms include seizures, agonal respiration, and for those patients who suffer an episode at night during sleep are witnessed as having labored respiration, agitation, loss of urinary bladder control, and not uncommonly recent memory loss (perhaps due to brain anoxia). Many patients who have the disease can appear to be otherwise very healthy and active, vigorously engaging in exertional activity or exercise. Physical examinations are almost always normal. Physicians who first work up these patients have a strong tendency to believe that the syncopal attacks are benign and of vaso-vagal origin. Many patients underwent a tilt-table test which was positive, they were treated accordingly and subsequently died suddenly. As seen in other clinical-electrocardiographic syndromes, there are different presentations of the disease.

There exist asymptomatic individuals in whom the atypical ECG is detected during routine examination. This ECG cannot be distinguished from that of symptomatic patients (Fig. 5). In other patients, the characteristic ECG is recorded during screening after the sudden death of a family member with the disease. On the other hand, there is the group of symptomatic patients who have been diagnosed as suffering syncopal episodes of unknown cause, or vaso-vagal origin, or have a diagnosis of idiopathic VF. Some of these patients are diagnosed at follow-up, when the ECG changes spontaneously from normal to the typical pattern of the syndrome (Fig. 6). This is also the case for those individuals in whom the disease is unmasked by the administration of an antiarrhythmic drug given for other arrhythmias, for instance atrial fibrillation.

Recent studies indicate that patients displaying the ECG characteristics of the syndrome and who have already had symptoms (aborted sudden death or syncope) have a

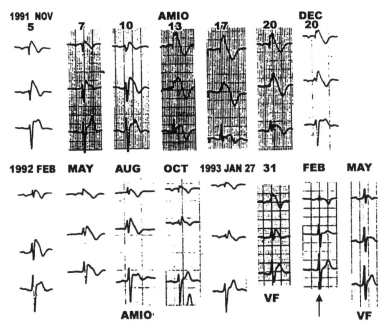

Fig. 6. ECG leads V1, V2, and V3 are shown from a single patient to illustrate the variability of the ECG pattern during follow-up. Please note that the ECG can be extremely abnormal (top tracings) but sometimes completely normal (bottom tracing of February 1993).

similar incidence of arrhythmia and sudden death as patients in which the ECG manifestation must be unmasked with a sodium channel blocker.

Up to 40% of individuals will develop a new or a first episode of polymorphic VT or sudden death during a 2–3 year follow-up. As we will discuss below, such is not the case in asymptomatic individuals.

DIAGNOSIS

The diagnosis of the syndrome is easily obtained by electrocardiography as long as the patient presents the typical ECG pattern (Fig. 1B) and there is a history of aborted sudden death or syncopes caused by a polymorphic VT. It is difficult to forget such a typical ECG. The ST segment elevation in V1 to V3 with the right bundle branch block pattern is characteristic. The ST changes are different from the ones observed in acute septal ischemia, pericarditis, ventricular aneurysm and in some normal variants like early repolarization *(36)*. There are though, ECG's which are not as characteristic, and they are only recognized by a physician who is thinking of the syndrome. There are also many patients with a normal ECG in whom the syndrome can only be recognized a posteriori when the typical pattern appears in a follow-up ECG or after the administration of ajmaline, procainamide or flecainide (Fig. 7).

Additional diagnostic problems are caused by the changes in the ECG induced by the autonomic nervous system and by other influences. The study by Myazaki et al. *(37)* was the first one to show the variability of the ECG pattern in the syndrome. Adrenergic stimulation decreases the ST segment elevation (Fig. 8) whereas vagal stimulation

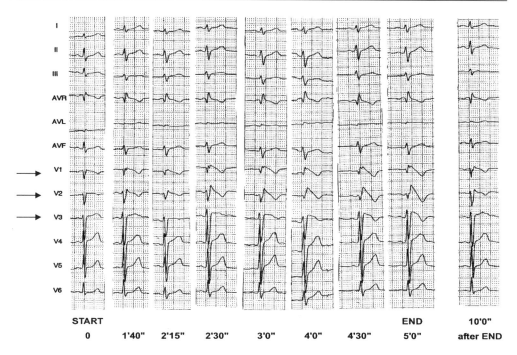

Fig. 7. Effects of the intravenous administration of ajmaline on the ECG.

worsens it. The administration of class Ia, Ic, and III drugs increase the ST segment elevation. Exercise decreases ST segment elevation, but in some patients it may increase immediately after exercise. The changes in heart rate induced by atrial pacing are accompanied by changes in the degree of ST segment elevation. When the heart rate decreases, the ST segment elevation increases and when the heart rate increases the ST segment elevation decreases.

RIGHT BUNDLE BRANCH BLOCK

It is unclear whether the right bundle branch block in this syndrome is real or whether it represents an early repolarization of right ventricular epicardium. The clinical and electrophysiological data suggest that both possibilities exist. Some ECGs clearly show a right bundle branch block after normalization of the ST segment (Fig. 8C). There is frequently a prolongation of the HV interval in these patients, which supports an abnormality of the conduction system. On the other hand, we can find ECGs without a right bundle branch block when the ST segment elevation is corrected. Moreover, not all patients have a prolongation of the H-V interval. It is likely that the different ECG patterns result from different ion channel defects. The dispersion of repolarization that forms the substrate for VT/VF can develop with a defect in any one of a number of ion channels and pathophysiologies, as discussed later.

The polymorphic VT can often be induced in these patients by programmed electrical stimulation of the heart, suggesting a reentrant mechanism. Two mechanisms are thought to underlie this syndrome: phase 2 reentry and circus movement reentry.

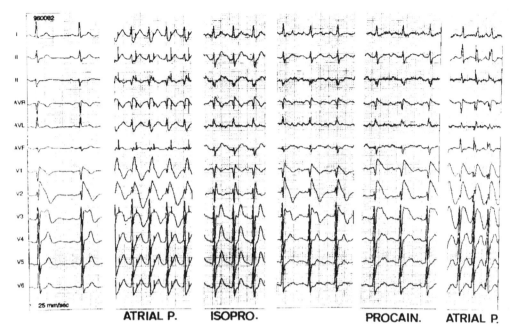

Fig. 8. The different panels illustrate the modulation of ST segment elevation which can be obtained by atrial pacing, isoproterenol infusion, and intravenous procainamide in a patient with the syndrome. Atrial stimulation worsens the right bundle branch block in **(B)** and results in T wave alternans. Acceleration of heart rate by isoproterenol, on the contrary, results in normalization of the ST segment, although an incomplete right bundle branch block can still be observed. **(D)** shows the return to the control situation. In **(E)** procainamide increases ST elevation, and atrial **(F)** after procainamide results again in bizarre ECG changes and T wave alternans.

Approximately 10% of patients with the syndrome exhibit paroxysmal atrial fibrillation. This arrhythmia may start at a rather young age, suggesting a possible genetic cause *(38)*. It is possible that similar genetic defects alter atrial and ventricular cellular electrophysiology in these patients.

RELATION WITH OTHER SYNDROMES
AND THE PSEUDO-SYNDROME

A possible relation between the syndrome under discussion and other syndromes, particularly right ventricular dysplasia has been suggested. Isolated case reports, particularly from Italy *(39)*, have suggested that in some patients with an electrocardiogram typical of the syndrome, some pathologic data suggested right ventricular dysplasia. The recent discovery of the genetic abnormalities of the Brugada syndrome in the gene SCN5A located in chromosome 3 *(19)* argues against such a relationship, because the loci thus far linked to right ventricular dysplasia are located on other chromosomes *(15–18)*. It is possible that some patients manifest two different diseases at the same time, and there also exists ECGs which look similar to Brugada syndrome, but which are not caused by the disease (pseudo-Brugada syndrome). Ikeguchi and coworkers (personal communication) have studied a patient with Wolff-Parkinson-White syndrome that was successfully

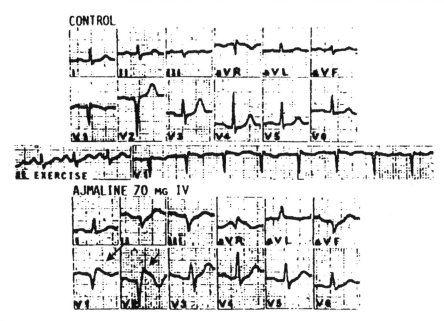

Fig. 9. ECG changes induced by intravenous ajmaline in a patient with serologic Chagas' disease but no manifest myocarditis. The changes are very similar to those observed in Brugada syndrome. The question arises about the possibility of two simultaneous diseases in the same patient, but the ECG abnormalities may be the same final pathway of alteration of the function of the sodium channels which is genetically determined in Brugada syndrome and could be acquired in Chagas' disease.

treated by means of radiofrequency catheter ablation. The patient died suddenly two years after ablation. Analysis of the ECGs of this case shows that he also suffered from the Brugada syndrome. It is not unthinkable, therefore, that some patients may suffer from right ventricular dysplasia and Brugada syndrome at the same time.

Other diseases may result in ECG's manifestations similar to the Brugada syndrome. For instance, it is interesting to observe the figures published from Buenos Aires in 1982 (Fig. 9) *(40)*. In patients with Chagas' disease Chiale et al. showed that the intravenous administration of ajmaline was of value to uncover latent conduction disturbances, but also what they called "latent disease." In patients with positive serology severe conduction disturbances occurred in one-third after the administration of iv ajmaline. In 8% of patients they observed the appearance of ventricular arrhythmias and in 7% elevation of the ST segment in the right precordial leads (Fig. 9). The question arises of the relation between Chagas' disease and Brugada syndrome in these patients. Chiale and coworkers actually considered the ajmaline challenge as a nonspecific test capable of detecting myocardial damage. In light of the recent discovery of the genetic defect underlying the Brugada syndrome, the question also arises about the possible occurrence of damage to the sodium channel by Chagas' disease. Although there exist major differences between Chagas' disease and Brugada syndrome, the final common pathway leading to sudden death may be the same: Damage to the sodium channel (infectious in Chagas' disease, genetic in Brugada syndrome) with conduction and repolarization disturbances leading to electrical chaos and ventricular fibrillation.

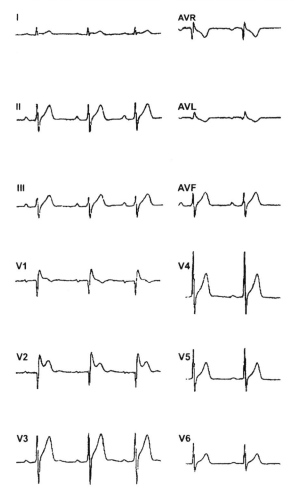

Fig. 10. ECG of a patient with Steinert's disease showing some similarities to Brugada syndrome.

Other conditions may result in ECGs simulating Brugada syndrome: Steinert's disease (Fig. 10), pectus excavatum, and mediastinal tumors *(41)*. These should be excluded before diagnosing Brugada syndrome.

ELECTROPHYSIOLOGIC AND HEMODYNAMIC FINDINGS

During invasive electrophysiologic investigations sinus node function has been normal in the large majority of the patients. However, isolated patients have manifest sinus node disease and are pacemaker dependent. As already discussed, about 10% of patients has paroxysmal atrial fibrillation. There exist no detailed studies on the ability to induce this arrhythmia by programmed electrical stimulation.

All published studies agree on the inducibility of polymorphic VT by programmed electrical stimulation in symptomatic patients *(1,6,13)*. About 80% of patients resuscitated from VF are inducible by giving 1 or 2 ventricular premature beats during ventricular pacing. In the group of patients with syncope, the inducibility rate is about 60%. In asymptomatic individuals with an abnormal ECG the inducibility rate is 33%. In some patients three premature stimuli are required. The induced arrhythmia is sustained in practically all cases, results in hemodynamic collapse and has to be terminated by an external DC shock. It can be criticized that polymorphic VT or VF induced by programmed stimulation is a nonspecific finding, because these arrhythmias can sometimes be induced in patients with a normal heart *(42)*. There exist, however, major differences between the two situations: 1. The clinical context, with symptomatic patients with Brugada syndrome having suffered from spontaneous ventricular arrhythmias. 2. The percentage of patients inducible to a sustained polymorphic ventricular arrhythmia in Brugada syndrome (33 to 80% depending on the group) as compared to individuals without the syndrome where a sustained polymorphic VT or VF is only exceptionally induced.

The same studies coincide in the frequent finding of conduction disturbances in patients with the disease. The H-V interval is prolonged in about half of the patients. The prolongation is not marked, rarely exceeding the 70 ms, but being clearly abnormal in this population with an average age of 40 yr. The H-V prolongation explains the slight prolongation of the P-R interval during sinus rhythm. We have found that programmed ventricular stimulation and the H-V interval have a prognostic value. Noninducible patients with a normal H-V interval have a better prognosis than inducible patients and patients with a prolonged H-V interval. That is true both in symptomatic and asymptomatic individuals. However, the recurrence rates in symptomatic individuals are too high not to implant a cardioverter-defibrillator *(43)*.

Hemodynamic studies in patients who underwent right and left heart catheterization were found to be normal. In SUDS patients with or without the typical ECG also had normal findings. The coronary arteries are normal and the right and left ventricular function and contractility also.

PROGNOSIS AND TREATMENT

This syndrome has a very poor prognosis when left untreated: We have recently shown that more than one-third of patients who suffer syncopal episodes or are resuscitated from near-sudden death develop a new episode of polymorphic VT within approximately two years *(43)*. Unfortunately, the prognosis of asymptomatic individuals with typical ECG is also poor. In spite of not having any previous symptoms, one-third of these individuals presents a first polymorphic VT or VF within two years of follow-up as well (Fig. 11). The observations on prognosis of patients with Brugada syndrome from Europe is virtually identical to that for SUDS patients in Thailand who show the abnormal ECG pattern. The cumulative proportion of VF or cardiac arrest occurred in approx 60% of the patients within one year and 40% were likely to die suddenly if untreated.

These data are of extreme importance for the delineation of treatment policies of these patients. Because antiarrhythmic drugs (amiodarone or beta-blockers) do not protect against sudden cardiac death *(32,43)*, the only available treatment is the implantable cardioverter-defibrillator. This device effectively recognizes and treats the ventricular arrhythmias. When provided with the implantable defibrillator total mortality in patients with Brugada syndrome has been 0% with up to 10 yr follow-up. These results are not surprising. These patients are young and usually devoid from other diseases. Because the heart is structurally normal, and there is no coronary artery disease, these patients do not die from heart failure or complications of ischemic events. Thus, they are the most ideal

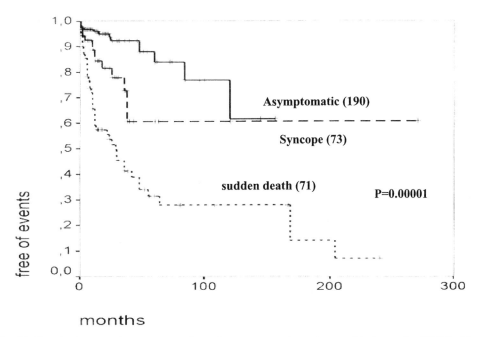

Fig. 11. Survival curves in symptomatic and asymptomatic patients with the typical ECG. About 30% of patients in both categories develop a recurrence of the first episode of polymorphic VT at about two yr mean follow-up.

candidates for treatment with an implantable cardioverter-defibrillator. All symptomatic patients should receive this device.

On the other hand, major concerns arise in the treatment of asymptomatic individuals. Data from electrophysiologic investigations may help us to predict prognosis. We have recently shown that of 190 asymptomatic individuals 16 died suddenly or presented their first VF with successful resuscitation during a follow-up of 27 mo *(43)*. There were 136 patients in whom programmed electrical stimulation was performed. Of them 45 were inducible and 91 not. In the noninducible group only one patient (1%) presented ventricular fibrillation, whereas that happened in 6 of the 45 inducible patients (14%). Unfortunately programmed stimulation was not available in 9 patients who died suddenly. That group of 9 patients represents a major limitation to assess the real prognostic value of programmed ventricular stimulation in asymptomatic individuals with Brugada syndrome. Actually, and as also confirmed by Priori et al. *(44)* the best predictor of event in asymptomatic individuals is a spontaneous abnormal ECG. From the 190 asymptomatic individuals 111 had a spontaneous abnormal ECG and 79 had an abnormal ECG uncovered by drug challenge. All 16 events occurred in the group with a spontaneous abnormal ECG giving an incidence of 14% sudden death during follow-up. Other data that are associated to a poorer prognosis is male sex, but not a family history of sudden death.

At present, we believe four different groups of patients can be distinguished:

1. Symptomatic individuals with the disease who require an implantable cardioverter-defibrillator. Symptomatic patients with transient normalization of the ECG during follow-up have the same prognosis as compared to patients with a permanently abnormal ECG.

2. Asymptomatic patients with a spontaneously abnormal ECG should be given the option of a defibrillator irrespective of the results from electrophysiological investigations.
3. Asymptomatic individuals with an abnormal ECG uncovered only after drug challenge but also with inducible sustained polymorphic ventricular arrhythmias, who probably must also be given the option of a defibrillator, particularly if there is a family history of sudden death, and that also for psychological reasons.
4. Asymptomatic individuals with an abnormal ECG only after drug challenge and no inducible ventricular arrhythmias who should not be treated but followed-up carefully for development of symptoms suggesting arrhythmias (particularly syncope).

Again in this last group a family history of sudden death, particularly when many members have died suddenly at a young age, may make it necessary to protect carriers of the disease for psychological reasons. One has to realize, however, that these recommendations may rapidly change depending upon the availability of new data.

REFERENCES

1. Brugada P, Brugada J. Right bundle branch block, persistent ST segment elevation and sudden cardiac death: A distinct clinical and electrocardiographic syndrome. J Am Coll Cardiol 1992;20:1391–1396.
2. Bjerregaard P, Gussak I, Kotar SL, et al. Recurrent syncope in a patient with prominent J-wave. Am Heart J 1994;127:1426–1430.
3. Yan GX, Antzelevitch C. Cellular basis for the electrocardiographic J wave. Circulation 1996;93:372–379.
4. Priori SG, Diehl L, Schwartz PJ. Torsade de pointes. In: Podrid PJ, Kowey PR, eds. Cardiac Arrhythmia. Baltimore, MD: Williams and Wilkins, 1995;951–963.
5. El-Sherif N. Polymorphic ventricular tachycardia. In ref. 4, pp. 936–950.
6. Brugada P, Brugada J. A distinct clinical and electrocardiographic syndrome: right bundle branch block, persistent ST segment elevation with normal QT interval and sudden cardiac death. PACE 1991;14:746.
7. Osher HL, Wolff L. Electrocardiographic pattern simulating acute myocardial injury. Am J Med Sci 1953;226:541–545.
8. Eideken J. Elevation of RS-T segment, apparent or real in right precordial leads as probable normal variant. Am Heart J 1954;48:331–339.
9. Levine HD, Wanzer SH, Merrill JP. Dialyzable currents of injury in potassium intoxication resembling acute myocardial infarction or pericarditis. Circulation 1960;6:920–928.
10. Roesler H. An electrocardiographic study of high take-off of the R(R)-T segment in right precordial leads. Altered repolarisation. Am J Cardiol 1960;6:920–928.
11. Calo AA. The triad secondary R wave, RS-T segment elevation and T waves inversion in right precordial leads: a normal electrocardiographic variant. G Ital Cardiol 1975;5:955–960.
12. Martini B, Nava A, Thiene G, et al. Ventricular fibrillation without apparent heart disease. Description of six cases. Am Heart J 1989;118:1203–1209.
13. Nademanee K, Veerakul G, Nimmannit S, et al. Arrhythmogenic marker for the sudden unexplained death syndrome in Thai men. Circulation 1997;96:2595–2600.
14. Vatta M, Dumaine R, Varghese G, et al. Genetic and biopphysical basis of sudden unexplained nocturnal death syndrome (SUNDS), a disease allelic to Brugada syndrome. Hum Mol Genet 2002;11:337–345.
15. Rampazzo A, Nava A, Erne P, et al. The gene for arrhythmogenic right ventricular cardiomyopathy maps to chromosome 14q23–Q24. Hum Mol Genet 1994;3:959–962.
16. Rampazzo A, Nava A, Erne P, et al. A new locus for arrhythmogenic right ventricular cardiomyopathy (ARVD2) maps to chromosome 1q42–Q43. Hum Mol Genet 1995;4:2151–2154.
17. Severini GM, Krajinovic M, Pinamonti B, et al. A new locus for arrhythmogenic right ventricular dysplasia on the long arm of chromosome 14. Genomics 1996;31:193–200.
18. Rampazzo A, Nava A, Miorin M, et al. ARVD4, a new locus for arrhythmogenic right ventricular cardiomyopathy, maps to chromosome 2 long arm. Genomics 1997;15:45(2):259–263.
19. Chen Q, Kirsch GE, Zhang D, et al. Genetic basis and molecular mechanisms for idiopathic ventricular fibrillation. Nature 1998;392:293–296.
20. Geisterfer-Lowrance AAT, Kass A, Tanigawa, et al. A molecular basis for familial hypertrophic cardiomyopathy: A beta-cardiac myosin heavy chain gene missense mutation. Cell 1990;62:999–1006.

21. Thierfelder L, Watkins H, MacRae C, et al. Alpha-tropomyosin and cardiac troponin T mutations cause familial hypertrophic cardiomyopathy: A disease of the sarcomere. Cell 1994;77:701–712.

22. Bonne G, Carrier L, Bercovici J, et al. Cardiac myosin binding protein-C gene splice acceptor site mutation is associated with familial hypertrophic cardiomyopathy. Nat Genet 1995;11:438–440.

23. Watkins H, Conner D, Thierfeld L, et al. Mutations in the cardiac myosin binding protein-C gene on chromosome 11 cause familial hypertrophic cardiomyopathy. Nat Genet 11:434–437.

24. Poetter K, Jiang H, Hassanzadeh S, et al. Mutations in either the essential or regulatory light chains of myosin are associated with a rare myopathy in human heart and skeletal muscle. Nat Genet 1996;13: 63–69.

25. Kimura A, Harada H, Park JE, et al. Mutations in the cardiac troponin I gene associated with hypertrophic cardiomyopathy. Nat Genet 196;16:379–382.

26. Watkins H, Rosenzweig A, Hwang DS, et al. Characteristics and prognostic implications of myosin missense mutations in familial hypertrophic cardiomyopathy. N Engl J Med 1992;326:1108–1114.

27. Watkins H, McKenna WJ, Theirfelder L, et al. Mutations in the genes for cardiac troponin T and alpha-tropomyosin in hypertrophic cardiomyopathy. N Engl J Med 1995;332:1058–1064.

28. Towbin JA. The role of cytoskeletal proteins in cardiomyopathies. Curr Opin Cell Biol 1998;10: 131–139.

29. Tohyou Y, Nakazawa K, Ozawa A, et al. A survey in the incidence of right bundle branch block with ST segment elevation among normal population. Jpn J Electrocardiol 1995;15:223–226.

30. Namiki T, Ogura T, Kuwabara Y, et al. Five-year mortality and clinical characteristics of adult subjects with right bundle branch block and ST elevation. Circulation 1995;93:334.

31. Hata Y, Chiba N, Hotta K, et al. Incidence and clinical significance of right bundle branch block and ST segment elevation in V1–V3 in 6- to 18-year-old school children in Japan. Circulation 1997;20:2310.

32. Brugada J, Brugada R, Brugada P. Right bundle branch block and ST segment elevation in leads V1–V3: A marker for sudden death in patients with no demonstrable structural heart disease. Circulation 1998;97:457–460.

33. Farre J, unpublished observations.

34. Kasanuki H, Ohnishi S, Ohtuka M, et al. Idiopathic ventricular fibrillation induced with vagal activity in patients without obvious heart disease. Circulation 1997;95:2277–2285.

35. Proclemer A, Facchin D, Fedruglio GA, Nucifora R. Fibrillazione ventricolare recidivante, blocco di branca destra, persistent sopraslivellamento del tratto ST in V1–V3: Una nuova syndroma aritmica? Descrisione di un caso clinico. G Ital Cardiol 1993;23:1211–1218.

36. Kambara H, Phillips J. Long-term evaluation of early repolarisation syndrome (normal variant RS-T segment elevation). Am J Cardiol 1976;38:157–161.

37. Miyazaki T, Mitamura H, Miyoshi S, Soejima K, Aizawa Y, Ogawa S. Autonomic and antiarrhythmic modulation of ST segment elevation in patients with Brugada syndrome. J Am Coll Cardiol 1996;27:1061–1070.

38. Brugada R, Tapscott T, Czernuszewic GZ, et al. Identification of a genetic locus for familial atrial fibrillation. N Engl J Med 1997;336:905–911.

39. Corrado D, Nava A, Buja G, et al. Familial cardiomyopathy underlies syndrome of right bundle branch block, ST segment elevation and sudden death. J Am Coll Cardiol 1996;27:443–448.

40. Chiale PA, Przybylski J, Liano RA, et al. Electrocardiographic changes evoked by ajmaline in chronic Chagas' disease without manifest myocarditis. Am J Cardiol 1982;49:14–20.

41. Tarin N, Farre J, Rubio JM, Tunon J, Castro-Dorticos J. Brugada-like electrocardiographic pattern in a patient with a mediastinal tumor. PACE 1999;22:1264–1266.

42. Brugada P, Green M, Abdollah H, Wellens HJJ. Significance of ventricular arrhythmias initiated by programmed ventricular stimulation: Importance of the type of ventricular arrhythmia induced and the number of premature stimuli required. Circulation 1984;69:87–92.

43. Brugada J, Brugada R, Antzelevitch C, Towbin J, Nademanee K, Brugada P. Long-term follow-up of individuals with the electrocardiographic pattern of right bundle branch block and ST segment elevation in precordial leads V1 to V3. Circulation 2002;105:73–78.

44. Priori S, Napolitano C, Gasparini M, et al. Natural history of Brugada syndrome. Insights for risk stratification and management. Circulation 2002;105:1342–1347.

20 Clinical Evaluation, Risk Stratification, and Management of Congenital Long QT Syndrome

Anant Khositseth, MD
and Michael J. Ackerman, MD, PhD

CONTENTS

INTRODUCTION
CASE VIGNETTES
CLINICAL EVALUATION
DIAGNOSIS OF LQTS
RISK STRATIFICATION
MANAGEMENT
CASE VIGNETTES REVISITED
REFERENCES

INTRODUCTION

Once considered an extremely rare and lethal arrhythmogenic peculiarity, the congenital long QT syndrome (LQTS) is understood today as a primary cardiac channelopathy that is far more common but less commonly lethal than previously recognized. The molecular breakthroughs of the 1990s led by the research laboratories of Drs. Mark Keating, Jeff Towbin, Silvia Priori, and others revealed the fundamental underpinnings of LQTS. Now, hundreds of mutations scattered amongst five cardiac channel genes account for approx two-thirds of LQTS. Further, LQTS is a "Rosetta stone," providing an important molecular model for ventricular arrhythmogenesis. Despite these tremendous advances, the bench-top discoveries have not yet translated to the patient's bedside in the form of a standard, routine molecular diagnostic test.

The cornerstone of the clinical evaluation for LQTS remains a time honored careful personal and family history and meticulous inspection of the 12-lead electrocardiogram (ECG) to detect the hallmark of LQTS, prolongation of the QT interval. In this chapter, three case vignettes will be used to highlight the challenges faced by a clinician when trying to unmask this potential silent killer. Then, the clinical evaluation will be discussed focusing on the objective tools available: 12-lead ECG, 24-h Holter, exercise stress testing with and without microvoltage T-wave alternans analysis, catecholamine provo-

From: *Contemporary Cardiology: Cardiac Repolarization: Bridging Basic and Clinical Science*
Edited by: I. Gussak et al. © Humana Press Inc., Totowa, NJ

cation tests, and mutational analysis of the known LQTS genes. Next, risk stratification in LQTS will be discussed. Once a patient is deemed to harbor the clinical and/or genetic substrate for LQTS, it is critical to try to determine whether or not he/she possesses a ticking time bomb just waiting for the necessary trigger to detonate. On the other hand, perhaps, the individual has a dud destined for asymptomatic longevity. Clearly, the profound heterogeneity of LQTS calls for individualized patient management. For example, should the duds be prohibited from all competitive sports? As will be evident in this chapter, the LQTS evaluation poses a tremendous diagnostic challenge to discern which asymptomatic family members are affected and who among the affected individuals harbor a ticking time bomb. Finally, the current treatment and lifestyle recommendations will be provided and the clinical evaluation for the case vignettes presented at the beginning of the chapter will be reviewed.

CASE VIGNETTES

Case #1: What Is a Diagnostic QTc?

JPA is a 15-yr-old female referred for a second opinion following the diagnosis of possible LQTS. At a preparticipation sports physical, an innocent murmur was heard, an ECG demonstrated a QTc of 450 ms, and subsequent exercise testing reported that the QT interval failed to shorten appropriately during exercise. By history, the patient and family history was completely negative. No ECGs were performed on the parents. The patient was diagnosed with "borderline QT prolongation, possible LQTS," placed on once-a-day atenolol beta-blocker therapy, and restricted from all competitive sports.

Case #2: Does My 13-yr-Old Have What Killed My 17-yr-Old Son? Evaluation of Sudden Unexplained Death.

SH was a 17-yr-old previously healthy male found dead in bed. Standard medico-legal autopsy was negative. His younger brother was brought for a second opinion to determine whether or not he was at risk. This 13-yr-old boy was asymptomatic, his QTc was 430 ms, Holter recorded no significant ventricular ectopy, and exercise stress test was unremarkable. Would you perform any additional tests or dismiss as normal?

Case #3: To Implant or Not to Implant? That Is the Question.

NCK is an asymptomatic 18-yr-old female whose sister died following a near-drowning, her sentinel event for LQTS. Because of the swimming-triggered cardiac event, a molecular autopsy was conducted revealing a defect in *KCNQ1/KVLQT1* (LQT1). Molecular testing confirmed this mutation in NCK. Her QTc is 450 ms. Should she receive a prophylactic ICD?

These three cases highlight several aspects in the clinical evaluation, risk stratification, and management of LQTS and the approach to each case will be summarized at the chapter's conclusion.

CLINICAL EVALUATION

LQTS Disease Classification

Two inherited forms of LQTS with different modes of inheritance have been described: The Romano-Ward syndrome (RWS) and the Jervell and Lange-Nielsen syndrome

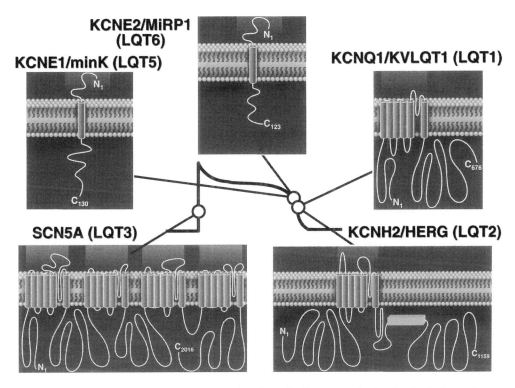

Fig. 1. LQTS: a cardiac channelopathy. Depicted are the linear topologies for the 5 channel genes implicated in LQTS. The gene responsible for LQT1, *KCNQ1* (commonly known as *KVLQT1*), resides on chromosome 11p15.5 and encodes a 676-amino acid protein comprising the alpha subunit of the I_{Ks} potassium channel. The gene responsible for LQT2, *KCNH2* (commonly known as *HERG*), resides on chromosome 7q35–36 and encodes a 1159-amino acid protein comprising the alpha subunit of the I_{Kr} potassium channel. The gene responsible for LQT3, *SCN5A*, resides on chromosome 3p21–24 and encodes a 2016-amino acid protein comprising the alpha subunit of the I_{Na} sodium channel. LQT4 has been linked to chromosome 4q25–27 but the gene remains elusive. The gene responsible for LQT5, *KCNE1* (commonly known as *minK*), resides on chromosome 21q22.1 and encodes a 130-amino acid beta subunit of the I_{Ks} potassium channel. The gene responsible for LQT6, *KCNE2* (commonly known as *MiRP1*), resides on chromosome 21q22.1 and encodes a 123-amino acid beta subunit of the I_{Kr} potassium channel.

(JLNS). RWS was first described separately by Romano *(1)* and Ward *(2)* in the early 1960s after observing families with similar presentations including prolongation of the QT interval, syncope, and sudden death. RWS is the most common inherited form of LQTS and is transmitted as an autosomal dominant trait. The incidence is speculated to be 1 in 5000 to 1 in 10,000 persons. To date, 6 LQTS loci, 5 LQTS genes encoding the alpha or beta subunits of cardiac ion channels, and hundreds of mutations have been identified: LQT1—chromosome 11p15.5, *KCNQ1 (KVLQT1)*, LQT2—chromosome 7q35–36, *KCNH2 (HERG)*, LQT3—chromosome 3p21–24, *SCN5A*, LQT4—chromosome 4q25–27, gene still unknown, LQT5—chromosome 21q22.1–22.2, *KCNE1* (MinK), and LQT6—chromosome 21q22.1–22.2, *KCNE2* (MiRP1) (Fig. 1) *(3–6)*.

Mutations in the gene encoding the cardiac ryanodine receptor *(RyR2)* have been identified in catecholaminergic polymorphic ventricular tachycardia (CPVT1) and mutations in the gene encoding the cardiac inwardly rectifying potassium channel (*KCNJ2* or Kir2.1) cause Andersen's syndrome that may include QT interval prolongation in its phenotype *(7–9)*. At this time, there is no evidence that either *RyR2* or *KCNJ2* mutations underlie isolated LQTS hence their exclusion from the LQT# subtypes. At present, 50 to 70% of families with RWS have one of the known LQTS genotypes *(6)*.

JLNS was first described in 1957 in a Norwegian family in which four of six children had prolonged QT intervals, congenital sensorineural hearing loss and recurrent syncope, three of whom died suddenly *(10)*. In contrast to RWS, JLNS is associated with congenital deafness. The incidence is extremely rare (1 to 6 cases per 1 million population). Initially understood as an autosomal recessive disorder, JLNS is now appreciated to be a syndrome where the auditory phenotype (deafness) is autosomal recessive but the cardiac phenotype is autosomal dominant. Thus, parents of JLNS actually have RWS but interestingly, the parents are most often asymptomatic. The patient with JLNS has inherited abnormal alleles (either *KVLQT1* or *KCNE1*) from both parents. The specific mutation can be the same (usually in consanguineous families) or different (compound heterozygosity).

Clinical Presentations

LQTS may remain dormant with a lifelong asymptomatic course or present with sudden cardiac death during infancy. Up to 40% of patients with heritable LQTS are asymptomatic at the time of diagnosis and this number may be an underestimate with the increasing recognition of genotype positive, asymptomatic individuals *(4,11,12)*. Conversely, 5–10% of LQTS patients present with cardiac arrest as their sentinel event. Unfortunately, this sentinel event is sometimes their first and last one. Syncope is the most frequent symptom occurring commonly between age 5 and 15 yr. The risk of cardiac events is higher in males until puberty and higher in females during adulthood *(13)*. However, females appear more vulnerable to LQTS-related cardiac events overall. In general, approx 60% of patients present with activity- or emotion-related symptoms primarily syncope, seizures, or palpitations. Eighty-five percent of cardiac events are related to physical activity or emotional stress. *To be certain, a fight-flight-fright-triggered faint must be considered potentially ominous until proven otherwise and a meticulous LQTS evaluation must be conducted.*

Some of the phenotypic heterogeneity in LQTS is now understood because of the underlying genetic heterogeneity particularly with respect to gene-specific triggers for cardiac events (Fig. 2) *(14)*. For example, patients with the most common genetic subtype (LQT1, *KCNQ1/KVLQT1*) have predominantly exertional-triggered symptoms. Interestingly, swimming appears to be a common LQTS trigger and prior to genotyping, it was observed that approx 15% of syncopal presentations in LQTS occurred during swimming *(15)*. Subsequently, swimming surfaced as a gene-specific arrhythmogenic trigger associated almost exclusively with LQT1 *(16–20)*. Ackerman et al. *(17)* first reported a case involving a 10-yr-old boy successfully defibrillated from torsades de pointes after near drowning in a public school and subsequently identified an F339del-KVLQT1 mutation *(18)*. Subsequently, a molecular autopsy in a 19-yr-old woman who died after a near drowning revealed a AAP71–73del-KVLQT1 mutation *(20)*. With few exceptions to date, all patients, with either a personal history or an extended family history of a near drowning, have a defective *KVLQT1* gene facilitating strategic genotyping *(16,19)*.

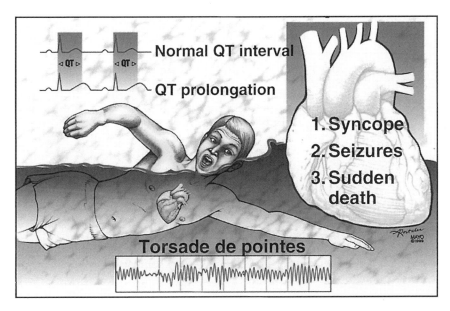

Fig. 2. Triggers to the long QT heart. Illustrated are the 2 essential elements necessary to precipitate a cardiac event. First, a cardiac channel defect (from Fig. 1) results in abnormal repolarization usually manifest on the surface ECG with QT prolongation. Second, a trigger is needed (in this case, swimming) to cause the stable but prolonged QT substrate to degenerate into the trademark arrhythmia of LQTS, TdP or polymorphic ventricular tachycardia. The outcome—syncope, seizures, or sudden death—depends on whether or not this dysrhythmia spontaneously terminates.

Auditory stimuli, such as a telephone ringing or an alarm clock sounding, is another common trigger in LQTS and may indicate the presence of a *HERG/KCNH2* (LQT2) defect *(14,16,21)*. Fifteen percent of the cardiac events occur during rest or sleep. Sleep/rest-triggered events seems most common in patients harboring a defective sodium channel *(SCN5A)* gene (LQT3) *(14)*. The underlying genotype has a profound influence on the clinical course *(22)*. LQT1 and LQT2 families comprise approx 50% of LQTS and have a much higher risk of cardiac events than patients with LQT3. However, the lethality of a given cardiac event appears to be greatest in LQT3. Fortunately, *SCN5A*-based LQTS (LQT3) is approx 10-fold less common than the potassium channel LQTS subtypes. Table 1 provides a generalized summary of genotype-phenotype relationships in LQT1, LQT2, and LQT3. Of course, these long QT genotypes do not read the papers published about them and there are numerous exceptions to how a particular genotype may or may not manifest its phenotype.

The 12-Lead Electrocardiogram

Despite tremendous research advances in elucidating the molecular underpinnings of LQTS, the 12-lead ECG remains the cornerstone in the LQTS evaluation and the chief screening tool. QT interval prolongation constitutes the hallmark of this syndrome (Fig. 2). The typical electrocardiographic features of LQTS include prolongation of the rate-corrected QT interval (QTc) as measured by Bazett's formula (QTc = QT interval/square root of RR interval) *(23)*.

Although there are numerous rate correction formulas, we continue to use Bazett's QTc. The QT interval is defined as the time interval between the onset of QRS and the

Table 1
Genotype-Specific Clinical Features

	LQT1	LQT2	LQT3
Inheritance	Autosomal dominant	Autosomal dominant	Autosomal dominant
Chromosome location	11p15.5	7q35	3p21
Gene	KCNQ1/KVLQT1	KCNH2/HERG	SCN5A
Gene function	I_{Ks}	I_{Kr}	I_{Na}
ECG pattern			
QTc	same	same	same
T wave abnormality	Prolonged T wave duration	Small or notched T wave	Delayed onset of T wave
Arousal-related cardiac events (%)	most common (85%)	common (67%)	less common (33%)
Event onset	Exercise	Rest/sleep	Rest/sleep
Gene-specific trigger	Swimming	Auditory stimuli	none
Cardiac events through age of 40 years			
≥ 1 event (%)	62	46	18
≥ 2 events (%)	37	36	5
Lethality of cardiac events (%)	4	4	20
Median age at first event (yr)	9	12	16

point at which the isoelectric line intersected a tangential line drawn at the maximal downslope of the positive T wave or at the maximal upslope of the negative T wave. This value is corrected for the heart rate by dividing it by the square root of the preceding RR interval (Bazett's QTc formula). Note, with a heart rate of 60 beats per minute (RR interval = 1 second), the QTc equals the QT interval. More rapid heart rates cause the calculated QTc to increase relative to the measured QT interval.

Lead II is generally the accepted lead for QTc calculation because the inscription of the T wave is usually discrete although the lateral precordial leads V5 and V6 are sometimes quite informative (15,24). Garson et al. (15) noted that lead II yielded the longest QT interval in 82% of patients. When sinus arrhythmia is present, an average QTc from the entire lead II strip (at least 3 consecutive determinations) must be determined (25,26). Simply taking the longest observed QTc will yield unacceptable false positive classifications.

Although the computer algorithms developed to analyze the ECG are generally useful and accurate, they are not acceptable in the evaluation of LQTS. We demonstrated that computer-generated ECG diagnostic interpretation read "normal ECG" for half of the family members with genotype positive LQT1 (27). The ECG must be directly visualized and QTc manually calculated by a physician with expertise in LQTS. Indeed, an ECG suggestive of LQTS is in the eye of the beholder and not all eyes or computer algorithms are created equal.

An alternative to manual calculation of the QTc is a simple nomogram in which only a ruler or caliper is needed for rapid identification of normal, borderline, and prolonged

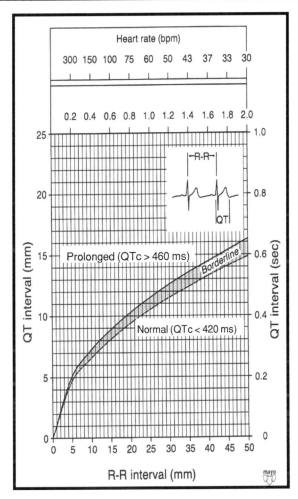

Fig. 3. Nomogram for manual QTc calculation. This simple nomogram requires only a ruler and enables the rapid classification of individuals with prolonged (≥ 460 ms), borderline (420–460 ms), and normal (< 420 ms) QTc. The 420 ms and 460 ms QTc lines are derived from plotting QT and R-R coordinates according to $QT = QTc \times RR^{1/2}$ (Bazett's formula). Assuming a paper speed of 25 mm/s (ECG standard), the physician can measure the QT and R-R interval in millimeters and plot these points on the left y-axis and bottom x-axis, respectively. The intersection of these points locates the QTc. Alternatively, if the patient is in sinus rhythm, the physician can plot the heart rate on the top x-axis instead of measuring the R-R interval. In either case (QT vs R-R or QT vs heart rate), if the intersection falls above the shaded region (QTc > 460 ms), the individual is likely to have the long QT syndrome (false positive ~ 5%) and should be referred to a cardiologist. If the intersection falls below the shaded region (i.e., QTc < 420 ms), the individual is probably normal (false negative < 2%). Note that five to ten percent of individuals with LQTS will fall within the borderline zone requiring a plot in this zone to be assessed carefully. Certainly, symptoms plus a plot in this borderline zone is compatible with the diagnosis of LQTS.

QTc (Fig. 3). The QTc lines of 420 ms and 460 ms have been drawn. Measuring the QT interval and RR interval with a ruler or caliper in millimeters, one can make a quick plot on the nomogram. A plot falling on or above the top line may be abnormal and an acquired or genetic cause should be investigated. A plot falling between lines of 420 ms and 460 ms is considered borderline and requires careful decision-making. Finally, a plot falling below the bottom line (420 ms) is unlikely to be LQTS. As a quick screen, the Bazette-derived QTc will be less than 460 ms if the QT interval is less than half of the preceding RR interval.

Figure 4 provides a diagnostic algorithm to assist the work-up when a QTc ≥ 460 ms is encountered. When exactly is a QTc too long is a question that continues to torment LQTS physicians and can plague the LQTS evaluation as depicted in case vignette 1. Before the molecular revelations in LQTS, a QTc of ≥ 440 ms was considered prolonged *(28)*. Subsequently, Vincent et al. *(25)* examined the QTc distribution in three families that were genotyped for the 11p15.5 locus for LQT1 and found that no genotype positive individuals had a QTc ≤ 410 ms and no unaffected (genotype negative) persons had a QTc ≥ 470 ms in men and ≥ 480 ms in women and that a significant number of patients were erroneously classified using the 440 ms cut-off. From a screening standpoint, if a QTc of 460 ms is used as a cutoff point, the positive predictive value is 92% and the negative predictive value is 94% *(4)*. Again for screening, we advocate designating QTc values ≥ 460 ms as prolonged and between 420 ms and 460 ms as borderline or equivocal to maximize the PPV and NPV as a *screening* test.

Figure 5 depicts QTc values in health and in LQTS. Below 400 ms, the interpretation is easy—Normal, no LQTS—with virtually 100% negative predictive value (*although we have documented a HERG patient with a QTc of 380 ms*). On the other end, a QTc ≥ 480 ms almost always indicates repolarization pathology owing to either acquired or congenital LQTS. However, the overlap zone (400–480 ms) is where great consternation occurs. Here, the physician must understand the normal QTc distribution in normal humanity vs the 1 in 5000 LQTS-affected persons. The significance of a QTc = 450 ms depends on the clinical history. IF 450 ms is documented in an incidental ECG from a teenage female (case vignette 1), this QTc should be NORMAL with an odds ratio of at least 1000:1. On the other hand, if congenital LQTS is established in a family and a relative has a QTc = 450 ms on his/her screening ECG, then the odds ratio is MUCH less favorable because approx 25% of genotyped LQTS patients have a resting QTc < 460 ms (Fig. 5). In fact, 5% to 10% of LQT1 patients had a QTc < 440 ms *(25)*.

Complicating matters further is the observation that LQTS individuals with a normal ECG (i.e., "low-penetrant" LQTS or "concealed" LQTS) can indeed have cardiac events including sudden death *(29)*. Data from the International Registry for LQTS show that 5% of 1345 family members who have a QTc < 440 ms had a cardiac arrest. Garson et al. *(15)* reported that 6% of 287 LQTS patients had a normal QTc. Moss et al. *(30)* reported that syncope and cardiac arrest can occur in approx 5% of LQTS family members who have an apparently normal QT interval. These observations have transformed the overlap zone into the nightmare zone. *Thus, a normal resting QTc (< 450 ms) in a genotype positive LQTS patient does NOT indicate a low-risk patient.* Understanding the overlap zone QTc is foundational to the LQTS evaluation and constitutes one of the major misunderstandings in the clinical evaluation of LQTS.

T-U Wave Abnormalities and T Wave Alternans

Besides manually calculating the QTc, sleuth-like inspection of the morphology of the T waves should also be conducted in a LQTS evaluation. Unusual T waves—wide-based

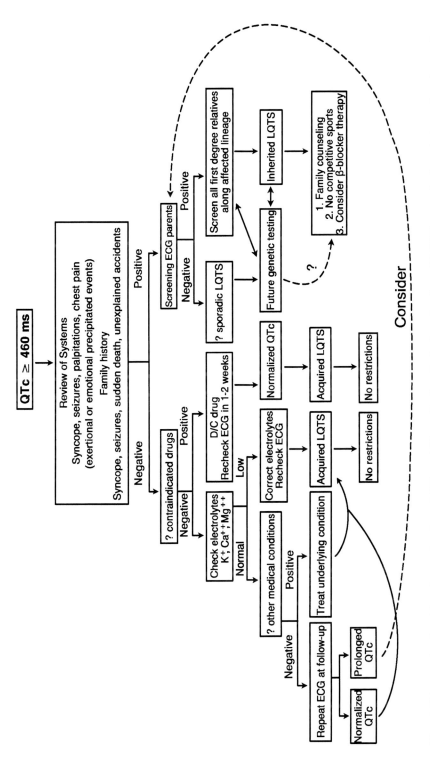

Fig. 4. Diagnostic algorithm for evaluation of QTc > 460 ms. In the clinical evaluation of LQTS, a meticulous independent inspection and calculation of the ECG is vital. Assuming a QTc approaching the upper limits of normal (QTc > 460 ms) is verified, then a sleuth-like review of the personal history and family history is central and critical. Depending on the clues turned up in the investigation, acquired mechanisms versus heritable mechanisms for the QT prolongation are sought. Because obvious QT prolongation in congenital LQTS can be transient, several ECGs may be necessary during the course of the evaluation.

455

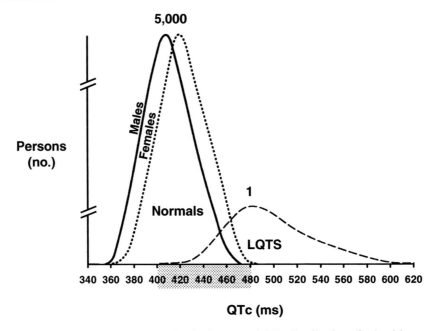

Fig. 5. Distribution of QTc in health and LQTS. Normal QTc distributions for healthy men (solid line) and women (dotted line) are shown as well as the distribution of QTc in LQTS (dashed line). The overlap zone between health and LQTS is indicated in the dotted rectangle. Importantly, the y-axis shows that the QTc distributions are not drawn to scale for the healthy population and the LQTS population. For every one person present in the LQTS profile, there are at least 5000 persons present in the normal male and female QTc profile.

slowly generated, notched, bifids, biphasic, low amplitude humps and bumps on the downslope limb, indistinct termination due to U waves, sinusoidal oscillation, or simply a delayed inscription of normally appearing T waves may lead to the diagnosis of LQTS despite a normal or borderline QTc *(31–33).* These T-wave abnormalities may be particularly evident in the precordial leads. However, great caution must be exercised during inspection of T-wave morphology because T-wave abnormalities can be observed in normal subjects as well although much less commonly than in LQTS patients (15% vs 62%) *(34).* Figure 6A shows a peculiar T wave leading to the diagnosis of LQTS and the subsequent molecular demonstration of a *HERG* defect whereas Fig. 6B shows a "funny" V2 tracing from a genotype-negative 12–yr-old boy in a known *HERG* family. *On their own, "funny" T waves in leads V2 right and V3 in children and adolescents do not equal LQTS.*

In addition, the T-wave morphology may be somewhat gene-specific providing another piece of evidence permitting strategic genotyping *(32,33).* The less common LQT3 patients tend to have a distinctive, late-appearing T wave clearly distinct from the low-amplitude, moderately delayed T wave observed in LQT2. Both of these T-wave profiles are different from the broad-based, prolonged T-wave pattern seen in LQT1. Recently, Lupoglazoff *(35)* classified a notched T wave as a grade 1 (G1) notch when it occurred at or below the apex whatever the amplitude, and as grade 2 (G2) when the protuberance occurred above the apex. G2 notches appear more specific and often reflects a HERG

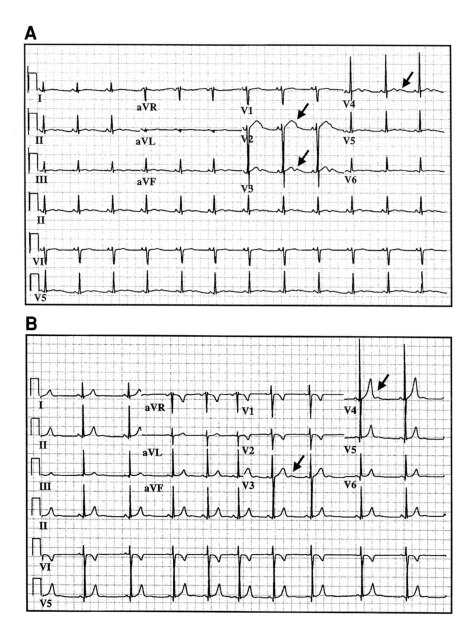

Fig. 6. Electrocardiograms with peculiar T wave morphology. (**A**) Teenager with LQT2 ECG obtained from a 16-yr-old male following a syncopal episode. Arrows indicate notched and bifid T waves in the precordial leads V2–V4. Mutational analyses subsequently confirmed a R366X-HERG mutation (LQT2). (**B**) Unaffected prepubertal boy of a known LQT2 family. Screening ECG obtained on a 12-yr-old boy as part of family evaluation of clinically suspected LQTS. Arrows indicate U waves in V3 and V4 that were considered indicative of LQTS particularly since patient had a previous syncopal episode. However, the boy was found subsequently to be negative for the family's N588D-HERG mutation.

LQT3 by ECG?

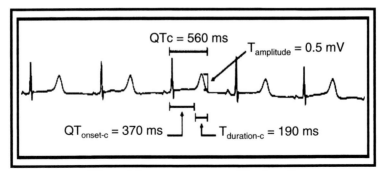

QTc = 560 ms

$T_{amplitude}$ = 0.5 mV

$QT_{onset-c}$ = 370 ms $T_{duration-c}$ = 190 ms

Should we use mexiletine?

Fig. 7. *LQT3*-specific ECG? Previous elegant studies by Moss and colleagues *(32)* and Zhang and colleagues *(33)* have demonstrated gene-specific ECG patterns. This ECG completely recapitulates the LQT3 morphology pattern. However, in this case, the ECG was obtained from a 12-yr-old boy with a F339del-KVLQT1 mutation (LQT1). While recognition of the ECG patterns is an excellent guide for strategic genotyping, treatment decisions should not be rendered based upon the ECG morphology.

(LQT2) genotype (Fig. 6A). *However, treatment decisions should NOT be based on an ECG-suspected LQTS genotype.*

Multiple genetic and acquired factors affecting ventricular repolarization limit the ability to accurately identify genotypes only by T-wave morphology *(32)*. Figure 7 shows a classic *SCN5A* (LQT3) ECG and the question has often been asked at meetings—should treatment include mexiletine? However, the displayed ECG was obtained from a patient with F339del-KVLQT1 (LQT1). Serial ECGs from the same patients have shown T-wave morphologies morphing between all of the ECG patterns. Again, the mandate for careful inspection of T-wave morphology is twofold:

1. Unmask a patient with concealed LQTS—i.e., a normal resting QTc with a peculiar T wave as shown in Fig. 6A.
2. Provide a starting point for the mutational analysis based upon the suggested ECG pattern.

In addition to QTc and T-wave morphology, macrovoltage and microvoltage T wave alternans (TWA) and QT dispersion (QTd) may be informative. TWA is characterized by beat-to-beat alternation of the morphology, amplitude, and/or polarity of the T wave and is a marker of major electrical instability and regional heterogeneity of repolarization and is likely to be associated with an increased risk of cardiac events *(36)*. QTd is defined as the difference between the maximal and minimal QT intervals in the 12 standard leads and may reflect spatial repolarization *(37)*. It has been described as an arrhythmic marker for LQTS. There is evidence that QT dispersion is increased in LQTS patients compared to normal controls *(38,39)*. Moenning et al. *(40)* has confirmed that a significant and independent difference in QT dispersion between mutation carriers and unaffected family members exists. However, a cut-off value of QT dispersion to distinguish LQTS from health is not available.

Holter Monitoring

In patients with a nondiagnostic resting QTc, Holter monitoring may aid in the evaluation of LQTS. Eggleling et al. *(41)* reported 5 of 14 LQTS patients with abnormal findings during a 24-h ambulatory ECG: 2 with TdP, 2 with TWA, and 1 patient with bradycardia owing to an intermittent sino-atrial (SA) block whereas all control subjects had normal ambulatory ECG recordings. Merri et al. *(42)* measured the interval from the R wave to the maximum amplitude of the T wave to represent the heart rate dependency of ventricular repolarization and reported that quantification of the dynamic relation between ventricular repolarization and RR cycle length can be obtained on a large number of Holter-recorded heart beats. Using this assessment of QT dynamicity, LQTS patients have an exaggerated delay in repolarization at long RR cycle lengths. Lupoglazoff et al. *(35)* suggests that Holter recording analysis is superior to the 12-lead ECG in detecting T-wave notches. Again, caution must be exercised with interpreting Holters in a patient with an equivocal history and a borderline QTc. *Here, a Holter-recorded maximum QTc exceeding 500 ms does NOT equal LQTS.* Presently, the normal distribution of 24-h maximal QTc values is poorly understood.

Exercise Testing

Exercise testing may enhance the diagnostic accuracy in LQTS patients with borderline QTc, as inadequate shortening of QTc with increasing heart rate has been observed *(43)*. Swan et al. *(44)* studied 19 LQTS patients and 19 healthy controls undergoing exercise testing. During the recovery phase of exercise, the QT interval lengthened abnormally and the inhomogeneity of repolarization increased in LQTS. LQT2 patients had a lesser degree of QT interval shortening than LQT3 patients in response to increasing heart rate *(45)*. Moreover, LQT1 patients displayed a diminished chronotropic response and exaggerated prolongation of QT interval after exercise. In contrast, the QT interval shortens more in LQT2 than in LQT1 patients when heart rate increases and the sinus nodal rate response is normal *(46)*.

The majority of these studies have been conducted in LQTS patients having a diagnostic QTc at rest and the value of exercise testing in a borderline QTc work-up has not yet been demonstrated. Induction of macrovoltage TWA during exercise is abnormal but is rarely seen in the LQTS evaluation. Whether or not exercise-induced microvoltage TWA will assist in the diagnosis or risk stratification of LQTS remains unclear.

Catecholamine Provocation

The cellular basis for the observed long QT interval is prolongation of the action potential duration, which renders the myocytes vulnerable to early afterrepolarizations (EADs). EADs provide a key initiating mechanism for developing torsade de pointes (TdP). Kawade et al. *(47)* demonstrated that isoprenaline or adrenaline infusions can induce TdP and inversion of the TU wave in LQTS patients. Sun et al. *(48)* demonstrated that epinephrine increased QT dispersion, suggesting that beta-adrenergic stimulation provokes arrhythmias in patients with LQTS by increasing spatial heterogeneity of ventricular repolarization.

Shimizu et al. *(49)* studied the effects of beta-adrenergic agonists in LQT1, LQT2, and LQT3 model of the LQTS and suggested that beta-adrenergic stimulation induces TdP by increasing transmural dispersion of repolarization in LQT1 and LQT2 but suppresses

TdP by decreasing dispersion in LQT3. Finally, Tanabe et al. *(50)* demonstrated that sympathetic stimulation produces a greater increase in both transmural and spatial dispersion of repolarization in LQT1 than in LQT2 but not in control subjects supporting the increased vulnerability to exertional triggers for individuals with LQT1.

These fundamental observations have been exploited recently in the development of an epinephrine provocation challenge for the diagnosis of concealed LQTS *(51)*. Ackerman et al. studied 37 patients with genotyped LQTS (19 LQT1, 15 LQT2, and 3 LQT3) and 27 control subjects at baseline and during gradually increasing rate of intravenous epinephrine infusion at 0.05, 0.1, 0.2, and 0.3 mcg/kg/min. 12-lead ECG was monitored continuously and QT, QTc, and heart rate were measured at each stage. During low dose epinephrine infusion (0.1 mcg/kg/min), all LQT1 patients manifest a paradoxical response to epinephrine with marked prolongation of the absolute QT interval (QT > 50 ms) whereas controls, LQT2, and LQT3 patients tended to shorten their QT intervals (Fig. 8). Epinephrine also triggered T wave alternans and/or nonsustained ventricular tachycardia in 3 of 37 LQTS vs no control subjects. In this study, the resting QTc was nondiagnostic (QTc < 460 ms) in half of the LQT1 patients although the QTc was borderline (> 440 ms) in half of the control subjects. A paradoxical QT response to low dose epinephrine may be pathognomonic for LQT1 distinguishing individuals with concealed LQT1 (normal resting QTc) from normals. Importantly, most of the epinephrine QT stress tests were conducted in the absence of beta-blockers. It is unknown whether or not this LQT1-specific paradoxical response to epinephrine will persist in the presence of beta-blockers. Epinephrine testing does not appear to unmask concealed LQT2 or LQT3.

Molecular Genetics of LQTS and Genetic Testing

At the present time, the molecular breakthroughs of the 1990s have not yet been translated into a routine, clinical molecular diagnostic test for LQTS. A select few LQTS research laboratories perform comprehensive mutational analysis of the five known LQTS genes and work with clinicians in an effort to try to provide a pseudo clinical test until a major technological advance occurs. Presently, the process of mutational analysis is laborious, expensive, and time consuming. Certainly, efforts at strategic genotyping can accelerate this process. For instance, documentation of a personal or family history of a swimming-triggered cardiac event points to LQT1 and a targeted screen for that specific family could yield their *KCNQ1*/KVLQT1 mutation within a week. However, as a general rule, it takes a laboratory 6–12 mo to analyze the five genes for 100 unrelated probands. The majority of mutations detected will be unique further underscoring the pronounced genetic heterogeneity underlying LQTS. To be sure, those families whose LQTS mutation is discovered have their gold standard diagnostic marker to determine unambiguously who does and does not harbor the family's LQTS defect. However, a putative pathogenic mutation will have been discovered for approx 50–60% of the LQTS probands. *Hence, a negative LQTS gene screen does not rule out the diagnosis of LQTS.* Thus, there is no role presently for molecular diagnostic testing in a research laboratory when the clinical evaluation of the proband or family remains equivocal.

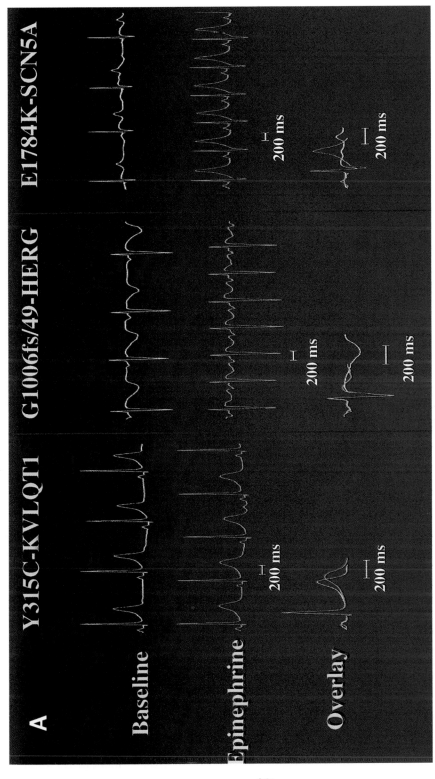

Fig. 8. Epinephrine QT stress test. Depicted are baseline ECG recordings and typical responses during low dose (0.05 to 0.1 mcg/kg/min) epinephrine QT stress testing in LQT1 (left panel), LQT2 (center panel), and LQT3 (right panel) in the absence of beta-blocker therapy. As shown in the overlay on the expanded time scale, LQT1 subjects uniformly exhibit a paradoxical response to epinephrine (i.e., the uncorrected QT interval lengthens) rather than QT-shortening that is seen in LQT2, LQT3, and normals (not shown). Epinephrine provoked QT prolongation is suggestive of an underlying LQT1 genotype and may help to unmask the patient with "concealed" LQTS.

Table 2
Schwartz Score for LQTS Diagnostic Criteria

Variable	Points
ECG findings	
QTc[a] (ms)	
480	3
460–470	2
450 (in males)	1
Torsades de pointes	2
T-wave alternans (macroscopic)	1
Notched T wave in 3 leads	1
Low heart rate for age[b]	0.5
Clinical History	
Syncope	
With stress	2
Without stress	1
Congenital deafness	0.5
Family History[c]	
Family members with definite LQTS[d]	1
Unexplained sudden cardiac death < age	0.5
30 yr among immediate family members	

[a]QTc calculated using Bazett's formula (QTc = QT/square root RR)
[b]Resting heart rate below the second percentile for age
[c]The same family member cannot be counted in both
[d]Definite LQTS is defined by a Schwartz score 4

DIAGNOSIS OF LQTS

Schwartz et al. *(52)* proposed the first diagnostic criteria for LQTS in 1985, that included the following major criteria: QTc > 440 ms, stress induced syncope, family members with LQTS, and minor criteria: Congenital deafness, episodes of T-wave alternans, low heart rate (in children), and abnormal ventricular repolarization. As discussed previously, more recent understanding of the overlap zone between LQTS and health has rendered this cut-off value of 440 ms a major limitation of the original Schwartz score.

A modified Schwartz score containing new criteria and a point system based upon a range of QTc values and the clinical/family history was formulated in 1993 (Table 2) *(53)*. The modified "Schwartz score" ranges from 0 to 9 and contains 3 diagnostic probabilities: 1: low probability of LQTS; 2 or 3: intermediate probability of LQTS; and 4: high probability of LQTS. Although the positive predictive value of a modified Schwartz score 4 approaches 100%, the presence of low penetrance LQTS or concealed LQTS continues to plague even a composite score.

Penetrance, defined as the ratio between patients with the clinical phenotype (QT prolongation, symptoms, and so on) and the total number of family member carriers of the mutation identified in the LQTS proband may be as low as 25% in LQTS. Priori et al. *(29)* also found that of 46 family members considered on clinical grounds to be normal, 15 (33%) were found to be gene carriers, so conventional clinical criteria had a sensitivity of only 38% in correctly identifying carriers of the genetic defect. *Thus, in the evaluation of first degree relatives of a definitely affected LQTS proband, it is no longer acceptable to exclude LQTS among individuals harboring an equivocal QTc.*

There are four clinical scenarios concerning to the diagnosis of LQTS. The first situation is the patient who presents with symptoms such as syncope, seizures, and cardiac arrest and a "Schwartz score" 4. Here, genetic testing is not necessary for the diagnosis. However, knowing the genotype may assist in the treatment plan owing to genotype specific LQTS disease.

The second scenario is a symptomatic patient who has a normal/borderline QTc (460 ms). The diagnosis based on clinical criteria is borderline or questionable (score = 2 or 3). In this situation, serial ECGs should be performed since the QTc value in LQTS patients may vary from time to time. Furthermore, a careful inquiry about family history of sudden death as well as screening ECGs from other family members may be informative. Exercise testing and Holter monitoring should be performed, although the positive predictive value is small. An epinephrine QT stress test looking for a paradoxical response (QT prolongation with low dose epinephrine) may unmask LQT1 patients. Finally, although the genetic testing is not yet widely available in many centers, genetic testing could be very helpful in making the diagnosis. The identification of a mutated LQTS gene would confirm the diagnosis and the management could be initiated properly. Again however, the failure to identify a mutation certainly does not rule out the diagnosis because 40% of LQTS remains genetically elusive.

The third scenario is an apparently asymptomatic relative of a definite LQTS proband. As we concluded earlier, it is no longer acceptable to exclude LQTS among family members of definitely affected patients because of an equivocal QTc. Here lies perhaps the greatest potential value of molecular diagnostic testing, the unambiguous classification of asymptomatic family members.

The last scenario is the screening ECG in asymptomatic patients found incidentally to have an equivocal QTc. As discussed earlier, normal healthy persons have overlapping QTc with LQTS patients, so one cannot rely only on the ECG to discriminate between health and LQTS with an overlapping QTc (Fig. 5). Moreover, there are many drugs and conditions that cause acquired prolongation of QT (Table 3). In this situation, strong reassurance can usually be given and no further investigation is needed generally except perhaps repeating the ECG and obtaining screening ECGs on the parents.

RISK STRATIFICATION

Risk stratification in LQTS is clinically vital and exceedingly difficult. The phenotypic expression of LQTS varies profoundly from asymptomatic longevity to premature sudden cardiac death despite medical therapy. The great challenge is to discern which of these divergent outcomes is most likely in each of our patients. Occurrence of a LQTS-related cardiac event like syncope before five years of age suggests a serious LQTS phenotype and syncope occurring in the first year of life is associated with an extremely poor prognosis *(54)*. Overall among LQTS patients, the risk of cardiac events is higher in males until puberty and higher in females during adulthood *(13)*. Males who are still asymptomatic at age 20 yr may be considered at a lower (but not zero) risk for sudden cardiac death. Females still have the same risk for cardiac events in adulthood and may be at increased vulnerability to an arrhythmic event during the postpartum period *(55)*.

Table 3
Causes of Acquired QT Prolongation

Drugs

Antiarrhythmics (amiodarone, bretylium, disopyramide, dofetilide, flecainide, ibutilide, N-acetylprocainamide, pirmenol, procainamide, quinidine, sematilide, sotalol, tedisamil)
Antibiotics/Antifungals/Antivirals (amantadine, amphotericin, azithromycin, chloroquine, clarithromycin, clindamycin, cotrimoxozole, erythromycin, fluconazole, foscarnet, gatifloxacin, grepafloxacin, halofantrine, itraconazole, ketoconazole, levofloxacin, moxifloxacin, pentamidine, sparfloxacin, spiramycin, TMP-SMX, troleandomycin)
Anticancer agents (arsenic trioxide, tamoxifen)
Anticonvulsants (fosphenytoin)
Antidepressants (amitriptyline, citalopram, desipramine, doxepin, fluoxetine, imipramine, maprotiline, sertraline, venlafaxine)
Antiemetics (chlorpromazine, compazine, dolasetron)
Antihistamines (astemizole, clemastine, diphenhydramine, hydroxyzine, terfenadine)
Antihypertensives (isradipine, moexipril, nicardipine)
Antipsychotics (chlorpromazine, haloperidol, mesoridazine, pimozide, quetiapine, risperidone, thioridazine, ziprasidone)
Gastrointestinal stimulants (cisapride)
Homeopathic agents (cesium chloride)
Lipid lowering agents (probucol)
Migraine treatments (naratriptan, sumatriptan, zolmitriptan)
Organophosphate insecticides
Sedatives (droperidol)

Electrolyte derangements

Acute hypokalemia (associated with diuretics, hyperventilation)
Chronic hypocalcemia
Chronic hypokalemia
Chronic hypomagnesemia

Medical conditions

Arrhythmias (complete atrioventricular block, severe bradycardia, sick sinus syndrome)
Cardiac (myocarditis, tumors)
Endocrine (diabetes, hyperparathyroidism, hypothyroidism, pheochromocytoma)
Neurologic (cerebrovascular accident, encephalitis, head trauma, subarachnoid hemorrhage)
Nutritional (acute weight loss, alcoholism, anorexia nervosa, liquid protein diet, starvation, obesity)

Among the known LQTS genotypes, individuals with LQT1 appear to be more frequent fainters who less commonly die whereas LQT3 individuals infrequently faint but appear to have the highest lethality rate per cardiac event *(14)*. The recessive variant is associated with very early clinical manifestations and a poorer prognosis than autosomal dominant Romano-Ward LQTS *(54)*. Marks et al. *(56)* reported a different genetic variant of LQTS manifesting syndactyly in addition to QT interval prolongation and observed a poor prognosis with this rare LQTS phenotype.

A history of cardiac arrest increases the probability of a cardiac arrest or sudden cardiac death at follow-up *(57)*. A negative family history for sudden cardiac death cannot be regarded as a predictor of favorable outcome, on the other hand, a family history of sudden cardiac arrest may indicate an increase risk to other family members *(54)*. A markedly prolonged QT interval (i.e., QTc > 600 ms) is associated with the greater risk for cardiac events but only a minority of LQTS patients manifest this degree of QT prolongation *(30)*. Unfortunately, there does not appear to be a linear relationship between clinical risk and degree of QT prolongation. Indeed, patients with a QTc < 440 ms can have syncope or even cardiac arrest (5% of family members of LQTS) *(58)*.

T-wave notching or humps appear to be more common in symptomatic patients and may be of prognostic significance *(34)*. QT dispersion may be associated with high risk. QT dispersion > 100 ms and a lack of shortening following a beta-blocker therapy are associated with risk factors for recurrent cardiac events *(39)*. Beat-to-beat repolarization lability may identify patients with sudden cardiac death and predict arrhythmia-free survival *(59)*. Various methods quantifying T-wave morphology have been developed based on observations that T-wave morphology is a reflection of repolarization wavefronts in the myocardium *(60)*. T-wave spectral variance (TWSV) index, a new method to assess beat-to-beat variability of the T wave, revealed increased heterogeneity of repolarization in patients prone to both VT and VF *(61)*. Macroscopic TWA on the 12-lead ECG is a marker of severe electrical instability in LQTS *(31,36)*. However, quantitation of the actual risk of sudden cardiac death associated with TWA is still uncertain and visible TWA is an infrequent sighting in the LQTS evaluation *(54)*. There appears to be no role for invasive electrophysiology studies in LQTS risk stratification as most LQTS patients are not inducible during programmed electrical stimulation *(62)*.

Microvoltage T wave alternans (μV-TWA) at low heart rate (HR) is a marker of arrhythmic risk in many conditions, but its significance in LQTS has not been established. μV-TWA is classified as abnormal if there is sustained alternans of at least 1.9 μV, lasting for at least one minute and consistently present while heart rate exceeds some patient-specific heart rate threshold value (< 110 beats/min), with noise 1.8 μV, alternans-to noise ratio 3, and ectopics 10% *(63)*. Kaufman et al. *(64)* observed sustained μV-TWA only among a minority of LQTS subjects and concluded that sustained μV-TWA was a specific (100%) but insensitive (18%) marker for LQTS, but it may hold promise as a predictor of individual susceptibility to arrhythmias. Using catecholamine provocation with dobutamine instead of exercise stress testing, we have demonstrated that μV-TWA occurs at lower heart rates in patients with LQTS than in healthy people but that it may fail to identify high-risk subjects *(65)*.

In contrast to catecholamine-induced μV-TWA, we have described and quantitated macroscopic nonalternating, beat-to-beat lability in T-wave amplitude and morphology during catecholamine stress testing with dobutamine (Fig. 9) *(66)*. This lability was quantified using a newly derived T-wave lability index (TWLI) based on a determination of the root-mean-square of the differences in T-wave amplitude at each isochronic point. The TWLI was significantly higher in LQTS and marked T wave lability (TWLI 0.095) was detected in all three LQTS genotypes (10/23), but in no control subjects. Importantly, all high-risk patients having either a history of out-of-hospital cardiac arrest or syncope plus at least one sudden death in the family had TWLI 0.095. Future studies are needed to determine whether or not such catecholamine provoked T-wave lability identifies patients harboring high-risk genetic substrates.

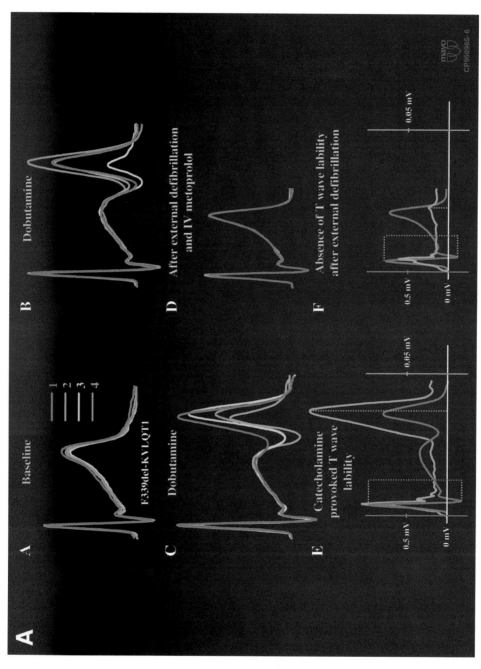

Fig. 9. Catecholamine provocation and T-wave lability **9A.** Presence of dobutamine provoked nonalternating, beat-to beat T-wave lability and quantification of TWLI. Four consecutive QRST complexes from lead V4 are overlayed to demonstrate T-wave lability. The sequence of the complexes is color-coded. **(A)** At rest, the T-wave morphology is nearly uniform, with only minimal fluctuation involving the magnitude of the peak of the T wave.

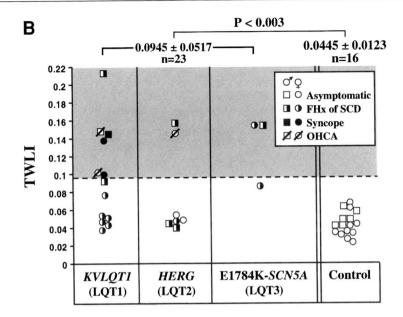

Fig. 9. *(Continued)* (**B and C**) During dobutamine infusion at 10 μg/kg/min, there is marked beat-to-beat T-wave variability particularly in the morphology of the second component of the T wave. (**D**) Ten minutes after defibrillation, the T-wave morphologies are essentially superimposable. (**E**) Quantification of T-wave lability present during dobutamine infusion at 10 μg/kg/min (**B and C**). The red curve shows signal averaged QRST complex. The green curve plots the root-mean-square differences for each isochronic point. The dotted vertical green line indicates the highest variability of repolarization. It is normalized for the span of the QRS complex (dotted vertical red line) to calculate TWLI. The time interval between the red and the green y-axis is 840 ms. Notice that the y-axis scale is expanded for the root-mean-square values. Here, the TWLI equals 0.148 indicating that the beat-to-beat T wave variability is nearly 15% of the magnitude of the total QRS voltage. Note that the maximum variability occurs after the peak of the T wave. (**F**) Corresponding data 10 min following defibrillation. The maximal T wave variability (dotted vertical green line) is reduced strikingly (TWLI = 0.026).

9B. Summary of TWLI in LQTS and in control. The study subjects are distinguished on the x-axis by LQTS genotype or control. Each individual's sex is indicated by square (males) or circles (females). Open symbols denote a negative personal and family history. Partially filled symbols indicate a positive family history SUD or aborted cardiac arrest. Filled symbols indicate a personal history of syncope. Finally, symbols with a slash through it identify those subjects who experienced an out-of-hospital cardiac arrest (OHCA). TWLI in LQTS patients is significantly higher than in normal subjects (0.0945 ± 0.0517 vs 0.0445 ± 0.0123, respectively; *p* < 0.003).

Table 4 summarizes the recent recommendations for risk stratification for sudden cardiac death in LQTS from the task force report on sudden cardiac death of the European Society of Cardiology *(54)*.

MANAGEMENT

All Symptomatic Patients with LQTS Require Treatment

The risk of sudden death without treatment is unacceptably too high. It has been estimated that the mortality without treatment is 20% in the first year after presenting with

Table 4
Recommendations for Risk Stratification Sudden Cardiac Death: Long QT Syndrome

	Recommendations	Level of evidence	Reference
Syncope	Class I	B	(30)
TdP/VF/CA	Class I	B	(30)
JLN recessive trait	Class I	B	(14,30)
LQT3 genetic variant	Class I	C	(14,22)
QTc > 600 ms	Class II a	C	(30)
Cardiac events in infants	Class II a	O	
Postpartum period	Class II a	C	(55)
Female sex	Class II a	C	(13)
Syndactyly and AV block	Class II a	C	(56)
T wave alternans (macroscopic)	Class II a	C	(36)
Family history	Class II b	O	
QT dispersion	Class II b	C	(39)
Programmed electrical stimulation	Class III	C	(62)

Class I = Conditions for which there is evidence and/or general agreement that a given procedure (risk stratification parameter) is useful and effective.

Class II = Conditions for which there is conflicting evidence and/or a divergence of opinion about the usefulness/efficacy of the procedure or treatment (or risk stratification parameter).

II a: weight of evidence/opinion is in favor of usefulness/efficacy.

II b: usefulness/efficacy is less well established by evidence/opinion.

Class III = Conditions for which there is evidence or general agreement that a given procedure/treatment is not useful/effective.

Evidence A = Data derived from multiple randomized clinical trials or meta-analyses.

Evidence B = Data derived from single randomized trials or non-randomized studies.

Evidence C = Consensus opinion of the experts.

Evidence O = Opinion of the Task Force Panel.

a LQTS-related event, syncope, seizures, or aborted cardiac arrest and 50% within 10 years of presentation.

On the other hand, the necessity for and approach to treating asymptomatic patients is less straightforward. In 1993, Garson et al. (15) reported that cardiac arrest was the sentinel event in 9% of LQTS patients. Further, 12% of patients who were asymptomatic at the time of diagnosis later developed symptoms including sudden death in 4% indicating the need for universal treatment of all LQTS patients, both symptomatic and asymptomatic. More recently, Priori et al. (67) suggested that all *young* asymptomatic patients should be treated because sudden death as the sentinel event has been documented too frequently. Schwartz (68) recommended treatment for the following asymptomatic LQTS patients: Neonates and infants, affected siblings of children who have died suddenly, patients with manifest T-wave alternans, patients with QTc > 600 ms, JLN-form of LQTS, and when there is anxiety or an explicit request for treatment in a family after thorough explanation.

Ackerman (4) recommended that after a patient with LQTS has been diagnosed, all first- and second-degree relatives must be screened, a cardiologist must be involved in the care of families with LQTS, symptomatic patients must be treated, and treatment options must be considered carefully in asymptomatic patients. We recommend that asymptomatic patients with LQTS should be provided LQTS therapy if

1. QTc > 550 ms.
2. LQT3 genotype.
3. Younger age at diagnosis (< 40 yr).
4. Family history of sudden cardiac death from LQTS.
5. Particular type of LQTS: Associated with congenital deafness (JLN) or associated with syndactyly.
6. T-wave alternans, TWLI > 9.5%.

To be sure, many patients with LQTS harbor a long QT dud rather than a ticking time bomb and are destined for asymptomatic longevity. In fact, there are many LQTS patients who require *no* therapy. However, until clinical testing reveals the virtually No Risk patient, near universal treatment will continue to be the prudent recommendation.

Debate will continue over when an asymptomatic patient is no longer young and has out-grown his/her LQTS risk such that no medical therapy is necessary. All LQTS investigators have a collection of patients who experienced their sentinel event in their 30s, 40s, 50s, and even 60s such that suggesting any age as a cut-off in the decision for prophylactic therapy in an asymptomatic patient seems arbitrary. Besides, this may be a mute point as the standard therapy for LQTS, i.e., beta-blocker therapy, may prolong life in older persons independent of its protective effect in LQTS providing an excuse/rationale for a universal treatment recommendation.

At a minimum, all LQTS patients must avoid drugs known to exacerbate the QT interval interval (Table 3). There are three excellent websites: www.qtdrugs.org, www.care.edu, and www.sads.org, that provide a more comprehensive list of potentially contraindicated medications. In addition, LQTS patients should ask their physician or pharmacist to perform a "QT safety check" on any intended prescription by searching a database like Micromedex to obtain recent information. For some, such drug exposure may be the only thing lying in wait to detonate their LQTS bomb. Occasionally, the patient will need a medicine that is on one of those contraindicated lists and the physician-patient must carefully consider the risks and benefits. If there is a reasonable alternative medication with similar efficacy, then the decision is simple. However, one area of great difficulty pertains to the treatment of concomitant depression. Here, most of the selective serotonin reuptake inhibitors (SSRIs) have documentation of a QT prolonging potential and are all on those lists of medications to avoid. In such instances, the physician must weigh carefully the evidence for this potential side effect and determine, in the context of treating the whole person, what constitutes the best risk-benefit decision.

Another prudent measure is the avoidance of competitive sports as competition brings together the key triggers that threaten the long QT heart, the fight-flight-fright response *(69)*. However, this competitive sports prohibition is arguably the single biggest issue facing the families of children and adolescents diagnosed with LQTS. There is no doubt that competitive sports pose no risk to some patients with LQTS. Unfortunately once again, clinical testing cannot determine which ones and hence the universal restriction. On the other hand, most LQTS experts support participation in recreational sports in moderate exertion in properly treated LQTS patients. Here, there is a bit of logical inconsistency behind prohibiting competitive sports whereas permitting recreational activities perhaps secondary to liability considerations. Clearly, there are known, predictable adverse health consequences for the obese, sedentary individual and encouraging an active, normal life for LQTS patients should be the goal.

The ultimate goal for the treatment of LQTS is to prevent sudden cardiac death secondary to a long QT heart that degenerates into polymorphic ventricular tachycardia and fails to spontaneously convert back to normal sinus rhythm. Currently, the treatment options for inherited LQTS included β-blocker therapy, implantable cardioverter-defibrillator (ICD), continuous pacing, a surgical procedure involving a left cervicothoracic sympathectomy, and genotype-directed therapy.

β-BLOCKER THERAPY

β-blocker therapy remains the principle therapy for most LQTS *(52,57)*. Although not a randomized study, β-blockers appear to decrease mortality from 71% in historical controls to 6% in a treated group *(68)*. A study from the Pediatric Electrophysiology Society demonstrated that β-blockers were effective in decreasing symptoms, ventricular arrhythmias, and sudden death *(15)*. Moss et al. *(57)* studied 869 LQTS patients treated with β-blocker noting a marked beneficial effect with a significant reduction in cardiac events including sudden death. It is generally thought that all beta-blockers are equally protective with propranolol 2–4 mg/kg/day, nadolol 0.5–1.0 mg/kg/day, metoprolol 0.5–1.0 mg/kg/day, and atenolol 0.5–1.0 mg/kg/day being most commonly used. These are not trivial doses of beta-blockers and a commonly observed mistake is inadequate dosing (homeopathic doses).

Unfortunately, β-blocker therapy does not eliminate the risk of sudden cardiac death completely *(70,71)*. Moss et al. *(57)* uncovered several risk factors for "breakthrough" cardiac events during prescribed β-blocker therapy. These factors were younger age (especially < 5 yr) and syncope or aborted cardiac arrest documented before drugs were started. Concerning death after starting β-blocker therapy; two-thirds of deaths were females, mean QTc value among fatal cases was slightly longer, β-blocker therapy mostly started before adolescence and 79% had one or more cardiac events before starting drugs. These results indicate that patients who had symptoms before β-blocker therapy have a high probability of having recurrent cardiac events (32% within 5 yr) despite being on β-blocker. Moreover, 14% of patients with an aborted cardiac arrest before β-blockers are expected to have recurrent cardiac arrest or death within five years while on therapy.

The appropriate or optimal dose of β-blockers in the treatment of LQTS is still uncertain. Noncompliance with β-blocker therapy is a risk factor for increased mortality in LQTS patients *(15)*. Compliance issues and adequacy of dose can be monitored by trough levels of drug in the case of propanolol, 24-h ambulatory monitoring to ensure a sufficient decrease in heart rate, exercise stress testing to demonstrate satisfactory blunting (~ 25–40%) in chronotropic response to exercise, and measuring QT dispersion. Priori et al. showed that a QT dispersion <100 ms during β-blockers was 80% sensitive and 82% specific in discriminating patients responsive to β-blockers from nonresponders *(39)*. Thus, the persistence of QT dispersion > 100 ms after β-blocker therapy is one possible marker denoting high risk and the need to proceed to other modalities of treatment.

Since some patients probably do not need beta-blockers (again we do not know which ones), all beta-blockers are likely to appear similarly effective. However, we have reviewed beta-blocker therapy failures in genotyped LQTS probands and found that 75% of the breakthrough events occurred while the patient was taking atenolol (unpublished data). In a previous study on the long-term follow-up of 37 patients treated with beta-blockers and continuous pacing, there were 6 compliant individuals with a sudden death or aborted sudden death and 5 of the 6 were on 50–200 mg/day of atenolol *(71)*. Whether or not these patients were dosed once or twice-a-day is not known. Nonetheless, although perhaps the best tolerated beta-blocker, atenolol may not afford adequate protection at least for symptomatic LQTS patients. At a minimum, proper dosing schedules must be adhered to carefully for atenolol as the pharmacokinetic properties of atenolol dictate a twice-a-day regimen rather than once-a-day. While many patients tolerate beta-blockers without difficulty, a significant minority find the side effects of fatigue, decreased attention, and depressed affect an unacceptable daily trade-off for the medicine's intended once in a lifetime treatment effect, prevention of sudden death.

The precise mechanism underlying the protective effect of β-blocker therapy in LQTS remain unclear. Activation of the β-adrenergic receptor elicits a signal transduction cascade that increases cyclic adenosine monophosphate (cAMP) and activates cAMP-dependent phosphorylation events mediated by protein kinase A. Both these intracellular second messengers seem to enhance the function of several types of cardiac ion channels including the I_{Na}, L-type calcium, potassium and even chloride channels. Interestingly, HERG, the potassium channel responsible for LQT2, has a cyclic nucleotide-binding domain. Investigators have postulated that cAMP may also activate HERG *(72)*. Recall that activation of HERG increases the net outward current and provides increasing repolarization force. In LQTS, a mutant ion channel disrupts the delicate balance normally occurring with enhanced sympathetic tone. Such a perturbation in the cardiac potassium channels (LQT1 and LQT2) could allow a predominant effect of adrenergic influence on the L-type calcium channel, facilitating calcium channel-mediated EADs. Conceivably, β-blockers may restore the balance of channel forces by interrupting the β-adrenergic receptor-mediated enhancement of L-type calcium channels.

Because of this possible mechanism, calcium channel blockers such as verapamil may be acceptable alternative pharmacotherapy for patients unable to tolerate β-blocker therapy (for example, those with asthma). To date, no studies have compared β-blockers with calcium channel blockers in the treatment of LQTS. Experimentally, however, verapamil has been demonstrated to eliminate or reduce EADs significantly and suppress TdP in patients with LQTS who underwent challenge with epinephrine infusion *(73)*. Shimizu et al. *(74)* showed in a canine model that chromanol 293B (an I_{Ks} blocker) was not sufficient to induce TdP but that the addition of a β-agonist was highly arrhythmogenic, likely by increasing transmural dispersion of repolarization. Shimizu et al. *(75)* also demonstrated that the addition of propranolol completely reversed the effect of epinephrine in prolongation of the QT interval and increasing the dispersion in LQT1 patients.

In conclusion, β-blocker therapy is effective in the treatment of LQTS, but fails to eliminate the risk of sudden death. Depending on the clinical presentation (aborted cardiac arrest as sentinel event for example), occurrence of breakthrough events despite compliance and adequate dosing, or experiencing unacceptable side effects, other LQTS therapies might be indicated such as an ICD, pacemaker, or in very rare cases, a left cervicothoracic sympathectomy.

Implantable Cardioverter-Defibrillator (ICD) Therapy

Gronefeld et al. *(76)* reported a 29-yr-old female with LQTS who was treated with propranolol and also received an ICD as primary prevention. During the next 17 mo, the patient was asymptomatic. After skipping her propranolol for three days, she had several syncopal spells: A total of 55 nonsustained runs of ventricular tachycardia and 16 sustained episodes that were correctly identified and successfully terminated by the device.

Groh et al. *(77)* reported 35 cases of LQTS in ICD to evaluate the use, efficacy, and safety of this device. Most of these patients had aborted sudden cardiac death before the implantation of ICD and the remaining presented with syncope or symptomatic ventricular arrhythmia. In this high-risk group, 60% of the patients had at least one appropriate ICD discharge during a mean follow-up of 31 mo. No deaths occurred during follow-up. However, the ICDs were not free of complications: pneumothorax (6%), postpericardiotomy syndrome (3%), and prolonged incisional pain (3%). A main concern about the ICD especially in the pediatric population is the emotional stress associated with the fear of device and pain associated with the initial ICD discharge, which can trigger arrhythmia. The size of device itself may limit its use in very small children.

In conclusion, the ICD device can protect sudden death in high-risk LQTS patients but it does not alter the underlying substrate leading to arrhythmia. ACC/AHA practice guideline recommends *(78)* the use of the ICD in LQTS patients who have recurrent syncope, sustained ventricular arrhythmia or sudden aborted cardiac arrest despite adequate drug therapy (secondary prevention). Furthermore, primary prevention ICD therapy should be considered when

1. The initial presentation involves aborted cardiac arrest.
2. There is a strong family history of sudden cardiac death.
3. Compliance or intolerance to β-blocker therapy is a concern.
4. When the underlying genotype is LQT3.

Of these considerations for primary ICD therapy, the latter suggestion is most controversial. Based upon studies from the International LQTS Registry, LQT3 is associated with fewer cardiac events but higher lethality per cardiac event and beta-blockers did not appear to have any protective effect *(22,57)*. Thus, there does not appear to be an established pharmacologic therapy to reduce the sudden death risk associated with LQT3. Initial studies with mexiletine demonstrated that the QTc shortened in LQT3 patients *(45)*. However, no studies have demonstrated a reduction in sudden death in LQT3. At the present time then, only ICD therapy can provide such protection.

PACEMAKER THERAPY

Viskin et al. *(79)* demonstrated that spontaneous arrhythmias in the congenital LQTS are often pause dependent. Overall, LQTS patients have slower resting heart rates than normal subjects, particularly LQT3 patients. Moreover, β-blocker therapy can cause profound bradycardia and sinus pauses. For these reasons, cardiac pacing in conjunction with β-blocker therapy has been shown to be beneficial in preventing pause-dependent TdP *(70,71)*. However, cardiac pacing should be used as an adjunct to β-blocker therapy, not as a sole therapy, in treatment of LQTS patients who have preexisting atrioventricular block or evidence of pause-dependent arrhythmias. Furthermore, concomitant beta-blocker therapy and continuous pacing has failed to reduce the sudden death risk in symptomatic patients significantly *(71)*. *Thus, if a pacing strategy is considered, the implanted device should include an ICD.*

LEFT CERVICOTHORACIC SYMPATHETECTOMY

The concept of imbalance in cardiac sympathetic innervation in LQTS *(80)* (overactivity of the left stellate ganglion and decreased right stellate ganglion activity) gave rise to the left cervicothoracic sympathetectomy. Moss et al. *(81)* first reported left cervicothoracic sympathetic ganglionectomy to treat symptomatic LQTS patients refractory to β-blockers. Schwartz *(68)* reported 123 patients who underwent left cervicothoracic sympathetic denervation with a mean follow-up period of 10 yr. All of these patients were unresponsive to or did not tolerate β-blocker therapy. A marked decrease in the number of patients with cardiac events (99% to 45%) and in the number of cardiac events per patient (21 ± 31 to 1 ± 3) after the surgical procedure was observed. Most of the patients who still had cardiac events after surgery had only one, usually during the first six mo. The total incidence of sudden death was 8% in 10 yr and the five-year survival rate was 94%. Despite the apparent success associated with the left cervicothoracic sympathectomy, this surgical procedure is performed rarely in the management of LQTS.

GENE-SPECIFIC THERAPY

Future therapeutic approaches to LQTS may someday involve gene-specific or mutation-specific strategies. Schwartz et al. (45) first demonstrated that the sodium channel blocker, mexiletine, significantly shortened the QTc and normalized the morphology of the T wave in patients with SCN5A mutations (LQT3). In contrast, LQT2 patients had no change in the QTc with mexiletine. In this study, patients with SCN5A defects were also demonstrated to have significant shortening of their QT intervals with increased heart rate.

Given that patients with SCN5A defects are more likely to have syncope and sudden death during sleep and bradycardia *(14)*, LQT3 patients might be best treated with mexiletine and if needed, atrial pacing instead of β-blocker therapy which results in bradycardia and may cause detrimental events in these patients. However, QT shortening cannot be equated with reduction in risk of sudden death. There is no data currently demonstrating that mexiletine either decreases the number of cardiac events or improves survival.

The potential role of sodium channel blockers like mexiletine in LQTS are not completely understood and may not be specific only to LQT3. Shimizu et al. *(74,82)* used an arterially perfused canine left ventricular wedge preparation and developed pharmacologically induced animal models of LQT1, LQT2, and LQT3, using chromosomal 293B, d-sotalol and ATX-II respectively. In these LQTS models, mexiletine effectively reduced dispersion and prevented TdP in both LQT2 and LQT3 *(82)*. In addition, mexiletine abbreviated the action potential duration of M cells more than that of epicardium and endocardium, thus diminishing transmural dispersion and the effect of isoproterenol to induce TdP in LQT1 models *(74)*. Mexiletine may have an adjunctive role with β-blocker therapy and its beneficial or long-term effects warrant further investigation.

Regarding potassium channel targeted interventions, Compton et al. *(83)* showed that increasing extracellular potassium levels to about 1.5 mEq/L above baseline with spironolactone, potassium chloride intravenous infusion, and oral potassium chloride supplementation resulted in a 24% reduction in the QTc in seven patients with LQT2, compared with 4% in five healthy control subjects and resolved the characteristic notched T wave abnormality. Shimizu et al. *(75,84)* demonstrated the benefit of nicorandil, an opener of the ATP-sensitive potassium channel, in a canine model of LQT1 and LQT2. Nicorandil reduced repolarization dispersion and prevented TdP in models of LQT1 and LQT2 but not LQT3. Nicorandil has also been reported to be effective in a patient with LQTS whose syncopal attacks were refractory to β-blocker therapy.

Currently, β-blocker therapy and ICD therapy are the chief treatment modalities in LQTS. As the arrhythmogenic mechanisms underlying the various LQTS genotypes are dissected, perhaps β-blocker therapy will be one day replaced by genotype or mutation-specific potassium channel-targeted interventions for patients with LQT1 and LQT2 or sodium channel-targeted interventions for those with LQT3.

CASE VIGNETTES REVISITED

Having considered the clinical evaluation, risk stratification, and management of congenital LQTS, the 3 case vignettes are now revisited and the approach to each case summarized.

Case #1: What Is a Diagnostic QTc?

JPA is a 15-yr-old female referred for a second opinion following the diagnosis of possible LQTS. At a preparticipation sports physical, an innocent murmur was heard, an ECG demonstrated a QTc of 450 ms, and subsequent exercise testing reported that the QT interval failed to shorten appropriately during exercise. By history, the patient and family history was completely negative. No ECGs were performed on the parents. The patient was diagnosed with borderline QT prolongation, possible LQTS, placed on once-a-day atenolol beta-blocker therapy, and restricted from all competitive sports.

Analysis: An incidental QTc of 450 ms will be normal with an odds ratio of approximately 1000-to-1. If any further evaluation is needed, ECGs from the parents is perhaps the most helpful. In this case, the mother's QTc was 410 ms and the father's QTc was 390 ms. JPA was dismissed as normal with no restrictions. If a diagnosis of LQTS were present, atenolol if selected as the beta-blocker must be dosed twice-a-day.

Case #2: Does My 13-yr-Old Have What Killed My 17-yr-Old Son? Evaluation of Sudden Unexplained Death

SH was a 17-yr-old previously healthy male found dead in bed. Standard medico-legal autopsy was negative. His younger brother was brought for a second opinion to determine whether or not he was at risk. This 13-yr-old boy was asymptomatic, his QTc was 430 ms, Holter recorded no significant ventricular ectopy, and exercise stress test was unremarkable. Would you perform any additional tests or dismiss as normal?

Analysis: An unexplained, autopsy-negative sudden death demands careful scrutiny. The autopsy report must be carefully reviewed. Here, it remained uninformative. A meticulous family history must be taken. In this case, 4 physician encounters later it was uncovered that the decedent's mother fell from the top of a 3-meter diving board decades ago. Based upon this clue, the mother and surviving son were evaluated by echocardiography (negative), electrocardiograms (QTc = 420 ms and 430 ms in mother and son), 24-h ambulatory monitoring (negative), and exercise stress testing (negative). Finally, an epinephrine QT stress test elicited a paradoxical response to epinephrine in the mother (Fig. 8). Mutational analysis established the LQT1 genotype in the mother and surviving son. A molecular autopsy confirmed the *KVLQT1* mutation in the decedent *(85)*.

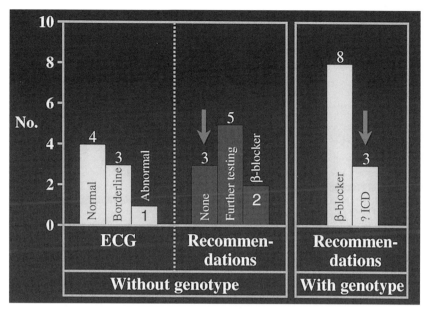

Fig. 10. Impact of molecular diagnostic testing. Summarized are the impressions and recommendations from eight electrophysiologists regarding the ECG from an 18-yr-old sibling of a LQTS proband who presented with an ultimately fatal near drowning as her sentinel event. Molecular autopsy identified a KVLQT1 mutation. The profound impact of the molecular diagnostic test is seen. This sibling's QTc was 448 ms with normal appearing T waves (not shown). Accordingly, without the genotype information, only 1 of the 8 electrophysiologists felt that the ECG was abnormal and 2 of the 8 recommended prophylactic beta-blocker therapy. With revelation that she in fact possessed the 9 base pair deletion resulting in an in-frame deletion of 3 amino acids in the cytoplasmic N-terminal region of KVLQT1 (i.e., mutation positive), all 8 would now recommend beta-blocker therapy and 3 would strongly consider a prophylactic ICD implant. The point—correctly or incorrectly, the genetic test alone changed the recommended intervention profoundly from dismiss as normal in 3 to implant a defibrillator in 3.

Case #3: To Implant or Not to Implant? That Is the Question.

NCK is an asymptomatic 18-yr-old female whose sister died following a near-drowning, her sentinel event for LQTS. Because of the swimming-triggered cardiac event, a molecular autopsy was conducted revealing a defect in KVLQT1/KCNQ1 (LQT1). Molecular testing confirmed this mutation in NCK. Her QTc is 450 ms. Should she receive a prophylactic ICD?

Analysis: Figure 10 summarizes the theoretical impact that molecular diagnostic testing had for NCK *(20)*. Eight cardiac electrophysiologists examined her screening electrocardiogram. Four considered her ECG normal, 3 borderline, and 1 abnormal. Without the genetic test result, 3 would have dismissed as normal and 2 would have placed NCK on beta-blockers. However, upon learning that she shares her deceased sister's LQT1 genotype, all 8 insisted on beta-blocker therapy and 3 would consider a prophylactic ICD. Thus, the genetic test would have had a profound impact on her management ranging from 3 dismissing as normal without the information to 3 considering an ICD implant with the genetic test result.

For NCK, molecular testing provided the gold standard diagnostic marker to establish that she harbors the LQT1 substrate but does it risk stratify? Unquestionably, NCK needs

LQTS therapy but does she need a prophylactic ICD? NCK was asymptomatic for 18 yr on no medications and now has been asymptomatic for 2 more years on beta-blocker therapy. Despite the tragic death of her sister, NCK's *asymptomatic* state, QTc of 450 ms, and LQT1 genotype would suggest that beta-blocker therapy should provide adequate protection *(57)* and that an ICD is not indicated based upon her positive family history alone.

REFERENCES

1. Romano CGG, Pongiglione R. Aritmie cardiache rare dell'eta'pediatrica. II. Accessi sincopali per fibrillazione ventricolare parossistica. Clin Peditr (Bologna) 1963;45:656–683.
2. Ward OC. A new famillial cardiac syndrome in children. J Irish Med Assoc 1964;54:103–106.
3. Ackerman MJ, Clapham DE. Ion channels—basic science and clinical disease. N Engl J Med 1997;336(22):1575–1586.
4. Ackerman MJ. The long QT syndrome: ion channel diseases of the heart. Mayo Clin Proc 1998;73(3): 250–269.
5. Keating MT, Sanguinetti MC. Molecular and cellular mechanisms of cardiac arrhythmias. Cell 2001;104(4):569–580.
6. Splawski I, Shen J, Timothy KW, et al. Spectrum of mutations in long-QT syndrome genes. KVLQT1, HERG, SCN5A, KCNE1, and KCNE2. Circulation 2000;102(10):1178–1185.
7. Marks AR, Priori S, Memmi M, Kontula K, Laitinen PJ. Involvement of the cardiac ryanodine receptor/ calcium release channel in catecholaminergic polymorphic ventricular tachycardia. J Cell Physiol 2002;190(1):1–6.
8. Plaster NM, Tawil R, Tristani-Firouzi M, et al. Mutations in Kir2.1 cause the developmental and episodic electrical phenotypes of Andersen's syndrome. Cell 2001;105(4):511–519.
9. Jongsma HJ, Wilders R. Channelopathies: Kir2.1 mutations jeopardize many cell functions. Curr Biol 2001;11(18):R747–R750.
10. Jervell A L-NF. Congenital deaf-mutism, functional heart disease with prolongation of the QT interval, and sudden death. Am Heart J 1957;54(59–68).
11. Moss AJ. Long QT Syndromes. Curr Treat Options Cardiovasc Med 2000;2(4):317–322.
12. Schwartz PJ. Clinical applicability of molecular biology: the case of the long QT syndrome. Curr Control Trials Cardiovasc Med 2000;1(2):88–91.
13. Locati EH, Zareba W, Moss AJ, et al. Age- and sex-related differences in clinical manifestations in patients with congenital long-QT syndrome: findings from the International LQTS Registry. Circulation 1998;97(22):2237–2244.
14. Schwartz PJ, Priori SG, Spazzolini C, et al. Genotype-phenotype correlation in the long-QT syndrome: gene-specific triggers for life-threatening arrhythmias. Circulation 2001;103(1):89–95.
15. Garson A, Jr, Dick M, 2nd, Fournier A, et al. The long QT syndrome in children. An international study of 287 patients. Circulation 1993;87(6):1866–1872.
16. Moss AJ, Robinson JL, Gessman L, et al. Comparison of clinical and genetic variables of cardiac events associated with loud noise versus swimming among subjects with the long QT syndrome. Am J Cardiol 1999;84(8):876–879.
17. Ackerman MJ, Porter CJ. Identification of a family with inherited long QT syndrome after a pediatric near-drowning. Pediatrics 1998;101(2):306–308.
18. Ackerman MJ, Schroeder JJ, Berry R, et al. A novel mutation in KVLQT1 is the molecular basis of inherited long QT syndrome in a near-drowning patient's family. Pediatr Res 1998;44(2):148–153.
19. Ackerman MJ, Tester DJ, Porter CJ. Swimming, a gene-specific arrhythmogenic trigger for inherited long QT syndrome. Mayo Clin Proc 1999;74(11):1088–1094.
20. Ackerman MJ, Tester DJ, Porter CJ, Edwards WD. Molecular diagnosis of the inherited long-QT syndrome in a woman who died after near-drowning. N Engl J Med 1999;341(15):1121–1125.
21. Wilde AA, Jongbloed RJ, Doevendans PA, et al. Auditory stimuli as a trigger for arrhythmic events differentiate HERG-related (LQTS2) patients from KVLQT1-related patients (LQTS1). J Am Coll Cardiol 1999;33(2):327–332.
22. Zareba W, Moss AJ, Schwartz PJ, et al. Influence of genotype on the clinical course of the long-QT syndrome. International Long-QT Syndrome Registry Research Group. N Engl J Med 1998;339(14): 960–965.

23. Bazett HC. An analysis of the time-relations of electrocardiograms. Heart 1920;7:353–370.
24. Garson A, Jr., Kertesz NJ, Towbin JA. Improved electrocardiographic identification of the long QT syndrome. J Am Coll Cardiol 2001;37(Suppl A):467A.
25. Vincent GM, Timothy KW, Leppert M, Keating M. The spectrum of symptoms and QT intervals in carriers of the gene for the long-QT syndrome. N Engl J Med 1992;327(12):846–852.
26. Allan WC, Timothy K, Vincent GM, Palomaki GE, Neveux LM, Haddow JE. Long QT syndrome in children: the value of rate corrected QT interval and DNA analysis as screening tests in the general population. J Med Screen 2001;8(4):173–177.
27. Miller MD, Porter C, Ackerman MJ. Diagnostic accuracy of screening electrocardiograms in long QT syndrome I. Pediatrics 2001;108(1):8–12.
28. Moss AJ, Schwartz PJ, Crampton RS, Locati E, Carleen E. The long QT syndrome: a prospective international study. Circulation 1985;71(1):17–21.
29. Priori SG, Napolitano C, Schwartz PJ. Low penetrance in the long-QT syndrome: clinical impact. Circulation 1999;99(4):529–533.
30. Moss AJ, Schwartz PJ, Crampton RS, et al. The long QT syndrome. Prospective longitudinal study of 328 families. Circulation 1991;84(3):1136–1144.
31. Schwartz PJ, Malliani A. Electrical alternation of the T-wave: clinical and experimental evidence of its relationship with the sympathetic nervous system and with the long QT syndrome. Am Heart J 1975;89(1):45–50.
32. Moss AJ, Zareba W, Benhorin J, et al. ECG T-wave patterns in genetically distinct forms of the hereditary long QT syndrome. Circulation 1995;92(10):2929–2934.
33. Zhang L, Timothy KW, Vincent GM, et al. Spectrum of ST-T-wave patterns and repolarization parameters in congenital long-QT syndrome: ECG findings identify genotypes. Circulation 2000;102(23): 2849–2855.
34. Malfatto G, Beria G, Sala S, Bonazzi O, Schwartz PJ. Quantitative analysis of T wave abnormalities and their prognostic implications in the idiopathic long QT syndrome. J Am Coll Cardiol 1994;23(2): 296–301.
35. Lupoglazoff JM, Denjoy I, Berthet M, et al. Notched T waves on Holter recordings enhance detection of patients with LQT2 (HERG) mutations. Circulation 2001;103(8):1095–1101.
36. Zareba W, Moss AJ, le Cessie S, Hall WJ. T wave alternans in idiopathic long QT syndrome. J Am Coll Cardiol 1994;23(7):1541–1546.
37. Napolitano C, Priori SG, Schwartz PJ. Significance of QT dispersion in the long QT syndrome. Prog Cardiovasc Dis 2000;42(5):345–350.
38. Day CP, McComb JM, Campbell RW. QT dispersion: an indication of arrhythmia risk in patients with long QT intervals. Br Heart J 1990;63(6):342–344.
39. Priori SG, Napolitano C, Diehl L, Schwartz PJ. Dispersion of the QT interval. A marker of therapeutic efficacy in the idiopathic long QT syndrome. Circulation 1994;89(4):1681–1689.
40. Moennig G, Schulze-Bahr E, Wedekind H, et al. Clinical value of electrocardiographic parameters in genotyped individuals with familial long QT syndrome. Pacing Clin Electrophysiol 2001;24(4 Pt 1): 406–415.
41. Eggeling T, Osterhues HH, Hoeher M, Gabrielsen FG, Weismueller P, Hombach V. Value of Holter monitoring in patients with the long QT syndrome. Cardiology 1992;81(2–3):107–114.
42. Merri M, Moss AJ, Benhorin J, Locati EH, Alberti M, Badilini F. Relation between ventricular repolarization duration and cardiac cycle length during 24-hour Holter recordings. Findings in normal patients and patients with long QT syndrome. Circulation 1992;85(5):1816–1821.
43. Vincent GM, Jaiswal D, Timothy KW. Effects of exercise on heart rate, QT, QTc and QT/QS2 in the Romano-Ward inherited long QT syndrome. Am J Cardiol 1991;68(5):498–503.
44. Swan H, Toivonen L, Viitasalo M. Rate adaptation of QT intervals during and after exercise in children with congenital long QT syndrome. Eur Heart J 1998;19(3):508–513.
45. Schwartz PJ, Priori SG, Locati EH, et al. Long QT syndrome patients with mutations of the SCN5A and HERG genes have differential responses to Na+ channel blockade and to increases in heart rate. Implications for gene-specific therapy. Circulation 1995;92(12):3381–3386.
46. Swan H, Viitasalo M, Piippo K, Laitinen P, Kontula K, Toivonen L. Sinus node function and ventricular repolarization during exercise stress test in long QT syndrome patients with KvLQT1 and HERG potassium channel defects. J Am Coll Cardiol 1999;34(3):823–829.
47. Kawade M, Ohe T, Kamiya T. Provocative testing and drug response in a patient with the long QT syndrome. Br Heart J 1995;74(1):67–70.

48. Sun ZH, Swan H, Viitasalo M, Toivonen L. Effects of epinephrine and phenylephrine on QT interval dispersion in congenital long QT syndrome. J Am Coll Cardiol 1998;31(6):1400–1405.

49. Shimizu W, Antzelevitch C. Differential effects of beta-adrenergic agonists and antagonists in LQT1, LQT2 and LQT3 models of the long QT syndrome. J Am Coll Cardiol 2000;35(3):778–786.

50. Tanabe Y, Inagaki M, Kurita T, et al. Sympathetic stimulation produces a greater increase in both transmural and spatial dispersion of repolarization in LQT1 than LQT2 forms of congenital long QT syndrome. J Am Coll Cardiol 2001;37(3):911–919.

51. Ackerman MJ, Khositseth A,Tester DJ, Hejlik J, Shen WK, Porter CJ. Epinephrine induced QT interval prolongation: a gene-specific paradoxical response in congenital long QT syndrome. Mayo Clin Proc 2002;77:413–421.

52. Schwartz PJ. Idiopathic long QT syndrome: progress and questions. Am Heart J 1985;109(2):399–411.

53. Schwartz PJ, Moss AJ, Vincent GM, Crampton RS. Diagnostic criteria for the long QT syndrome. An update. Circulation 1993;88(2):782–784.

54. Priori SG, Aliot E, Blomstrom-Lundqvist C, et al. Task Force on Sudden Cardiac Death of the European Society of Cardiology. Eur Heart J 2001;22(16):1374–1450.

55. Rashba EJ, Zareba W, Moss AJ, et al. Influence of pregnancy on the risk for cardiac events in patients with hereditary long QT syndrome. LQTS Investigators. Circulation 1998;97(5):451–456.

56. Marks ML, Trippel DL, Keating MT. Long QT syndrome associated with syndactyly identified in females. Am J Cardiol 1995;76(10):744–745.

57. Moss AJ, Zareba W, Hall WJ, et al. Effectiveness and limitations of beta-blocker therapy in congenital long-QT syndrome. Circulation 2000;101(6):616–623.

58. Schwartz PJ, Zaza A, Locati E, Moss AJ. Stress and sudden death. The case of the long QT syndrome. Circulation 1991;83(4 Suppl):II71–II80.

59. Atiga WL, Calkins H, Lawrence JH, Tomaselli GF, Smith JM, Berger RD. Beat-to-beat repolarization lability identifies patients at risk for sudden cardiac death. J Cardiovasc Electrophysiol 1998;9(9): 899–908.

60. Zareba W. New electrocardiographic indices of risk stratification. J Electrocardiol 2001;34:332.

61. Steinbigler P, Haberl R, Nespithal K, Spiegl A, Schmucking I, Steinbeck G. T wave spectral variance: A new method to determine inhomogeneous repolarization by T wave beat-to-beat variability in patients prone to ventricular arrhythmias. J Electrocardiol 1998;30(Suppl): 137–144.

62. Bhandari AK, Shapiro WA, Morady F, Shen EN, Mason J, Scheinman MM. Electrophysiologic testing in patients with the long QT syndrome. Circulation 1985;71(1):63–71.

63. Hohnloser SH, Klingenheben T, Li YG, Zabel M, Peetermans J, Cohen RJ. T wave alternans as a predictor of recurrent ventricular tachyarrhythmias in ICD recipients: prospective comparison with conventional risk markers. J Cardiovasc Electrophysiol 1998;9(12):1258–1268.

64. Kaufman ES, Priori SG, Napolitano C, et al. Electrocardiographic prediction of abnormal genotype in congenital long QT syndrome: experience in 101 related family members. J Cardiovasc Electrophysiol 2001;12(4):455–461.

65. Nemec J, Ackerman MJ, Tester DJ, Hejlik J, Shen WK. Catecholamine-provoked microvoltage T wave alternans in genotyped long QT syndrome. Pacing Clin Electrophysiol 2003;in press.

66. Nemec J, Hejlik J, Shen WK, Ackerman MJ. Catecholamine-induced T wave lability in congenital long QT syndrome: a novel phenomenon associated with syncope and cardiac arrest. Mayo Clin Proc 2003; in press.

67. Priori SG, Maugeri FS, Schwartz PJ. The risk of sudden death as first cardiac event in asymptomatic patients with the long QT syndrome. (abstract). Circulation 1998;98 suppl I:777.

68. Schwartz PJ. The long QT syndrome. Curr Probl Cardiol 1997;22(6):297–351.

69. Maron BJ, Isner JM, McKenna WJ. 26th Bethesda conference: recommendations for determining eligibility for competition in athletes with cardiovascular abnormalities. Task Force 3: hypertrophic cardiomyopathy, myocarditis and other myopericardial diseases and mitral valve prolapse. J Am Coll Cardiol 1994;24(4):880–885.

70. Eldar M, Griffin JC, Van Hare GF, et al. Combined use of beta-adrenergic blocking agents and long-term cardiac pacing for patients with the long QT syndrome. J Am Coll Cardiol 1992;20(4):830–837.

71. Dorostkar PC, Eldar M, Belhassen B, Scheinman MM. Long-term follow-up of patients with long-QT syndrome treated with beta-blockers and continuous pacing. Circulation 1999;100(24): 2431–2436.

72. Curran ME, Splawski I, Timothy KW, Vincent GM, Green ED, Keating MT. A molecular basis for cardiac arrhythmia: HERG mutations cause long QT syndrome. Cell 1995;80(5):795–803.

73. Shimizu W, Ohe T, Kurita T, et al. Effects of verapamil and propranolol on early afterdepolarizations and ventricular arrhythmias induced by epinephrine in congenital long QT syndrome. J Am Coll Cardiol 1995;26(5):1299–1309.

74. Shimizu W, Antzelevitch C. Cellular basis for the ECG features of the LQT1 form of the long-QT syndrome: effects of beta-adrenergic agonists and antagonists and sodium channel blockers on transmural dispersion of repolarization and torsade de pointes. Circulation 1998;98(21):2314–2322.

75. Shimizu W, Kurita T, Matsuo K, et al. Improvement of repolarization abnormalities by a K+ channel opener in the LQT1 form of congenital long-QT syndrome. Circulation 1998;97(16):1581–1588.

76. Gronefeld G, Holtgen R, Hohnloser SH. Implantable cardioverter defibrillator therapy in a patient with the idiopathic long QT syndrome. Pacing Clin Electrophysiol 1996;19(8):1260–1263.

77. Groh WJ, Silka MJ, Oliver RP, Halperin BD, McAnulty JH, Kron J. Use of implantable cardioverter-defibrillators in the congenital long QT syndrome. Am J Cardiol 1996;78(6):703–706.

78. Gregoratos G, Cheitlin MD, Conill A, et al. ACC/AHA guidelines for implantation of cardiac pacemakers and antiarrhythmia devices: a report of the American College of Cardiology/American Heart Association Task Force on Practice Guidelines (Committee on Pacemaker Implantation). J Am Coll Cardiol 1998;31(5):1175–1209.

79. Viskin S, Fish R, Zeltser D, et al. Arrhythmias in the congenital long QT syndrome: how often is torsade de pointes pause dependent? Heart 2000;83(6):661–666.

80. Schwartz PJ, Locati E. The idiopathic long QT syndrome: pathogenetic mechanisms and therapy. Eur Heart J 1985;6 Suppl D:103–114.

81. Moss AJ, McDonald J. Unilateral cervicothoracic sympathetic ganglionectomy for the treatment of long QT interval syndrome. N Engl J Med 1971;285(16):903–904.

82. Shimizu W, Antzelevitch C. Sodium channel block with mexiletine is effective in reducing dispersion of repolarization and preventing torsade des pointes in LQT2 and LQT3 models of the long-QT syndrome. Circulation 1997;96(6):2038–2047.

83. Compton SJ, Lux RL, Ramsey MR, et al. Genetically defined therapy of inherited long-QT syndrome. Correction of abnormal repolarization by potassium. Circulation 1996;94(5):1018–1122.

84. Shimizu W, Antzelevitch C. Effects of a K(+) channel opener to reduce transmural dispersion of repolarization and prevent torsade de pointes in LQT1, LQT2, and LQT3 models of the long-QT syndrome. Circulation 2000;102(6):706–712.

85. Ackerman MJ, Tester DJ, Driscoll DJ. Molecular autopsy of sudden unexplained death in the young. Am J Forensic Med Pathol 2001;22(2):105–111.

21

Prolonged Repolarization and Sudden Infant Death Syndrome

Peter J. Schwartz, MD

CONTENTS

INTRODUCTION

Sudden Infant Death Syndrome (SIDS) remains the leading cause of sudden death during the first year of life in the western world and produces devastating psychosocial consequences in the families of the victims.

SIDS is defined as the sudden unexpected death of any infant or young child, which is unexpected by history and in which a thorough postmortem examination fails to identify an adequate cause of death. A death-scene investigation has been recommended as a requirement for diagnosis.

Despite a large number of theories, mostly focused on abnormalities in the control of respiratory or cardiac function, the causes of SIDS remain unknown. The suggestions over the years that cardiac mechanisms and specifically life-threatening arrhythmias *(1,2)* might account for a significant portion of cases of SIDS have been controversial.

This chapter describes the rationale and the origin of the cardiac hypothesis that some SIDS cases might be because of ventricular fibrillation associated with prolonged repolarization, summarizes the results of our 20-yr-long prospective study with ECG recordings in 34,000 infants *(3)*, discusses our new findings *(4,5)* which provide the first

From: *Contemporary Cardiology: Cardiac Repolarization: Bridging Basic and Clinical Science*
Edited by: I. Gussak et al. © Humana Press Inc., Totowa, NJ

molecular evidence linking SIDS to the Long QT Syndrome (LQTS), and addresses the unusual one-sided controversy *(6)* that followed publication of the prospective study *(3)*.

THE QT HYPOTHESIS

Many hypotheses have been proposed to explain SIDS but none has yet been proven. There is a consensus that SIDS is multifactorial *(2,7)*, an important concept which implies that a sudden and unexpected death in infancy may be caused by different causes. A logical corollary is that the validity of one mechanism is not negated by the validity of another. What really matters is to dissect out those mechanisms accounting for significant portions of those infant deaths that are currently labeled as SIDS, largely because of our inability to identify a more specific disease or cause. It should be remembered that SIDS is a diagnosis of exclusion: when we cannot explain, on the basis of current knowledge and after a thorough and expert postmortem examination, why an apparently healthy infant has been found dead then the diagnosis becomes that of SIDS.

Most SIDS cases probably result from an abnormality in either respiratory or cardiac function *(7,8)*, or in their neural control, that may be transient in nature but sufficient to initiate a lethal sequence of events.

As to the so-called apnea hypothesis, its final test was carried out in the large, NIH-funded, prospective study CHIME on over 1000 infants who during the first six months of life were observed with home cardiorespiratory monitors for a total of almost 720,000 hr of home monitoring *(9)*. The conclusion of the study was that even extreme events (including apnea of at least 30 s or heart rate below 50 b/min for at least 10 s) are not likely to be precursors of SIDS. The accompanying editorial by Alan Jobe *(10)* puts the issue in the proper perspective and reminds that the current cost in the US *for monitoring alone is about $24 million per year for preterm infants, not including physicians fees and other ancillary medical costs and not including monitors for term infants thought to be at increased risk for SIDS.* Jobe concludes that *this report disproves the assumption that infants thought to be at increased risk of SIDS have more cardiorespiratory events than healthy infants and is consistent with the conclusion that such events are not precursors to SIDS. This study justifies a severe curtailing of home monitoring to prevent SIDS.*

As to the cardiac hypothesis, in my original reasoning, shared by Peter Froggatt, a pioneer in the role of cardiac mechanisms in infant deaths *(11)*, I gave weight to the fact that in the Western world the leading cause of mortality in age 20–65 is sudden cardiac death *(12)*, and that the mechanism involved is almost always a lethal arrhythmia, ventricular fibrillation. It would be odd if sudden cardiac death, and therefore lethal arrhythmias, would not contribute at all to some infant sudden deaths.

It was thus that in 1974, in a funded NIH grant application *(13)*, and in 1976 *(1)*, I proposed that some cases of SIDS might have been caused by a mechanism similar to that responsible for the sudden death of the patients affected by LQTS, a leading cause of sudden death below age 20 *(14,15)*. One such mechanism might have been a developmental abnormality in cardiac sympathetic innervation predisposing some infants to lethal arrhythmias in the first year of life *(1)*. Another likely mechanism might have been the same genetic alterations that only recently have been shown to cause LQTS *(14,15)*. The only clinically detectable marker for these mechanisms is a QT interval prolongation on the electrocardiogram (ECG).

Following my 1976 editorial *(1)*, the hypothesis that QT interval prolongation might play a role in the genesis of SIDS received considerable attention but—despite some very early support by Maron et al. *(16)*—it was rapidly, and perhaps prematurely, discarded on the basis of a series of apparently negative results *(17–21)*. The arguments against the role of prolonged QT in SIDS had glaring weaknesses previously discussed in detail, and the interested reader is referred to these publications *(2,22)*. Here, I will just provide a brief comment.

Most of these so-called negative studies were performed in populations of very small size or in infants defined as "at increased risk for SIDS," like the siblings of SIDS victims *(18,20)* or the so-called near-miss or aborted SIDS *(17,19)*, who were not found to have QT prolongation. Conclusions drawn from these studies are quite unlikely to be relevant to the assessment of the risk for SIDS associated with QT interval prolongation. It is essential to remember that for diseases characterized by a very low incidence, such as SIDS, any risk factor will yield a high number of false positives. In the case of SIDS, even assuming a risk as high as two per thousand, any factor that would increase risk by five times would still leave 99% of false positives! This means that whenever investigators study 100 of these allegedly high risk infants, they can expect only one of them (1%) to subsequently die of SIDS; the fact that this one SIDS victim does not show a proposed marker of risk obviously has no implications whatsoever for the relevance of that marker. It follows that the absence of a given marker, prolonged QT interval in our case, among subjects at high risk for SIDS only indicates that this factor is not important in the specific patient(s) under study; moreover, extrapolation to the general population and to the true SIDS victims is simply unwarranted. These considerations, based on elementary statistics, seemed to escape many SIDS investigators.

THE ITALIAN STUDY ON NEONATAL ELECTROCARDIOGRAPHY AND SIDS

To test the hypothesis of a relationship between QT interval prolongation and SIDS, in 1976 we designed a prospective study based on the recording of a standard ECG in 3–4-d-old infants. Given the low incidence of SIDS (0.5–1.5 per 1000 live births), we had to prospectively collect neonatal ECGs in a very large population and to subsequently follow these infants for one year to assess the occurrence of SIDS or deaths for other causes. The results of this study were published in 1998 *(3)* and, partly because of the accompanying editorial *(23)* and partly because of the media attention, were widely publicized. For this reason, here I will simply summarize the main facts and findings.

Twelve-lead ECGs were recorded in 34,442 neonates born in nine maternity hospitals. The QT interval was measured on the ECGs of all infants that died and on the ECGs of a random sample of 9725 infants taken from the entire study population. All measurements were performed by investigators blind to the survival status of the infant. The study lasted 19 yr.

Of the 34,442 infants enrolled, 33,034 (96%) completed the one-year follow-up. The lost-to-follow-up were due to change of residence. The mean QTc (QT interval corrected for heart rate) was 400±20 ms and it did not differ between males and females (401±19 vs 400±20 ms). The normal and symmetrical distribution of the QTc in our population made the 97.5[th] percentile value of QTc correspond to 440 ms, two standard deviations above the mean. Consequently, and for the purpose of the study, we considered a value greater than 440 ms as a prolonged QTc.

During the one-year follow-up there were 34 deaths: 24 due to SIDS and 10 due to other causes. All postmortem examinations of SIDS victims were negative and failed to

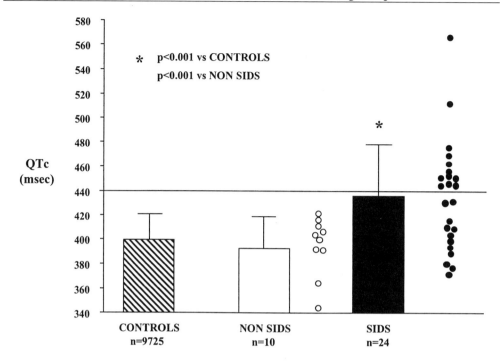

Fig. 1. Mean QT interval corrected for heart rate (QTc) in control infants, in Sudden Infant Death Syndrome victims (SIDS) and in victims for other causes (NON-SIDS). The line represents the 97.5[th] value of QTc in the whole population and corresponds to 440 ms, 2 standard deviations above the mean. The filled and the open circles represent the individual values of QTc of the SIDS victims and of the non-SIDS victims, respectively *(3)*.

document an adequate cause of death. No SIDS victim had a family history of LQTS or sudden death.

The mean QTc was 435±45 ms in the SIDS group, significantly longer than that of the non-SIDS victims (392±26 ms, $p<0.05$) and of that of healthy controls (400±20 ms, $p<0.01$, Fig. 1). Of greater importance, the analysis of the individual values of QTc in the two groups of victims (Fig. 1) showed that 12/24 (50%) infants who died for SIDS had a QTc greater than 440 ms, whereas all the infants who died for other causes had a QTc shorter than 440 ms.

Since heart rate in the neonatal period is relatively high, the traditional Bazett's formula might not be appropriate to correct QT interval for short cycle lengths. Accordingly, we also divided the RR intervals in 17 classes with progressively increasing values (20 ms stepwise) and for each class we calculated the percentile distribution of the corresponding absolute values of QT interval (from the 2.5[th] to the 97.5[th]). Figure 2 shows that the individual values of 12/24 (50%) SIDS victims were located above the 97.5[th] percentile, whereas all the values of the non-SIDS victims were below the 90th percentile.

On the basis of our results the absolute risk of SIDS in infants with a normal QTc is 0.37 per thousand, while that of infants with a QTc $\geq$ 440 ms is 15 per thousand. The odds ratio for SIDS associated with a prolonged QTc (>440 ms) is 41.3 (95% CI 17.3–98.4), significantly greater than that of infants with a normal QTc.

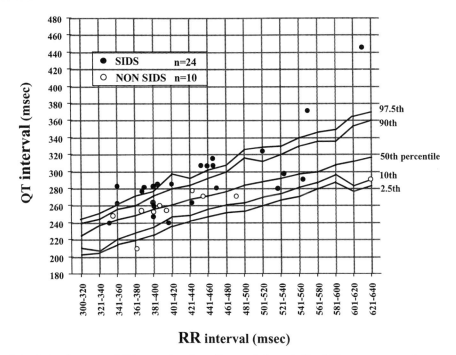

Fig. 2. Relation between QT interval and cardiac cycle length. Each line represents the percentile values of uncorrected QT intervals at the corresponding range of RR intervals. The filled and the open circles represent the individual values of QTc of the SIDS victims and of the non-SIDS victims, respectively *(3)*.

This large prospective study based on more than 34,000 infants provided the demonstration that QT interval prolongation, on the standard ECG recorded on the 3rd–4th d of life, is a major risk factor for SIDS.

QT PROLONGATION AND LIFE-THREATENING ARRHYTHMIAS

The evidence for a strong association between SIDS and QT interval prolongation, a marker of reduced cardiac electrical stability, suggests that in some infants there may be an increased susceptibility to life-threatening arrhythmias.

Experimental and clinical studies have shown that QT interval prolongation favors the occurrence of lethal arrhythmias and is associated with increased risk for sudden death in several clinical conditions *(24,25)* and also in apparently healthy individuals *(26)*. Among these conditions the most relevant to SIDS undoubtedly is LQTS *(14,15)*.

The presence of false positives (2.5%), i.e., infants with prolonged QT interval who did not die of SIDS, probably has at least two causes and one implication.

Among the causes, the first and most important is the high probability of cases of "spurious QT prolongation" (i.e., an infant with a normal QT interval who on day 3–4 has a measurement just above the cut-off point and who on subsequent measurements would show normal values). In this regard it is always worth remembering that QT measurement is gross and that a few milliseconds errors are unavoidable. The second is the fact that 440 ms is an arbitrary cut-off (a very reasonable one, placed at 2 SD above normal and thus encompassing the upper 97.5th percentile of the normal population) which does not imply at all that infants above that value are affected by LQTS.

The implication is that other factors in the postnatal period contribute to the lethal event. This is consistent with the concept of QT prolongation acting as an arrhythmogenic "substrate" which requires a trigger for the occurrence of life-threatening arrhythmias. The best known "triggers" for lethal arrhythmias in the setting of QT prolongation are represented by release of catecholamines secondary to activation of the sympathetic nervous system and by factors (e.g., hypokalemia or drugs that block the I_{Kr} current, as many antibiotics, antihistaminics, and prokinetics such as cisapride) that further prolong the QT interval (14,27). It is interesting to note, and we do it here for the first time, that the prone sleeping position may be one of these triggers. Indeed, this recently discovered risk factor for SIDS (28) is associated with signs of increased sympathetic and decreased vagal activity to the heart—an established risk factor for arrhythmic death (29).

Clinical Implications

Our article (3) ended by mentioning two rather obvious, but nonetheless troublesome, clinical implications, and it was largely this section that ignited the most recent controversy.

One was that the highly significant association between QT prolongation and occurrence of SIDS unavoidably raises the issue of the potential value of a routine neonatal ECG screening. The low incidence of SIDS in the general population (< 0.1%) forces a low predictive value for any factor associated with the event, and QT prolongation (1.5%) is no exception even though its relative risk of 41 is strikingly higher than any previously reported. Despite this limitation, a simple electrocardiographic screening might contribute to identity a portion of the infants at high risk for SIDS.

The second complex issue is the management of the infants found to have a prolonged QTc. Our study contained no data to justify new therapeutic recommendations; however, the association between prolonged QT interval and SIDS should allow some cautious speculation. The lethal arrhythmias favored by QT prolongation are usually triggered by sudden increases in sympathetic activity. In the first year of life this may be often elicited by multiple conditions (2) including sudden noise, exposure to cold, REM sleep, apnea leading to a chemoreceptive reflex, arousals, and probably the prone position. In LQTS antiadrenergic interventions are quite successful (14). Data from almost 1000 LQTS families indicate that treatment with beta-blockers has reduced mortality below 3% (14). This information is relevant to the prevention of SIDS in newborns with a prolonged QT interval. It also provides a ready therapy for those infants serendipitously identified, by neonatal ECG screening, as definitely affected by the LQTS and offers a valid option for the yet unproven but reasonable possibility of reducing risk in the neonates with a prolonged QT interval.

Practically, whenever infants at risk because of QT prolongation are identified early on, preventive therapy could be considered and then instituted for a few months. Normalization of the QT interval during development will allow rapid withdrawal of therapy in the unavoidably large number of false positives, but will allow also the continuation of therapy in the minority of infants with a persistent QT prolongation in whom beta-blockers are likely to be life-saving. The number of false positives could be greatly reduced by performing the screening ECG in the 3rd–4th week of life.

AN UNUSUAL RESPONSE

There are several ways to discuss one's own data. A difficult one, but probably the best in the long term, is to take into account the points of view reflecting the most common criticisms. An unprecedented unilateral attack *(6)* offers a unique chance for a candid discussion.

Our original article *(3)* was published with an accompanying editorial written by two expert pediatricians, Towbin and Friedman *(23)*. They concluded *"Schwartz and colleagues present compelling evidence that the long QT syndrome should be considered an important factor in the pathogenesis of SIDS. They are to be commended for conducting this forward-thinking, long-term prospective study (involving nearly 20 yr of data) of a tragic disorder. Over time, their work will almost certainly help to improve the outcome of infants at risk."*

This editorial not only was insufficient to prevent the subsequent reaction *(6)* headed by Jerold Lucey, the Editor-in-Chief of *Pediatrics*, but seems to have actually triggered it.

Disagreement is essential for scientific development, and it is not uncommon for Editors to publish opinions strongly against a given theory or a given study. Whenever this happens, the author of the criticized study is always given a chance to reply, often in the same issue and always with the same space; this behavior is a golden rule in scientific journals but the present case was an exception.

In April 1999, Lucey published an article in which, having *decided that the article warranted a more forceful critique*, he solicited the opinions on our study of seven of his reviewers.

ARGUMENTS AGAINST THE QT HYPOTHESIS

Here, I will review the main arguments used in the forceful critique by the team assembled by Lucey.

Martin and colleagues *(33)* criticized our conclusion that the cause of death in the SIDS victims with a prolonged QT interval is likely to be an arrhythmia. They stated: *There is no evidence for lethal arrhythmias as precipitating events in infants who have died of SIDS while on cardiorespiratory monitors (33).*

The issue of *"no evidence for arrhythmias"* calls into question their understanding of the implications of SIDS being a multifactorial disease. The infants who are on cardiorespiratory monitors represent a population with a specific selection bias; namely, to have been discovered by the parents during an apparently life-threatening event. As carefully discussed almost 20 yr ago *(8)*, most near miss infants enter in this category because of an episode of apnea. A respiratory death is slow and allows time for struggle and cyanosis, whereas death by ventricular fibrillation is fast and silent. There are simply more statistical chances that a mother will find her baby dying a respiratory than a cardiac death, and this will allow her to interrupt the deadly process and the end-result will be a new near miss. Thus, it is likely that most true near misses would have died a respiratory death, and it is expected that these infants would show some respiratory abnormality. The fact that an infant considered at increased risk because of an apneic episode does not have ventricular arrhythmias should not surprise a competent clinician; why should he have cardiac arrhythmias if his risk comes from a respiratory abnormality?

Martin et al. continue with the following criticism: *Ventricular arrhythmias have not been described in patients who have been evaluated after survival of an acute life-threatening event (33).*

This comment implies an inadequate understanding of the arrhythmias associated with a prolonged QT interval. These arrhythmias, mostly torsade de pointes ventricular tachycardia degenerating into ventricular fibrillation, are of very short duration. They either convert spontaneously to sinus rhythm within 20–30 s or proceed toward ventricular fibrillation leading to loss of consciousness and sudden death within a few minutes. In the first case, if the patient is a grown-up he will have syncope and faint and this will not escape attention; however, if the patient is an infant lying in his crib where he is going to fall? A transient, nonfatal episode will almost always go unnoticed. In the second case, only a fortuitous set of circumstances may allow the parents to observe and attempt to interrupt a lethal episode that would be over in 3–5 min; the point here is that when prolonged ventricular tachycardia deteriorates into ventricular fibrillation the infants almost never survive and would not be available for further monitoring. Those more likely to survive are the infants who have life-threatening episodes for respiratory abnormalities and in the subsequent monitoring there is no reason to expect ventricular tachyarrhythmias. Finally, it is extremely unusual for patients affected by LQTS to have ventricular arrhythmias outside their life-threatening episodes; they are almost always in sinus rhythm and then, all of a sudden, they may have a run of torsade de pointes and faint or die.

Guntheroth *(34)* states that *the most damning problem is the lack of independent confirmation in the past 22 yr. In fact, there have been four prospective studies (21,35–37) that have contradicted the Italian data.* We would worry indeed if someone had performed a study similar to ours and found significantly different results; the point is that no one—with the partial exception of Southall—had even come close to what we did. Guntheroth's statement is simply not correct, as shown by the following review of the four studies quoted by him.

Southall et al. *(21)* studied 7254 infants, 15 of whom subsequently died of SIDS. Even though they concluded for no difference between SIDS victims and controls, 6 of the 15 (40%) infants who died of SIDS had a QTc equal or greater than the value corresponding to the 90th percentile of their own population. This incidence is four times higher than expected and implies an Odds Ratio for SIDS of 6, significantly greater than that of infants with a normal QTc. Their erroneous conclusion was reached because the authors compared the means of the two groups (victims and survivors), an analysis appropriate if SIDS had one cause only and quite wrong when dealing with multifactorial diseases. The detailed arguments for the methodologically correct approach to Southall's data have been presented elsewhere *(22)*. Another significant problem lies in the fact that his study was performed on day 2 when the physiologic fluctuation in the QT is still high and when many infants who 1–2 d later will have a normal QT may still show a prolonged QT interval *(38)*. This results in a spuriously high number of infants with QT prolongation which of course reduces the power of the study and the possibility of correctly assessing the relative risk associated with a prolonged QT interval.

The other three studies *(35–37)* are simply not relevant. The study by Weinstein and Steinschneider *(35)*, was a retrospective analysis of eight SIDS victims studied as part of an investigation on apnea and whose QT interval was found similar to that of other infants. It is critical to note that these infants were studied at a temperature of 90°F.

Heating modifies sympathetic activity and may revert to normal a neurally mediated QT prolongation. The study by Schaffer et al. *(36)* is based on one (!) SIDS victim with a normal QT. The study by Gillette and Garson *(37)* is on three SIDS victims with a normal QT but Guntheroth failed to correctly inform the readers that one of the three was the single victim already described by Schaffer!

This brief overview shows how the validity of the QT hypothesis is not affected by the arguments commonly used in the literature.

THE MOLECULAR LINK

Potential Causes for QT Prolongation in Infants

We have provided evidence that a prolonged QT interval increases the risk of SIDS *(3)*. A major question, however, remained. Why should an infant have a QT prolongation? Which mechanisms would be involved? It is clear that inability to provide rational explanations to these questions would weaken the QT hypothesis.

We have proposed three different mechanisms that might be involved in the genesis of QT interval prolongation in some newborns. The first is a developmental abnormality in cardiac sympathetic innervation *(1)*. The second is a *de novo* mutation in one of the LQTS genes. The third involves cases of LQTS with low penetrance *(39)*.

The first mechanism is partly based on the fact that an imbalance in cardiac sympathetic innervation with left dominance, experimentally produced by removing the right stellate ganglion, prolongs the QT interval and increases susceptibility to ventricular fibrillation in several conditions, including three weeks old puppies with normal hearts *(40)*. The sympathetic innervation of the heart continues to develop after birth and becomes functionally complete by approximately the sixth month of life *(41)*. The right and left sympathetic nerves may occasionally develop at different rates and lead temporarily to a harmful imbalance. A sudden increase in sympathetic activity, particularly when involving the arrhythmogenic left sided nerves *(42)*, might easily trigger a lethal arrhythmia in these electrically unstable hearts. Infants with these characteristics would be more vulnerable during the first few months of life and the higher risk for SIDS could be identified by the observation of a prolonged QT interval.

As the other two possibilities, more easily testable, involve LQTS and some related concepts of genetics, it becomes necessary to summarize here some critical points concerning the information available on the genetics of LQTS. LQTS is a familial disease, which may nonetheless present also sporadic cases (no apparent familial involvement) and is characterized by QT prolongation and high risk for sudden death, usually under stressful conditions but also during sleep *(14)*. LQTS has genetic heterogeneity and genes located on chromosomes 3, 7, 11, and 21 have been identified *(15)*. A potential difficulty for linking LQTS to SIDS is that the latter is not a familial disease. Two concepts are highly relevant here. The first is that among sporadic cases of LQTS *de novo* (spontaneous) mutations have been found in the two genes, *HERG* and *KvLQT1*, which encode the potassium channels for I_{Kr} and I_{Ks}, two of the major repolarizing currents, and in the cardiac sodium channel gene *SCN5A*. A *de novo* mutation, by definition, is not found among the parents. The second is represented by the demonstration of "low penetrance" in LQTS *(39)*. Penetrance is defined as the ratio between gene-carriers and individuals showing the full phenotype of the disease. A low penetrance implies that clinical diagnosis

A   **Age 44 days - No therapy**

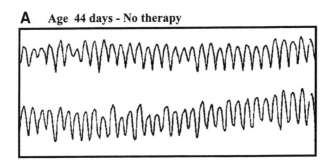

B   **Age 44 days - QTc: 648msec - No therapy**

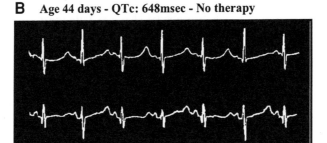

C   **Age 3 years - QTc: 510msec - Propranolol + Mexiletine**

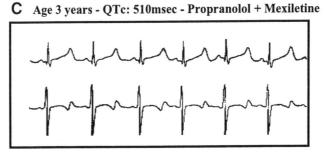

Fig. 3. ECG leads DII and V2, showing ventricular fibrillation at hospital admission **(A)**; QT interval prolongation observed the same day after restoration of sinus rhythm **(B)**; and ECG recorded at the last follow-up visit **(C)** *(4)*.

is often inadequate and that many affected individuals may appear completely normal at clinical examination.

We now have the evidence that the second of these three possibilities may indeed account for some cases of SIDS and thus explain prolongation of the QT interval in some SIDS victims with parents who have a completely normal QT interval.

Molecular Evidence

We have recently reported two independent cases which demonstrate that *de novo* mutations in LQTS genes may manifest as, and be indistinguishable from, typical cases of near-miss for SIDS or as SIDS itself *(4,5)*.

In the first case, a seven-wk-old infant was found cyanotic, apneic, and pulseless by his parents *(4)*. He was rushed to a nearby hospital while his father was attempting CPR;

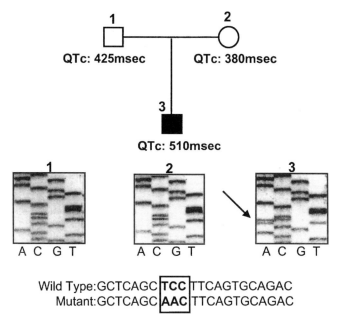

Fig. 4. Family tree and results of the molecular screening. DNA sequences of the exon 16 of *SCN5A* gene demonstrate the presence of two abnormal bands (arrow), determining a heterozygous mutation in the proband, absent in the parents *(4)*.

in the emergency room an ECG showed ventricular fibrillation (Fig. 3). Thus, this infant presented as typical "near-miss" for SIDS. After defibrillation, the ECG revealed a major QT prolongation (QTc 648 ms), LQTS was diagnosed and therapy was instituted by combining beta-blockade and the sodium channel blocker mexiletine. A critical point is that the QT interval of both parents was normal, paternity being confirmed. Molecular screening identified a mutation on *SCN5A*, the cardiac sodium channel gene responsible for the LQT3 subtype of LQTS *(15)*. This disease-carrying mutation was not present in the mother nor in the father; paternity was confirmed, thus establishing that this was a *de novo* mutation (Fig. 4).

The documentation of ventricular fibrillation at arrival in the emergency room is quite important given the frequent statements such as *no one has recorded ventricular arrhythmias in infants at risk for SIDS (34)*. Had the infant died, a certainty without cardioversion, the absence of an ECG and the normal QT of both parents would have ruled out any suspicions of LQTS and would have prompted the classic diagnosis of SIDS. Thus, infants who have similar *de novo* mutations, involving one of the ionic channels controlling ventricular repolarization, may have a prolonged QT interval at birth. Some of them may die because of ventricular fibrillation already *in utero*, and thus become stillbirths, or during the first few months of life and without an available ECG they would be labeled as SIDS victims. Others would probably begin to have syncopal episodes or nonfatal cardiac arrests during their childhood and would only then be diagnosed as sporadic cases of LQTS.

In the second case *(6)*, a 4-mo-old infant was found dead in her crib. She was lying in the supine position, the room temperature was appropriately cool for early summer, the parents do not smoke. A thorough postmortem examination was negative and the

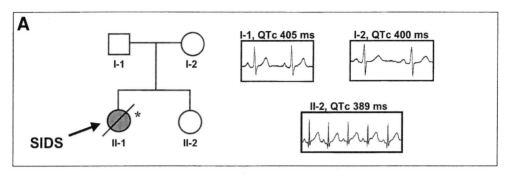

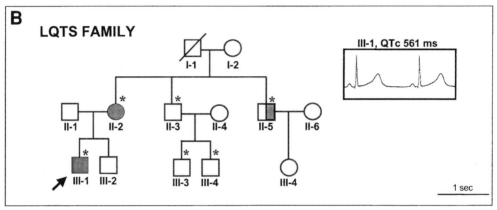

Fig. 5. Pedigrees and ECG tracings of the two families with P117L mutation included in the present study. **(A)** shows the pedigree of the SIDS family. ECG tracings of the parents (I-1 and I-2) and the sister (II-2) of the proband showing a normal QT interval (lead D2) are reported on the right. **(B)** shows the pedigree of the LQT1 family with the P117L mutation. On the left, lead D2 ECG recording obtained in the proband (III-1). Arrows indicate probands. Gray symbol indicates the SIDS victim. Filled symbols represent individuals presenting with syncope and prolonged QT interval. Half-filled symbols represent individuals with QT interval prolongation and no symptoms. Asterisks indicate carriers of the P117L mutation.

diagnosis of SIDS was made. When postmortem molecular screening was performed we identified a point mutation leading to replacement with leucine of a highly conserved proline at position 117 of the KvLQT1 protein. Both the parents of the victim and her sister had normal QT intervals and no one had the P117L mutation. Paternity was confirmed, thus establishing that this was a *de novo* mutation. The same identical mutation is present in one of the LQTS families followed at our institution (Fig. 5). This case provides the first evidence that in a child whose death was classified as SIDS, according to all current standards, postmortem molecular screening can help to reach the diagnosis of an arrhythmogenic disease, LQTS.

The significance of these findings exceeds by far that commonly associated with single case reports because they represent proof of concept for the link between LQTS and SIDS. They do indeed provide the first unequivocal demonstration that life-threatening events in infancy and actual unexpected sudden deaths in infancy, with all the characteristics for SIDS or for near miss for SIDS, can depend on a *de novo* mutation in one of the

LQTS genes thus escaping recognition in the parents and lead to sudden death because of ventricular fibrillation.

The major difference between negative and positive findings is not always fully appreciated. A very large number of negative findings is required in order to dismiss the possible involvement of a given mechanism. By contrast, a single positive finding is sufficient to demonstrate that a given mechanism *can* be operant; then, what remains to be assessed is the frequency with which this mechanism is operant. In the case of prolonged QT interval and SIDS, an initial quantitative information has already been suggested by our large prospective study showing that 50% of SIDS victims had a prolonged QT interval in the first few days of life. It has of course to be remembered that a QTc exceeding by a few milliseconds the upper limit of normal values (440 ms) does not imply the diagnosis of SIDS. Even with very conservative estimates, however, it is not unreasonable to expect that LQTS-related cases of SIDS might be in the range of 15–20%.

In this regard, useful information has been very recently provided by Ackerman et al. *(43)*. They examined tissue from 93 SIDS victims searching from mutations on *SCN5A* and found functionally important mutations in two cases. Towbin and Ackerman, commenting on their own study and on an additional *de novo* mutation in *SCN5A (44)* leading to arrhythmias and sudden death in infancy (not a SIDS case, as LQTS was diagnosed on the first day of life due to malignant arrhythmias), stated "*We can definitely conclude that SCN5A mutations are significant causes of SIDS*" *(45)*. The study by Ackerman et al. stimulates three considerations. The first is that mutations in *SCN5A* account for approximately only 10% of all genotyped LQTS patients. The second is that, even in the best laboratories, only 50–60% of patients with a clinically definitive diagnosis of LQTS are successfully genotyped; this point alone suggests that whatever percentage of SIDS victims will be positively genotyped for LQTS it will be likely to represent approximately half of the individuals with actual LQTS mutations. The third is that the population under study was racially biased against the probability of finding LQTS mutations as 34 of the 93 SIDS victims were black (36.5%), and LQTS among blacks seems particularly rare. If the analysis had been limited to the 58 white infants (there was 1 Hispanic) then the incidence of *SCN5A* mutations would have been 3.4%.

In conclusion, there is now definitive evidence for one of the mechanisms that we had hypothesized to be involved in SIDS *(3–5,43)*. The findings support the concept of widespread neonatal ECG screening and indicate that at least this subset of infants at high risk for sudden infant death can be diagnosed early on and that their impending death can probably be prevented.

MEDICO-LEGAL IMPLICATIONS

The findings reported above, besides the fairly obvious clinical implications, carry significant medico-legal implications. The existence of these legal implications explains in part the otherwise puzzling opposition by many to the QT hypothesis.

The all issue centers around what would happen if the medical community accepts the fact that a certain number (never mind if 10% or 25%) of future SIDS victims might be identified by neonatal electrocardiography and that, due to the understanding of the lethal mechanisms involved, high chances would exist to prevent sudden death in these infants. The still prevailing concept of the impossibility of identifying infants at truly high and specific risk for SIDS has the undeniable advantage that no one has to be blamed, except a cruel fate. The acceptance of the QT hypothesis would change all that. The final turning point is represented by our demonstration that it is possible to make the diagnosis of LQTS even in a dead infant already labeled as SIDS and in whom no ECG was ever made *(5)*. Parents of SIDS victims or, more appropriately, their physicians may now begin to ask for a postmortem molecular screening. What will happen whenever, as in our case, the molecular diagnosis will reveal LQTS as the cause of death? The bereaved parents, and their lawyers, will start asking new questions and above all why had they not been informed of the very rare possibility (probably 1 in 3000) that their baby might have been affected by a deadly but curable disease which could have rather easily be unmasked by a simple ECG.

The complexities do not end here. If a neonatal ECG is performed, someone will have to assume the responsibility of deciding whether the QT is normal, borderline, or abnormal, and then to suggest what to do. In a litigation-prone society it is not difficult to realize that the possibility of having to examine a large number of infantile ECGs and having to then express an opinion on the duration of the QT interval is regarded as anathema by anyone who might become embroiled in the process. This is, I believe, the true reason behind the otherwise incomprehensible hostility generated in the pediatric world anytime it was suggested, or whenever actual data support the concept, that neonatal electrocardiography might be useful for the identification of those infants who are at risk for an early arrhythmic death.

ADDENDUM

The findings reported above have already had consequences. Some European countries have begun to consider the possibility of introducing in their National Health Services the performance of an ECG during the first month of life in all newborns, as part of a cardiovascular screening program.

Should neonatal screening indeed be introduced as part of National Health Services, then hospital cardiologists—most of whom are utterly unfamiliar with neonatal ECGs—would be asked to read these tracings. The European Society of Cardiology has realized the potential complications for European cardiologists and for health care, and has acted accordingly by instituting a Task Force for the creation of guidelines for the interpretation of the neonatal ECG *(46)*. The main objective of the Task Force was to provide such guidelines focusing on the most clinically relevant abnormalities, on the ensuing management and referral options. This document represents the official position of the European Society of Cardiology on this subject.

ACKNOWLEDGMENTS

My studies on SIDS are partially supported by the Fondation Leducq grant *Molecular epidemiology of hereditary arrhythmogenic disorders.*

REFERENCES

1. Schwartz PJ. Cardiac sympathetic innervation and the sudden infant death syndrome. A possible pathogenetic link. Am J Med 1976;60:167–172.
2. Schwartz PJ. The quest for the mechanism of the sudden infant death syndrome. Doubts and progress. Circulation 1987;75:677–683.
3. Schwartz PJ, Stramba-Badiale M, Segantini A, et al. Prolongation of the QT interval and the sudden infant death syndrome. N Engl J Med 1998;338:1709–1714.

4. Schwartz PJ, Priori SG, Dumaine R, et al. A molecular link between the sudden infant death syndrome and the long QT syndrome. N Engl J Med 2000;343:262–267.

5. Schwartz PJ, Priori SG, Bloise R, et al. Molecular diagnosis in a child with sudden infant death syndrome. Lancet 2001;358:1342–1343.

6. Lucey JF. Comments on a sudden infant death article in another journal. Pediatrics 1999;103:812.

7. Schwartz PJ, Southall DP, Valdes-Dapena M, eds. The sudden infant death syndrome. Cardiac and respiratory mechanisms and interventions. Ann NY Acad Sci 1988;533:474.

8. Schwartz PJ. The sudden infant death syndrome. In: Reviews in Perinatal Medicine. Scarpelli EM, Cosmi EV, eds. New York: Raven Press, 1981;475–524.

9. Ramanathan R, Corwin MJ, Hunt CE, et al. The Collaborative Home Infant Monitoring Evaluation (CHIME) Study Group: Cardiorespiratory events recorded on home monitors: Comparison of healthy infants with those at increased risk for SIDS. JAMA 2001;285:2199–2207.

10. Jobe AH. What do home monitors contribute to the SIDS problem? JAMA 2001;285:2244–2245.

11. Froggatt P. A cardiac cause in cot death: a discarded hypothesis? Ir Med J 1977;70:408–414.

12. Lown B. Sudden cardiac death: the major challenge confronting contemporary cardiology. Am J Cardiol 1979;43:313–328.

13. NIH Grant HDO8796 1975/1978: Experimental Reproduction of Long QT Syndrome and SIDS.

14. Schwartz PJ, Priori SG, Napolitano C. Long QT syndrome. In: Cardiac Electrophysiology. From Cell to Bedside. III Edition. Zipes DP and Jalife J, eds. Philadelphia: WB Saunders Co., 2000;597–615.

15. Priori SG, Barhanin J, Hauer RNW, et al. Genetic and molecular basis of cardiac arrhythmias: impact on clinical management. Part I and II. Circulation 1999;99:518–528; Part III Circulation 1999;99:674–681, and Eur Heart J 1999;20:174–195.

16. Maron BJ, Clark CE, Goldstein RE, Epstein SE. Potential role of QT interval prolongation in sudden infant death syndrome. Circulation 1976;54:423–430.

17. Kelly DH, Shannon DC, Liberthson R. The role of the QT interval in the Sudden Infant Death Syndrome. Circulation 1977;55:633–635.

18. Steinschneider A. Sudden infant death syndrome and prolongation of the QT interval. Am J Dis Child 1978;132:688–691.

19. Haddad GG, Epstein MAF, Epstein RA, Mazza NR, Mellins RB, Krongrad E. The QT interval in aborted sudden infant death syndrome infants. Pediat Res 1979;13:136–138.

20. Montague TJ, Finley JP, Mukelabai K, et al. Cardiac rhythm, rate and ventricular repolarization properties in infants at risk for Sudden Infant Death Syndrome: Comparison with age- and sex-matched control infants. Am J Cardiol 1984;54:301–307.

21. Southall DP, Arrowsmith WA, Stebbens V, Alexander JR. QT interval measurements before sudden infant death syndrome. Arch Dis Child 1986;61:327–333.

22. Schwartz PJ, Segantini A. Cardiac innervation, neonatal electrocardiography and SIDS. A key for a novel preventive strategy? Ann NY Acad Sci 1988;533:210–220.

23. Towbin JA, Friedman RA. Prolongation of the QT interval and the sudden infant death syndrome. N Engl J Med 1998;338:1760–1761.

24. Schwartz PJ, Wolf S. QT interval prolongation as predictor of sudden death in patients with myocardial infarction. Circulation 1978;57:1074–1077.

25. Algra A, Tijssen JGP, Roelandt JRTC, Pool J, Lubsen J. QTc prolongation measured by standard 12-lead electrocardiography is an independent risk factor for sudden death due to cardiac arrest. Circulation 1991;83:1888–1894.

26. Schouten EG, Dekker JM, Meppelink P, Kok FJ, Vandenbroucke JP, Pool J. QT interval prolongation predicts cardiovascular mortality in an apparently healthy population. Circulation 1991;84:1516–1523.

27. Napolitano C, Schwartz PJ, Brown AM, et al. Evidence for a cardiac ion channel mutation underlying drug-induced QT prolongation and life-threatening arrhythmias. J Cardiovasc Electrophysiol 2000;11:691–696.

28. Dwyer T, Ponsonby AL, Blizzard L, Newman NM, Cochrane JA. The contribution in the prevalence of prone sleeping position to the decline in Sudden Infant Death syndrome in Tasmania. JAMA 1995;273:783–789.

29. Schwartz PJ, La Rovere MT, Vanoli E. Autonomic nervous system and sudden cardiac death. Experimental basis and clinical observations for post-myocardial infarction risk stratification. Circulation 1992;85(Suppl. I):I77–I91.

30. Guntheroth WG, Wedgwood RJ, Benditt EP, eds. Discussion in Sudden Death in Infants (First Conference), Public Health Service Publication n° 1412, Government Printing, p. 6, 1963.

31. Steinschneider A. Prolonged apnea and the sudden infant death syndrome: clinical and laboratory observations. Pediatrics 1972;50:646–654.
32. Firstman R, Talan J. The Death of Innocents. New York: Bantam Books, 1997.
33. Martin RJ, Miller MJ, Redline S. Screening for SIDS: a neonatal perspective. Pediatrics 1999;103: 812–813.
34. Guntheroth WG, Spiers PS. Prolongation of the QT interval and the sudden infant death syndrome. Pediatrics 1999;103:813–814.
35. Weinstein SL, Steinschneider A. QTc and R-R intervals in victims of the sudden infant death syndrome. Am J Dis Child 1985;139:987–990.
36. Schaffer MS, Trippel DL, Buckles DS, Young RH, Dolan PL, Gillette PC. The longitudinal time course of QTc in early infancy. Preliminary results of a prospective sudden infant death syndrome surveillance program. J Perinatol 1991;11:57–62.
37. Gillette PC, Garson A Jr. Sudden cardiac death in the pediatric population. Circulation 1992;85(Suppl I):I64–I69.
38. Walsh ZS. Electrocardiographic intervals during the first week of life. Am Heart J 1963;66:36–43.
39. Priori SG, Napolitano C, Schwartz PJ. Low penetrance in the long QT syndrome. Clinical impact. Circulation 1999;99:529–533.
40. Stramba-Badiale M, Lazzarotti M, Schwartz PJ. Development of cardiac innervation, ventricular fibrillation and Sudden Infant Death Syndrome. Am J Physiol 1992;263:H1514–H1522.
41. Gootman PM, ed. Developmental Neurobiology of the Autonomic Nervous System. Clifton, NJ: Humana Press, 1986.
42. Schwartz PJ. QT prolongation, sudden death, and sympathetic imbalance: the pendulum swings. J Cardiovasc Electrophysiol 2001;12:1074–1077.
43. Ackerman MJ, Siu BL, Sturner WQ, et al. Postmortem molecular analysis of SCN5A defects in Sudden Infant Death Syndrome. JAMA 2001;286:2264–2269.
44. Wedekind H, Smits JP, Schulze-Bahr E, et al. De novo mutation in the SCN5A gene associated with early onset of sudden infant death. Circulation 2001;104:1158–1164.
45. Towbin JA, Ackerman MJ. Cardiac sodium channel gene mutations and sudden infant death syndrome: confirmation of proof of concept? Circulation 2001;104:1092–1093.
46. Schwartz PJ, Garson A Jr., Paul T, et al. Guidelines for the interpretation of the neonatal electrocardiogram. A Task Force of the European Society of Cardiology. Eur Heart J 2002;23:1329–1344.

22

Short QT Interval
ECG Phenomenon and Clinical Syndrome

Ihor Gussak, MD, PhD,
Charles Antzelevitch, PhD,
Daniel Goodman, MD,
and Preben Bjerregaard, MD, DMSc

CONTENTS

INTRODUCTION
CURRENT PERSPECTIVE
POSSIBLE MECHANISMS AND ARRHYTHMOGENIC POTENTIAL
LIMITATIONS
REFERENCES

INTRODUCTION

Although many factors influence the duration of ventricular repolarization and the detailed appearance of ECG (Table 1), regional differences in the configuration of action potentials across the myocardial wall are considered to be major determinants of the three-dimensional pattern of ECG waves and intervals. The QT interval is a surrogate electrocardiographic index of ventricular repolarization. Its duration under normal conditions is mainly determined by expression, properties, and balance of the repolarizing forces inward sodium and calcium, and outward potassium and chloride currents (**intrinsic** cardiac properties).

QT interval is also a function of the heart rate and is affected by various **extracardiac** factors, such as:

1. Serum electrolytes (K^+, Na^+, Ca^{2+}).
2. Acid-base balance.
3. Autonomic nervous system.

The gradual adjustment of the QT duration to the heart rate is a normal adaptive electrophysiological response and the incremental or decremental effects range within predictable physiological limits.

From: *Contemporary Cardiology: Cardiac Repolarization: Bridging Basic and Clinical Science*
Edited by: I. Gussak et al. © Humana Press Inc., Totowa, NJ

Table 1
The List of Intrinsic and Extracardiac Electrophysiological Factors That Determine
and Modulate the Electrocardiographic Contour and the Duration
of the Ventricular Repolarization

Intrinsic cardiac factors:
    Shape and duration of the action potentials and their heterogeneity
    Numbers of depolarizing cells participating in generation of the repolarizing currents
    Degree of electrotonic transmission and cell-to-cell coupling conductance
    Primary asynchrony of the repolarization
    Secondary asynchrony of the repolarization due to asynchrony of depolarization
Extracardiac factors:
    Neurotransmitters
    Electrolytes
    Temperature

The upper limit of normal for the QT interval is addressed in numerous studies and is well defined, and its prolongation has been used as an ECG marker to identify patients at risk for sudden arrhythmogenic death. However, there is no consensus on the *lower limit* of normal for the QT interval or its clinical significance. Persistently short QT interval is clinically most often encountered in patients with hypercalcemia *(1,2)*, and until recently it has not been considered a sign of an increased risk for arrhythmias *(5,6)*. Although a link between short QT and electrical instability of the heart is not as yet firmly established, there is some evidence that a short QT interval may at times be associated with an increased risk for arrhythmic events.

CURRENT PERSPECTIVE

Predefined ECG Criteria and Incidence of the Short QT Interval

Whether a QT interval is unusually short, becomes apparent when it is seen in the context of the study by Rautaharju et al. *(7)*. They examined the QT interval in 14,379 *healthy individuals* and established a formula by which the duration of the QT interval can be predicted (QTp): QTp (ms)=656/(1+Heart Rate/100). In their study, the incidence of a QT interval shorter than 88% of the predicted value was 2.5% (360 of 14,379), whereas a QT duration less than 80% of the predicted value was seen in only 0.03% (4 of 14,379; all females). Since two standard deviations below the mean is 88% of QTp *(7)* it would seem reasonable to consider this value of the QT duration as the lower limit of normal for QT interval *(5,6)*.

In another large-scale database of 336,675 ECGs from 113,811 *drug studies subjects* of both sexes and primarily adult, healthy volunteers (D. Goodman, unpublished data) reasonably similar numbers were found. QT intervals shorter than 88% and 80% of predicted value was seen in 0.11% and 0.006% of the population (no gender difference was noted), respectively.

Clinical Presentation: ECG Phenomenon vs Clinical Syndrome

Recently, two forms of abnormally short QT interval have been described:

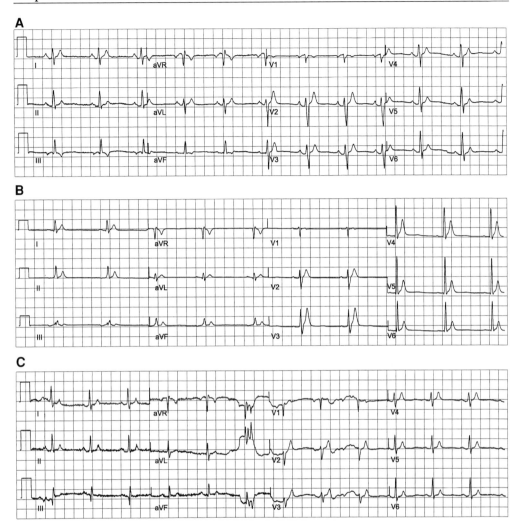

Fig. 1. Idiopathic familial initially short QT interval. **(A)** Twelve-lead ECG from 17-yr-old patient with QT interval duration of 71% of a predictive value. Note: QT interval duration: 280 ms; heart rate: 69 bpm; predictive value of the QT interval: 393 ms; QTc (by Bazzet's formula): 300 ms. **(B)** Twelve-lead ECG from 21-yr-old brother with QT interval duration of 66% of a predictive value. Note: QT interval duration: 272 ms; heart rate: 58 bpm; predictive value of the QT interval: 415 ms; QTc (by Bazzet's formula): 267 ms (half standard). **(C)** Twelve-lead ECG from 51-yr-old mother with QT interval duration of 69% of a predictive value. Note: QT interval duration: 260 ms; heart rate: 74 bpm; predictive value of the QT interval: 377 ms; QTc (by Bazzet's formula): 289 ms.

1. Idiopathic (persistently) short QT interval.
2. Paradoxical deceleration-dependent shortening of the QT interval (DDSQTI).

Idiopathic Persistently Short QT Interval

Recently, we have presented different clinical cases where unexplained (idiopathic) very short QT interval was associated with serious arrhythmias *(5)*. This first clinical

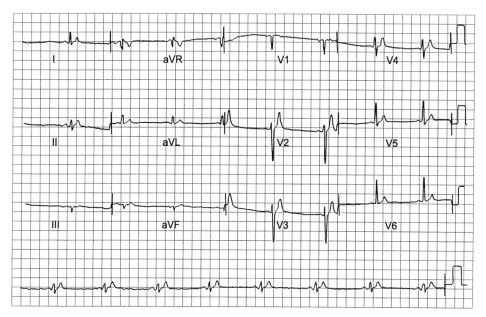

Fig. 2. Twelve-lead ECG obtained from 37-yr-old victim of sudden cardiac death. Note: QT interval of 266 ms; heart rate of 52 bpm; predictive value of the QT interval of 431; QT interval of 63% of predictive value; QTc (by Bazzet's formula) of 248 ms.

report of an idiopathic familial persistently short QT interval *(5)* described three members of one family—two siblings and their mother (but not father who had a normal QT interval)—who demonstrated identical ECG phenomenon: an idiopathic abnormally short QT interval (Fig. 1). All QT intervals in these relatives were less than 80% of predicted value (QTp). The 17-yr-old female patient had a QT of 280 ms, which was 71% of the QTp. Her brother had a QT of 272 ms, which was 66% of the QTp. Her mother had a QT interval of 260 ms or 69% of QTp.

In the 17-yr-old patient, the short QT interval was associated with several episodes of paroxysmal atrial fibrillation requiring electrical cardioversion. It was noteworthy that there was no correlation between the QT interval duration and the cardiac cycle length, even during atrial fibrillation. There were also two episodes of dizziness and palpitations reported by the mother, but no documented arrhythmias.

In 1996, Dr. Josep Brugada obtained the ECG recording in otherwise healthy 37-yr-old Caucasian female with a history of syncopal episodes who died suddenly, while awaiting further diagnostic work-up. Her QT was almost twice shorter than normal (Fig. 2) *(5)*.

Paradoxical (Deceleration-Dependent) Shortening of the QT Interval

Another form of short QT, the dramatic paradoxical deceleration-dependent shortening of the QT interval (DDSQTI) has been described in a 4-yr-old African-American girl with complications related to her premature birth, including developmental delay and several episodes of cardiac arrest *(6)*. An episode of severe transient bradyarrhythmia was documented by Holter monitoring (Fig. 3). A unique feature of the rhythm strips was a paradoxical (deceleration-dependent) gradual shortening of the QT interval to 216 ms with accompanying transient T waves abnormalities.

Paradoxically shortened QT interval after a prolonged pause was described in two patients with prolonged RR interval and was interpreted as an abnormal adaptation of repolarization time to an abrupt increase in preceding RR intervals (8).

Clinical Significance

The clinical significance of a short QT interval becomes apparent when it is seen in the context of the study by Algra et al. (9). They reported that both a prolonged and a shortened mean QTc over 24 h was associated with a more than twofold risk of sudden death compared to patients in whom mean QTc was normal (400–440 ms). The relative risk of sudden death was 2.3 for patients with a prolonged mean QTc (>440 ms) and 2.4 for patients with shortened QTc (<400 ms). Another large-scale epidemiological study on the value of QT interval as a cardiac risk factor in middle aged people, revealed that a shortened QT interval predicts death in men with heart disease who smoke (10).

A few case reports demonstrating a strikingly short QT interval have been published in the literature; some of them have directed attention to this unusual ECG abnormality. Transient short QT interval was evident in the ECG obtained from a 7-yr-old patient with catecholaminergic polymorphic ventricular tachycardia (11). Marked shortening of the QT interval immediately after spontaneously terminated ventricular fibrillation was reported in patient with a long history of recurrent syncope (Fig. 4) (12). Shortening of the QT interval immediately preceding the onset of idiopathic spontaneous ventricular tachycardia was noted by Fei et al. (13).

The presence of an abnormally short QT interval in conjunction with arrhythmias in otherwise healthy subjects points to a causal relationship and the immediate question is whether this is a new clinical syndrome.

Thus far, it seems that, like in the case of Brugada Syndrome, the short QT interval as a special ECG phenomenon has been overlooked in the past. Interestingly, QT interval shorter than normal was reported by Aihara and his colleagues in 1990 in their first patients with Brugada Syndrome (14).

POSSIBLE MECHANISMS AND ARRHYTHMOGENIC POTENTIAL

Because little is known about the electrophysiologic feature of this syndrome, a discussion of possible mechanisms is speculative at best. Our current working hypotheses are:

1. Idiopathic persistently short QT interval is primary because of a congenital defect involving an intrinsic abnormality of ion channel function of the cardiac cell. Because the T wave remains upright and the interval between the peak and end of the T wave is not prolonged, we can assume that abbreviation of repolarization involves a homogeneous abbreviation of the action potential of the three predominant cell types spanning the ventricular wall, and that transmural dispersion of repolarization is not augmented. Abbreviation of the action potential may be owing to any number of factors including but not limited to:
   a. A change in the density or kinetics of inactivation and reactivation of the transient outward current (I_{to}); the latter may be more feasible since an increase in I_{to} density alone (although capable of importantly abbreviating the action potential secondary to

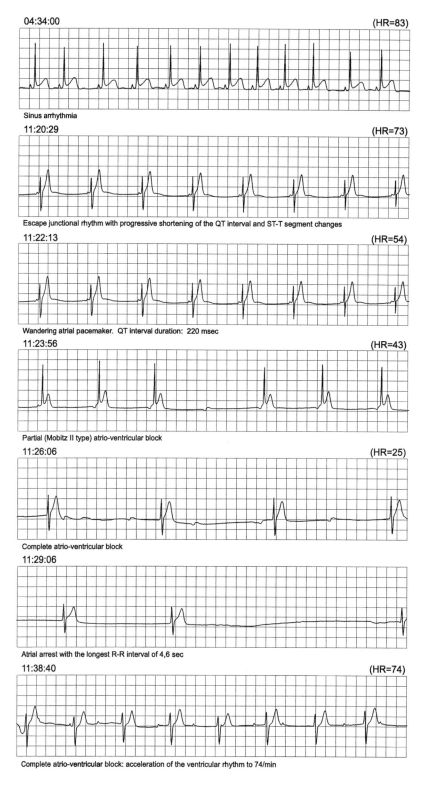

Fig. 3. Paradoxical (deceleration-dependent) shortening of the QT interval.

04:34:00: Sinus arrhythmia with normal QT interval.

11:20:29: Escape junctional rhythm with progressive shortening of the QT interval and tall T wave.

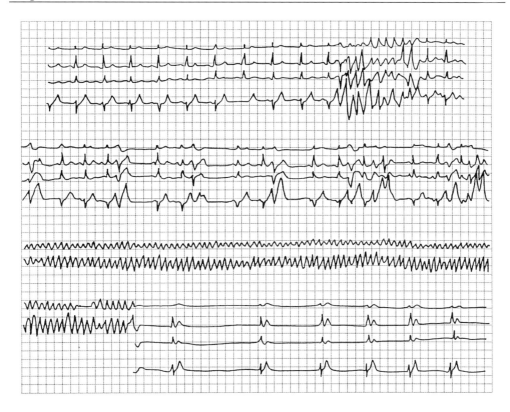

Fig. 4. An episode of self-terminating idiopathic ventricular fibrillation in 38-yr-old man. Note: a dramatic shortening of the QT interval immediately after the termination of the ventricular fibrillation.

loss of the action potential dome) would quickly deplete the cell of calcium needed to maintain contraction.

b. An increase in density or altered kinetics of activation and/or inactivation of I_{Kr}, I_{Ks}, $I_{K\text{-}ATP}$, and/or $I_{K,ACh}$.

c. Reduced density of late I_{Na} or I_{Ca}.

In all cases the abbreviation of action potential duration (APD) would be expected to be accompanied by a proportional abbreviation of refractoriness. The shorter refractory period would be expected to permit the establishment of reentrant circuits over a shorter path length owing to the abbreviated wavelength (refractory period times conduction velocity) of the reentrant wavefront. This may in turn contribute to a greater proclivity

---

Fig. 3. *(Continued)*

11:22:13: Wandering atrial pacemaker; QT interval duration: 220 ms; heart rate 54 bpm.

11:23:56: Escape (supraventricular) rhythm with partial (Mobitz II type) atrioventricular block.

11:26:06: Complete atrioventricular block with the shortest QT interval duration of 216 ms (third complex).

11:29:06: Atrial arrest with the RR interval of 4600 ms.

11:38:40: Complete atrioventricular block with acceleration of the ventricular rhythm to 76 bpm and normalization of the QT interval duration.

for the development of atrial and/or ventricular tachyarrhythmias. It is of interest that a short QT interval is a normal ECG feature in some animals including the rat, mouse, and kangaroo *(15,16)* because of their rapid ventricular repolarization *(16)*. Of note, kangaroo is also known for a high incidence of sudden cardiac death *(16)* (see Chapter 3).

2. Transient paradoxical shortening of QT interval is extracardiac in origin and is modulated by autonomic nervous system. The activation of the $I_{K,ACh}$ owing to unusually high vagal tone to the heart was proposed as a possible mechanism responsible for the DDSQTI *(6)*. Paradoxical shortening of the QT interval dependent on marked slowing of heart rate has been described in experiments addressing dose-dependent effects of ACh on the heart. High levels of ACh can inhibit I_{Ca} and activate $I_{K,ACh}$ resulting in abbreviation of ventricular repolarization *(17,18)*.

LIMITATIONS

Electrophysiologic and genetic data are not available for any of the patients discussed previously. Electrophysiological studies of such patients would be most helpful as would more complete investigations of family members. Owing to the limited availability of information, it is not clear whether we are dealing with a distinct clinical entity or an ECG phenomenon with a broad spectrum of etiologies. The casual association of this ECG signature with arrhythmic events warrants our attention.

REFERENCES

1. Commerford PJ, Lloyd EA. Arrhythmias in patients with drug toxicity, electrolyte, and endocrine disturbances. Med Clin North Am 1984;68:1051–1078.
2. Nierenberg DW, Ransil BJ. Q-aTc interval as a clinical indicator of hypercalcemia. Am J Cardiol 1979;44:243–248.
3. Nakagawa M, Takahashi N, Iwao T, et al. Evaluation of autonomic influences on QT dispersion using the head-up tilt test in healthy subjects. Pacing Clin Electrophysiol 1999;22:1158–1163.
4. DiFrancesco D, Ducouret P, Robison RB. Muscarinic modulation of the cardiac rate at low acetylcholine concentrations. Science 1989;243:669–671.
5. Gussak I, Brugada P, Brugada J, et al. Idiopathic short QT interval: a new clinical syndrome? Cardiology 2000;94(2):99–102.
6. Gussak I, Liebl N, Nouri S, Bjerregaard P, Zimmerman F, Chaitman BR. Deceleration-dependent shortening of the QT interval: a new electrocardiographic phenomenon? Clin Cardiol 1999;22:124–126.
7. Rautaharju PM, Zhou SH, Wong S, et al. Sex differences in the evolution of the electrocardiographic QT interval with age. Can J Cardiol 1992;8:690–695.
8. Takahashi N, Ito M, Ishida S, et al. Paradoxically shortened QT interval after a prolonged pause. PACE 1998;21:1476–1479.
9. Algra A, Tijssen JG, Roelandt JR, Pool J, Lubsen J. QT interval variables from 24 hour electrocardiography and the two year risk of sudden death. Br Heart J 1993;70(1):43–48.
10. Karjalainen J, Reunanen A, Ristola P, Viitasalo M. QT interval as a cardiac risk factor in a middle aged population. Heart 1997;77(6):543–548.
11. Leenhardt A, Lucet V, Denjoy I, Grau F, Ngoc DD, Coumel P. Catecholaminergic polymorphic ventricular tachycardia in children. A 7-year follow-up of 21 patients. Circulation 1995;91(5):1512–1519.
12. Kontny F, Dale J. Self-terminating idiopathic ventricular fibrillation presenting as syncope: a 40-year follow-up report. J Int Med 1990;227:211–213.
13. Fei L, Camm AJ. Shortening of the QT interval immediately preceding the onset of idiopathic spontaneous ventricular tachycardia. Am Heart J 1995;130(4):915–917.
14. Aihara N, Ohe T, Kamakura S, et al. Clinical and electrophysiologic characteristics of idiopathic ventricular fibrillation. Shinzo 1990;22 (Suppl. 2):80–86.
15. Campbell TJ. Characteristics of cardiac action potentials in marsupials. J Comp Physiol [B] 1989;158:759–762.

16. Gussak I, Chaitman BR, Kopecky SL, Nerbonne JM. Rapid ventricular repolarization in rodents: electrocardiographic manifestations, molecular mechanisms, and clinical insights. J Electrocardiol 2000;33(2):159–170.
17. Litovsky SH, Antzelevitch C. Differences in the electrophysiological response of canine ventricular subendocardium and subepicardium to acetylcholine and isoproterenol. A direct effect of acetylcholine in ventricular myocardium. Circ Res 1990;67:615–627
18. Yang ZK, Boyett MR, Janvier NC, MsMorn SO, Shui Z, Karim F. Regional differences in the negative inotropic effect of acetylcholine within the canine ventricle. J Physiol (Lond) 1996;492:789–806.

23 T-Wave Alternans
Mechanisms, Relevance, and Clinical Implications

Etienne Pruvot, MD
and David S. Rosenbaum, MD

CONTENTS

EPIDEMIOLOGY OF SUDDEN CARDIAC DEATH

Cardiovascular disease is the main cause of death in Western countries and account for more than half a million deaths annually in the USA. Sudden cardiac death (SCD) accounts for more than 50% of cardiovascular mortality and its incidence has been estimated as high as 0.1 to 0.2% in the overall population *(1)*. In approx 1/3 of cardiac patients, SCD is the first manifestation of coronary artery disease, and its incidence is increasing proportionally to the number of risk factors *(2)*.

The elaboration of intensive care units in the fifties has greatly improved the prognosis of patients suffering from an acute myocardial infarction (MI), with a twofold reduction in mortality rate from 30% to 13% during the in-hospital period *(3)*. Nowadays, with aggressive therapy of acute MI, short-term and long-term prognosis is improved with a < 6% mortality rate during the acute phase *(3,4)*. However, despite considerable progress in the management of cardiac patients, a substantial amount of this population is still

From: *Contemporary Cardiology: Cardiac Repolarization: Bridging Basic and Clinical Science*
Edited by: I. Gussak et al. © Humana Press Inc., Totowa, NJ

experiencing life-threatening events and SCD, particularly during the year following discharge from the hospital.

RISK STRATIFICATION OF POST-MI PATIENTS

Numerous invasive and noninvasive techniques have been developed over the years in order to identify patients at risk of late arrhythmic events such as ventricular tachycardia (VT) or fibrillation (VF). Reduced left ventricular ejection fraction (LVEF), over 10 VPC/hour during Holter monitoring, nonsustained VT and presence of pulmonary rales in intensive care units were the first parameters used for the prognosis assessment among patients hospitalized for an acute MI. Although some success in risk assessment has been achieved with noninvasive techniques, such as signal averaged ECG and heart rate variability analysis for instance, none of these (alone or combined) is known to offer a positive predictive value of future adverse events sufficient enough to preventively implant ICDs.

Over the last two decades, programmed ventricular stimulation (PVS) has been used to stratify post-MI patients at risks for late arrhythmic events. Originally thought to be as high as 80 to 90%, its sensitivity has dropped with the advent of follow-up data based on registry of patients with negative studies (5,6). Following an acute MI, patients with depressed LVEF are still at high risk of suffering from ventricular arrhythmias despite a negative study (6). Recent studies, however, have reported its utility as a risk stratification tool for ventricular arrhythmias after preselection by noninvasive means (6–8). In these primary prevention studies, post-MI patients with nonsustained VT and depressed LVEF (<0.35–0.4) were screened with PVS. Those with sustained ventricular arrhythmias were randomized to conventional drug therapy or to implantable cardioverter defibrillator (ICD), and followed for more than three years. The survival of patients treated with an ICD was clearly improved as compared to patients treated with conventional therapy, including those whose antiarrhythmic drug regimen was guided by VPS. In the MADIT study, the overall mortality in the ICD group was reduced by 54% as compared to the control group, but the proportion of patients with an ICD dying during follow-up remained as high as 16% (7). With a similar design, the MUSTT study was aimed at comparing patients with VPS-guided therapy, including antiarrhythmic drugs and ICD, to patients without conventional therapy. A clear benefit of ICDs over the two other groups was observed, with a risk reduction of SCD or arrhythmia as high as 76%. Among inducible patients not implanted with an ICD, the five-year rate of death from arrhythmia was 32%. Nowadays, those patients are systematically implanted with an ICD. Taking into account the MUSTT data, it appears that 68% of the patients with reduced LVEF and PVS-induced ventricular arrhythmias will not benefit from their ICD. Moreover, the MUSTT registry revealed a clear adverse prognosis among noninducible patients with depressed LVEF. The rate of arrhythmic events was nearly equal to the one of inducible patients not treated by ICDs (6). With the ongoing improvement in ICDs technology, the challenge does not appear to be the therapeutic approach anymore, but the appropriate identification of high risk patients. Risk stratification has to be accurate enough to identify as many patients as possible who are at risk for SCD, whereas avoiding as much as possible ICD implantation in those who will remain asymptomatic. This appears particularly true in light of the recent finding of the MADIT2 trial, whose purpose was to determine the benefit of ICD implantation in any patients with depressed LVEF following an acute MI

(9). No preselection with VPS was required. To prevent one SCD over two years, 17 ICDs had to be implanted, which left 16 patients with the burden but no clear benefit of ICD implantation.

BIOPHYSICS OF THE T WAVE

The scalar ECG is characterized by different waves reflecting depolarization and repolarization processes of myocardial cells, which lead to cardiac contractions. Among these, the T wave is of particular relevance, because it specifically reflects the repolarization process of the myocardium. The action potential of myocardial cells displays different phases of activation and inhibition of ionic currents. Calcium and potassium fluxes are of particular importance in the genesis of T waves because they are mainly responsible for the repolarization currents of the action potential. The myocardial wall is composed of three layers of cells described as the endocardium, the mid-myocardium (composed of M cells) and the epicardium. The myocardial wall is depolarized from the endocardium to the epicardium. The steep voltage gradient produced by phase 0 of the endo-, followed by the M cells and then by the epicardial cells inscribes the abrupt QRS wave of the ECG. The biophysical properties of the repolarization process of the three layers differ, which account for the genesis of the T wave of the ECG. M cells display the longest action potential, followed by endocardial, then by epicardial cells. As a consequence, the order of repolarization of the three layers does not follow that of depolarization. Epicardial cells repolarize first, followed by endocardial cells, then by M cells. This produces opposing voltage gradients on either side of the M cells, responsible for the inscription of the T wave on the ECG. Briefly, the T wave begins when the plateau of the epicardial action potential separates from that of the M cells. Opposite to the epicardium, with a little delay, the endocardium plateau deviates from that of the M cells generating an opposite voltage gradients that limits the amplitude of the T wave. The T wave ends when M cells are fully repolarized *(10).* From these considerations, it appears that any change in the ST segment and T-wave morphology will indicate changes in voltage gradients across the transmural wall. Moreover, any change in beat-to-beat ST and T-wave morphology (i.e., T-wave alternans) is indicative of a change in repolarization voltage gradient on an every-other-beat basis.

T-WAVE ALTERNANS AS A HARBINGER
OF SUDDEN CARDIAC DEATH

Electrical alternans is defined as repetitive beat-to-beat fluctuations of ECG amplitude within the QRS, ST, and T waves. This ECG pattern was first described by Herring in 1909 and was initially thought to be of little significance *(11).* Shortly after the introduction of the ECG, however, Sir Thomas Lewis recognized electrical alternans as a distinct clinical pathophysiological entity: "…alternans occurs either when the heart muscle is normal but the heart rate is very fast or when there is a serious disease and the rate is normal" *(12).* In 1948, Kalter and Schwartz reported a 62% mortality rate in patients with visibly apparent T-wave alternans *(13).* Then, T-wave alternans was subsequently observed in a surprisingly wide variety of clinical and experimental conditions associated with ventricular arrhythmias, including acute MI *(14,15),* electrolyte imbalances *(16,17),* Prinzmetal's angina *(18,19),* and Long QT syndrome *(20–22).*

In the 80s Cohen and coworkers *(23,24)* measured visually undetectable T-wave alternans using signal processing tools based on a power spectrum analysis of T wave indices. They established for the first time a quantitative relationship between T-wave alternans and susceptibility to VF. VF threshold and amplitude of surface T-wave alternans were compared in experimental settings including hypothermia, tachycardia and coronary artery ligation. A clear negative relationship was reported: as VF threshold decreased, T-wave alternans amplitude increased. Importantly, this peculiar pattern was generally not detectable by visual inspection of the ECG! In 1994, microvolt-level of alternans was established as a marker of susceptibility to SCD *(25)*, a finding which was subsequently reaffirmed by a number of clinical trials *(26–34)*.

OPTICAL MAPPING STUDIES ON THE MECHANISMS OF T-WAVE ALTERNANS

The first historical observations reported an increased susceptibility to ventricular arrhythmias in patients showing signs of T-wave alternans on surface ECG. Then, T-wave alternans was observed under a broad variety of conditions, from the most benign to the most dramatic ones, and as a consequence, did not appear to bear any prognostic value. It is with the advent of techniques allowing recording of the depolarization as well as the repolarization phases of the action potential that a clear understanding of the link between T-wave alternans, action potential duration (APD) variations and VF onset was made possible. Monophasic action potential (MAP) and optical mapping recordings are two typical examples. In this regard, optical mapping bears many advantages over MAP because it allows one to record simultaneously a much larger number of action potential at different resolution, ranging from single cells to nearly the whole heart. Optical mapping is based on the recording of fluorescent light emitted by voltage sensitive dyes in response to an excitation source. Voltage sensitive dyes have been used extensively to measure transmembrane potential in a variety of neuronal and cardiac preparations. These dyes bind to the cell membrane with high affinity and exhibit changes in fluorescence intensity which vary linearly with transmembrane potential *(35)*. Optically recorded action potential waveforms closely mimic the time course and morphology of action potential recorded using microelectrode techniques under various pharmacological and ionic interventions. A comprehensive review of cardiac and optical mapping techniques was published previously *(36)*.

Our optical mapping system is capable of recording high fidelity action potential from 256 simultaneous sites in beating intact hearts without the use of drugs that artificially suppress cardiac contraction *(26,37,38)*. Hearts are stained with the voltage-sensitive dye di-4-ANEPPS by direct coronary perfusion. Automated computer algorithms have been developed to analyze action potential activation, recovery, and morphology. Quantitative measurements of APD are possible because of the high temporal (0.3 to 1.0 ms) and voltage (0.5 to 2 mV) resolutions achieved with our data acquisition hardware and tandem lens imaging technology which optimizes action potential fidelity *(26,27,39)*. Because system noise is minimized, our filters are set at 0.01–1000 Hz, well outside the bandwidth of optically recorded ventricular action potentials, and thus do not distort their characteristics. Flexible magnification allows one to record potentials from a 17×17 mm (~1 mm resolution between recording sites) to a 4.5×4.5 mm (~350 μm resolution between recording sites) region of ventricle. Finally, action potential and ECGs are sampled to 512

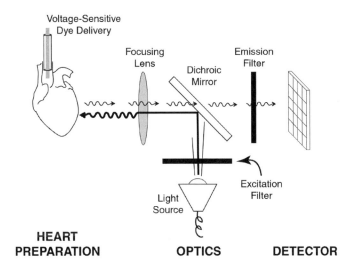

Fig. 1. Typical optical mapping system consisting of three major components: 1. The heart preparation; 2. A system of optics; and 3. A detector. An excitation filter is used to pass selected wavelengths of light from the light source to a dichroic mirror, which semiselectively reflects light of this wavelength and directs it toward the preparation. In response to excitation light, voltage-sensitive dye molecules bound to the heart cells fluoresce light in proportion to the membrane potential of the cell to which they are bound. Light emitted from the dye has a longer wavelength, and therefore passes through (it is not reflected) the dichroic mirror, undergoes a final stage of filtering, and is focused onto the detector.

MB circular memory buffer permitting continuous recordings of the initiation and evolution of any arrhythmias during premature stimulation of the heart.

Figure 1 shows a schematic of the system used in our laboratory. Beating and perfused hearts are immersed in a custom built Tyrode-filled Lexan chamber and positioned with a micromanipulator so that the mapping field (1×1 cm) is centered over the anterior surface of the left ventricle. To maintain surface temperature of the viable epicardium, the heart is immersed in the coronary effluent which is maintained at a constant temperature with a heat exchanger inside the chamber. By applying gentle pressure to the posterior surface of the heart with a moveable piston, hearts contract freely except for the surface within the mapping field. This design eliminates motion artifacts from optically recorded action potentials without altering electrophysiological properties and thus obviates the need for suppressing cardiac contraction with drugs known to influence action potential characteristics and reentrant excitation.

For the purpose of understanding the mechanisms leading to action potential alternans, Fig. 2 shows representative examples of parameters used to characterize activation, repolarization as well as APD from optically recorded waveforms. The first parameter of interest is the activation time (AT) which is defined as the time elapsed between a reference (e.g., stimulus artifact) and the maximum of the first derivative of optical action potential signals. This measure is a reliable marker of the depolarization of cardiomyocytes, and corresponds electrophysiologically to the maximum influx of sodium ions in response to the opening of sodium channels *(40)*. The second parameter of interest is repolarization time (RT), defined as the time elapsed from a reference and the maximum

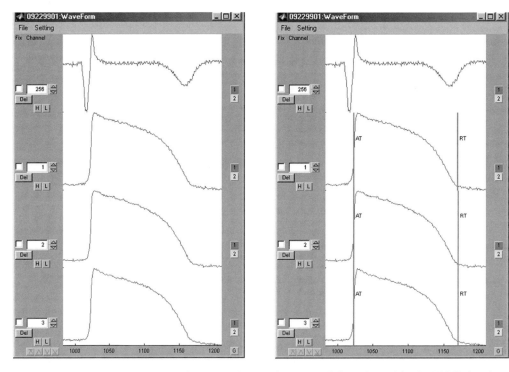

Fig. 2. Representative examples of three optical action potentials and one bipolar ECG simultaneously acquired from a grid of 256 photodiodes covering a surface of 1 cm^2 of the epicardium of a guinea pig Langendorff preparation. Each waveform was acquired at a sampling rate of 1 KHz, and represents the integral optical activity of an area of 625×625 μm. Signals are normalized to the same amplitude. AT and RT depict activation time and repolarization time annotations respectively. APD is measured by subtracting AT to RT values.

of the local second derivative of the action potential signal *(39,40)*. This measure has been shown to be less sensitive to motion artifacts and baseline drift, unlike algorithms based on absolute thresholds of action potential (e.g., APD$_{90}$) or on first derivative *(40)*. The third currently used parameter is action potential duration (APD) directly measured from subtracting AT to RT. Color gradient are used to display similar timing of the depolarization or repolarization processes for the 256 recording sites. Each color or shade represent an area of cardiomyocytes activated in a given amount of time (e.g., 5 ms, 10 ms, etc.), resulting in maps of synchronous (e.g., isochronal) activation and repolarization, known as contour maps. Figure 3 shows a typical example of AT and RT contour map as well as the resulting APD of a guinea pig heart paced at a CL of 400 ms and during delivery of a premature stimulus. Note the earliest activation and repolarization time near the pacing site for the premature stimulus, which is consistent with a propagating wave moving away.

RESTITUTION-BASED HYPOTHESIS FOR ALTERNANS

Action potential restitution kinetics appear to play a key role in the genesis of APD alternans at the level of single cell as well as at tissue level. Classically, APD restitution is measured after delivering an extrastimulus over a wide range of coupling intervals at

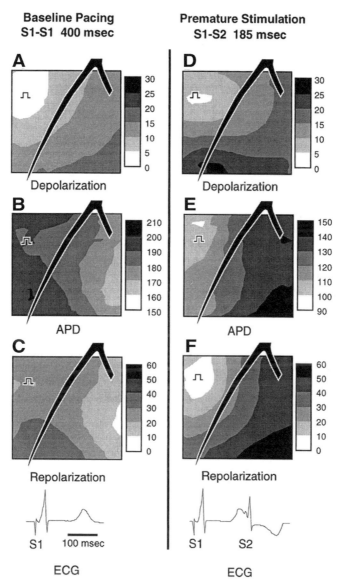

Fig. 3. Contour maps of depolarization (**A** and **D**), APD (**B** and **E**) and repolarization (**C** and **F**) during baseline pacing (left) and a premature stimulus (right). To the right of each map is a gray scale with corresponding numerical values in millisecond. APD during baseline pacing shows a right to left gradient, that nearly shifts 180° during delivery of a premature stimulus near refractory period. Inversion of repolarization is reflected in the ECG (bottom) by the inversion of T-wave polarity during the premature stimulus. Reproduced with permission *(39)*.

the end of a regular train of stimuli. As shown in Fig. 4, APD typically decreases monotonically and exponentially as a function of the previous diastolic interval (DI), which suggests some nonlinear behavior of the processes underlying action potential restitution kinetics.

Alternation of the T wave and of the membrane potential is provoked above a threshold heart rate, which most likely corresponds to a time interval that is shorter than the recovery

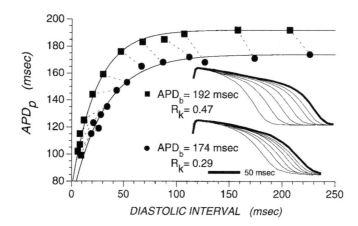

Fig. 4. Restitution curves generated from optical action potentials (inset) measured simultaneously from two ventricular sites. The bold action potentials were recorded during the last beat of the constant cycle length drive train, and the remaining potentials were recorded at progressively shorter S1–S2 coupling intervals. The site at which APD_b is longer (square) has a faster time course of restitution compared with the site at which APD_b is shorter (circle). The dashed lines connect data points recorded simultaneously during each S1–S2 coupling intervals tested. Reproduced with permission from *(39)*.

kinetics of one or more time-dependent currents *(41,42)*. Computer simulation studies have also highlighted the role played by the steepness of the APD restitution curve in the genesis of concordant alternans. Only cells and tissues whose APD restitution curves displayed a slope > 1 were able to alternate *(43–47)*. In experimental and virtual settings, the flattening of the APD restitution curve by changing the kinetics of one or more membrane currents prevented the development of concordant and discordant alternans *(48)*, but also VF initiation *(49)* as well as spiral wave breakups by stabilizing the reentrant circus *(49–51)*.

How does the steepness of the restitution curve affect alternans threshold? Why a slope > 1 appears to be a prerequisite condition for the onset of alternans? The restitution curve below the point of slope =1 produces major changes in APD for little changes in DI, which is a result of the nonlinear relation of the APD-DI couple. For that specific part of the curve, a little increment in heart rate during fast pacing rate will result in a small reduction in DIs, but in a dramatic decrease in APDs as shown in Fig. 4. According to the nonlinear APD-DI relation, the long DI following the short APD will in turn produce a long APD, initiating a sustained alternans of short DI-APD resulting in long DI-APD couples that can last nearly for ever. From an electrophysiological viewpoint, it is very likely that the membrane and cellular processes governing the repolarization of the short APD will have enough time to fully recover during the next long DI, allowing the expression of a fullblown APD. The APD-DI coordinate of slope =1 of the APD restitution curve defines the heart rate threshold at which APD alternans develops, where the threshold in bpm = 60 × (1000/APD + DI) *(48,52)*. Figure 4 also shows that restitution kinetics are heterogeneously distributed from base to apex across the guinea pig heart, with the base displaying the steeper kinetics, and theoretically the lowest threshold for alternans. This finding appears essential for the understanding of the spatial distribution of alternans reported experimentally *(26,27)*.

By looking at the parameters of the Luo-Rudy 1 model for instance, it appeared that APDs were alternating on a beat-to-beat basis because the pacing rate was above the restitution kinetics of at least two composite ionic currents: I_{x1}, a K current, and I_{CA}, mostly a Ca^{2+} current. Computer modeling allowing for more detailed analysis showed that both the opening gating variable of the I_{x1} and the closing gating variable of the I_{CA} during a long APD had not recovered yet at the time the following depolarization started, which may account for the self-perpetuating sequence of long-short APDs. Recently, a new model integrating some of the specific features that were lacking in previous ones refined our understanding of the ionic and intracellular processes leading to alternans *(43)*. APD alternans was clearly related to the steepness of the restitution curve. Any interventions flattening the action potential kinetics increased the threshold or prevented the development of alternans. A reduction in the time constant of the I_{CA} inactivation gating variable, an increase in the magnitude of I_{Na}, and any modification of the Na^+-Ca^{2+} exchanger current reduced alternans amplitude. I_K currents did not appear to play any significant role in alternans, although any increase of these currents suppressed alternans by reducing APDs and prolonging DIs *(43)*. Ionic processes involved experimentally in APD alternans will be discussed in the following paragraph.

CELLULAR AND SUBCELLULAR MECHANISMS OF ALTERNANS

An association between repolarization alternans and contraction alternans has been recognized for years. Since its first description, two main mechanisms were proposed for electro-mechanical alternans. The first one considers that repolarization alternans results from variations in myocytes mechanical loading via mechano-electrical feedback mechanisms *(53,54)*. Short DIs reduce diastolic filling, which results in a weaker contraction based on the Frank-Starling relationship, but also in short APD as a result of the mechano-electrical feedback. It also leaves a greater end-systolic volume for the next beat. The next DI is thus long, which allows a better filling resulting in a stronger contraction, in a longer APD but also in a lower end systolic volume, and so forth. Although this mechanism does not appear to be responsible for the APD and T-wave alternans observed in many arrhythmogenic conditions, some studies in intact and isolated hearts are consistent with this hypothesis. A detailed review on the mechanism and pathophysiological significance of cardiac alternans was reviewed elsewhere *(55)*.

The second theory states a common cellular mechanism for repolarization and contraction alternans. This hypothesis is supported by experimental observations reporting concomitant occurrence of action potential and pressure alternans at constant DIs *(41)* or by the observation of repolarization alternans during inhibited cardiac contractions *(41,56,57)*. Action potential and mechanical alternans in single cell and tissue preparations have been reported under various conditions for years *(58–62)*. Interventions such as acidosis, ischemia, reduced temperature, low bath Ca^{2+} concentration, known to alter cell restitution kinetics, lowered the heart rate threshold at which alternans appeared *(59)*.

Data supporting the hypothesis that T-wave alternans resulted from beat-to-beat changes of membrane and/or intracellular ionic processes are:

1. Alternation of membrane potential may be provoked by delivery of a critically coupled premature beat *(58)*.
2. Alternation of membrane potential is provoked experimentally with a regular pacing rate above a threshold value *(26)*.

3. Pharmacological probes that affect L-type Ca^{2+} currents are able to simultaneously affect APD and pressure alternans *(41,56,57)*.

In experimental conditions, L-type Ca^{2+} channel blockers have been able to prevent APD alternans and to reduce pressure alternans without suppressing it at concentration at which they mainly affect slow inward Ca^{2+} currents *(41,56,57)*. Caffeine, known to deplete Ca^{2+} content of the sarcoplasmic reticulum, has been shown to suppress both action potential and tension alternans experimentally, suggesting that both types of alternans are caused by fluctuations of Ca^{2+} transients *(41,57)*. Ryanodine, which suppresses sarcoplasmic reticulum Ca^{2+}, also suppressed repolarization and contraction alternans *(57)*.

Functional studies have shown that Ca^{2+} release from the sarcoplasmic reticulum is triggered by the free cytosolic Ca^{2+} produced by the L-type Ca^{2+} current (i.e., Ca^{2+}-induced Ca^{2+}-release) *(63)*. Therefore, it is not surprising that drugs that modulate L-type Ca^{2+} current may indirectly affect sarcoplasmic reticulum Ca^{2+} current, contraction, and action potential alternans. On the other hand, it is expected that conditions that impair ion channel function may also reduce the heart rate threshold required to elicit T-wave alternans. This may explain why T-wave alternans was accentuated by hypothermia *(26)* and why T-wave alternans is observed at relatively slow heart rate in patients at risk of SCD *(25,31,64)* but is provoked only by rapid heart rate in normal hearts.

The mechanisms that control Ca^{2+} handling are complex. Briefly, the activation of I_{CA} by the depolarization front releases free Ca^{2+} in proximity to the T tubule. The cytosolic Ca^{2+} binds to the ryanodine receptors of the sarcoplasmic reticulum which, in turn, releases abundant sarcoplasmic reticulum Ca^{2+} into the cytosol via the Ca^{2+}-induced Ca^{2+}-release mechanism (CICR) *(65)*. When I_{CA} is blocked, or during prolonged depolarization of membrane voltage, sarcoplasmic reticulum Ca^{2+} release can also be stimulated by inward Ca^{2+} current from the Na^{+}-Ca^{2+} exchanger (NCX) operating in "reverse mode." After each contraction, the large majority of Ca^{2+} is removed into the sarcoplasmic reticulum by the SR-Ca^{2+}-ATPase, some by sarcolemmal NCX, and a minor proportion by sarcolemmal Ca^{2+} ATPase *(66)*. During repolarization, the NCX works in its forward mode, and for each Ca^{2+} ion extruded from the cell, three Na^{+} ions are transported in *(67)*, resulting in a net depolarizing current that contribute to prolong APD. The free cytosolic Ca^{2+} has at least two important electrogenic feedback mechanisms for the control of sarcoplasmic reticulum Ca^{2+} release:

1. Sarcoplasmic reticulum Ca^{2+} release tends to inactivate the sarcolemmal I_{Ca2+} channels, resulting in a lowering of membrane voltage and in APD shortening.
2. Sarcoplasmic reticulum Ca^{2+} release enhances Ca^{2+} extrusion by NCX, resulting in an increase in membrane voltage and in APD lengthening.

Although many studies have highlighted the role played by Ca^{2+} in the genesis of APD alternans, none has pointed out the role precisely played by each component of Ca^{2+} handling. Sorting out the ionic mechanisms of action potential alternans presents a difficult "chicken and egg" problem because of the inter-dependence of membrane voltage and intracellular Ca^{2+}, as summarized previously.

Single cell and tissue recordings have now well established in different experimental settings that action potential, Ca^{2+} transients, and mechanical alternans are closely linked

(68). Thus, the first question to be solved is whether action potential alternans is the primary event that triggers Ca^{2+} transient and mechanical alternans or whether Ca^{2+} transients trigger action potential alternans. Data supporting the hypothesis that Ca^{2+} transients trigger voltage alternans are:

1. Keeping APD constant with voltage clamp, it was shown that mechanical and Ca^{2+} transients alternans can still occur in experimental preparations (69,70) and simulated cells *(70)*.
2. During alternans, peak current did not alternate, suggesting that I_{CA}, which triggers Ca^{2+} release from the sarcoplasmic reticulum, is not the key mechanism responsible for the development of electro-mechanical alternans *(71)*.
3. It has been recently reported in single cells that reducing the amount of ATP available for the sarcoplasmic reticulum macromolecular complex formed of ryanodine receptors, phosphatases and protein kinase, triggers alternans in conditions where it did not appear usually *(71)*.

Taking together these results and previous ones showing that mechanical alternans unlike action potential alternans is reduced but not abolished by Ca^{2+} channel blockers, it is likely that alternation in I_{CA} is not the primary event that drives APD, Ca^{2+} transients and mechanical alternans. Apart from I_{CA}, several repolarization currents are at least partially under the control of cytosolic free Ca^{2+}, such as the Ca^{2+}-activated Cl^- ($I_{Cl(CA)}$), the NCX as well as the delayed rectifier current (I_{Ks}). Any beat-to-beat variations in the amount of cytosolic free Ca^{2+} could theoretically promote or reduce alternans by modulating one of these currents. A field of research opens where the respective role played by the components governing cytosolic Ca^{2+} handling in the genesis of Ca^{2+} transients alternans have still to be determined.

On one hand, there are compelling data suggesting a role of Ca^{2+} handling in the genesis of action potential alternans. On the other hand, the steepness of the APD restitution and the spatial variation in APD restitution kinetics have been mandatory for the development of electrical alternans in animal and virtual experiments. For the time being, no one has reconciled both prevailing hypotheses. A limited amount of studies are providing some information about the role played by Ca^{2+} handling in action potential restitution kinetics. We know that L-type Ca^{2+} channel blockers flatten APD restitution curves on one hand, and prevent APD alternans, VF induction and convert VF to a periodic rhythm on the other hand *(49)*. Computer simulation studies have allowed us to go in more detail about the role played by ionic currents in the APD restitution curve, although these results may not fully apply to single cell or tissue preparations *(48)*. I_{Na} and I_K currents appear to control respectively the initial and terminal parts of the APD restitution curve, which is consistent with experimental findings in cardiac tissue *(48,72–74)*, while I_{CA} appears to control the intermediate steep part of the restitution curve. Any reduction in I_{CA} increased the alternans heart rate threshold or abolished APD alternans, although flattening the restitution curve and shortening APD for any given DI *(43)*.

Eventually, repolarization alternans can also result from a spatial dispersion of refractoriness that gives rise secondary to alternations in propagation. In this condition, repolarization alternans is considered as secondary to propagation alternans, which occurs when the time between consecutive activations is shorter than the total refractory period. This finding is supported by several early studies performed during acute ischemia,

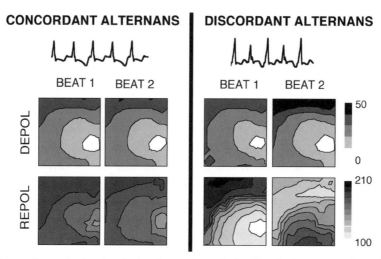

Fig. 5. Patterns of ventricular depolarization and repolarization during concordant (left, CL 200 ms) and discordant (right, CL 180 ms) alternans. Shown are 10-ms isochrone plots representing depolarization (depol) and repolarization (repol) within mapping array for 2 consecutive beats. Adapted from *(26)*.

where ECG alternans was generated by alternating conduction block into the ischemic zone *(75,76)*. However, the majority of patients at risk of arrhythmic events exhibits T-wave alternans in the absence of acute ischemia *(25,31,64)*. One could argue that ischemia develop at a subclinical level, however, there are compelling evidences that T-wave and APD alternans are rate-dependent phenomena, that do not require ischemia to come out.

MECHANISMS LINKING T-WAVE ALTERNANS TO VENTRICULAR ARRHYTHMIAS

Experimentally, two types of action potential alternans have been reported, i.e., concordant alternans and discordant alternans. Concordant alternans is defined as an homogeneous alternation of APD across the heart on an every-other-beat basis, without significant alternation in activation time (i.e., conduction velocity) *(26)*. The long action potential remains long while propagating across the heart, and is followed by a short action potential at all recording sites. Because voltage gradients are somewhat changed on an every-other-beat basis during repolarization, but not during depolarization, the T wave but not the QRS displays some degree of alternation on the surface ECG. Figure 5 right shows a typical example of an optical mapping recording of concordant alternans. Note that activation time is similar between even and odd beats. Despite a significant difference in repolarization time between even and odd beats, the orientation of the voltage gradient of repolarization remains the same for both beats, with the stimulation site being the first to repolarize. Dispersion of repolarization measured during concordant alternans was not different from values measured during no alternans *(26)*.

Discordant alternans, defined as islands of neighboring cells whose repolarization is spatially out of phase, is usually observed for faster pacing rate than concordant alternans *(26,48)*. In contrast to concordant alternans, during discordant alternans the pattern of repolarization varied substantially because the direction of repolarization reversed nearly

180° on consecutive beats, while the direction of depolarization remained the same. Figure 5 left shows a typical example of an optical mapping recording of discordant alternans. Note that activation time is similar between even and odd beats, however repolarization shows an 180° shift in gradient, that was not seen during concordant alternans.

Discordant alternans manifests itself on the surface ECG as some degree of QRS alternans because of conduction slowing, but more specifically as a marked alternans of the T wave shape and/or phase because of the 180° shift in repolarization gradient on an every-other-beat basis. Propagation is delayed regionally in islands of prolonged refractoriness. Dispersion of refractoriness increases far above baseline and concordant alternans values, which greatly enhanced the susceptibility to VF and VT (26,27). Unidirectional block of conduction has been reported in areas of most delayed repolarization, that were retrogradely activated, forming the first spontaneous beat of reentrant arrhythmias such as VT and VF (26,27).

Initiation of ventricular arrhythmias requires a certain amount of repolarization dispersion to favor unidirectional block of conduction, retrograde invasion of the refractory tissue, and reentry (26,77,78). Previous works have established this sequence in tissue with inhomogeneous electrophysiological property characterized by a fixed spatial dispersion of refractoriness (77,78). However, all arrhythmogenic diseases do not necessarily display the required amount of APD dispersion. In that case, an intermittent process is expected to alter nonuniformly APD, resulting in a transient spatial dispersion of refractoriness above the critical value. Discordant alternans might be one of the candidates, because it appears only above a given heart rate threshold. It is therefore unapparent at slow pacing rate. During discordant alternans, the patterns of repolarization reversed by 180° on alternating beats (26), markedly enhancing the amount of APD dispersion. Optical mapping recordings have been of great help in understanding the link between T-wave alternans, APD alternans and the susceptibility to ventricular arrhythmias. Figure 6 shows AT and RT contour maps of the last few beats before induction of a VF. Note the 180° reversal in repolarization gradient on alternating beats, consistent with discordant alternans. A further reduction of 10 ms in pacing CL produced an anterograde block as represented by the hatched area, that was retrogradely invaded, forming the first reentrant beat that lead to VF (26). When a similar protocol was used in an experimental setting where a linear lesion was created by laser, the resulting structural barrier produced an anchor for the reentrant wave, resulting in a monomorphic VT instead of a VF, but also reduced the threshold at which alternans appeared (27). In conclusion, discordant alternans provides a common pathway of enhancing gradient of refractoriness, that may enhance susceptibility to VF as well as VT, depending on the underlying anatomical characteristics of the tissue, i.e., presence or not of a structural barrier.

MECHANISMS LEADING TO DISCORDANT ALTERNANS

What are the mechanisms of discordant alternans? Two hypotheses prevail, which are not mutually exclusive. The first one states that discordant alternans develops because of a spatial gradient of APD restitution kinetics (26,27), whereas the second one states that discordant alternans develops because of marked slowing in conduction velocity (48,79). In other words, the first hypothesis states that the spatial heterogeneity of action potential restitution kinetics is the priming for the development of discordant alternans. Under

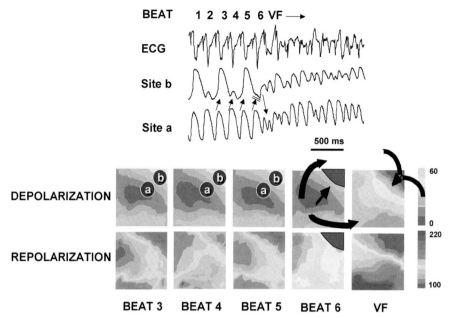

Fig. 6. Mechanism of initiation of VF during discordant alternans. Shown are 10-ms isochrone plots of depolarization and repolarization for beats that immediately preceded VF. Top: ECG and action potentials recorded from 2 ventricular sites marked on isochrone map (beat 3). Depolarization and repolarization times are referenced to stimulus artifact during pacing and to earliest activation time during first beat of VF. On beats 1 through 5, depolarizing wave front propagated uniformly from site of stimulation. However, patterns of repolarization differ substantially but reproducibly on alternans beats (compared beats 3 and 5). During beat 6, block occurred, as represented by hatched area in depolarization map. Block is shown in top panel by failure of propagation from site 1 to 3. After block occurred, pattern of depolarization reversed from site 1→ site 2 →site 3 to site 3→site 2→site 1, indicating first reentrant beat that led to VF. First beat of VF occurred 120 ms after pacing artifact of beat 6. Adapted from *(26)*.

some circumstances such as during fast pacing rate, discordant alternans can arise because the excitation front changes the phase of some cells but not others. Thus, the reversal in repolarization phase depends on the steepness of the restitution curves, which has to be >1, but also on where on the APD restitution curves the DI value preceding the excitation front arrives. The excitation front may result in long APDs for a specific restitution curve at a given location, and in short APDs for other ones. As a consequence, APDs will be spatially out of phase between neighboring islands of cells, i.e., discordant.

The first hypothesis is supported by results of experimental studies conducted on guinea pigs using optical mapping recordings. Figure 5 right shows optical mapping of activation and repolarization times during discordant alternans in a guinea pig. Although discordant alternans shows more crowding of AT isochrones at the base than during concordant alternans, it appears that reduction in conduction velocity is of little significance. Simulation studies have also reported that discordant alternans could be elicited during concordant alternans with the delivery of an ectopic beat in an homogeneous medium without significant change in conduction velocity *(79)*. Figure 7 top shows how an ectopic beat delivered opposite to the site of regular pacing collides with the "sinus " beat and produces the critical amount of spatial gradient of APD and DI that leads to phase reversal, and discordant alternans.

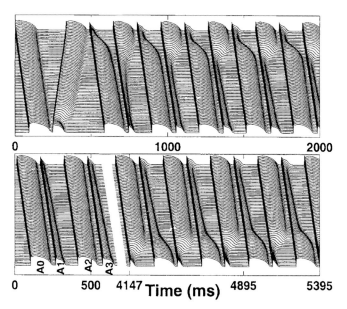

Fig. 7. Top: Ectopic focus scenario of discordant alternans initiation. The vertical axis denotes length of a cardiac cable (8 cm) and the horizontal axis denotes time. Action potential traces from 75 positions are shown. The cable was in quiescence until the first stimulation at the top end of the cable. A stimulus was given 310 ms after the arrival of the first excitation at the bottom end of the cable to simulate an ectopic focus firing. The ectopic excitation traveled up the cable and collided with the excitation from the second stimulus given at the top. Stimuli were thereafter given at 310-ms intervals at the top end of the cable to simulate sinus excitations. Although conduction velocity was essentially constant and the tissue was homogeneous, the increasing diastolic interval (DI) in the upward direction produced increasing action potential duration (APD) in the upward direction. This gradient, in turn, produced increasing DI and APD in the downward direction when the next sinus excitation traveled down the cable. This inversion continued and alternans was discordant. Bottom: Sinus node scenario of discordant alternans initiation. Orientation as in top panel. All stimuli were applied at the top end of the cable at 310-ms intervals following a long quiescence. The second stimulus followed the maximum possible APD, and DI was short. The short DI produced slow conduction that gave rise to increasing DI as the wavefront traveled down the cable, as seen in the mild increase in the DI preceding the excitation marked A1 and in the mild increase in APD (A1). The third stimulus followed a relatively long DI, producing maximum conduction velocity down the initial segments of the cable. Fast conduction coupled with APD increase down the cable on the previous beat produced decreasing DI and APD (A2) down the length of the cable. The reversal of DI spatial distribution (increasing down the cable for $S1_2$, decreasing for $S1_3$) was exaggerated as pacing continued, and gradually formed a node. The right part of the figure begins with the 13th excitation, and the top and bottom of the cable are clearly alternating out of phase. Reproduced with permission from *(79)*.

The second hypothesis comes originally from computer simulation studies, where discordant alternans following concordant alternans was observed in an homogeneous tissue whose restitution kinetics was uniform *(48,79)*. To proceed from concordant to discordant alternans, the pacing rate had to be short enough to engage conduction velocity restitution. In a manner similar to the APD-DI relation, conduction velocity restitution is defined as a reduction in the velocity of the wavefront as a function of the preceding DI interval. In some regions, the wavefront met short DIs resulting in a decrease in its regional velocity. Figure 7 bottom shows in an homogeneous cable how discordant alternans may arise from the interaction between conduction velocity and APD restitution kinetics during concordant alternans. The y-axis is the cable length in cm, and the x-axis is the time in ms. Pacing rate is above alternans threshold defined as the APD-DI coordinates of slope = 1 on the APD restitution curve. Figure 7 bottom shows that concordant APD alternans developed as soon as the fast pacing rate was initiated, while spatial alternans (i.e., discordant alternans) only appeared after a few beats. The explanation for the delayed appearance of discordant alternans is the following: Because of concordant alternans, the first long APD (A0) is followed by a short DI, resulting in a short APD (A1). Owing to the underlying conduction velocity restitution, A1 propagates somewhat slower than A0, which gives rise to increasing DI as the wavefront traveled down the cable, as seen in the mild increase in the DI preceding A1 and in the APD of A1 as seen in Figure 7 bottom. In other words, the wavefront of long APD having a maximum conduction velocity tends to catch the waveback of the preceding short APD with a reduced conduction velocity. The overall result is that long APDs progress spatially toward shorter values, whereas short APDs progress toward longer values, resulting in spatial alternans of APD, in other words discordant alternans.

From this example, it appears that conduction velocity may play a significant role in the genesis of discordant alternans by interacting with the APD restitution curve. As illustrated by Fig. 7 bottom, the amount of conduction velocity change across the cable is little, and does not appear to be more pronounced than what has been observed experimentally in guinea pigs (26). Clearly, the two hypotheses mentioned previously are not mutually exclusive. It is possible that heterogeneity of APD restitution between myocytes plays a critical role in discordant alternans in "normal" hearts with fast conduction velocity, but under circumstances where conduction velocity is slowed (e.g., by myocardial disease or antiarrhythmic drugs), conduction velocity restitution may play an additive role. As a matter of fact, recent studies mixing experimentations and simulations have shown that:

1. The amount of conduction velocity variation, as measured by the local variation in activation time, is little and in the range of 1–3 ms (80). Variation of activation time of this magnitude is likely to be obscured under most experimental circumstances.
2. That tissue heterogeneities are capable of pinning location of node (79), which may be responsible for the consistent pattern of base-to-apex distribution of discordant alternans seen in experimental setting (26).

Electrically uncoupling regions with different restitution kinetics also appears to play a significant role in the genesis of discordant alternans. The introduction of a structural barrier resulted in a reduction of the heart rate threshold at which discordant alternans developed, with a straightforward transition from no alternans to discordant alternans. As shown in Fig. 8, the structural barrier formed a portion of the line of separation between regions that were in opposite phase. When a fast pacing rate followed by an ectopic beat was used for arrhythmia induction, the structural barrier produced an anchor for the reentrant wave, resulting in a monomorphic VT instead of a VF. Figure 9 shows such an example. The extrastimulus blocked in the region of most delayed repolarization, that was retrogradely invaded, forming the first beat of a monomorphic VT. How did the structural barrier reduce the alternans threshold? We know that action potential restitution kinetics in guinea pigs are heterogeneously distributed across the heart in a base to

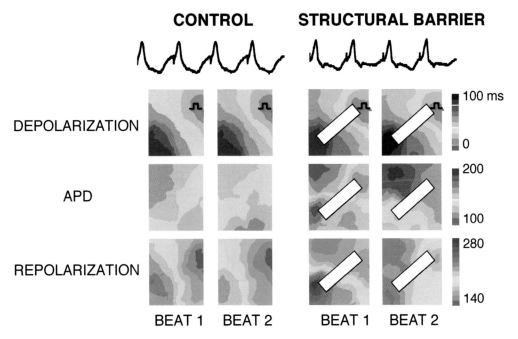

Fig. 8. Changes in ventricular repolarization caused by the structural barrier (SB). 10-ms isochrone maps represent patterns of depolarization, APD, and repolarization for 2 consecutive beats in absence (i.e., control) and presence of SB at an identical heart rate. Activation propagates as expected from site of stimulation (square pulse symbol) in all cases. SB produces large changes in magnitude and orientation of APD gradients (right middle panel) that were not present during control (left middle panel). This creates large spatial gradients of repolarization in presence of SB. These effects are evident on the ECG (top) as visible T-wave alternans is apparent with SB. Adapted from *(26)*.

apex fashion as shown in Fig. 4. The structural barrier was introduced transverse to this APD gradient, which insulated cells with different restitution kinetics and reduced their electrotonic coupling, a process known to enhance dispersion of repolarization *(81)*. We also know that the gradient of action potential restitution kinetics is the driving force for the genesis of discordant alternans *(26)*. Thus, any uncoupling (e.g., structural barrier) enhancing this gradient should reduce the alternans threshold, which appears to be the case in guinea pigs. From a clinical viewpoint, these findings are at utmost relevance, because they establish a link between susceptibility to ventricular arrhythmias and the electrophysiological state of the underlying cardiac tissue. Any increase in action potential heterogeneities produced by macroscopic (e.g., remote MI) and microscopic (e.g., fibrosis in cardiomyopathies) uncoupling will lower threshold of T-wave alternans and will enhance the likelihood of developing ventricular arrhythmias, which is precisely the case of patients with structural heart diseases *(25,29,32,33,64,82)*.

CLINICAL RELEVANCE OF T-WAVE ALTERNANS ANALYSIS

The first studies published on the performance of T-wave alternans as a risk stratification tool included patients suffering from various types of heart disease as well as

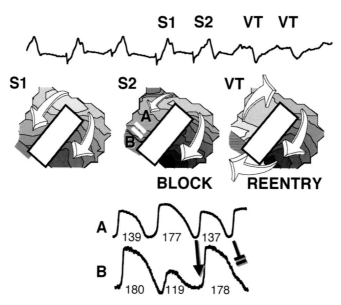

Fig. 9. Alternans-induced reentry in presence of a structural barrier (SB). Top, ECG lead showing initiation of reentry by introduction of a premature stimulus (S_2) in a heart with a SB (white box). Middle, 10-ms isochrone maps of depolarization for the beat preceding the S_2 and during the initiation of the arrhythmia. Notice that discordant alternans (action potential tracings, bottom panel) between mapping sites A and B creates a large gradient of repolarization that produces functional block (hatched area, middle isochrone plot) necessary for reentry around the SB. Adapted from *(26)*.

patients with and without ventricular arrhythmias *(25,30,64)*. In these preliminary studies, a positive T-wave alternans predicted results of PVS with an averaged sensitivity of 87% and specificity of 80%. Having a positive T-wave alternans test increased the risk of developing a ventricular arrhythmia at PVS by a factor of 5 to 8. During follow-up of high risk populations, T-wave alternans also predicted arrhythmic events or SCD as well as PVS, which is the gold standard for risk stratification of post-MI patients *(25,30,64)*.

In contrast to PVS, T-wave alternans analysis is not restricted to post-MI patients. Recent works have shown that T-wave alternans seems also to be a harbinger of SCD for nonischemic dilated cardiomyopathy *(83,84)*, as well as for electrical diseases such as the Long QT syndrome *(20–22)*. In the following paragraphs, the prognostic yield of T-wave alternans will be discussed in patients with (secondary prevention) and without (primary prevention) known ventricular arrhythmias.

There are only a few studies, cumulating approx 150 patients, that have looked at the performance of T-wave alternans analysis as a predictor of ventricular arrhythmias recurrence in post-MI patients *(32,85)*. In a population of 95 patients implanted with an ICD because of recurrent ventricular arrhythmias, a positive TWA test was the only independent predictor of arrhythmia recurrence *(32)*. Neither positive PVS, reduced LVEF, depressed baroreflex sensitivity, presence of late potentials nor decreased heart rate variability were independently related to arrhythmia recurrence *(32)*.

Table 2 gives an overview of the most recent studies that have looked at the prognostic value of T-wave alternans in patients without known ventricular arrhythmias *(86–88)*.

Table 2
Overview of the Performance of T-Wave Alternans Analysis for Risk Assessment
of Arrhythmic Events in Post-MI Patients Without Known Ventricular Arrhythmias[1]

	Patients (n)	LVEF (%)	Event During FU (%)	MV predictor of arrhythmic events	RR of events if +TWA	Event free if +TWA (%)	Event free if –TWA (%)
Ikeda et al. 2000	102	49 ± 9	15	Combined +TWA and +SAECG	17	70	98
Tapanainen et al. 2001	379	45 ± 10	5	+SAECG	NS	100	96
Ikeda et al. 2002	850	51 ± 13	8	+TWA, LVEF<40%	11	92	99

[1]In two studies performed by the same group *(86,87)*, the risk of suffering from an arrhythmic event after a positive T-wave alternans test, alone or in combination with late potentials, was increased by more than X10. In contrast, in the Tapanainen study *(88)*, a positive T-wave alternans test had no significant power to predict future arrhythmic event during follow-up. FU, follow-up; LVEF, left ventricular ejection fraction; MV, multivariate; NS, non significant; RR, risk ratio; +SAECG, positive signal averaged ECG; TWA, T-wave alternans analysis; –TWA, negative TWA; +TWA, positive TWA.

Taken altogether, these studies have followed during 1 to 2 yr approx 1500 patients with mild left ventricular dysfunction following an acute MI. All patients had been treated with the usual revascularization procedures (thrombolysis, PCI, CABG). Conventional risks markers were performed simultaneously to T-wave alternans analysis and compared together. Despite clear similarities between patients in term of clinical characteristics and LVEF, the results are conflicting in what concerns the prognostic value of T-wave alternans *(88)*. In two studies performed actually by the same group, the multivariate analysis revealed that a positive T-wave alternans test alone or in combination with late potentials was a strong independent predictor of SCD or resuscitated VF during follow-up, with a hazard ratio of 11 to 17, although late potentials alone were only predictive of sustained VT but not of VF or SCD *(86,87)*. In contrast, Tapanainen et al. reported no association between positive T-wave alternans testing and the risk of subsequent arrhythmic events *(88)*. Their multivariate analysis identified an indeterminate T-wave alternans test as well as the presence of other indices as independent predictors of adverse events. How can such contradictory results be? The only apparent differences between the studies of Ikeda et al. and Tapanainen et al. are:

1. More than 50% of the patients in the Tapanainen study had residual sign of ischemia at discharge of hospital while all patients in the Ikeda et al. study were successfully revascularized.
2. The time elapsed between MI and measures of prognostic indices ranged between 5 d to 3 wk in the study of Tapanainen et al. and 3 mo in the study of Ikeda et al.

We know from early experimental and clinical studies that residual ischemia is associated with an increase risk of adverse event after MI, which may explain why Tapanainen et al. did not find any prognostic value of T-wave alternans analysis and LVEF, but also why the inability of performing a treadmill test was the most significant predictor of cardiac death. Taken together, these conflicting results suggest that TWA analysis should not be performed too early after an acute MI, but at least 3 wk after the ischemic event, and that treatment of residual ischemia should be the primary goal before any risk assessment for ventricular arrhythmias in the post-MI setting.

CONCLUSIONS

Nearly a century ago, T-wave alternans was reported as a harbinger to SCD, but its role as a marker of arrhythmia susceptibility was first suggested 15 yr ago. T-wave alternans has opened a unique field of research, whose most recent results have clearly established the link between transient abnormal repolarization on an every-other-beat basis and susceptibility to ventricular arrhythmias and SCD in a broad variety of organic and electrical heart diseases. However, many questions remain unresolved. The subcellular mechanisms of action potential alternans, and more specifically the role played by the various components of intracellular Ca^{2+} handling, are not fully understood yet and deserve special attention because their understanding might open new curative or preventive strategies.

The clinical significance of a positive T-wave alternans test also deserves further studies, and needs to be prospectively compared to PVS-based conventional risk stratification in primary prevention studies. With respect to these open questions, the Alternans Before Cardioverter Defibrillator (ABCD) trial has been recently launched, whose goal is to prospectively compare the ability of T-wave alternans analysis and VPS to predict arrhythmic events following an acute MI.

ACKNOWLEDGMENTS

This work was supported by The Fondation Suisse de Bourses en Médecine et Biologie (FSBMB) and The National Institutes of Health grant RO1–HL54807.

REFERENCES

1. Goldstein S. Sudden death and coronary heart disease. Sudden death and coronary heart disease. Mt. Kisco, NY: Futura Publishing Co., 1974.
2. Myerburg RJ, Kessler KM, Castellanos A. Sudden cardiac death: epidemiology, transient risk, and intervention assessment. Ann Intern Med 1993;119(12):1187–1197.
3. Lee TH, Goldman L. The coronary care unit turns 25: historical trends and future directions. Ann Intern Med 1988;108:887–894.
4. Anonymous. Metoprolol in acute myocardial infarction. Mortality. The MIAMI Trial Research Group. Am J Cardiol 1985;56:15G-22G.
5. Tanel RE, Triedman JK, Walsh EP, et al. High-rate atrial pacing as an innovative bridging therapy in a neonate with congenital long QT syndrome. J Cardiovasc Electrophysiol 1997;8:812–817.
6. Buxton AE, Lee KL, DiCarlo L, et al. Electrophysiologic testing to identify patients with coronary artery disease who are at risk for sudden death. Multicenter Unsustained Tachycardia Trial Investigators. N Engl J Med 2000;342(26):1937–1945.
7. Moss AJ, Hall WJ, Cannom DS, et al. Improved survival with an implanted defibrillator in patients with coronary disease at high risk for ventricular arrhythmia. Multicenter Automatic Defibrillator Implantation Trial Investigators. N Engl J Med 1996;335:1933–1940.

8. Buxton AE, Lee KL, Fisher JD, Josephson ME, Prystowsky EN, Hafley G. A randomized study of the prevention of sudden death in patients with coronary artery disease. Multicenter Unsustained Tachycardia Trial Investigators. N Engl J Med 1999;341(25):1882–1890.

9. Moss AJ, Zareba W, Hall WJ, et al. Prophylactic implantation of a defibrillator in patients with myocardial infarction and reduced ejection fraction. N Engl J Med 2002;346(12):877–883.

10. Antzelevitch C, Yan GX, Shimizu W, Burashnikov A. Electrical heterogeneity, the ECG, and cardiac arrhythmias. In: Zipes DP, Jalife J, eds. Cardiac Electrophysiology. From Cell to Bedside. W.B. Saunders Company, 2000:222–238.

11. Herring H. Experimentelle Studien an Saugetieren uber das Electrocardiogramm. Z Exper Med 1909;7:363.

12. Lewis T. Notes upon alternation of the heart. Q J Med 1910;4:141–144.

13. Kalter HH, Schwartz ML. Electrical alternans. NY State J Medicine 1948;98:1164–1166.

14. Puletti M, Curione M, Righetti G, Jacobellis G. Alternans of the ST segment and T wave in acute myocardial infarction. J Electrocardiol 1980;13:297–300.

15. Salerno JA, Previtali M, Panciroli C, et al. Ventricular arrhythmias during acute myocardial ischaemia in man. The role and significance of R-ST-T alternans and the prevention of ischaemic sudden death by medical treatment. Eur Heart J 1986;7 Suppl A:63–75.

16. Reddy CV, Kiok JP, Khan RG, El Sherif N. Repolarization alternans associated with alcoholism and hypomagnesemia. Am J Cardiol 1984;53(2):390–391.

17. Shimoni Z, Flatau E, Schiller D, Barzilay E, Kohn D. Electrical alternans of giant U waves with multiple electrolyte deficits. Am J Cardiol 1984;54(7):920–921.

18. Kleinfeld MJ, Rozanski JJ. Alternans of the ST segment in Prinzmetal's angina. Circulation 1977;55:574–577.

19. Cheng TC. Electrical alternans. An association with coronary artery spasm. Arch Intern Med 1983;143:1052–1053.

20. Platt SB, Vijgen JM, Albrecht P, Van Hare GF, Carlson MD, Rosenbaum DS. Occult T wave alternans in long QT syndrome. J Cardiovasc Electrophysiol 1996;7:144–148.

21. Shimizu W, Yamada K, Arakaki Y, Kamiya T, Shimomura K. Monophasic action potential recordings during T-wave alternans in congenital long QT syndrome. Am Heart J 1996;132:699–701.

22. Burattini L, Zareba W, Rashba EJ, Couderc JP, Konecki J, Moss AJ. ECG features of microvolt T-wave alternans in coronary artery disease and long QT syndrome patients. J Electrocardiol 1998;31 Suppl: 114–120.

23. Adam DR, Smith JM, Akselrod S, Nyberg S, Powell AO, Cohen RJ. Fluctuations in T-wave morphology and susceptibility to ventricular fibrillation. J Electrocardiol 1984;17:209–218.

24. Smith JM, Clancy EA, Valeri CR, Ruskin JN, Cohen RJ. Electrical alternans and cardiac electrical instability. Circulation 1988;77(1):110–121.

25. Rosenbaum DS, Jackson LE, Smith JM, Garan H, Ruskin JN, Cohen RJ. Electrical alternans and vulnerability to ventricular arrhythmias. N Engl J Med 1994;330:235–241.

26. Pastore JM, Girouard SD, Laurita KR, Akar FG, Rosenbaum DS. Mechanism linking T-wave alternans to the genesis of cardiac fibrillation. Circulation 1999;99:1385–1394.

27. Pastore JM, Rosenbaum DS. Role of structural barriers in the mechanism of alternans-induced reentry. Circ Res 2000;87(12):1157–1163.

28. Narayan SM, Smith JM. Differing rate dependence and temporal distribution of repolarization alternans in patients with and without ventricular tachycardia. J Cardiovasc Electrophysiol 1999;10:61–71.

29. Gold MR, Bloomfield DM, Anderson KP, et al. A comparison of T-wave alternans, signal averaged electrocardiography and programmed ventricular stimulation for arrhythmia risk stratification. J Am Coll Cardiol 2000;36(7):2247–2253.

30. Hohnloser S, Cohen RJ. T wave alternans and left ventricular ejection fraction, but not QT variability index, predict appropriate ICD discharge. J Cardiovasc Electrophysiol 1999;10: 626–627.

31. Hohnloser SH, Klingenheben T, Zabel M, Li YG, Albrecht P, Cohen RJ. T wave alternans during exercise and atrial pacing in humans. J Cardiovasc Electrophysiol. 1997;8:987–993.

32. Hohnloser SH, Klingenheben T, Li YG, Zabel M, Peetermans J, Cohen RJ. T wave alternans as a predictor of recurrent ventricular tachyarrhythmias in ICD recipients: prospective comparison with conventional risk markers. J Cardiovasc Electrophysiol 1998;9(12):1258–1268.

33. Klingenheben T, Zabel M, D'Agostino RB, Cohen RJ, Hohnloser SH. Predictive value of T-wave alternans for arrhythmic events in patients with congestive heart failure. Lancet 2000;356(9230): 651–652.

34. Kitamura H, Ohnishi Y, Okajima K, et al. Onset heart rate of microvolt-level T-wave alternans provides clinical and prognostic value in nonischemic dilated cardiomyopathy. J Am Coll Cardiol 2002;39(2): 295–300.

35. Loew LM. Mechanisms and principles of volatage-sensitive fluorescence. In: Rosenbaum DS, Jalife J, eds. Optical Mapping of Cardiac Excitation and Arrhythmias. Futura Publishing, 2001:33–46.

36. Rosenbaum DS, Jalife J, eds. Optical Mapping of Cardiac Excitation and Arrhythmias. New York, NY: Futura Publishing, 2001.

37. Diehl RR, Linden D, Chalkiadaki A, Diehl A. Cerebrovascular mechanisms in neurocardiogenic syncope with and without postural tachycardia syndrome. J Auton Nerv Syst 1999;76(2–3):159–166.

38. Akar FG, Laurita KR, Rosenbaum DS. Cellular basis for dispersion of repolarization underlying reentrant arrhythmias. J Electrocardiol 2000;33 Suppl:23–3133 Suppl:23–31.

39. Laurita KR, Girouard SD, Rosenbaum DS. Modulation of ventricular repolarization by a premature stimulus. Role of epicardial dispersion of repolarization kinetics demonstrated by optical mapping of the intact guinea pig heart. Circ Res 1996;79(3):493–503.

40. Rosenbaum DS, Kaplan DT, Kanai A, et al. Repolarization inhomogeneities in ventricular myocardium change dynamically with abrupt cycle length shortening. Circulation 1991;84(3):1333–1345.

41. Hirayama Y, Saitoh H, Atarashi H, Hayakawa H. Electrical and mechanical alternans in canine myocardium in vivo. Dependence on intracellular calcium cycling. Circulation 1993;88:2894–2902.

42. Luo CH, Rudy Y. A model of the ventricular cardiac action potential. Depolarization, repolarization, and their interaction. Circ Res 1991;68:1501–1526.

43. Fox JJ, McHarg JL, Gilmour RF Jr. Ionic mechanism of electrical alternans. Am J Physiol 2002;282(2):H516–H530.

44. Nolasco JB, Dahlen RW. A graphic method for the study of alternation in cardiac action potentials. J Appl Physiol 1968;25(2):191–196.

45. Vinet A, Chialvo DR, Michaels DC, Jalife J. Nonlinear dynamics of rate-dependent activation in models of single cardiac cells. Circ Res 1990;67(6):1510–1524.

46. Courtemanche M, Glass L, Keener JP. Instabilities of a propagating pulse in a ring of excitable media. Phys Rev Letters 1993;70(14):2182–2185.

47. Koller ML, Riccio ML, Gilmour RF Jr. Dynamic restitution of action potential duration during electrical alternans and ventricular fibrillation. Am J Physiol 1998;275(5 Pt 2):H1635–H1642.

48. Qu Z, Garfinkel A, Chen PS, Weiss JN. Mechanisms of discordant alternans and induction of reentry in simulated cardiac tissue. Circulation 2000;102(14):1664–1670.

49. Riccio ML, Koller ML, Gilmour RF Jr. Electrical restitution and spatiotemporal organization during ventricular fibrillation. Circ Res 1999;84(8):955–963.

50. Garfinkel A, Kim YH, Voroshilovsky O, et al. Preventing ventricular fibrillation by flattening cardiac restitution. Proc Natl Acad Sci USA 2000;97(11):6061–6066.

51. Qu Z, Kil J, Xie F, Garfinkel A, Weiss JN. Scroll wave dynamics in a three-dimensional cardiac tissue model: roles of restitution, thickness, and fiber rotation. Biophys J 2000;78(6):2761–2775.

52. Pruvot E, Jacquemet V, Vesin JM, et al. Action potential alternans in a mono-cellular model based on Beeler-Reuter kinetics. In: Virag N, Blanc O, Kappenberger L, eds. Computer Simulation and Experimental Assessment of Cardiac Electrophysiology. Armonk, NY: Futura Publishing, 2001:69–77.

53. Kurz RW, Mohabir R, Ren XL, Franz MR. Ischaemia induced alternans of action potential duration in the intact-heart: dependence on coronary flow, preload and cycle length. Eur Heart J 1993;14: 1410–1420.

54. Murphy CF, Lab MJ, Horner SM, Dick DJ, Harrison FG. Regional electromechanical alternans in anesthetized pig hearts: modulation by mechanoelectric feedback. Am J Physiol 1994;267: H1726–H1735.

55. Euler DE. Cardiac alternans: mechanisms and pathophysiological significance. Cardiovasc Res 1999;42(3):583–590.

56. Saitoh H, Bailey JC, Surawicz B. Alternans of action potential duration after abrupt shortening of cycle length: differences between dog Purkinje and ventricular muscle fibers. Circ Res 1988;62:1027–1040.

57. Saitoh H, Bailey JC, Surawicz B. Action potential duration alternans in dog Purkinje and ventricular muscle fibers. Further evidence in support of two different mechanisms. Circulation 1989;80: 1421–1431.

58. Rubenstein DS, Lipsius SL. Premature beats elicit a phase reversal of mechanoelectrical alternans in cat ventricular myocytes. A possible mechanism for reentrant arrhythmias. Circulation 1995;91:201–214.

59. Lab MJ, Lee JA. Changes in intracellular calcium during mechanical alternans in isolated ferret ventricular muscle. Circ Res 1990;66(3):585–595.

60. Hirata Y, Toyama J, Yamada K. Effects of hypoxia or low PH on the alternation of canine ventricular action potentials following an abrupt increase in driving rate. Cardiovasc Res 1980;14(2):108–115.

61. Allen DG, Lee JA, Smith GL. The consequences of simulated ischaemia on intracellular Ca2+ and tension in isolated ferret ventricular muscle. J Physiol 1989;410:297–323.

62. Spear JF, Moore EN. A comparison of alternation in myocardial action potentials and contractility. Am J Physiol 1971;220(6):1708–1716.

63. Beuckelmann DJ, Wier WG. Mechanism of release of calcium from sarcoplasmic reticulum of guinea-pig cardiac cells. J Physiol (Lond) 1988;405:233–255.

64. Estes NA, Michaud G, Zipes DP, et al. Electrical alternans during rest and exercise as predictors of vulnerability to ventricular arrhythmias. Am J Cardiol 1997;80:1314–1318.

65. Meissner G. Ryanodine receptor/Ca2+ release channels and their regulation by endogenous effectors. Annu Rev Physiol 1994;56:485–508.

66. Bassani RA, Bassani JW, Bers DM. Relaxation in ferret ventricular myocytes: unusual interplay among calcium transport systems. J Physiol 1994;476(2):295–308.

67. Reeves JP, Hale CC. The stoichiometry of the cardiac sodium-calcium exchange system. J Biol Chem 1984;259(12):7733–7739.

68. Laurita KR, Singal A, Pastore JM, Rosenbaum DS. Spatial heterogeneity of calcium transients may explain action potential dispersion during T-wave alternans. Circulation 1998;I-187.

69. Orchard CH, McCall E, Kirby MS, Boyett MR. Mechanical alternans during acidosis in ferret heart muscle. Circ Res 1991;68(1):69–76.

70. Chudin E, Goldhaber J, Garfinkel A, Weiss J, Kogan B. Intracellular Ca(2+) dynamics and the stability of ventricular tachycardia. Biophys J 1999;77(6):2930–2941.

71. Huser J, Wang YG, Sheehan KA, Cifuentes F, Lipsius SL, Blatter LA. Functional coupling between glycolysis and excitation-contraction coupling underlies alternans in cat heart cells. J Physiol 2000;524 Pt 3:795–806.

72. Varro A, Lathrop DA. Sotalol and mexiletine: combination of rate-dependent electrophysiological effects. J Cardiovasc Pharmacol 1990;16(4):557–567.

73. Lathrop DA, Varro A. The combined electrophysiological effects of lignocaine and sotalol in canine isolated cardiac Purkinje fibres are rate-dependent. Br J Pharmacol 1990;99(1):124–130.

74. Lathrop DA, Varro A, Schwartz A. Rate-dependent electrophysiological effects of OPC-8212: comparison to sotalol. Eur J Pharmacol 1989;164(3):487–496.

75. Downar E, Janse MJ, Durrer D. The effect of acute coronary artery occlusion on subepicardial transmembrane potentials in the intact porcine heart. Circulation 1977;56:217–224.

76. Konta T, Ikeda K, Yamaki M, et al. Significance of discordant ST alternans in ventricular fibrillation. Circulation 1990;82:2185–2189.

77. Kuo CS, Munakata K, Reddy CP, Surawicz B. Characteristics and possible mechanism of ventricular arrhythmia dependent on the dispersion of action potential durations. Circulation 1983;67:1356–1367.

78. Allessie MA, Bonke FI, Schopman FJ. Circus movement in rabbit atrial muscle as a mechanism of tachycardia. II. The role of nonuniform recovery of excitability in the occurrence of unidirectional block, as studied with multiple microelectrodes. Circ Res 1976;39:168–177.

79. Watanabe MA, Fenton FH, Evans SJ, Hastings HM, Karma A. Mechanisms for discordant alternans. J Cardiovasc Electrophysiol 2001;12(2):196–206.

80. Fox JJ, Riccio ML, Hua F, Bodenschatz E, Gilmour RF, Jr. Spatiotemporal transition to conduction block in canine ventricle. Circ Res 2002;90(3):289–296.

81. Tan RC, Joyner RW. Electrotonic influences on action potentials from isolated ventricular cells. Circ Res 1990;67(5):1071–1081.

82. Kaufman ES, Mackall JA, Julka B, Drabek C, Rosenbaum DS. Influence of heart rate and sympathetic stimulation on arrhythmogenic T wave alternans. Am J Physiol 2000;279(3):H1248–H1255.

83. Sakabe K, Ikeda T, Sakata T, et al. Comparison of T-wave alternans and QT interval dispersion to predict ventricular tachyarrhythmia in patients with dilated cardiomyopathy and without antiarrhythmic drugs: a prospective study. Jpn Heart J 2001;42(4):451–457.

84. Sakabe K, Ikeda T, Sakata T, et al. Predicting the recurrence of ventricular tachyarrhythmias from T-wave alternans assessed on antiarrhythmic pharmacotherapy: a prospective study in patients with dilated cardiomyopathy. Ann Noninvasive Electrocardiol 2001;6(3):203–208.

85. Kavesh NG, Shorofsky SR, Sarang SE, Gold MR. The effect of procainamide on T wave alternans. J Cardiovasc Electrophysiol 1999;10(5):649–654.

86. Ikeda T, Sakata T, Takami M, et al. Combined assessment of T-wave alternans and late potentials used to predict arrhythmic events after myocardial infarction. A prospective study. J Am Coll Cardiol 2000;35(3):722–730.

87. Ikeda T, Saito H, Tanno K, et al. T-wave alternans as a predictor for sudden cardiac death after myocardial infarction. Am J Cardiol 2002;89(1):79–82.

88. Tapanainen JM, Still AM, Airaksinen KE, Huikuri HV. Prognostic significance of risk stratifiers of mortality, including T wave alternans, after acute myocardial infarction: results of a prospective follow-up study. J Cardiovasc Electrophysiol 2001;12(6):645–652.

INDEX